STRATEGIC HEALTH PLANNING:

Methods and Techniques Applied to Marketing and Management

Developments in Clinical Psychology

Glen R. Caddy, series editor
Nova University

MMPI-168 Codebook, by Ken R. Vincent, Iliana Castillo, Robert I. Hauser, H. James Stuart, Javier A. Zapata, Cal K. Cohn, and Gregory O'Shanick, 1984

Integrated Clinical and Fiscal Management in Mental Health: A Guidebook, by Fred Newman and James Sorensen, 1986

The Professional Practice of Psychology, edited by Georgiana Shick Tryon, 1986

Clinical Applications of Hypnosis, edited by Frank A. DePiano and Herman C. Salzberg, 1986

Full Battery Codebook, by Ken R. Vincent, 1987

Developments in the Assessment and Treatment of Addictive Behaviors, edited by Ted D. Nirenberg, 1987

Feminist Psychotherapies, edited by Mary Ann Douglas and Lenore E. Walker, 1988

Child Multimodal Therapy, by Donald B. Keat II, 1990

Psychophysiology for Clinical Psychologists, by Walter W. Surwillo, 1990

Strategic Health Planning: Methods and Techniques Applied to Marketing and Management, by Allen D. Spiegel and Herbert H. Hyman, 1991

In Preparation:

Behavioral Medicine: International Perspectives (Vol. 1–3), edited by D.G. Byrne and Glenn R. Caddy

Language and Psychopathology, by Stephen Schwartz

The MMPI: A Contemporary Normative Study of Adolescents, edited by Robert C. Colligan and Kenneth P. Offord

STRATEGIC HEALTH PLANNING:

Methods and Techniques Applied to Marketing and Management

Allen D. Spiegel

State University of New York

Herbert H. Hyman

Hunter College, CUNY

ABLEX PUBLISHING CORPORATION
NORWOOD, NEW JERSEY

Third Printing 1998

Printed in the United States of America

Library of Congress Cataloging-in-Publication Data

Spiegel, Allen D.
    Strategic health planning : methods and techniques applied to
marketing and management / by Allen D. Spiegel and Herbert H. Hyman
        p. cm.—(Developments in clinical psychology)
    Includes Bibliographical references and index.
    ISBN 0-89391-742-7 (cloth).—ISBN 0-89391-892-X (paper)
    1. Health Planning. 2. Strategic planning. I. Hyman, Herbert
Harvey. II. Title. III. Series.
RA393.S673 1991   90-26054
                                             CIP

Ablex Publishing Corporation
355 Chestnut Street
Norwood, New Jersey 07648

P

Table of Contents

About the Authors   *xvii*

Preface   *xix*

1 • AN INTRODUCTION TO STRATEGIC HEALTH PLANNING   *1*
Changing Times and Tides   *1*
Demise of Federal Planning Legislation   *2*
Strategic Health Planning Advances   *3*
What Is the Business of This Business?   *4*
Characteristics of Strategic Planning   *5*
A Comparison of Strategic and Comprehensive Health Planning   *7*
External and Internal Environmental Assessment   *9*
Providers Must Cope   *9*
  Prospective Payment System   *9*
  Monitoring Quality of Care   *9*
  High Technology   *10*
  Competition   *10*
  Hospital Occupancy   *11*
  Professional Staff Competition   *11*
  Alternative Care   *11*
  Consumer Self-Care   *11*
Four Pressing Specific Issues   *12*
  AIDS   *12*
  Home Health Care   *12*
  Physician Surplus—Nursing Shortage   *13*
  Cost Containment   *14*
Planning and the Turbulent Environment   *14*
Constrictions on Planning   *16*
Significant Health Planning Trends   *17*
A Caveat About Methods and Techniques   *18*
Planning Pitfalls   *21*

Objectives as Linchpins   *23*
Take Time to Formulate Objectives   *25*

2 • IDENTIFYING THE STRATEGIC PROBLEM: NEEDS, DEMANDS,   *29*
ASSESSMENT, AND RESOURCES ANALYSIS
Environmental Dynamics   *29*
Planning With Limited Resources and Service Reductions   *30*
Power of External Actors on Planning   *31*
Environmental, Community, and Market Assessment   *32*
A MOSAIC Assessment   *32*
Basics Re Need Assessment   *34*
Attributes of Need Assessment   *36*
Concepts of Health   *37*
Need/Demand or Vice Versa   *38*
Needs Assessment Methods   *39*
  Key Informant Survey   *39*
  Community Survey   *42*
  Demographic Analysis   *45*
  Inferential Indicators   *47*
  Programmatic Data   *49*
  Index of Well-Being   *51*
  Duke—UNC Health Profile   *56*
  Sickness Impact Profile   *59*
  Sentinel Health Events   *61*
  HSRI's Quadrant Method for Estimating Mentally Ill Population   *70*
Demand Assessment Methods   *72*
  The Formula Approach   *72*
  The Stochastic Method   *74*
  Markov Chain Process   *75*
  Quality of Life Index   *79*
  Criteria Mapping   *82*
  Functional Status Index   *86*
Sources of Data   *88*
  Additional Data Sources   *89*
Computers and Data   *94*
  Management and Computer Decisions   *94*
  Basic Software Programs for Strategic Planners   *95*
Considerations Regarding Data Sources   *96*
Obstacles to the Receiving of Technical Information   *98*
The Value of Statistics   *98*

3 • RESOURCES MEANS MANPOWER, MATERIALS, AND MONEY   *103*
Rationing Resources   *104*
  Making Rationing Decisions   *104*
  Media-Driven Humanitarianism   *106*
  Rationing Guidelines   *107*
  Attitudes Toward Rationing   *108*

Methods of Resource Allocation   *109*
  Resource Allocation Methodology [RAM]   *109*
  Drug Abuse Prevention Program   *115*
  Resources Allocation Simulation in Model Locality   *116*
  Computer Simulation of Emergency Room Use   *116*
  Computer Mapping of Resources   *117*
  Self-Administered Questionnaires   *118*
  Structural Method for Increasing Resources   *120*
Peoplepower, Manpower, and Personnel   *121*
  Physician Hiring Process   *121*
  Medical Planning and Impact Analysis   *122*
  GMENAC Study of Physician Resources   *122*
  Responses to Personnel Supply Projections   *125*
  Efficient and Productive Use of Personnel   *128*
  Looking for People Power   *132*
Facilities   *132*
  Issues Concerning For-Profit Hospitals   *133*
  Methodology for Determining Capital Resources   *134*
  Forecasting Bed Need Methodology   *135*
  Mental Health System for the District of Columbia   *138*
Impact of Nursing Shortages on Facility Resources   *140*
Coordination of Planning Medical Resources   *142*
Equipment and Supplies   *143*
  High Technology Equipment Issues   *143*
  Routine Equipment and Supplies   *144*
Funding   *144*
  Flexibility and Innovation   *145*
  Resource Classification Taxonomies   *145*
  Collection of Inventory Data   *146*
  Key Word Technique   *147*
  Possible Resource/Potential Source Checklist   *148*
  Common and Uncommon Resources   *151*
  Implication of Policies for Resource Allocation   *151*

4 • GENERATING AND CONSIDERING ALTERNATIVE   *159*
    COURSES OF ACTION
Orientation to Creativity and Innovation   *159*
Ground Rules for Generating Alternatives   *161*
Lateral vs Vertical Thinking—Convergent or Divergent Paths   *162*
Breaking Away from Conformity   *162*
Elements of Creative Behavior   *163*
Barriers to Creativity and Innovation   *164*
Techniques for Generating Alternatives   *166*
  Brainstorming   *166*
  Questioning Checklists   *167*
  SCAMPER   *168*
  Why? Why? Why?   *168*

Five W's and an H   *168*
Charting, Mindmapping and Spidergram   *169*
Free Association or Thought Stream   *171*
Explain the Difficulty   *171*
Techniques for Groups   *171*
Slip Writing   *171*
Nominal Group Technique   *172*
Focus Groups   *172*
Phillips 66   *172*
Forced Association   *173*
Visual Synetics   *174*
Synetics   *175*
Delphi   *176*
Conceptualization   *176*
Innovator Computer Program   *176*
Is There a Best Technique?   *180*
Examining the Alternatives   *180*
Basic Criteria in CEA, CBA, and CUA   *181*
Cost Measurement Terminology   *182*
Cost-Benefit Analysis   *183*
Purposes and Limitations   *184*
Steps in CBA   *185*
CBA Examples   *185*
Whither CBA?   *191*
Cost Effectiveness Analysis   *191*
CEA Limitations   *191*
Steps in CEA   *192*
CEA Examples   *192*
Cost Utility Analysis   *196*
Value Distinctions and Choices   *197*
Creativity Exercise—Possible Solutions   *198*

5 • LIMITING AND RANKING OPTIONS: SELECTING PRIORITIES   *203*
Priority Setting Examples   *203*
WHO Plan for Health   *203*
Health Policy Agenda for the American People   *204*
Healthy People Priorities   *204*
Priorities in Public Health   *205*
Strategic Directions for Governing Boards   *207*
CEO Priorities   *208*
Consumer Priorities   *208*
Individual and Irrational Priorities   *208*
Changing Priorities Over Time   *209*
Goals and Priority Determination   *209*
Determination of Priorities   *209*
Criteria for Priority Determination   *210*
Components of the Process   *211*

Priority-Setting Methodologies   *212*
   The Simplex Method   *212*
   The Nominal Group Process   *217*
   Criteria Weighting Method   *221*
   The Hanlon Method   *224*
   Delphi Forecasting   *229*
Additional Methods for Setting Priorities   *232*
   Size of Need Gap   *232*
   Cluster Method of Prioritizing   *233*
   Preference Surveys   *235*
   Timing of Implementation and Priorities   *236*
   Social Area Analysis Method   *237*
   Potentially Productive Years of Life Lost [PPYLL]   *241*
   Computer Graphic Mapping Method to Identify Priorities   *243*
Priorities Now Compared to Then   *248*

6 • IMPLEMENTATION   *251*
A Humbling Observation   *251*
Implementation Strategies   *252*
Risk Factors and Implementation   *253*
Implementation in Action   *254*
   Smoking Cessation   *254*
   Freestanding Ambulatory Surgery Center   *254*
Setting Goals in Implementation   *255*
From A to B to C: Implementing Change   *255*
   Changing Behavior   *255*
   Overcoming Resistance to Change   *256*
   Changing Three Hospitals Into One   *256*
Constraints/Barriers/Pressures Toward Change   *257*
Implementing Health Care Marketing Activities   *259*
   Health Marketing Surges   *259*
   Marketing Basics   *259*
   Culture of Corporate Business   *261*
   Governing Board and CEO Directions   *262*
   Problems in Marketing   *263*
Product Lines, Market Segmentation, and Market Research   *264*
   Product Line Management   *264*
   Market Segmentation   *265*
   Market Research   *269*
Linking Marketing, Changing Behavior, and Implementation   *273*
   Ambulatory Care   *273*
   Home Health Care   *274*
   Long-Term Care   *275*
   Wellness Centers   *275*
   Nurse Entrepreneuring   *277*
Implementation Methods and Techniques   *277*
   Implementation Worksheet   *277*

Action Plan for AIDS Education   *279*
Flow Diagrams   *282*
Referral Network Diagram   *285*
Referral and Decision Network   *285*
Timeline [Gantt Chart]   *289*
Who/What/When Computer Software Program   *289*
Program Evaluation Review Technique [PERT]   *294*
Role Gridding   *297*
Gaming and Simulation   *300*
Sociopolitical Interactions in Implementation   *304*
Models of Health Care Governance   *305*
Classification of Sociopolitical Actors   *307*
Competitive vs. Cooperative Bargaining   *307*
Manipulation of Community Involvement   *308*
One Hospital's Trials and Tribulations   *308*
Task Forces, Work Groups, and Sociopolitics   *309*
Techniques for Meetings and Presentations   *310*
Sociopolitical Tradeoffs in Planning   *310*
Public Interests vs. Private Interests   *314*
Significant or Urgent Health Problems?   *315*
Implementation Imperatives   *316*

7 • EVALUATION   *323*
Why Do Evaluation?   *324*
Evaluation and Marketing   *325*
Managed Health Care Plan Market Survey   *325*
Hospital Market Evaluation   *326*
Marketing To Industry   *330*
Marketing and Regulation   *330*
Procedures for Evaluation   *330*
Monitoring As Evaluation   *332*
Generic Measurement Concepts   *333*
Evaluation Terminology Classifications   *335*
Generic Statistical Approaches   *336*
Evaluation Designs—Simple to Complex   *337*
Preexperimental Designs   *338*
True Experimental Designs   *338*
Quasi-Experimental Designs   *339*
Problems in Evaluation   *340*
Reliability and Validity   *341*
Evaluation Measurements, Methods, and Techniques   *343*
Knowledge, Attitudes, and Behavior   *344*
Structure, Process, and Outcome Evaluation   *345*
Management Use of S-P-O   *345*
S-P-O in "Soft Services"   *348*
Mainly Outcome Evaluations   *348*
Indicators as Measurements   *352*

Administrative Data Indicators   *353*
BED Instead of DOC   *353*
Poor Quality Indicators   *354*
Data for Indicators   *354*
Objectives of Indicators   *357*
Health Concept and Indicators   *357*
Shortcomings of Poverty Indicators   *358*
Quality of Life Indicators   *359*
Utility Value of Life   *362*
Access to Services Indicators   *362*
Sentinel Health Events (Occupational)   *362*
Comparison of National Health Indicators   *369*
Measurement Using Indexes   *369*
Years Lost, Well Years and Healthy Days   *370*
Functional Status Index for ESRD   *370*
Cross National Index Comparison   *370*
Rehabilitation Index   *371*
Tracer Method as Index   *372*
Measurement By Criteria, Checklist, Guidelines, Standards, And So On   *372*
Checklists for Evaluation   *374*
Strategic Planning Checklist in Retardation   *374*
Corporate Critical Success Factors   *375*
Nursing Care for Long Stay Patients   *376*
Computer and Manual Criteria for Auditing Quality of Care Guidelines   *376*
What Are Clinical Trials All About? Questions?   *381*
Business Checklists   *382*
Hospitalization for Suicide   *382*
Scales as Measurement Tools   *382*
Types of Scales   *382*
Performance Appraisal Systems   *384*
Ward Atmosphere Scale   *386*
Scales Rate Doctors Who Use Computers   *386*
Arthritis Impact Measurement Scale   *387*
Survey Techniques in Evaluation   *387*
Types of Surveys   *386*
Mail, Telephone, and Personal Survey Comparison   *389*
Computer-Assisted Telephone Interview   *389*
Surveys of Health Status   *390*
Surveys of Mental Illness   *397*
Patient Satisfaction Surveys   *400*
Evaluations of Programs   *405*
Distinctions Between Evaluation and Research   *406*
Steps in Program Evaluation   *406*
Evaluation of Utilization Review Program   *407*
Self-Care Program to Reduce Utilization   *408*
Utilization Focused Evaluation   *408*
Technology Assessment Iterative Loop [TAIL]   *409*

National Long-Term Care Channeling Demonstration   *410*
Access to Primary Care at Lower Cost   *411*
Evaluation Reports Do Spread the Words   *412*
A New Cycle of Evaluation   *414*

Author Index   *423*

Subject Index   *432*

List of Exhibits

1-1	Stages of Health Planning	*3*
1-2	Strategic Planning Process	*7*
1-3	Planning Trends: Historical and National Legislation	*19*
2-1	Primary Components of the Environmental Assessment	*33*
2-2	Components of the Community and Market Assessment	*34*
2-3	MOSAIC Strategic System Network	*35*
2-4	Scales and Definitions for Functional Level Classification	*52*
2-5	Function-Level Classification and Measured Values	*53*
2-6	Computation of Function Status Index	*55*
2-7	Computation of Value-Adjusted Life Expectancy	*56*
2-8	Duke–UNC Health Profile: A Health Status Instrument	*57*
2-9	Sickness Impact Profile Categories and Selected Items	*60*
2-10	Summary of Sickness Impact Profile (SIP) Structure and Content with a Scoring Example	*61*
2-11	Unnecessary Disease, Disability, and Untimely Death: Indexes Based on Rates	*63*
2-12	Quadrant Method for Estimating the Seriously/Chronically Mentally Ill Population	*71*
2-13	Probabilistic Distribution of Daily Census, Pediatrics	*75*
2-14	Transition Matrix for Buyers of Three Types of Automobiles	*76*
2-15	Markov Chain Forecast for Long-Term Care by Place and Level of Care	*77*
2-16	Markov Chain Results: New Clients	*78*
2-17	Quality of Life Index for Colostomy Patients	*80*
2-18	Mean Values for Overall QLI Score and Subscores	*82*
2-19	Sample Portion of Chest Pain Criteria Map	*83*
2-20	Estimated Risk and Map Scores for Selected Patients	*84*
2-21	Chest Pain Criteria Map Scores for Admitted Patients	*85*
2-22	Functional Status Index	*87*
2-23	Functional Outcomes: Response Patterns in Medical and Surgical Patients	*89*
2-24	Examples of Data by Type and Sources	*90*
2-25	Considerations Regarding Sources of Data—Examples	*97*
3-1	A Public Health Care Model: Problems; Intervention; Effects	*112*

3-2	Four Health Care Indices in Resource Allocation Method (RAM)	*113*
3-3	General Form of RAM Allocation Formula	*114*
3-4	Resource Analysis Worksheet	*115*
3-5	Market Penetration Rates by Zip Code: Boston	*118*
3-6	Acute Myocardial Infarction Death Rates by County, Alabama	*119*
3-7	Supply and Potential Spatial Accessibility of General Practitioner Services in Abitibi-Temiscamingue, Canada	*120*
3-8	Five Defining Characteristics of Health Care Plans	*121*
3-9	Medical Manpower Planning/Impact Analysis Flow Process	*123*
3-10	Combination of Skills Identified by Employers as Meeting Their Needs	*127*
3-11	A Patient Care Unit Example—Portable Acute Hemodialysis	*131*
3-12	Factors Used in Assessing the Need for Modernization/Renovation/Replacement	*136*
3-13	Nebraska Mental Health Service System Model	*137*
3-14	California Community Mental Health Program Model	*137*
3-15	Organization of Proposed Mental Health System	*138*
3-16	District Hospitals and Community Mental Health Centers	*139*
3-17	Comparison: Current Mental Health System vs. Proposed System	*141*
3-18	Step-by-Step Inventory Development Procedure	*146*
3-19	Outpatient Health Resources Collection Form and Guidelines	*147*
3-20	Key Word List for Potential Resources	*148*
3-21	Possible Resources and Potential Sources	*149*
3-22	Common and Uncommon Resources	*152*
4-1	Creativity Exercises	*160*
4-2	A Dilemma for the Mice in Council	*160*
4-3	A Self-Interrogation Checklist of W's and H's	*169*
4-4	Free Association via Charting	*170*
4-5	Concept Mapping and Cluster Grouping	*177*
4-6	Innovator Computer Pull-Down Menus	*178*
4-7	Examples of Computer Brainstorming Using Innovator Software	*179*
4-8	CEA, CBA, CUA: Costs and Benefits Formulations	*182*
4-9	CBA: Hip Replacement vs. Ulcer Drug vs. Spina Bifida Screening	*186*
4-10	CBA: Parenteral Nutrition—Hospital vs. Home	*188*
4-11	CBA: Four Technical Information Components and Costs	*189*
4-12	Potential Savings in Medicaid Abuser Control Program	*190*
4-13	CEA: Six Strategies to Reduce Neonatal Mortality	*193*
4-14	CEA: Decision Tree Outcomes for Direct Antigen Testing	*195*
4-15	CEA Values and Sensitivity of Predictive Testing	*195*
5-1	Simplex Questions on Community Health	*213*
5-2	Simplex Questions on General Social Concerns	*214*
5-3	Simplex Questions on Strategic Health Planning Concerns	*215*
5-4	Simplex Questions on Political Concerns	*216*
5-5	Nominal Group Task Statement Forms	*219*
5-6	Nominal Group Vote Tally Sheet Example	*220*
5-7	Nominal Group Final Rank Tally Sheet Example	*221*
5-8	Criteria Weighting: Determining Significance Levels for Community Health Issues Criteria	*223*
5-9	Criteria Weighting: Significance Level Rating of Importance of Three Proposals	*224*

5-10   Mortality Rates for Four Disease Conditions: Indian Reservation, South Dakota
     and the U.S.   232
5-11   Single Health Event Disease Occurrences by Major Diagnoses and Selected
     Groups: New York State Residents   234
5-12   Priority Alternative Options for a Deficit-Ridden Facility   235
5-13   Priority Rank on Each Need Category and Total Need for 15 Mental
     Health Areas   239
5-14   Program Development Priorities by Need and Resources for 15 Mental
     Health Areas   239
5-15   Seven Indicators of Alcohol-Related Mortality   240
5-16   Ten Leading Causes of Death and Rank by Potentially Productive Years
     of Life Lost [PPYLL]   242
5-17   Business Participation in Health Care Politics by State   244
5-18   Alcohol-Related Chronic Health Problems Index, New Mexico   245
5-19   Alcohol-Related Casualties Index, New Mexico   246
5-20   Cancer of the Trachea, Bronchus, and Lung, Georgia   247
6-1   Marketing Segmentation Nursing Home Action Plan   268
6-2   Advantages and Disadvantages of Survey Methods   271
6-3   Health Care Marketing Techniques by Implementation Variables   271
6-4   Niches, Parameters, and Differentiators for Long-Term Care Providers   276
6-5   Steps in the Development of Implementation Strategy   278
6-6   Generic Implementation Worksheet for a Countrywide Detection
     and Treatment Center   278
6-7   Strategic Health Planning Activity Worksheet   279
6-8   Seven-Step Approach in AIDS Education   280
6-9   Flow Diagram for New Outpatients   283
6-10   Patient Incident Investigative Process: Veterans Administration   284
6-11   Problem-Solving Technique Via a Flow Chart   286
6-12   Referral Network: Unwed Teenage Pregnant Girls   288
6-13   What Happens to Vocational Rehabilitation Disability Referrals?   290
6-14   Modernization Time Schedule: Veterans Benefits Department   292
6-15   Who/What/When People View   293
6-16   Who/What/When Project View   293
6-17   Who/What/When Daily Calendar   294
6-18   Program Implementation Using PERT (Program Evaluation
     and Review Technique)   295
6-19   PERT Network for Developing an Open Heart Surgery Unit   296
6-20   Role Gridding Model: State Mental Health Department Drug Abuse Program   298
6-21   Input and Output Data from Health Services Simulation   301
6-22   GamePlan Computer Menu and Summary of Cards   304
6-23   Four GamePlan Corporate Sociocultural Descriptions   306
6-24   Meetings, Groupings, and Presentation Techniques   311
7-1   Ten Tips for a Successful Survey   326
7-2   Hospital Market Survey Description and Questions for General Public, Recent
     Patients, Physicians, and Industry   327
7-3   Evaluation Do's and Don'ts   331
7-4   Four Levels of Measurement and the Statistics Appropriate to Each Level   337

7-5	Variations in Evaluation Designs	*338*
7-6	Measures of Structure, Process, and Outcome	*345*
7-7	Selected Performance Measures	*346*
7-8	Structural and Process Variables Enhancing Organizational Performance	*347*
7-9	Comparison of HCFA and Alternative Approaches for Analyzing Medicare Patient Outcomes	*350*
7-10	Process, Outcome, and Impact Evaluation in Drug Abuse Prevention	*353*
7-11	Indicators and Criteria for Important Aspects of Care, By Type of Care	*355*
7-12	Social Indicators Highly Correlated with Need for Mental Health Services	*358*
7-13	Medicaid Eligibility: Criterion, Indicators, and Measures	*361*
7-14	Sentinel Health Events—Occupational	*362*
7-15	Reintegration to Normal Living Index: Survey Statements	*372*
7-16	Checklist for Evaluating Mental Retardation Planning	*374*
7-17	Criteria for Evaluating Nursing Care	*377*
7-18	COOP Chart to Measure Physical Function	*378*
7-19	Quality Screening Criteria	*379*
7-20	Comparisons of Five Health Status Measures	*393*
7-21	Short Form Health Survey: Medical Outcomes Study	*395*
7-22	Duke—UNC Functional Social Support Questionnaire	*396*
7-23	Measures Used in 13 Studies to Assess Prevalence of Mental Illness Among Homeless Persons	*398*
7-24	Short Screening Instrument for Depression	*400*
7-25	Checklist for Better Written Communications	*413*

About the Authors

Allen D. Spiegel is a professor of preventive medicine and community health, College of Medicine, Health Science Center at Brooklyn, State University of New York. Previously, he was a special research fellow at Brandeis University; a health education associate with The Medical Foundation, Inc., in Boston; and chief of the radio and TV unit of the New York City Health Department.

His education includes degrees from Brooklyn College (A.B.; B.S. Equivalent), New York University (Special Diploma in Radio & TV), Columbia University (M.P.H.) and the Heller School at Brandeis University (Ph.D.).

Dr. Spiegel is active as a consultant and speaker to a wide variety of medical, health, and social welfare organizations on topics such as community mental health, strategic health planning, public/patient/ physician health communications, medical sociology, and health care organization and administration.

A prolific author, Dr. Spiegel has more than 100 articles to his credit in addition to more than 20 books including:

Perspectives in Community Mental Health
Medicaid: Lessons for National Health Insurance
The Medicaid Experience
Curing and Caring
Basic Health Planning Methods
Rehabilitating People with Disabilities into the Mainstream of Society
Medical Technology, Health Care and the Consumer
Home Healthcare: Home Birthing to Hospice
Cost Containment and DRGs: A Guide to Prospective Payment
Home Healthcare (Second ed.)

Since 1968, **Herbert H. Hyman** has been a professor of health planning and administration, Graduate Program of Urban Affairs and Urban Planning, Hunter College, City University of New York. He has a doctorate from the Heller School of Brandeis University, Waltham, Massachusetts.

Dr. Hyman has written or co-authored six books on health and human resources subjects with emphasis on health regulation, health planning methods, implementation of health planning, and health systems planning. All his books have been widely adopted for use in graduate college curriculums.

In addition, Dr. Hyman has served as a consultant to federal, state, and municipal governments as well as to private corporations. During the 1988/1989 academic year, he was awarded a Fulbright scholarship to Israel where he taught health planning and health administration courses at Tel Aviv University's Recanati School of Business.

Preface

Since the beginning of the 1980s, health planning has been in a turmoil and decidedly more so as the federal government switched its planning initiatives. Even prior to the turbulent 1980s, hospitals began to emphasize strategic health planning patterned after corporate business planning. Today, strategic health planning is consistent with the concentration on privatization of health care services and the corporate model that stresses the bottom line and earning profits. Health services in general, and specifically hospitals, are engaged in a highly competitive marketplace fighting for patients and profits. Amidst the competitive marketplace, the federal government's use of Diagnosis Related Groups (DRGs) as a reimbursement mechanism and the Peer Review Organizations (PROs) as a quality and utilization watchdog fuels the dynamic environment. These happenings can lead to the situation where services may be eliminated that do not attract enough customers to at least break even in the profit-and-loss column. Trends such as these have triggered a surge in concern about strategic health planning.

Although strategic health planning applies the concepts of rational planning, the emphasis is quite varied. Concerned with survival, health care providers seek to discover the target audience for their services and to market those services to that population group. Strategic health planning does focus on market segmentation, marketing, and promotion. This book does explain the similarities and differences between comprehensive health planning and strategic health planning.

Within the framework of a six-step strategic planning process, this book provides an extensive and comprehensive compilation of methods and techniques for each aspect of planning. Obviously, the collection is not complete, but the myriad of approaches do suggest guideposts for strategic planners to effectively and efficiently complete their assignments. Special attention is given to marketing and promotion in the chapter on implementation and throughout the book in the numerous examples and exhibits.

This book can be useful to those concerned with identifying and resolving the problems existing in the delivery of health care services. Trustees, chief executive officers, department administrators, and staff planners will find that this text can assist them in the following manner: in pinpointing needs in their geographic service areas; in garnering resources in terms of staff, material, and money; in creating and selecting priority alternative options; in implementing the activities; and in evaluating the outcomes. In an environment of spirited competition, it is vital that decision makers base their choices on more than educated guesses and intuition. Facts, trends, demographic analysis, and real needs are all part of the fodder for decisions included in our concept of strategic health planning. No other source book assembles in one place the range of the methods and techniques supplied in this volume.

Educational faculty members may find our text appropriate for teaching students in a variety of health care-related programs about the strategic health planning process. Being educators ourselves, we certainly feel that the book presents a wealth of material suitable for instructional purposes.

Both of us have served as consultants to government and private health care organizations and conducted research in health planning, regulation, health care organization/administration and evaluation. We are fully aware of the resources required for a commitment to institutional strategic health planning. Our book can help organizations to reduce their input of resources in a number of ways. For those working on specific ad hoc planning problems, our book serves up a compendium of methods and techniques to pick and choose from to select the ones best suited to your special difficulty. For those concerned with particular topics, the broad range of illustrative examples and exhibits offer models that can be copied, adopted, or adapted to your own needs and objectives. For those requiring additional detailed information, all the chapters are well documented with relevant sources. For those who require data on certain topics located throughout the book, an extensive table of contents and index allows for intelligent gathering of pertinent material. Lastly, for those who wish to nibble here and there and skim through strategic health planning, we hope that our book attracts your attention and holds your interest as the pieces stand by themselves. In a dynamic field such as strategic health planning, we sought to provide the jumping off place from where others can extend and enlarge the scope of the methods and techniques we have presented.

We also wish to acknowledge the major contribution of Grant Abrams, our research associate, who diligently tracked down elusive articles and journals to review and evaluate. Medical reference librarians at the Health Science Center at Brooklyn also provided indispensable assistance in managing the flow of information and in resolving problems. In addition, Lois Hahn proved to be a veritable powerhouse of help with the mechanical aspects of communicating with the computer in the formation of our manuscript. Furthermore, Molly Kessert, Cheryl Moore, Jennifer Rothstein, and Cynthia Skeete assisted with typing and assorted tasks. We sincerely thank all who contributed to our endeavor with the humble realization that a project such as this is not completed in isolation and silent meditation.

Allen D. Spiegel
Herbert H. Hyman

1

An Introduction to Strategic Health Planning

CHANGING TIMES AND TIDES

Health planning has been subjected to buffeting twists and turns in health policy decisions since the heydays of popularity in the early 1960s. In discussing U.S. health policy expectations and realities, Ginzberg [1988] examines the following 10 policy areas "bedeviled by confusion or, in less charged terms, where current beliefs are out of sync with reality:"

Cost containment
Physician supply
Private insurance
Long-term care
Prevention
Wasteful and ineffective care
Rationing expensive care
The procompetition solution
Health maintenance organizations
Canadian Health Care System model

Ginzberg's comments about each of the policy areas sums up his analysis: Costs continue to rise; there is undoubtedly waste in the system; 260 to 270 physicians per 100,000 by the year 2000 may be a surplus, a balance, or a shortage; HMOs appear to be a big white hope regarding the provision of care; neither competition or regulation holds much promise individually; private insurance hasn't benefited from the self-insurance trend; long-term care is still unresolved; to deny high-tech medicine to individuals is not feasible; effective prevention methods are not consistent with democratic values; and the U.S. population is about 10 times larger than Canada's and dislocations in that system may get more serious.

Continuing in a somewhat negative vein on similar and related issues, former Colorado

Governor Richard D. Lamm [1988] throws down the gauntlet in the following eight-count indictment against American public health policy:

1. America spends more per capita for health care than any other nation, yet our health statistics are among the worst in the industrial world.
2. We give little or no thought to how we can maximize the money we spend on health care.
3. Unacceptable and wide discrepancies exist in medical practice between various geographic areas in America.
4. The health care industry wrongly leads us to believe they are the only [or at least the best] way to good health.
5. We are not wise enough to turn off the machines we were smart enough to invent.
6. Defensive medicine is costing America billions of dollars that add dramatically to our health care costs.
7. Our society intimates that we can "cure" death and thus misallocates billions of dollars, badly needed elsewhere, in our social spending.
8. Health care overspending has become an economic cancer to the American economy.

Lamm's summary: "Our health care system is costing us too much and producing too little."

Despite the deep-seated health policy issues raised by both Ginzberg and Lamm, most people still feel that they are getting good care and respect and trust their physicians.

DEMISE OF FEDERAL PLANNING LEGISLATION

On October 3, 1986, the National Health Planning and Resources Act [PL 93–641] was rescinded. That Act's demise completed a 12-year experiment that appeared to fail, ending more than 20 years of federal involvement in health care planning. Mueller [1988] provides a political explanation for the failure of PL 93–641. He claims that the Act failed to constrain costs or to provide a framework for a projected national health insurance program anticipated by the framers of the law. During that 12-year period, the supporters of the Act weakened in their resolve while the political environment and strategies for containing costs also radically changed. In concert, President Ronald Reagan's opposition and the shift from neutrality to opposition by the American Hospital Association and the American Medical Association combined to overturn the weakened supporters of the Act. In addition, studies raised questions about the degree of public support and confidence in the Health Systems Agencies [HSAs] suggesting that the American public was skeptical about health planning in general [Mick & Thompson, 1984]. More importantly, the strategic movement from reliance on regulation to stimulating competition provided a significant alternative for containing spiraling medical costs. A prospective payment system [PPS] using the diagnosis related groups [DRGs] reimbursement mechanism, expansion of Health Maintenance Organizations [HMOs], and consumer emphasis on prevention and the use of ambulatory medical services became significant alternatives to the failed cost containment efforts of PL 93–641's reliance on certificate-of-need regulation to curtail medical costs.

At the same time, significant changes occurred within the hospitals' environment. On the one hand, hospital income was dropping due to lowered occupancy rates, shorter hospital stays,and DRG limits on inpatient charges. On the other hand, pressures were being placed on hospitals to maintain the quality of care. Professional Review Organizations [PROs] and the heightened emphasis by the Joint Commission on the Accreditation of Healthcare Organizations [JCAHO] on quality assurance urged hospitals to do more with less income. These two forces placed hospitals in an atmosphere where survival, not growth, becomes the primary concern.

A new environment has emerged that is quite different from prior situations—the so-called "medical-industrial-complex." In fact, Stoline and Weiner [1988] detailed the major trends in their physician's guide to the new medical marketplace and the health care revolution. This changing environment and the demise of PL 93–641 prompted revisions to make planning theory consistent with the new environment of challenge and competition. PL 93–641's concern for access to care, availability, continuity, quality, and affordability of care were no longer the relevant emphases. Cost containment pre-empted all of these as the most important factor troubling Congress, the executive branch, and the general public. Exhibit 1-1 shows the evolution of health planning from the 1900s depicting the shift to a market emphasis. However, Budrys' [1986, p. 133] study of 20th-century developments in planning for the nation's health concludes that there is a consensus that the health care delivery system is in crisis, but there is a lack of consensus on how to solve the problems.

STRATEGIC HEALTH PLANNING ADVANCES

Although people interchangeably use the terms "strategic planning," "long-range planning," and "strategic management," Yoo and Digman [1987] disagree and note a distinction. "Strategic management is more than strategic planning since another essential ingredient, *strategic control,* should be included" [authors' emphasis]. That control distinction is probably most often subsumed in the literature relative to strategic planning. However, planners should be alert to the management control issue in planning as the discussion continues.

Pomrinse [1983] attributes the failure of hospitals to survive on the lack of a strategic plan to move expeditiously in a dynamic changing market. He states that the failure to aggregate capital is the primary cause of hospital closings. Usually, that lack of capital results from a hospital's poor leadership, a failure to maintain technological adequacy, and a consequent loss of hospital staff and patient population. As Pomrinse notes:

> In the health field, with its rapidly changing technology, the need for timely employment of human and financial capital is even more obvious. If an organization cannot perform this function adequately, it will founder and fail.

Exhibit 1-1. Stages of Health Planning.

Stages	Time Period	Major Concern	Control
Private Sector	1900–Late 1950s	Quality of Care	Professional
Public Sector Initial Stage	Late 1950s to Early 1970s	Access to Care	Administrative Grounded in Volunteerism
Public Sector Advanced Stage	Early 1970s to End of 1970s	Cost Containment	Administrative Combined with Regulation
Regionalization of Health Planning	1980–	Managerial Efficiency	Market

Source: From *Planning for the nation's health: A study of 20th century developments in the U.S.,* by G. Budrys, p. 4a, 1986, Greenwood Press. Reprinted by permission.

Two other health researchers [Kennedy & Dumas, 1983] examined five variables related to hospital closures: hospital size, occupancy rate, type of ownership, length of stay, and expenditures per patient-day. In their study of hospital closures in three states, they found that only two of these variables correlated with closure: size and occupancy. Maryland,the state with the highest occupancy rate and largest average hospital size, had only one hospital closure during the 1960–1980 period. Together, Pennsylvania and Arizona experienced 52 closures during this period. Both had lower occupancy rates and smaller-sized hospitals than Maryland.

Based on this study, Kennedy and Dumas [1983] hypothesize that "small hospitals lacking medical school affiliation, with less powerful and committed boards of trustees, limited services, limited levels of technology, and less skilled managerial staffs are at greater risk of closure than are hospitals without these characteristics."

Obviously, this struggle for survival results in competition among hospitals and between health care providers and places a premium on marketing and strategic planning.

Smith [1987] extensively discusses the meaning of strategic management while Evashwick and Evashwick [1988] define the fine art of strategic planning in precise language:

> Strategic planning is the process of assessing a changing environment to create a vision of the future; determining how the organization fits into the anticipated environment based on its institutional mission, strengths, and weaknesses; and then setting in motion a plan of action to position the organization accordingly.

Winners in this process and product competition are more likely to survive and even grow if they recruit top physician personnel, engage in mergers that are likely to reduce competition, provide more comprehensive services, and develop satellite services near higher socioeconomic communities [Kennedy & Dumas, 1983]. In a publication from the American Hospital Association, Peters [1985] details a strategic planning process for hospitals.

Strategic planning and/or strategic management is the new emphasis in health planning. It is an old concept with new heightened immediacy. Strategic planning is based on corporate market planning in which the emphasis is on maximizing profits through control of a market segment. Identification of that market segment leads to the strategic formulation of methods of interdiction with those consumers interested in the products being offered. Hospitals, for example, are faced with the dual problem of being both comprehensive to meet the needs of the general public and of being selective and known as *the* hospital that offers specialized services in sports medicine, pain control, open heart surgery, or whatever, better than any of its competitors. Whether they are operating at a primary, secondary, or tertiary level of care, hospitals are currently offering a comprehensive array of services. What distinguishes one from the other? Why should a patient or a physician be associated with one or the other? To the point, McDevitt's [1987] survey of 80 hospitals showed that most "have not yet made the critical transition from the traditional production orientation to the more progressive marketing orientation."

WHAT IS THE BUSINESS OF THIS BUSINESS?

To unconfuse or demystify the consumer, initially a hospital must know its own mission. Organizational development theory posits that as an organization evolves, the sharp focus on achieving the original goals and objectives dims. Organizations become more concerned with maintaining or conserving the status quo. In sum, organizations shift from being goal-oriented to maintenance-oriented. In fact, the very success and growth of hospitals through the 1960s and early 1970s resulted in many of them forgetting their original goals. Even in the shorter term, this holds true. In studying the goal statements of several mid-western hospitals over a three-year period, Timmel and Brozovich [1981] found a distinct pattern. Goal and project statements all utilized a "management by objectives" framework, and were well written, "but there was no defined scope, sequence, nor any discernible connection between the goals in years one, two and three." In an era of cost consciousness and federal oversight of both expenditures and provision of quality care, health care providers, hospital trustees and administrators must step back and examine themselves. To do this, Simyar, Lloyd-Jones, and Caro [1988, p. 7] suggest asking three basic questions:

> Where are we now?
> Where do we wish to go?
> How will we get there?

Simplistic as these questions appear, when health care officials begin to try and answer them, the questions become complex and may create confusion in those trying to respond to them.

In strategy formulation, the main question is "What is the business of this business?" [Drucker, 1974, p. 99]. Do the trustees, for example, of a 200-bed community hospital want to specialize in some service such as sports medicine, preventive medicine, or diabetes control? Are they satisfied with their present role as an undistinguished but good community hospital? Are they willing to change the structure of their hospital, the type of traditional trustees, the patient population, the marketing techniques, and the methods of raising funds? Do they know who their competitors are, the size of the market or population requiring services, or the new regulatory measures? Answering these basic questions leads to a profound soul searching by health care providers. Yet, this soul searching is required for the formulation of a strategic plan.

CHARACTERISTICS OF STRATEGIC PLANNING

Cartwright [1987] stresses that "planning involves judgment as well as technique" in dealing with four fundamental types of problems: simple problems, compound problems, complex problems, and metaproblems. Obviously, not every problem benefits from a "quick fix" and planning may be doomed because "too much is expected of it or because not enough is put into it." Going further in the discussion about the lost art of planning, Cartwright suggests the following four rationales for trying to resurrect the art of planning:

- Using the wrong planning strategy is not just misguided. It can be disastrous.
- A rational approach to solving a simple problem is not the same as a rational approach to making improvements relative to a complex problem. It is a mistake to describe any planning strategy as *the rational strategy* [author's emphasis].
- Any planning strategy that is rigidly linear or sequential is limited in applicability. Doubling-back or forward may be required to account for emerging developments.
- Complex and meta-problems can't be separated from implementation. Monitoring and adaptation with a succession of ameliorating actions rather than a single solution may be required.

Within these rationales, Cartwright points out that one-dimensional planners may wish to hew too closely to their comfortable process, comprehensive, and/or bureaucratic strategies to force closure on problems. Two proverbs are cited as disclaimers: The best is sometimes the enemy of the good; and it is sometimes cruel to be kind.

Major attributes that distinguish strategic from other forms of health planning have been identified by Clemenhagen and Champagne [1984]:

- A market-driven and market-based approach.
- More emphasis on qualitative than quantitative analysis.
- Development under the direct control of the chief executive officer without delegation.
- Strategy must be clearly stated and persuasively sold throughout the institution.
- Final planning goals, objectives, and programs must be vigorously implemented.
- Middle management must be carefully prepared to engage in strategic planning.
- Emphasis of data collection and analysis is on the "nuts and bolts" of the health institution's business.
- Strategic planning is integrated with other management functions.
- Strong focus is on the gaining and sustaining of a competitive advantage.

Simyar et al. [1988] identify the following eight steps in the strategic health planning process:

1. Identifying the organization's current position including present mission, long-term objectives, strategies, and policies.
2. Analyzing the environment.
3. Conducting an organizational audit.
4. Identifying the various alternative strategies based on the relevant data.
5. Selecting the best alternative.
6. Gaining acceptance of the chosen strategy.
7. Preparing long-range and short-range plans to support and carry out the strategy.
8. Implementing the plan and conducting an ongoing evaluation.

Exhibit 1-2 depicts another strategic planning process that also reveals similarities. Whitman [1988] uses the technique to identify the right services to offer.

Dyson and Foster [1983] delineate the following characteristics of an effective strategic planning system. Interestingly, Yoo and Digman [1987] regard these attributes as similar to their concept of strategic management:

Clear statement of objectives
Integration
Catalytic action
Richness of formulation
Depth of evaluation
Treatment of uncertainty
Resources planned
Data
Iteration in the process
Assumptions
Quantification of goals
Control measures
Feasibility of implementation

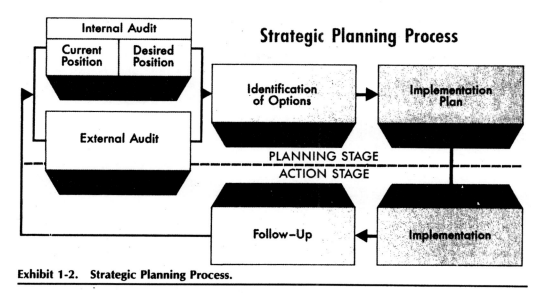

Exhibit 1-2. Strategic Planning Process.

Source: From "Identifying the right services to offer," by J. J. Whitman, 1988, *Provider, 14*[4], 10–13. Reprinted with permission of the American Health Care Association.

While obviously related, these varying characteristics will allow for gathering the components of strategic planning together for comparative analysis.

A COMPARISON OF STRATEGIC AND COMPREHENSIVE HEALTH PLANNING

An examination of the various strategic planning process leads to the curious finding that the methodology is not much different from comprehensive health planning.

A study of this process clearly reveals the similarity between strategic and comprehensive planning as outlined by Spiegel and Hyman [1978]. Despite the semantic differences, problems are still identified; resources are still inventoried; alternatives are still generated; priorities are still selected; choices are still implemented; and there is still an ongoing evaluation.

In a critical review of the planning literature from the 1960s through the 1980s plus the results of personal interviews with planning practitioners, Kaufman and Jacobs [1987] further examine the distinctions between strategic and comprehensive public planning. Their examination begins with the following basic steps in strategic planning as outlined by Sorkin, Ferris, and Hudak [1984]:

- Scan the environment.
- Select key issues.
- Set mission statements or broad goals.
- Undertake external and internal analyses.
- Develop goals, objectives, and strategies for each issue.
- Develop an implementation plan to carry out strategic actions.
- Monitor, update, and scan.

From the planning literature, Kaufman and Jacobs concluded: "We find that the critiques and suggestions embodied in strategic planning are long-standing, well-developed, and well-known . . . corporate strategic planning is distinctive in bringing these points together into a coherent planning process model." From telephone interviews with 15 planners across the U.S. who practiced strategic planning, Kaufman and Jacobs reported typical comments: "I don't see the strategic planning process as significantly different from what I learned in planning school." "Strategic planning is like pouring old wine into new bottles." Respondents were both favorable and unfavorable toward strategic planning. "All, however, found that strategic planning was not significantly different from good comprehensive planning; it was different in emphasis, they said, but not different in kind" [Kaufman & Jacobs, 1987].

If these similarities exist in both processes, what are the differences between the two concepts? Philosophically, strategic planning focuses on organizational survival through ensuring selection of those services that bring profits to the operations. While strategic planning results in providing services for the welfare and health of the public, the services are selective in terms of which segments of the population will benefit. Services are primarily offered that create profits. Specific differences have been identified by proponents of strategic planning [Kaufman & Jacobs, 1987]:

- Oriented more toward action, results, and implementation.
- Broader and more diverse participation in the planning process.
- Emphasis on understanding the community in its external context, determining the opportunities and threats to a community via an environmental scan.
- Embraces competitive behavior on the part of communities.
- Emphasizes assessing a community's strengths and weaknesses in context of opportunities and threats.

On the other hand, comprehensive health planning is concerned with the health and medical needs of the entire population, regardless of the profit and loss statement. This general orientation of benefiting the entire population regardless of profit gives most providers their nonprofit status. Of course, that is in direct contrast to the outcome of strategic planning where profits are the prime consideration and the needs of the population secondary.

Comprehensive health planning takes a broad umbrella look at the terrain. Resources of all health care providers, rather than each one as a separate entity, are examined to determine the total range of resources available to meet the population's defined needs. Cooperative activities rather than competition are fostered. Coordination of services is a vital function in implementation of comprehensive health planning recommendations. Emphasis is on quality of care, access, availability of services, and continuity of care. While attention is paid to cost, it is of secondary importance in this planning process.

Strategic planning must determine whether there is a large enough base of consumers in need of and ready to use the offered services. Additionally, there has to be a consideration of whether the organization's leadership, resource base, and structure are capable of rendering those services. In essence, health care providers move from a service-based orientation to a profit-motivated one, from serving a general public regardless of internal needs and profits to a selective population that will guarantee organizational survival through generating profits.

In addition, Rohrer and Levey [1987] identify a further difference: "Strategic planning is generally directed from the apex of the organization. In government, a similar structure would have the state in control of the planning process, as opposed to a situation where the agency merely serves as a referee among competing interest groups."

Thus, whereas the steps in strategic planning and comprehensive planning are similar, the philosophical emphases are quite distinct.

These conflicting alternative concepts highlight the different emphases in the planning process. Strategic planning engages in selective need assessment analysis, evaluates the strengths and weaknesses of other health care providers, and competes for market shares. This process stresses an examination of both the external and internal environment.

EXTERNAL AND INTERNAL ENVIRONMENTAL ASSESSMENT

At least 10 components are included in Hawley's [1988] environmental assessment: the economy, demographics, morbidity and mortality statistics, reimbursement, financing, and legislation, technology and research, health care delivery, cost and utilization, human resources, medical ethics, and social attitudes and lifestyle factors.

Internal environment review includes elements such as mission statements, goals, and objectives, historical organizational review, operating data, staffing, facilities, and space [Whitman, 1988]. This is the so-called SWOT internal analysis of *s*trengths, *w*eaknesses, *o*pportunities, and *t*hreats [Hawley,1988].

PROVIDERS MUST COPE

Health care providers have been forced to pay attention to a number of trends and policy issues that impact on their potential for survival and growth. These have been mentioned earlier and are expanded upon here.

Prospective Payment System

Implementation of DRGs as a prospective payment price setting reimbursement method to cover Medicare inpatients placed hospitals and other health care providers in the role of profit-making corporations. With a contract to provide a given medical service at a predetermined price, providers earn a profit if services can be rendered at a cost lower than the preset reimbursement. Conversely, providers suffer a loss if expenses exceed the payment. Large enough losses may eventually bankrupt the facility or the provider. For this reason, health care providers may be forced to be selective in both the patient mix and the services provided.

Monitoring Quality of Care

A further pressure on a provider's capacity to survive is the federal government's monitoring of the quality of care given to Medicare patients. Importantly, Medicare beneficiaries may represent about 30–35 percent of a hospitals' patient population. Professional review organizations, created by federal legislation, ensure that Medicare patients are not short-changed or overserviced in their treatment. PROs pay close attention to a hospital's quality of care and the cost of those services. In some cases, private businesses also formed coalitions to monitor and to publish cost data about physicians and institutions. For example, the Midwest Business Group on Health found that "just collecting health care utilization data helps trim costs" and that "providers improve their efficiency simply because they are being watched." Calling this the "sentinel effect," these private users are placing great importance on improved data collection and monitoring [Drury, 1984]. Through the pressure generated by these processes, providers are forced to study the diagnostic/treatment activities of their services. Indirectly, physicians and other providers who deviate from expected federal norms and standards will be called to account by both health care administrators and PROs. PROs can withhold payment for services improperly offered and even exclude errant providers from the Medicare program.

High Technology

Providers are increasing their use of high technology equipment and computers for diagnosis, treatment, and administrative purposes. This trend will have a revolutionary impact on the health care environment in future years. Physicians are already depending on computers for the management of sophisticated diagnostic/treatment equipment in the clinical setting. For example, in conjunction with ultrasound, electron-microscopy, or any other imaging process, the microcomputer is used to predict the chance of a given tumor being malignant. Video images can show the blood flow through a patient's heart.

In terms of diagnosis, independent computer systems create the capacity to interact through local area networks [LANs]. Vast amounts of patient data become accessible to the practitioner. Computer-stored medical records can eliminate much of the subjectivity involved in medical history taking, patient analysis, and treatment prescription.

Networking, combined with larger data storing capabilities, give managers the ability to collect, correlate, and evaluate financial information with clinical information. Indeed, that capability is necessary for survival under the DRG system and is a vital part of modern strategic planning. Also, as the smaller computers interact with larger mainframe machines, regional data become available to the manager and enable administrators to evaluate markets, simulate models, and make forecasts [Cummings & Cowart, 1986].

These sophisticated tools may provide increasingly accurate measures and speed up the work of physicians and administrative staff. However, high technology utilization does add to the costs of operations. Under DRGs, those added costs may or may not be reimbursable and may represent a drain on potential profits and undermine an organization's effectiveness if not used efficiently.

Competition

Competition between health care providers appears to be a short-term dynamic that eventually will lead to a new balance of services being offered by providers. During this chaotic period of an agency's experimentation with new services, mergers, joint ventures or establishing off-site satellites, inefficient and poorly planned changes may fail, leading to bankruptcies and closures. As a result of competition for survival, providers will be caught up in the dilemma of targeting potential profitable market services while trying to maintain comprehensive existing services, including those that do not make a profit. Sound planning and effective implementation practices supported with adequate resources are essential if health care providers are to have a better than 50 percent chance of succeeding. Eventually, the winners may gobble up the losers, resulting in larger but more stable organizations available to the public.

Hospital Occupancy

Total nonfederal hospital beds increased by six percent while the number of hospitals decreased by 200 between 1975 and 1985. At the same time, hospital occupancy rate dropped from 75 percent to 65 percent during this period [USDHHS, NCHS, 1988]. This implies a volatile situation in which some hospitals are growing larger at the expense of those which fail. That situation provides an opportunity for hospitals to offer new services in currently unused space and produce additional cash flow to replace current cash losses.

Professional Staff Competition

Not only is the external environment throwing providers into defensive postures, but the internal environment is doing likewise. Rivalry among professional staff and competition for authority and status is also producing a volatile situation. Nurses are upgrading their educational and training experiences to compete with physicians in providing basic medical services previously rendered only by physicians. Licensed practical nurses are vying with registered nurses for improved professional status, responsibility, and pay by upgrading their training. In the health care provider's quest for improving efficiency, substituting lower cost professional services for higher cost care is an enticing strategy. Indirectly, that strategy promotes and encourages the professional rivalries growing within the agency's setting.

Alternative Care

Providers are also under pressure to reduce services that can appropriately be provided in an alternative setting. Certain surgical procedures can be undertaken in a physician's office or ambulatory setting that were formerly provided only within the hospital. These are only two examples of services that are being moved outside the hospital's walls to the possible detriment of the hospital's fiscal well-being.

Consumer Self-Care

Consumers are slowly responding to the constant advertising campaigns to take more responsibility for their own health and mental well-being. Promotion of positive health practices of proper dieting, exercising, sleeping, and drinking alcoholic beverages in moderation are taking hold. One outcome of this is improvement in the population's health status. One consequence of a healthier population is that there may be less need for physician and hospital inpatient services. A dramatic result is seen in the decrease in the heart disease death rate per 100,000 persons, age-adjusted: from 307 in 1950 to 180 in 1985, a 40 percent reduction [USDHHS, NCHS, 1988]. While this is a plus factor for the population, the decrease does represent part of the dynamic changes occurring in our society to which health care providers must adjust.

All of these trends have been proceeding for a considerable time period and are expected to continue into the near term. Until a new equilibrium takes place in the changing dynamics of health care providers, organizations would do well to engage professionals with expertise to help administrators develop short- and long-range strategic plans.

FOUR PRESSING SPECIFIC ISSUES

At least four pressing specific health issues have emerged which require a response from health care providers. These are AIDS, home health care, physician surplus and nurse shortage, and a frenzied legislative climate concerned with containing health care costs.

AIDS

AIDS [Acquired Immune Deficiency Syndrome] has become the most invidious and potentially dangerous disease to strike the United States in years. Immense attention is given to AIDS in the mass media and especially by the federal Surgeon General's Office. Statistics clearly show the large increase in the number of AIDS cases. Since 1981, the federal Centers for Disease Control [CDC] received reports of 112,000 AIDS cases and projected 365,000 U.S. cases by 1992. Fifty-five percent of all persons with AIDS reported during the 1982–1987 period have died. CDC estimates the number of cases of HIV infection to be between 945,000 and 1.4 million. One report estimates 900,000 deaths from AIDS in the year 2013 [Voelker, 1989].

Males account for more than 90 percent of the cases. Among males, in almost 93 percent of the cases, AIDS was transmitted by homosexual and bisexual intercourse, and through intravenous drug use. Transmission by heterosexual intercourse and blood transfusion represent less than four percent of the cases. While two states, New York and California, account for 66 percent of all AIDS cases, the syndrome has spread to virtually every state to become a national problem. Of course, AIDS requires extensive medical care in hospitals, at home, and in hospices. With the expected number of AIDS cases increasing rapidly in the coming years, strategic planning has a vital role to play. Certainly, the great influx of new cases will place increased pressures on hospitals for bed space and on professional personnel to render care. This is already an acute problem for facilities in metropolitan centers such as New York City and San Francisco. In efforts to keep up-to-date, DeHovitz and Altimont [1989] provide an 800+ page guide for health care administrators, *The AIDS Manual*, twice annually.

Home Health Care

Home health care is one of the fastest growing components of the health industry. It is estimated that $5 billion will be spent on home health care in 1987 [Freudenheim, 1988]. Impetus for increased utilization of home health services has been spurred by the DRG form of prospective payment for Medicare hospitalized patients. Since a hospital is limited to a preset amount of reimbursement for each diagnosed illness, it behooves the hospital to discharge patients as soon as possible. Prior to DRGs, patients who may have remained in the hospital for several additional days of recuperation are now discharged as quickly as possible [Spiegel, 1987].

Often, patients require extended medical care, but Medicare will not reimburse hospitals because that care can be provided on an outpatient basis. This has resulted in the growth of home health care. Many believe that the cost of comparable care on a home health basis is 30 to 70 percent lower than hospital inpatient care. New and sophisticated lighter and easier-to-manage high technology medical care modalities make it possible to set up a minihospital in the home. In 1983, a home health agency could only treat 30 different diagnostic categories. In 1987, the agencies can now deal with more than 900. Providers can even use "interactive telemonitoring" to communicate with patients and adjust medications and nutritional needs by remote control with quality monitoring at a central communication station [Spiegel, 1990].

Recognizing the potential profits to be made in home health care, about 2,000 hospitals have established home health agencies within their facility. Physicians are also beginning to recognize the importance of home health care as a treatment modality. However, medical economists believe the profits now being generated by high technology home health care advances will be short-lived because of Medicare's reimbursement practices and the need of hospitals to prorate their costs over a smaller inpatient base. This will necessitate an acceleration of hospital costs in spite of DRG reimbursement cost caps and will most likely offset any savings accrued through the use of home health care services. Again, strategic planning would be vital to help monitor medical expenditures and the changing environment favoring home health care by both the consuming public and health care professionals.

Physician Surplus—Nursing Shortage

There is a growing surplus of physicians in the United States at the same time that a shortage of registered nurses [RNs] exists. In 1975, there were 385,000 active physicians in the United States or 174 per 100,000 population [USDHHS, NCHS, 1988]. By 1985, this had increased to 535,000 and 220 per 100,000 population. It is projected that this number will increase to almost 700,000 by the year 2,000 and 260 per 100,000 population.

This increase in the number of physicians has many ramifications for health care in terms of access, quality, availability, and costs. There will certainly be more physicians voluntarily practicing in communities where few or no physicians previously worked, resulting in a better geographic distribution. With more American educated physicians, the quality of care to which Americans are accustomed may also improve. Physicians will also begin competing with each other for patients by offering high-quality care at competitive prices. Offsetting these gains, medical costs generated by physicians through their own fees and the use of expensive equipment, inpatient hospital services, drugs, and allied medical personnel can be expected to go much higher.

If physicians were responsible for only 50 percent of the estimated $442 billion in medical expenditures in 1985, each of the 490,000 actively practicing physicians annually generates about $425,000 worth of medical services. Mathematically, the physician glut could readily speed health care providers, especially hospitals, into potential bankruptcy. Certainly, Medicare, Medicaid, private commercial health care carriers, and Blue Cross/Blue Shield insurers cannot afford to continue to reimburse for those escalating medical costs.

In a provocative article peering into the future, Fifer [1987] predicts that physicians will have a more defined role in hospital management because of the mutual need for each other due to greater competition among medical facilities. He predicts that "medical staff will participate in both policy formulation and professional management within the hospital becoming involved in strategic planning and assuming 'professional manager' roles in technology assessment, product line management, and cost-effective clinical decisions."

While a physician surplus is predicted with changing roles in hospitals, substantial nursing shortages of 13 percent and more also exist [Tolchin, 1988]. There are about 1.6 million practicing nurses. Yet there is also an estimated shortage of 200,000 to 300,000 nurses to meet hospital and other health care needs. At the same time, enrollment in nursing schools declined about 10 percent since 1974. This leads to a bidding war for nurses, but hospitals are constrained by DRG reimbursement patterns in the salaries offered to nurses.

Strategic planning must deal simultaneously with two opposite types of professional personnel issues, a physician surplus and a nursing shortage.

Cost Containment

Cost containment is an issue that strategic health planners will have to face by predicting and reacting to anticipated governmental actions to control medical costs. DRGs and the use of PROs are only two of the most potent and recent efforts undertaken by the federal government to reduce medical costs [Spiegel & Kavaler, 1986]. In fact, Pinkney [1989] reports that $3–5 billion in cuts are expected annually in federal health programs.

Traditionally, consumers and unions have fought to keep medical costs from being shifted to the general public. This resistance may be changing. A powerful lobby, the American Association of Retired Persons [AARP], endorsed, with reservations, a Congressional catastrophic medical plan that shifted the cost from government to the senior citizens themselves to pay for drugs and other high-cost hospital bills. However, an avalanche of protest led to Congress repealing the catastrophic plan.

Many corporations are shifting some of the burden of paying for medical costs to their employees through deductibles, co-insurance, and reduced benefit options. If this trend continues, does it mean that the federal government has reached the limits of its capacity to raise revenue for medical benefits?

Given the huge national domestic and trade debts, there is little room for expanding present health benefits programs. What will this mean for the capacity of health care providers to grow and meet the needs of its patient population? What impact will this have on the quality and availability of care? What are the implications for the ability of health care providers to meet the costs of treating the poor and the uninsured? More than ever, health care providers will have to engage in strategic planning for their own future survival and possible growth. Strategic planners will have to determine whether their past missions and goals are still viable in a fast-changing health environment.

These four pressing specific issues will impact heavily on providers and how and to whom they provide care. Strategic planning is a critical process to assist health care personnel to deal with these vital issues while determining the real impact on health care operations.

PLANNING AND THE TURBULENT ENVIRONMENT

Planning is a necessary tool in an environment of continuing turbulence. With so many factors and trends occurring at the same time, an organization that does not plan can easily lose track of what is relevant to its own future and what is illusionary. Agencies should be aware of what the health care actors are doing and the impacts of the ensuing drama. Large national nonhealth-related corporations are moving into the provision of hospital care, home health care, nursing home facilities, hospice services, and many other types of health care services. In a concern for equity, Congress is closely monitoring hospitals via increased regulation. Essentially, federal regulations require health care providers to do more with less. At the same time, consumers demand more information and ask more questions concerning hospital and physician diagnostic and treatment practices. People want to know more about risks of entering a medical facility or undergoing a physician-ordered procedure. Individuals are taking less for granted and are showing less faith in health care professionals. A variety of voluntary associations also question health care providers and professionals. These organizations want to know why specific procedures cost so much and if the procedures are being ordered for the patient's benefit or to legally protect professionals from lawsuits. Industrial and commercial corporations with a large financial stake in health benefit plans are demanding more input into the policies and practices of health care providers. Granting all these intertwined forces at work, a turbulent, dynamic, and unpredictable environment exists and health care providers must cope to survive. Experience and intuition can no longer suffice as the basis for major policy and practice decisions. Too many variables must be weighed and balanced and too many specialists and actors concerned with the future well-being of the organization must be involved to help sort out all the events taking place. Of course, these specialists add to the very turbulence and dynamics they are being asked to resolve.

Just to maintain a parity with competitors, health care providers must engage in some form of planning. In fact, some view planning as simply a process to speed up the learning process in an environment where success comes from the ability to learn faster than competitors about items such as new markets, new technologies, and cost-cutting measures [DeGeus, 1988]. As one health care agency engages in strategic planning to determine where it is, where it wants to go, and how to get there, competing health providers may be looking at that agency to identify market segments and/or poorly designed services that they can provide better to lure patients to their agency's services. To stand still in this dynamic environment is to slowly die. Health care providers must know a great deal more than they have in the past. Organizations must be more precise in what they want to do and know how to market their services to obtain their desired share of the potential target population. There is no longer an open spigot from which the money flows. Health care providers must work hard to achieve fiscal stability while realizing that competitors are working just as hard to undo what the organization is trying to achieve.

Strategic planning becomes critical for the agency's survival, for providing services to the targeted communities, and for keeping current on what is happening in the organization's external and internal environments.

There was a time when Lindblom's [1959, 1979] disjointed incrementalism was the way most corporate executives engaged in planning. Relying on their intuition and past experiences, executives picked the brains of a few experts when making decisions to improve their organization's operations. That is no longer feasible. Planning "by the seat of your pants," that is, by trial and error, leads to disaster if you guess wrong. For a few minor decisions, this style of planning may still be as good as any, but it is no longer relevant for engaging in long-term planning and decision making. These major decisions require more than experience and intuition. Sophisticated decision making requires a firm knowledge base, an understanding of the pertinent political and economic currents affecting the institution, an availability of resources and their costs, and much more.

On the other hand, comprehensive health planning is just that: too comprehensive to be relevant in a constantly changing environment. It costs too much in time, effort, and funds to develop an in-depth knowledgeable plan. There is simply too much to know for comprehensive health planners to take into account in making plans, setting goals, and determining priorities. Comprehensive planning is somewhat like the scientist peering through his/her microscope. In the very process of observing the phenomena, patterns and environmental conditions change before our very eyes. As an illustration, Harlem Hospital in New York City opened after 10 years of planning and construction. On the day the hospital opened, it was obsolete. If it takes a year or more to develop a comprehensive health plan, how relevant are the goals and objectives when new dynamics are at work: an AIDS epidemic, a shortage of nurses, or the enactment of a DRG reimbursement program. Environmental factors changed so rapidly that a new plan or a major portion of the old one will have to be reworked to integrate the new variables. Admirable as comprehensive health planning is, the process may really no longer be feasible or relevant in a market-dominated environment. However, Rohrer and Levey [1987] "argue that comprehensive planning for long-term care programs is again necessary because of the inadequate performance of that sector in health care." Others may also support comprehensive health planning in areas such as regulation, control, and decentralization.

Strategic health planning does appear to be that compromise between incremental and comprehensive health planning. By targeting a service population and enunciating a narrow mission, the health care provider can limit the scope of examination to a specific part of the health care universe. Providers need not be everything to everybody. Organizations can select a small part of the population and develop relevant services that are second-to-none. But, before agencies can determine which part of the population to focus on, the provider's planning staff should engage in an overview of the entire population. Planners must discover the main currents stirring in the environment so the decision to pick and choose can be informed, responsible, and feasible. Strategic health planners study the target population in depth, but always within the context of what is happening in the overall community. In short, a strategic plan provides a limited but relevant glimpse of the overall environment, focusing on a detailed and in-depth scrutiny of the particular targeted segments of the population. In this way, health care providers keep abreast of the rapid changes in the total environment while evaluating the positive or negative impact on their specialized services.

In sum, by keeping track of the gestalt environment, providers maintain a flexibility to shift their course of action, their goals, objectives, and service populations. In this manner, strategic health planning embraces the best of incrementalism and comprehensive planning, the specific and the general.

CONSTRICTIONS ON PLANNING

An extensive review of the literature on strategic health planning by Files [1988a, 1988b] points to one clear conclusion. Health care providers are in the "very early stages of effective strategy formulation—and even that involvement is limited." She goes on to state that few providers "incorporate strategic planning as an integral part of the day-to-day executive management process." Rather, providers engage in episodic planning for some parts of the organization.

One of the limiting factors for this slow start is the lack of staffing required to carry out strategic planning. Typically, one or two staff are assigned part-time to such an activity. Planning represents only a part of the staff's professional responsibilities. As Files implied, most of the planning is responsive planning to crises or demands made on the executive branch by hospital departments for changes in personnel, equipment, and space. Therefore, there is little time left over for the planning staff to engage in strategic planning.

Availability of data is another limiting factor. Building up a database to engage in strategic planning is time consuming and costly. Collection of data should be a continuous rather than an episodic process. Few health care providers have the capacity to engage in an extensive data-gathering process. Data are usually collected and analyzed for specific departmental services. Certificate-of-need proposals generally require demographic data and informational support for the population's need for the new service or new equipment. However, even those data are too limited to engage in strategic health planning for the organization as a whole.

A third limiting factor is the capacity of the executive staff to engage in integrated strategic planning. Without continuous input from executives, it is unlikely that the planning staff will have the power and influence to obtain the cooperation of the many professionals required to carry out strategic planning. There must be a visible commitment in time and effort by top management for strategic planning to succeed. Relman [1989] points out the need for "a broad strategy linking reforms in payment and financing with improvements in the delivery of care."

Directly related to the third limiting condition is the need to identify the values and the mission of the health care provider. New environments mandate that providers reassess what they stand for. If an agency is losing patients to competing community providers in the area, should that organization continue its mission of serving undifferentiated community needs? Should the agency specialize? Should the agency merge with a larger provider and become a subsidiary satellite? Should the agency change values from a concern with ready accessibility to everyone regardless of ability to pay, to a goal of self-reliance in which only individuals with financial means will be served? If yes, would that mission include senior citizens who rely on Medicare?

In the reality of a new environment, health care providers may already have subconsciously modified value emphases from open accessibility to self-reliance because of an inability to survive on federal reimbursement rates. However, until the agency's top management pauses to examine where it is and where it wishes to go, the administrators may not be aware that their mission and values changed to take into account a new reality. As an example, Schroeder, Zones, and Showstack [1989] pinpoint the unresponsiveness of "academic medicine" to the numerous vexing problems in providing health care to the public.

A fifth limiting condition refers to the external constraints of federal legislative and regulatory actions and the competition of other hospitals. DRGs and PROs impose both legislative and regulatory constraints on choices available to strategic planners. Predetermined pricing shifts the burden for an agency's fiscal soundness to the organization's administration. PROs' monitoring of utilization and the quality of services shifts the burden to medical and professional staff to meet a minimum set of federal standards and protocols in providing treatment. Errant decisions will endanger an agency's fiscal health.

At the same time, strategic planning must take into account the strengths and weaknesses of competitors. In addition, a host of other external factors must be taken into account such as a community's local zoning laws, the degree to which consumers are organized to monitor a hospital's activities, and the decisions made by unions and corporations regarding health benefit plans.

All of these internal and external conditions will have an impact on where a health care provider intends to go and whether it can get there. Piecemeal planning, which providers are accustomed to doing, will no longer work, at least for the long term.

SIGNIFICANT HEALTH PLANNING TRENDS

With the passage of time and the stimulus from major federal legislation, health planning has undergone significant changes. A number of trends emerged with the implementation of the National Health Planning and Resources Development Act of 1974 [PL 93–641]. Trends are undergoing radical change with the inception and acceptance of strategic health planning as the primary process for assisting hospitals and other health care providers to determine their futures. Seven changes resulting from the emergence of strategic health planning follow:

1. Increased consumer involvement in health planning decisions has virtually ceased. Acting as consumers, an agency's board of trustees now make most of these decisions. Grass roots consumers are involved only in terms of their membership in health organizations which monitor the activities of health care providers.

2. Regional planning is no longer accepted as the major type of planning undertaken by communities. Even where health planning agencies continue to exist, regional plans are used primarily by the state to determine the need for certificate-of-need proposed changes. Strategic health planning reversed the trend toward regional planning and replaced it with a focus on hospital or facility planning.
3. Comprehensive health plans are no longer developed by communities. Strategic health plans are comprehensive only with respect to the mission, goals, and priorities of the individual health care provider.
4. Strategic health planning has not changed the major role the federal government continues to play in funding health care costs, especially hospital costs. Nevertheless, this increasing emphasis on federal financing has slowed considerably. Federal budget deficits in combination with the President's ideological position regarding financing medical costs, resulted in the slowdown in federal reimbursement for health care.
5. With the demise of comprehensive health planning organizations, a number of planning staff from these agencies found positions as hospital planners. However, the needs of hospital planning are far less than those of a regional planning agency. Yet, with a need by hospitals and other providers to reevaluate their mission, it appears that most health care organizations are inadequately staffed to carry out a strategic health plan except for the largest agencies.
6. In the process of strategic planning, coordination and integration of services plays a lesser role, except where it concerns the health care provider's staff itself or meets a need in strategic health planning. Survival and growth of the organization are the main concerns of strategic planning and not whether improved coordination and integration occur.
7. Strategic health planning is dominated by the private sector with little or no input from government. Of course, planners must still be aware of the limitations and potential impact of governmental regulations and legislation on strategic planning goals and objectives.

These seven trends are illustrated in Exhibit 1-3 and can be seen easily by following the changes across each of the trends.

A CAVEAT ABOUT METHODS AND TECHNIQUES

This book details various methods and techniques for strategic health planners to use in specific work situations. Most of the methods are considered basic to the profession. However, health planners are encouraged to add, delete, adapt, or in some other way change the methods to suit their own particular situation. Readers may discover a number of methods and techniques appropriate to the strategic health planning process. Basically, consider this book the starting point and not the end-all for health planners. Most importantly, health planners should realize that methods are tools to direct planning into the scientific mold.

This book divides the health planning process into six steps that are constant with both the strategic planning process and the comprehensive health planning process. Other planning processes may segment into fewer or more than the six steps used in this text. Regardless of the number of steps used, the processes all have the same logic: setting a conceptual framework, diagnosing the situation within that framework, setting goals, implementing them, and finally, evaluating their outcomes. This is a circuitous process that is self-perpetuating through the final evaluation step that resolves and creates a new round of suggestions to further improve the situation. Planning processes with more or fewer steps simply aggregate or disaggregate these

Exhibit 1-3. Planning Trends: Historical and National Legislation.

Trend Factors		Legislation						
	Hill-Burton	Facilities Planning	Community Mental Health Act	Regional Medical Planning	Comprehensive Health Planning	Certificate of Need "1122"	National Planning PL 93-641	Strategic Planning
Citizen Involvement	Provider elite consumer	Slight increased consumer involvement	Provider elite grass roots consumers	Provider elite grass roots consumers	Wide range of consumer & provider involvement	"A" Elite consumer provider involvement "B" Broad consumer involvement	Broad consumer involvement	Minimal citizen involvement
Toward Regional Planning	Regional planning	Regional planning	Subregional planning	Regional planning	Regional planning	Project planning	Regional/state planning	Minimal regional planning
Comprehensive Planning	Stressed facility planning	Facilities planning	Facilities, services, manpower planning	Broad mandate ad hoc planning	Broac mandate project functional planning	Subregional planning	Extensive services & facilities planning	Facilities planning
Toward Federal Funding Inputs & Controls	Increased federal funding and control	Federal funding; input but no control	Strong federal funding and control	Strong federal funding and control	Vacillating federal controls & funding	Indirect federal controls & increased funding	Strong federal funding and control	Strong federal funding control

(continued)

Exhibit 1-3. (Continued)

					Legislation			
Trend Factors	**Hill-Burton**	**Facilities Planning**	**Community Mental Health Act**	**Regional Medical Planning**	**Comprehensive Health Planning**	**Certificate of Need "1122"**	**National Planning PL 93-641**	**Strategic Planning**
Adequate Planning Staffs	Adequate expert staff	Competent staff of limited size	Competent staff of limited size	Adequate professional staff	Professional staff of limited size	Adequate professional staff	Very adequate competent staff	Competent staff of limited size
More Coordination & Integration of Services	Minimal activity in this area	Limited coordination; no integration	Increased activity re mental hlth. services	Limited coordination; no integration of RMP projects	Coordination of services; no integration	Some coordination; limited integration	Increase in coordination & integration of services & facilities	No community coordination; mergers etc. integrating health services
Toward Private Government Partnership	Private dominance; some govt. influence	Private dominance; no federal influence	Public planning; private activation; balanced partnership	Little government influence	Limited local but strong federal government influence	Increased government influence at all levels	Balanced federal private partnership	Private control; government monitoring

Source: Updated and modified from *Health Planning & Public Accountability Workbook* by A.D. Spiegel and H.H. Hyman, 1976, p. 22, Rockville, MD: Aspen Publishers, Inc., Copyright 1976. Reprinted by permission.

basic steps to provide more or less detail at each step in the process. Because of the dynamics of the rapidly changing environment with which health care providers are involved, strategic health planning should ideally be viewed as one of the relevant models of a rational planning process. Through continuous study and evaluation, the goals and objectives of health care providers may remain realistic and in tune with the current status of the internal and external environment.

Methods and techniques in this book are described in each of the following six chapters and pertain in that specific chapter to that particular phase of the planning process. However, this should not constrict health planners from using different methods in any of the other phases of the planning process. For example, the Delphi method can be used in setting priorities, in data assessment, in generating alternatives, and in evaluation. Each time, the technique may be used a little differently, but the fundamentals remain the same. As each method is described, do not constrict that technique's use to the given example. Be alert to other situations where that method could be used or adapted.

Strategic health planning is not as neatly ordered as in the six steps cited in this book. Such organization makes for a logical flow of ideas, but planning does not always occur logically. Planners might start anywhere in the planning process, especially when their efforts are initiated by a significant and/or urgent crisis. Evaluation activities may yield data to cause a health planner to begin another investigation. Nevertheless, the total planning process will eventually occur to cover all the steps required for a reasonable conclusion, even if in abbreviated form.

PLANNING PITFALLS

In a rather amusing discussion of why planning fails, Goodes [1988] identifies 10 pitfalls that planners must watch out for and avoid. A recitation of these failures will soon reveal the obvious fact that beneath the humor the pitfalls are common knowledge. Yet, strategic health planners may do little to avoid the known difficulties. Therefore, a reminder of the obvious may be pertinent.

You Can't Drive A Car without A Driver. No strategic planning process will succeed unless there is commitment and leadership from the top. This requires the chief executive's active involvement in the strategic planning process. President Kennedy's active commitment to landing a man on the moon was most responsible for that achievement. Likewise, President Reagan's commitment to his economic philosophy resulted in one of the biggest and longest periods of prosperity in American history.

You Can't Start Out Unless Everyone Is In the Car. It is not enough to involve the top leaders. Those at the bottom, who will be responsible for the day-to-day activities of implementing the goals of the plan, must also be involved. Through their active participation, it becomes their plan too—a plan they want to succeed. Involvement in strategic health planning must come from those at the top, in the middle, and at the bottom of the organizational ladder.

The Plan as an End In Itself. Those involved in planning must not become so enamored with the design of the completed plan that the written plan becomes an end in itself. A plan is meaningless unless it is implemented, and implementation requires an action plan. Legislators who designed the 1974 comprehensive health planning act were fully cognizant of this fact.

Mandates required the planning agencies to develop a five-year long-term health plan as well as an annual implementation plan for achieving those long-term goals.

The Road without Milestones. Too often, plans are developed without any way of identifying whether they are succeeding. One way to deal with this pitfall is to develop a plan with milestones or major achievements. After all, before a new wing of a hospital can be constructed, it requires the important milestone of an architectural design. That is followed by raising funds to pay for the design—another important milestone. Finally, there is the actual construction and the acceptance of patients. A plan needs events that show progress. Strategic health plans should be developed with milestones clearly indicated.

Allowing Assumptions to Become Facts. Planners generally make assumptions in developing their plans. However, assumptions should not be accepted as facts. One can assume that a hospital's occupancy rate will increase if it is able to recruit a well-known specialist for its pediatric unit. In reality, there may be pertinent facts that prevent that assumption from fulfilling the planner's prediction. Only as the assumption is supported by real facts does the true meaning emerge. Those caught up in the strategic planning process should avoid the tendency to accept assumptions as facts.

You Can't Drive the Car In Six Different Directions at Once. Strategic plans must have an internal consistency between the plan's goal and its implementation. Internal organizational differences in perception or ideology can interpret the same plan's goals differently. A vice president for financial affairs may want to conserve the limited reserves of the hospital for a "rainy day." A vice president for marketing may see the need to expand the hospital's ambulatory care services with satellites in specific neighborhoods. Each perceives the road to success in opposite terms; one in conserving resources and the other in expanding and spending.

Confusing Hopes with Objectives. One may hope the plan will succeed or that the community will perceive the health care provider in a better light. These are hopes. Planners should aim for objectives that are specific and measurable outcomes. An increase in the pediatric occupancy rate by 50 percent is a measurable objective.

You Can't Drive A Car To San Francisco In One Day, and You Can't Drive to London at All. Strategic health planning is the scientific art of the possible. Through diagnostic evaluation of the internal and external environments, supported by facts, goals will be set that are neither too high nor too low. A goal set too high leads to disillusionment; a goal set too low leads to complacency. A realistic goal is one that is achievable with hard work. That effort results in the eventual success of achievement leading to a feeling of real accomplishment and a sense of worth. If 10 hospitals are already providing a similar treatment procedure, an 11th hospital that seeks to capture 50 percent of the patients from the other 10 may be aiming far too high.

When You Give Out the Rewards, Make Sure You Know What the Rewards Are For. To encourage people to continue to work toward the final goal, rewards should be commensurate with the achievement of the intermittent milestone and not be considered a successful stopping point. Only when all the milestones are achieved and the long-term goal completed can congratulations be given all around. Hospital officials who congratulated each other at a groundbreaking may have been premature. If fund raising faltered, or a city zoning ordinance impeded construction, or a particular building material was no longer available, that hole in the ground would remain exactly that. A preliminary milestone was reached, but the long-term goal was not achieved. Incentives and rewards should encourage completion of the long-term goal and not allow implementors to stand pat or feel complacent when a milestone or two are achieved.

You Can't Drive the Car All By Yourself. Strategic health planning works best when everyone is involved rather than a small cadre of planners and others interested in such planning. This requires communicating up and down the hierarchical ladder so everyone knows what is happening. "Planning and checking, explaining and revising, checking up and communicating back—these are all different ways of saying 'information systems.' In a real sense, an entire organization is an information system waiting to be tapped. And tap it managers must, because planning is not only an unceasing process, it is, when well done, a constantly informed one" [Goodes, 1988].

While there may be other pitfalls, health planners should certainly be alert to these critical situations. By explicitly identifying pitfalls, planners and their colleagues will not only avoid them, but will become more aware of how they can prevent their occurrence in the first place.

OBJECTIVES AS LINCHPINS

Specification of objectives is the linchpin of any health planning activity. There is a direct correlation between the preciseness of an objective and ensuing activities of health planners. However, too often objectives are fuzzy and ill-conceived. Consequently, the implementation that ensues also becomes fuzzy and ill-conceived. To be acceptable and valid, Bergwall, Reeves, and Woodside [1984, p. 80] feel that objectives should meet the following straightforward criteria:

- The organization should have the authority to undertake the objective.
- Objectives should be legal and consistent with the ethical and moral values of the affected community.
- Objectives must be acceptable to those responsible for carrying them out.
- Objectives should identify results or conditions to be achieved rather than activities to be performed.
- Objectives should be limited in time so as to provide milestones of achievement.
- Objectives should be stated in terms of what is to be done rather than in terms of what is to be avoided.
- Objectives should be designed to cover a single end result.
- Objectives should readily indicate baseline data.
- Objectives should be written in quantifiable terms that are easily measured in terms of established standards.
- Objectives should indicate the minimum level of achievement or standard that is acceptable.
- Objectives should fit within the framework of the overall goals and policies of the program.
- Objectives should be realistic and attainable.
- Objectives should be consistent with resources available and anticipated.
- Objectives should have minimum side effects resulting from their achievement.

In setting objectives, it is essential that planners begin working from goal statements. If objectives are written that simply identify expected results of a health care provider's ongoing activities, it may well be impossible to identify potential areas of improvement or new program areas. This is particularly critical for providers in the current turbulent environment. One of the primary functions of strategic health planning is to identify new program needs and to monitor for improvements.

Objectives generated from goal statements will most likely result in some objectives that are easily measurable and some which are more subjective and less amenable to statistical or exacting measure. Measuring an objective such as "improved hospital morale" is more difficult than "a 25 percent increase in the occupancy rate of the pediatric ward." However, the fact that some objectives are more easily or objectively measured does not diminish the importance of the other goals. Relative importance of objectives should not be determined by whether or not they can be objectively measured. To do so would give them undue emphasis in the planning and evaluation process. If "improved hospital morale" is vital to meeting a given goal, then that objective should be used to give direction to the hospital's program activities. In that case, the planning staff should find the most reliable objective measure of "improved hospital morale" that can be used to evaluate its outcome. Measures could include noting smiling employees or those saying "Good Morning" on arriving.

Writing objectives in the proper language can greatly enhance the development of an evaluation design. In fact, evaluation relates specifically to the measures identified in the objectives. An outstanding authority on preparing objectives [Mager, 1975] contends that every objective should identify the performance required, the criterion of acceptable performance, and the conditions under which that performance is to take place. In addition, Mager opts for as much behavioral specification as possible in the performance. Evaluation then becomes a matter of pinpointing ways of gathering the data specifically identified in the objective.

In stating objectives, all the results and conditions that should be attained over the next year to achieve the goal should be clearly stated. Those results that cannot be achieved in a year should have a time frame specified when they are expected to be completed.

Following are examples of objectives to achieve the goal: "By 1992, increase the occupancy rate of the hospital from 76 percent to 90 percent:"

1. By 1990, increase inpatient admissions from the emergency room by five percent.
2. By 1991, reduce the number of pediatric beds by 15, or three percent of the hospital's complement of certified beds.
3. By June 1991, convert 15 obstetric beds to a new alcohol detoxification unit to be initiated by December 1991.
4. By 1992, increase the number of open-heart surgical procedures from 135 to 200 cases per year.

Each of these objectives by itself may not achieve the overall goal of raising the hospital's occupancy rate from 76 percent to 90 percent by 1992. However, each of these milestone objectives, and others not stated, makes an additive contribution to the totality of movement toward the achievement of the overall goal.

An analysis of objective number 1 will illustrate how it fares in meeting the criteria list of essential elements previously discussed [Bergwall et al., 1984, p. 80].

With respect to this objective, the hospital has legal authority to carry it out, and the objective is consistent with the community's ethical and moral values. Regarding acceptability, those entrusted with expansion of emergency room admissions are committed to this objective. Results to be achieved are identified in measurable terms and within a time-frame consistent with the overall goal. Further, the objective is stated in positive terms of what is to be done rather than what is to be avoided. A single end result is covered, although several different objectives may be required to achieve this overall goal. Baseline data can be derived from emergency room statistics. A 5 percent increase in admissions from emergency room cases represents the minimal level of acceptable achievement. This objective fits within the framework of the overall hospital goal to increase the occupancy rate. While it appears the objective is realistic and attainable, there is some question whether the assumption of how to do this is open to question. At issue is the assumption that a marketing campaign can be developed to encourage community residents to use the hospital's emergency room rather than another facility. Resources have been made available by the board of trustees to allow for increased use of emergency room facilities. There appear to be no negative side effects in achieving this objective.

Thus, except for the assumption of how the objective will be achieved, all criteria of this objective statement have been met.

TAKE TIME TO FORMULATE OBJECTIVES

It cannot be stressed too strongly that adequate time should be devoted to the development of clearly stated objectives with performance, criterion, and conditions delineated. Strategic and comprehensive health planners will find the time and energy well spent. Once the objectives are specifically detailed, the remainder of the planning process is able to move ahead steadily and successfully without getting mired in muddy waters.

REFERENCES

Bergwall, D.F., Reeves, P.H., & Woodside, N.B. (1984). *Introduction to health planning*. Washington, DC: Information Resources Press.

Budrys, G. (1986). *Planning for the nation's health. A study of 20th century developments in the U.S.* New York: Greenwood Press.

Cartwright, T.J. (1987). The lost art of planning. *Long Range Planning*, *20*(2), 92–99.

Clemenhagen, C., & Champagne, F. (1984). Medical staff involvement in strategic planning. *Hospital & Health Services Administration*, *29*(4), 79–94.

Cummings, S., & Cowart, R. (1986). Micros and medicine. Financial and regulatory pressures are spurring a wider PC role in administration and treatment. *PC Week*, *3*(4), 51–54.

DeGeus, A.P. (1988). Planning as learning. *Harvard Business Review*, *88*(2), 70–74.

DeHovitz, J.A., & Altimont, T.J. (1989). *The AIDS manual*. Owings Mills, MD: National Health Publishing.

Drucker, P.F. (1974). *Management, tasks, responsibilities, practices*. New York: Harper & Row.

Drury, S. (1984). Playing the numbers game: Coalitions sponsoring data collection. *Business Insurance*, *18*(2), 3.

Dyson, R.G., & Foster, M.J. (1983). Making planning more effective. *Long Range Planning*, *16*(6), 68–73.

Evashwick, C.J., & Evashwick, W.T. (1988). The fine art of strategic planning. *Provider*, *14*(4), 4–6.

Fifer, W.R. (1987). The hospital medical staff of 1997. *Quality Review Bulletin*, *13*(6), 194–197.

Files, L.A. (1988a). Strategy formulation in hospitals. In F. Simyar & J. Lloyd-Jones (Eds.), *Strategic management in the health care sector* (pp. 48–60). Englewood Cliffs, NJ: Prentice-Hall.

Files, L.A. (1988b). Strategy formulation in hospitals. *Health Care Management Review*, *13*(1), 9–16.

Freudenheim, M.H. (1988). The boom in home health care. *New York Times*, p. D1.

Ginzberg, E. (1988). US health policy—Expectations and realities. *Journal of the American Medical Association, 260*(24), 3647–3650.

Goodes, M.R. (1988). Seizing the competitive initiative: Strategic planning in the health care field. In F. Simyar & J. Lloyd-Jones (Eds.), *Strategic management in the health care sector* (pp. 136–142). Englewood Cliffs, NJ: Prentice-Hall.

Hawley, C. (1988). An environmental assessment is key. *Provider, 14*(4), 14–20.

Kaufman, J.L., & Jacobs, H.M. (1987). A public planning perspective on strategic planning. *American Planning Association Journal, 53*(11), 23–33.

Kennedy, L., & Dumas, M.B. (1983). Hospital closures and survivals: An analysis of operating characteristics and regulatory mechanisms in three states. *Health Services Research, 18*(4), 489–512.

Lamm, R.D. (1988). An eight-count indictment against America. *Medical Group Management Journal, 35*(4), 21–24.

Lindblom, C.D. (1959). The science of muddling through. *Public Administration Review, 19*(2), 79–88.

Lindblom, C.E. (1979). Still muddling, not yet through. *Public Administration Review, 39*(6), 517–526.

Mager, R.F. (1975). *Preparing instructional objectives.* Belmont, CA: Fearon Publishers, Inc.

McDevitt, P. (1987). Learning by doing: Strategic marketing management in hospitals. *Health Care Management Review, 12*(1), 23–30.

Mick, S.S., & Thompson, J.D. (1984). Public attitudes toward health planning under the Health Systems Agencies. *Journal of Health Politics, Policy and Law, 8*(4), 782–800.

Mueller, K.J. (1988). Federal programs to expire: The case of health planning. *Public Administration Review, 48*(3), 719–725.

Peters, J. (1985). *A strategic planning process for hospitals.* Chicago, IL: American Hospital Publishing, Inc.

Pinkney, D.S. (1989). Cuts in federal programs expected to continue. *American Medical News, 32*(11), 7.

Pomrinse, S.D. (1983). Comments on hospital closings in New York City. *Health Services Research, 18*(4), 571–581.

Relman, A.S. (1989). The national leadership commission's health care plan. *New England Journal of Medicine, 320*(5), 314–315.

Rohrer, J.E., & Levey, S. (1987). Strategic planning for long-term care. *Journal of Public Health Policy, 8*(3), 359–368.

Schroeder, S.A., Zones, J.S., & Showstack, J.A. (1989). Academic medicine as a public trust. *Journal of the American Medical Association, 262*(6), 803–812.

Simyar F., Lloyd-Jones, J., & Caro, J. (1988). Strategic management: A proposed framework for the health care industry. In F. Simyar & J. Lloyd-Jones (Eds.), *Strategic management in the health care sector: toward the year 2000* (pp. 6–17). Englewood Cliffs, NJ: Prentice-Hall.

Smith, D.P. (1987). One more time: What do we mean by strategic management? *Hospital & Health Services Administration, 32*(5), 219–233.

Sorkin, D.L., Ferris, N.B., & Hudak, J. (1984). *Strategies for cities and counties. A strategic planning guide.* Washington, DC: Public Technology, Inc.

Spiegel, A.D. (1987). *Home health care* (2nd ed.). Owings Mills, MD: National Health Publications.

Spiegel, A.D. (1990). High technology home health care: Doing right for the wrong reason. In M.J. Mehlman & S.J. Younger (Eds.), *High technology health care in the home.* Owing Mills, MD: National Health Publishing.

Spiegel, A.D., & Hyman, H.H. (1978). *Basic health planning methods.* Rockville, MD: Aspen Systems.

Spiegel, A.D., & Kavaler, F. (1986). *Cost containment and DRGs: A guide to perspective payment.* Owings Mills, MD: National Health Publications.

Stoline, A., & Weiner, J.P. (1988). *The new medical marketplace: A physician's guide to the health care revolution.* Baltimore, MD: Johns Hopkins University Press.

Timmel, N., & Brozovich, J. (1981). Managing through values. *Hospital Forum, 24*(3), 31–39.

Tolchin, M. (1988, April 18). Health worker shortage is worsening. *New York Times.*

U.S. Department of Health and Human Services (USDHHS), Alcohol, Drug Abuse and Mental Health Administration. (1981). *Prevention planning workbook, Volume I* (DHHS Pub. No. (ADM) 81–1062). Washington, DC: Government Printing Office.

U.S. Department of Health and Human Services (USDHHS), Alcohol, Drug Abuse and Mental Health Administration. (1981). *Prevention planning workbook, Volume 1* (DHHS Pub. No. (ADM) 81–1062). Washington, DC: Government Printing Office.

Voelker, R. (1989). Model predicts huge jump in AIDS in coming years. *American Medical News, 32*(48), 4–5.

Whitman, J.J. (1988). Identifying the right services to offer. *Provider, 14*(4), 10–13.

Yoo, S., & Digman, L.A. (1987). Decision support system: A new tool for strategic management. *Long Range Planning, 20*(2), 114–124.

2
Identifying the Strategic Problem: Needs, Demands, Assessment, and Resources Analysis

Initially, the strategic planning process focuses on methods to identify key targets for institutional opportunities to meet health needs in their geographic areas. To pinpoint problem health issues and therefore potential opportunities, institutional planners must survey not only their immediate, but also the forces in the national arena which impact on their localities. That task requires an environmental assessment of factors such as the national and local economies, demographic changes, technology and research, morbidity and mortality statistics, social and lifestyle characteristics. Additionally, an environmental assessment includes an understanding of the following [Hawley, 1988]:

- Changes in the Gross National Product [GNP]
- Inflation and interest rates
- Employment trends
- Cancer, heart, stroke, AIDS, and substance abuse morbidity and mortality trends
- Needs of the poor
- Fitness and wellness trends
- Working mothers
- Technological innovations in nutrition, pharmaceuticals, and genetic engineering.

ENVIRONMENTAL DYNAMICS

Occurring at a faster rate than anticipated, health care providers are facing dynamic changes in their environment. Conner and Newman [1987] note the activities creating turmoil:

- An increasing surplus of beds, hospitals, and physicians
- Payors taking away any leverage of rate increases to compensate for lost volume
- Increasing competition for patients and loyal physicians
- Greater emphasis on quality indicators.

Furthermore, managed health care plans now render services to about 60 percent of the 160 million Americans with employer-sponsored health insurance. Kramon [1988] points out that 16 percent of employees are enrolled in health maintenance organizations: 11 percent in preferred provider organizations and 32 percent in fee-for-service plans with controls on the patient's use of the hospital. Those employer-sponsored plans exert great pressures on health care providers to manage their organizations more efficiently and to expand into alternative health care modalities. At the same time that more is being asked of health care providers, the organizations have less authority, control, and financial resources to meet their responsibilities. This catch–22 dilemma requires an examination of the local and national environments to determine how health care providers can best deal with the new responsibilities thrust upon them.

In the 1960s and 1970s, there was tremendous growth in federal funding of health programs, particularly funds for hospitalization and long-term care needs of senior citizens and the poor; Medicare and Medicaid were enacted in the 1960s. In the 1980s, these growing expenditures slowed considerably with a likely continuation of this slowdown through the 1990s. Nevertheless, Congress continues to be concerned about funds being spent in a legal and effective manner to alleviate the illnesses of people. Responses to this concern require answers offered in quantitative and measurable terms.

Congress also seeks to determine how the health status of the United States has fared over time. Over the decades, there has been demonstrable improvement in most of the medical indicators used to plot trends in the nation's health. Crude death rates, infant mortality under one year, the heart disease death rate, cerebrovascular deaths, and disability days per person have all exhibited dramatic drops from the 1950s to the mid–1980s [USDHHS, 1988, Tables 21, 22, 44, 64, 84, 106]. Only cancer deaths appear resistant to intervention. These changes are accompanied by a reduction in average length of hospital stay, a lowered hospital occupancy rate, and fewer days of care per 1,000 persons in a hospital.

If health care providers and physicians have been so effective, how much more positive change can be expected in the future? Have we reached the point where future, small reductions in mortality and morbidity statistics will require enormous inputs of new resources? It is obvious that the national emphasis on cost containment may only result in incremental increases in health expenditures in the future. Federal legislation to insure against catastrophic health care and pharmaceutical costs for the elderly affirms the point. Coleman [1988] noted that the elderly were to be billed for almost all of the expected $30 billion to pay for those expanded benefits during the initial five years. Strong negative reactions to the additional payments caused Congress to repeal the catastrophic care act.

PLANNING WITH LIMITED RESOURCES
AND SERVICE REDUCTIONS

In essence, health care providers are being asked to plan and to operate in a medical environment that is very strange to them. Planning must evolve in an atmosphere of limited resources and service reductions. A fish-bowl world will have regulators looking over the shoulders of health officials to ensure that proper decisions are made and that the medical care benefits that government and private insurers are paying for are truly rendered. On that point, Wagstaff [1989] surveyed British literature and detailed econometric studies related to the National Health System [NHS]. He found that the market aspect was more important than the institutional details.

Health care providers are being asked to be efficient rather than effective. Agencies are being asked to do more with the current medical technology rather than to look forward to new technology coming on board. Organizations are being asked to assure a continuing high quality of care while receiving reduced reimbursement. They are being asked to compete with neighboring health care providers for patients, staff, and financial resources rather than to maintain a cooperative relationship. Providers are being asked to change their "patterns of practice" as a result of the public spotlight of monitoring by consumer groups and business coalitions. While the changes are called for, the providers have less authority to act as decisively as they had in the past.

POWER OF EXTERNAL ACTORS ON PLANNING

Health care providers working in the public spotlight can be illustrated by the activity of the Greater Detroit Area Health Council [Gottlieb, 1986]. In 1983, the Council embarked on a plan to ensure access to medical care for all people living within the Greater Detroit Area. Membership of the Council includes 150 of the largest business corporations, labor unions, medical societies, and insurance carriers in the region, along with consumer groups and governmental agencies. After much deliberation, the Council determined that the most important medical priority was the financing of health care for the poor. While recognizing the dominant responsibility of the federal government, the Council did identify several groups among the poor who could be assisted by health care providers in the region. By their actions, the Council, an external public body, forced hospitals in the area to pay attention to their concerns and stated goals. In the process, the Council impacted on the hospitals' decision-making power. As Gottlieb states:

> Providers . . . understand that their ability to compete effectively is severely hampered by the burden of under-compensated care. Most providers realize that if those currently carrying a disproportionate share of the burden do not survive, the burden will simply be transferred to them. Nonprofit providers also recognize that their tax-exempt status and their community support are at risk if they do not find some way of carrying out their charitable community service roles.

In another example, Herzlinger [1985] shows how business tackles health care costs. She found that few, if any, companies desired to get involved in providing direct medical services for their employees. Instead, the employers preferred other measures to cut costs. One measure involved business' motivating employees to enroll in health maintenance organizations. Another stimulated senior executives to serve on the governing boards of health care providers. Business executives perceived HMOs to provide a wider variety of services including preventive care, to have lower costs, and to require no or minimal payments by their employees. On the other hand, when asked the best strategy for reducing medical costs by 10 percent, 34 percent of the business executives felt their involvement in coalitions would result in this change; another 28 percent wanted to negotiate directly with health care providers; and 24 percent believed that

HMOs could exert the greatest influence in achieving a positive outcome.

These two examples show the strong influence of external local actors. Hopefully, that influence will yield a positive involvement in the decision-making authority of local health care providers. In addition, these examples stress the need for health care providers to conduct an environmental assessment.

ENVIRONMENTAL, COMMUNITY, AND MARKET ASSESSMENT

Carrying out an environmental assessment is a time-consuming dedicated venture. Resources, expertise, and commitment from the institution's leadership are required as well as from the strategic planning staff. Exhibit 2-1 reveals the multidimensional information needed to undertake an environmental analysis to gain an understanding of the forces affecting the institution's regional domain.

It is unlikely that any health care institution's planning staff will have the resources to investigate all facets of the 10 areas in Exhibit 2-1. Planners will have to collect the national data required to frame the analysis and to identify potential impacts on the service area. Many health care providers do not have to cope with issues related to the unionization of interns and residents. Many areas of the country are not affected by medical ethical questions dealing with care of AIDS patients. Institutions can therefore be selective in determining what aspects of the assessment to emphasize.

On the other hand, Exhibit 2-2 illustrates the principal components of the community and market assessment that should be required of any strategic health plan. Local providers must know their local demographic trends, economic conditions, and morbidity/mortality trends. Agencies must know their competitors, their market share, and their strengths and weaknesses. Detailed information is required about the community's service needs and the resources available, with special emphasis on the local supply of physicians, nurses, and allied health professionals. Furthermore, providers must know about the utilization trends in the local regions, the case-mix, patient characteristics, and inpatient use trends.

A MOSAIC ASSESSMENT

Another way of perceiving the same strategic assessment process is dubbed MOSAIC by Scotti [1988, p. 153]. Exhibit 2-3 shows the first three steps in the strategic information base—the formulation of what the institution wants and can do. Identification of the "mission" requires an environmental assessment that answers the question, "What will we do?" Responses become the potentials or possibilities of what the health care provider's mission might be. A mission statement spells out the institution's basic reason for being or serving the community. In concrete terms, Scotti [1988, p. 152] lists characteristics included in a mission statement: "major functions [patient care, research, education], service mix [surgery, obstetrics, pediatrics], primary client groups [by age, disease category, religion], community need, and desired public image."

From this mission statement, appropriate objectives are identified and answer the question, "What should we do?" Answers require an explicit or implicit statement of the organization's philosophy with respect to social obligations and related moral principles. For example, Catholic hospitals generally view abortion as a sin and believe that they have no social obligation to encourage that medical service. However, as part of their social obligation, Catholic

/

Primary Components of the Environmental Assessment

THE ECONOMY

Review of national economy and trends in business and industry and how they affect health care:
- changes in GNP
- national debt
- inflation
- interest rates
- monetary issues
- employment trends
- poverty level

DEMOGRAPHICS

Review of major demographic trends and how they affect the health care sector:
- population growth trends
- influence of population subgroups: elderly, baby boomers, minorities, single parents, etc.
- life expectancy trends

MORBIDITY & MORTALITY STATISTICS

Review of major trends in illness and disease and how they affect health care:
- cancer
- heart disease
- stroke
- AIDS
- substance abuse, etc.

REIMBURSEMENT, FINANCING & LEGISLATION

Review of major trends in health care reimbursement, financing, and legislation:
- Medicare/Medicaid reimbursement issues and projected changes
- growth of managed health care initiatives
- actions by insurance carriers
- other legislative concerns

TECHNOLOGY & RESEARCH

Review of clinical research and technological breakthroughs and their impact on health care delivery:
- nutrition
- pharmaceuticals
- genetic engineering

HEALTH CARE DELIVERY

Review of major trends in the design, development, organization and structure of health care services:
- diversification
- vertical integration
- growth strategies
- new services
- competition, etc.

SOCIAL & LIFESTYLE

Review of major social attitudes and lifestyle factors that impact health care delivery:
- needs of the poor
- fitness/wellness trends
- convenience
- working mothers
- consumer preferences, etc.

COST & UTILIZATION

Review of major trends in health care costs and utilization:
- LTC use trends
- costs and inflation trends

HUMAN RESOURCES

Review of major trends impacting the availability and distribution of health care professionals:
- physician supply
- nurse supply
- professional issues
- unionization

MEDICAL ETHICS

Review of major ethical issues facing health care providers:
- treatment of handicapped infants
- nutrition/hydration issues
- euthanasia/living wills
- informed consent
- care for the poor
- genetic engineering
- care of AIDS patients, etc.

Exhibit 2-1. Primary components of the environmental assessment.

Source: From "An environmental assessment is a key," by C. Hawley, 1988, *Provider, 14*(4), 14–20. Reprinted with permission of the American Health Care Association.

SERVICE AREA CHARACTERISTICS	COMPETITOR ANALYSIS
► Service area definition ► Demographic trends and projections: population growth trends, birth rate, etc. ► Economic conditions: poverty data, local economy, employment/business trends ► Morbidity/mortaility statistics	► Identify key competitors: hospitals, SNFs ► Analyze strengths and weaknesses of institution and competitors on basis of services, cost, reputation, location, etc. ► Market share trends for institution and major competitors over past five years. Breakdown by service and patient characteristics where possible
COMMUNITY HEALTH NEEDS AND RESOURCES	UTILIZATION TRENDS
► Community needs assessment: identify major service needs and/or oversupply; discuss needs of the poor and elderly ► Inventory of community health ser- vices and facilities including hospitals, clinics, LTC facilities, home care, hospice, etc. ► Human resources—local supply of physicians, nurses, and other health professionals	Past 3–5 Year Trends in Community: ► Health cost trends and comparative rates across institutions ► Inpatient use trends: admissions days, occupancy, average length of stay ► Patient characteristics by: age/sex, payor mix, service groupings, patient origin ► Case-mix trends ► Provide health care utilization forecasts for institution and major competitors

Exhibit 2-2. Components of the community and market assessment.

Source: From "An environmental assessment is a key," by C. Hawley, 1988, *Provider, 14*(4), 14–20. Reprinted with permission of the American Health Care Association.

hospitals may provide charitable obstetrical services for poor families along with follow-up home health care services after the baby and mother have returned home.

In MOSAIC, "S" stands for strategy and answers the question, "What can we do?" Of course, responses take into account the institution's resources currently available and those that can be secured in the future. A strategy is based on a resource profile of what the provider did in the past in terms of service, recruiting, and marketing and what it can do in the future to meet the new objectives. An environmental assessment provides the basic data permitting an analysis and interpretation to answer the three basic questions in the formulation stage of MOSAIC.

BASICS RE NEED ASSESSMENT

A number of techniques can be used to assess the needs of the community. Assessment techniques are particularly useful in helping health care providers to discover populations requiring special health assistance or in identifying unmet medical needs in specific geographic areas. These assessment methods can also assist institutions in establishing health status baselines for a community or a specific subgroup. Health status baselines enable providers to evaluate the impact of an institution's intervention in improving weak points while reinforcing areas of strength. Measurements of health status after the intervention provide the comparative data.

In addition to health status, assessment methods can also deal with a community's acute care and long-term care bed needs and quality of life measures. Satin and Monetti [1985] explain the use of census tract predictors to determine need assessment in physical, psychological, and social functioning areas.

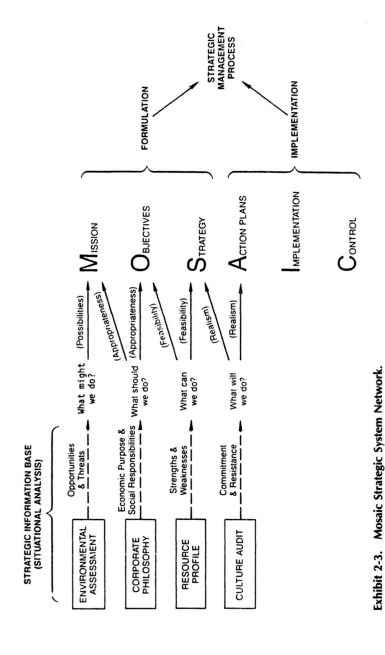

Exhibit 2-3. Mosaic Strategic System Network.

Source: From "Cultural Factors in Choosing a Strategic Posture: A Bridge Between Formulation and Implementation," by D.J. Scotti, Chapter 13 in *Strategic Management in the Health Care Sector: Towards the Year 2000*, F. Simyar and J. Lloyd-Jones (editors), 1988, Englewood Cliffs, NJ: Prentice-Hall. Reprinted by permission.

All of these need assessment techniques and methods serve at least the following purposes:

1. Identification of a baseline against which future changes can be measured.
2. Evaluation of the needs of the community, the strengths, weaknesses, and the potential areas of opportunity.
3. Analysis of changes over time.
4. Comparisons among subpopulations in the catchment area, either at a point in time or between two or more time periods.

Specific issues affect all needs assessment methods: validity, reliability, precision, and accuracy. Another problem concerns the distinction between techniques that determine "need" and those that concentrate on "demand."

Generally, a variety of needs assessment techniques seek to segment populations and individuals according to health status prior to symptomatic awareness.

ATTRIBUTES OF NEED ASSESSMENT

Methods used to measure health status should be "sensitive" enough to identify minor changes in the population or individuals. Thus, sensitivity is a critical variable in the selection of needs assessment methods.

Validity is another attribute. Usually, validity is defined as the capability of the method to actually measure a general or specific health status measure such as morbidity or mortality. If a needs assessment method categorized "poverty" as a proxy health status indicator, does that indicator truly measure the need for health services? As an indicator, poverty might correlate with morbidity or mortality as compared to income or social class categories. However, poverty may also be a measure of poor housing, limited education, or lack of opportunity for self-improvement. In fact, poverty might be a better indicator for mental health than for health. In sum, needs assessment methods should not use data to pinpoint health status indicators that may be invalid or ambiguous.

Reliability, as an attribute, refers to the consistency and/or dependability of the measurement technique. There is a consideration of the variety of data to be collected by the method to be used. In turn, reliability relates to the type of questions asked, the actual wording, and the placement order in the instrument. Reliability deals with the interpretation given to responses with the interpretative consistency between the interviewers. Similarly, respondents should be constant in understanding the questions. It is possible that a status indicator may be valid, but the reliability is doubtful. Respondents may give different answers to the same questions in the instrument. Therefore, it is necessary that the indicators and instruments be valid and reliable to guarantee the predictive ability of the method to measure health status.

A fourth attribute refers to the accuracy of methods. Accuracy is directly linked to the validity and reliability of the technique. If the method is either invalid or unreliable, the accuracy of the indicators will also be erroneous. A final index measure will be inaccurate if data for measures used to aggregate a health status index are unavailable or inconsistent in their accessibility: available for one ethnic group but not another; for one population area and not another; or based on different compilations. If the same respondents vary widely in their answers to the same question at different times, particularly if nothing warranted the different responses, the accuracy of the index will be problematical [Parkerson, Gehlboch, & Wagner,

1981; Sackett, Chambers, MacPherson, Goldsmith, & McCauley, 1977; Bergner, Bobbit, & Carter, 1981].

Additional health status measurement attributes worth pondering include the following: the precision of measurement; the ease of collection and availability of data; and the relative ease of mathematical computations to calculate the status indices or measures. An index must be precise enough to detect variability among subgroups in a population or discover changes over time in the status of a population. Although accurate, a measure could be couched in vague terminology or in numerical ranges making it impossible to detect minor differences within a population. A locality could exhibit a low morbidity rate for heart diseases as compared with United States data. Yet, if the vague index is unable to pinpoint differences among segments of the population residing in the area, a significant subgroup in the locality with a high morbidity rate could be overlooked.

Data must be readily available and collected in an efficient, cost-effective manner for health status indices to be used on a routine basis. A major obstacle to utilizing an individual survey technique is the high cost per interview, and few health care providers can afford such expenditures. If survey data are not collected on a routine periodic basis—one year, two years, or more—the value is diminished. Methods to keep track of a population's health status must be simple and relatively inexpensive. Partially financed and coordinated by the federal National Center for Health Statistics, the State Cooperative Health Statistics Program is a step in the right direction.

Another attribute indicates that the health status index mathematics should be easy for strategic planning staff to manipulate. Planners may not have high-level training in either mathematics or in statistics. Many planners measure success in new services and programs without using statistical calculations and complicated formulae. Of course, computer software programs are available that calculate sophisticated statistical analyses at the touch of a button.

In addition to these attributes, Bergner [1985] believes that health status indices should take into account five dimensions:

1. Genetic foundations or inherited characteristics that form the basic structure on which all other aspects of health status must build.
2. Biochemical, physiologic, or anatomic condition, which includes disease, disability, or handicap, whether obvious or not.
3. Functional condition, which includes performance of all the usual activities of life, such as working, walking, and thinking.
4. Mental condition, which includes self-perception of mood and emotion.
5. Health potential of the individual, which includes longevity, functional potential, and the prognosis of disease and disability.

CONCEPTS OF HEALTH

Abanobi [1986] raises serious questions about the content validity of three distinct concepts of health: the medical, holistic, and wellness models. To be acceptable, a concept of health must be comprehensive including both the negative and positive aspects of health status. Both the medical and wellness models are too limited as each excludes the main factors of the others. On the other hand, the holistic model is broad enough in concept to include both factors. However, the problem with the holistic model is the difficulty in making the concept operational to carry out empirical validation studies. In sum, "the lack of a universally accepted 'generic' concep-tualization and operational definition of health results in problems of consistency and com-parability" [Abanobi, 1986]. While this is a limitation, it should not deter the implementation of a strategic health planning process using the available tools and data.

NEED/DEMAND OR VICE VERSA

Need is generally defined as "the amount of medical services, which in the opinion of medical professionals, should be consumed by members of a community if they are to become or remain as healthy as possible given existing medical knowledge." *Demand*, on the other hand, refers to the amount of medical services community members want to consume at certain prices as reflected by their tastes and preferences for all goods and services available to them" [USDHHS, 1981, p. 12].

A child with bruised hands cannot grasp a baseball, and has a specific need that inhibits one of the child's primary activities. A college student with a broken leg cannot move about to attend classes and take care of his educational responsibilities. An individual with diabetes also has specific needs, although the illness may not be debilitating enough to restrict daily activity. In addition, De La Rosa [1989] elaborates on health care needs of Hispanics, Young [1989] on geriatric age-defined needs, and Zylke [1989] on maternal and child health needs. All of these situations fall into definable types of potential health care needs.

Need is changed to a demand when the individual seeks medical assistance due to increased severity. A demand is not generated if mother cares for the child's burned hands with home remedies. If the person with diabetes does not seek medical care, there is no demand. Obviously, this means that the need for health care services generally exceeds any overt de-mands made upon the health care delivery system. On the other hand, individuals may demand services but not receive care for the following reasons: not able to afford the service; not able to get to the service at a convenient time and place; service is simply not available; or religious beliefs may prevent the use of specific medically needed services.

This relationship between need and demand is the crux of strategic planning. Health care providers must have accurate information about the nature of the medical need in their health service areas.

Connections between need and demand garner attention, but the link is tenuous. Systems analysts delve into variables impacting upon the need/demand dyad such as individual accessi-bility to care, availability of services, the cost of services, the quality offered, the continuity of care, and the individual's acceptability of the service. These factors are an integral part of the health care delivery system. Indeed, these variables sharply influence people with needs to take action to turn that need into a demand for service. At one time, health care providers believed that an equilibrium existed between need and demand as the available resources were used by individuals coming for care. With new insights and fresh data, an awareness developed that many groups had unmet needs and were unable to secure services. Those groups include senior citizens, the homeless, single-parent mothers, housebound disabled, AIDS victims, and work-ing adults. All of these and others represent strategic targets of opportunity for health care providers. Who has what type of needs? How many people are there? Where are they located? How often do they use medical facilities? What facilities? How sick are they? Who will care for them? Who will pay for the medical services? Answers to these and many other questions can be obtained by a variety of assessment methods and techniques.

NEEDS ASSESSMENT METHODS

A variety of techniques can determine both need and demand. Each method has advantages and disadvantages. One point to keep in mind while discussing these need- and demand-based methodologies is that they are fundamentally ideologically based. Pillemer [1984] argues that even though appearing to be scientific, the techniques are not as valid as they would appear:

> This lack of validity is due to the subjective value decisions which must be made in level-of-care decisions, to the inherent inability of any methodology to incorporate certain key variables into the quantitative need equation, and to the fact that even the most carefully designed need-based planning target must pass severe political hurdles before it can be implemented.

Pillemer contends that demand-based methodologies employ current utilization norms in the calculations. That may be undesirable because current utilization patterns may be changing. Of even more importance, it is probable that the current utilization patterns are exactly what needs to be changed.

Regarding need-based methods, Pillemer identifies three major difficulties:

- Inevitability of having to use faulty normative assumptions to make decisions.
- Insufficient data resulting from the existence of unaccounted-for-variables.
- Difficulties emanating from the influence of political decision making.

Various approaches to needs assessment have been catalogued [USDHHS, 1981, pp. 27–58]. Generally, health assessments embrace three main areas: the environment, lifestyle, and health services utilization. Indicators for each of these areas have been developed and are reported in the annual *Health: United States* series, published by the National Center for Health Statistics [USDHHS, 1990]. Environmental indicators in the series refer to variables such as toxic agents, accident prevention, and fluoridation. Lifestyle indicators include smoking control, improved nutrition, and physical fitness, among others [Andersen, Aday, & Chen, 1986]. Deficiencies in these three factors may have a major impact on the level of the health status of the population as measured by death, disease, disability, discomfort, and dissatisfaction measurements. Strategic planners for health care providers can use these national and/or regional measures to compare with their own communities and discover discrepancies in medical and health services for those groups requiring substantial improvement. Following are needs assessment methods that can measure the factors affecting a community's health status.

Key Informant Survey

Description. Essentially, the key informant technique is a survey of individually knowledgeable people such as police, clergy, clinic directors, school officials, program clients, and politicians. These key informants are asked about their perceptions of the nature and extent of the existing or potential medical and/or health-related problems in the community.

Purpose. This survey is an effort to locate and identify the at-risk populations and to specify the needs for health care services among those populations.

Resources Required for a Key Informant Survey. Generally, this is a simple, quick, and inexpensive technique to gather initial data about area problems and needs. Depending upon local variables, a key informant survey could be completed in 20 to 60 days.

Compared to other techniques that collect primary data, the key informant technique is inexpensive. Major factors affecting the cost are the number of informants used and the interview method. In calculating expenditures, the following need to be considered:

- Personnel costs
- Reproduction costs for interview instruments and reports
- Mileage, parking, and other travel expenses
- Telephone, typing, and miscellaneous office expenses.

Personnel costs include staff members, consultants, or community residents required to collect and analyze the data, and to prepare reports. A key informant survey in which 25 to 50 people are to be interviewed could require the following person-day estimates by each task in the process.

- Research design and planning: 3 to 5 person-days
- Selecting key informants: 3 person-days
- Constructing an instrument or interview guide: 6 to 8 person-days
- Pilot testing: 3 to 6 person-days
- Training interviewers: 3 to 6 person-days
- Making appointments with informants: 2 person-days
- On-site interviews with informants: 14 to 18 person-days (travel time must be taken into account)
- Data reduction and analysis: 5 to 7 person-days
- Report writing: 5 to 8 person-days.

Advantages. Where time and cost are major factors or where initial information is needed, the simplicity and quick turnaround possible with this technique will appeal to providers. This technique is useful in facilitating communication among concerned agencies and individuals. Input is gathered from a diverse group of informants providing the special perspective of each person.

Disadvantages. Information collected may be subjective and impressionistic, reflecting the bias of the informants or a limited viewpoint of the problems. In addition, informants may not be aware of persons not visible to them. Key informant data are not easily amenable to systematic analysis. Furthermore, the data lack stand-alone validity and require verification by consultation with other sources.

Steps in Implementation. Usually, there are seven steps involved in a key informant survey:

1. *Describe the goals and objectives of the survey.* An essential first step is to describe the goals and objectives of the key informant survey. Questions that need to be answered should be outlined in detail. Importantly, there has to be a determination about how the forthcoming data will be used, making it possible to construct an instrument to provide relevant information.
2. *Develop criteria for selection of key informants.* To identify the number and types of

informants needed, the target populations and subject area need to be examined. Individuals have to be selected who are likely to come into contact with or otherwise be knowledgeable about the population and the problems. Selection criteria could be based on formal and/or informal affiliations within the affected community.

3. *Identify key informants.* Potential key informants may be identified by contacting schools, social service agencies, local governments, health, and medical treatment programs, local police, and health care providers. Agencies and individuals should be asked to suggest other agencies and individuals to contact. During the interviews, informants should be asked to provide key persons to speak with.

4. *Develop a data collection methodology.* Data collection techniques should reflect the restraints imposed by available resources and types of data needed. Planners must determine:

- Data collection methods
  —Face-to-face interview
  —Telephone interview
  —Group interview
  —Mail survey
  —Delphi approach
- Structure of the interview
  —Structured with instrument that obtains the same type of information from each respondent
  —Structured with flexible interviewer's guide
  —Unstructured and open-ended with no attempt to secure the same type of information from each respondent
- Type of questions to be asked (if a structured approach is used)
  —Open-ended design to allow the respondent freedom of expression on the issues
  —Forced choice where responses are limited to prestated alternatives.

For the purpose of a key informant survey, the structured, face-to-face interview with open-ended questions is recommended. This approach should have the lowest nonresponse rate, permit specific questions to be answered, and still allow the respondent to provide relevant information and details that might otherwise be overlooked.

5. *Construct the instrument or interviewer's guide.* Goals and objectives of the survey determine the data that will be needed. Often, it is advantageous to outline the type of reports and tables desired before data collection begins. Instruments should ask *only* for information that will actually be used. Questions should be asked in a logical, well-ordered manner, and difficult or sensitive questions should be asked last.

6. *Select and train staff.* Interviewers should have good communication skills, be sensitive to local community issues, and should be carefully trained in key informant survey techniques.

7. *Analyze the data.* Unless your key informant survey is unusually large, the most appropriate data analysis techniques are probably manual tally as opposed to computer analysis and content analysis. In all likelihood, the easiest way to develop an analytic framework is to review each open-ended question answered by the first informant and list all the distinct points, opinions, and estimates using meaningful categories. Then, proceed to the next

informant's questionnaire, tallying any points that are repeated and adding any new points and different opinions or questions. After all the data have been tabulated, it may be useful to bring a few of the informants together for an evaluation meeting. Findings can be discussed and new insights may emerge. In addition, the review meeting may also increase the communication, cooperation, and referrals between the health care providers, the community agencies,and the key informants.

Community Survey

Description. An interview or self-administered questionnaire is used to collect data on sociodemographic characteristics, on problems and needs, and on knowledge and attitudes related to the needs of various community populations and pressing community issues. If properly administered, the community survey is a sophisticated method that yields objective, scientific data. Problems may occur relative to sampling and the validity of self-reported information.

Purpose. This technique attempts to identify and refine the affected community populations while specifying their needs as well as the most effective means to reaching those populations.

Resources Required. Depending on the sample size, the amount of information to be collected, and the method for collecting the data, this technique can be expensive and time-consuming. Factors influencing the cost are the size of the sample and the method of administration. Door-to-door surveys tend to be very expensive. Self-administered questionnaires mailed out or used in group settings such as schools or hospitals can cost less and may even be quite inexpensive. In developing cost estimates, the following elements need to be considered:

- Personal costs
- Reproduction costs for instruments and reports
- Mileage, parking, and travel if interview or other site work is involved
- Telephone charges for telephone interviews or follow-up calls
- Postage for mail questionnaires
- Form editing, key punching, and computer time, if necessary.

Staff members, consultants, or community resources are required to collect the data, analyze the data, and to write reports. Person-day estimates by task areas for a community survey of 1,000 respondents follow:

- Research design, planning, and administration: 10 to 20 person-days
- Sample selection: 3 to 8 person-days
- Construction of instrument: 8 to 12 person-days
- Pilot testing: 3 person-days
- Training of interviewers, if necessary: 2 person-days for trainer and 1 person-day each for interviewers
- Data collection, by type
  —Door-to-door survey: 100 to 500 person-days (travel time must be taken into account)
  —Face-to-face interviews in an institutional setting: 60 to 200 person-days (travel time may be involved)

—Telephone interviews: 50 to 150 person-days

—Mail questionnaire: 3 to 15 person-days of processing time; 3 to 10 person-days for follow-up contacts

—Self-administered questionnaires in institutional setting: 10 to 30 person-days (estimated for 20 groups of 50; travel time may be involved)

- Data reduction and analysis (using a computer)

—Editing of forms: 15 to 50 person-days

—Key punching with verification: 3 to 40 person-days (major factor is form length)

—Computer programming: 2 to 10 person-days

—Computer processing (not requiring the skills of a programmer): 1 to 5 person-days

—Data analysis and interpretation: 3 to 15 person-days

- Data reduction and analysis (performed manually)

—Editing of forms: 3 to 50 person-days

—Data reduction: 3 to 90 person-days

—Data analysis and interpretation: 3 to 15 person-days

- Report writing: 2 to 15 person-days.

Computer equipment and/or facilities are required for analysis of data from surveys with large sample sizes. Assistance may be obtained though the state government, local universities, banks, and private companies. Universities tend to be the least expensive and private companies tend to be the most expensive. Using existing computer analysis packages such as SPSS (Statistical Package for the Social Sciences), SAS (Statistical Analysis System), and BMD-P (Bio Medical Data Programs) is usually significantly more economical than developing specialized programs for special study purposes.

Depending on the methodology selected and the sample size, the community survey can be more time consuming than the other techniques. Turnaround time may range from 1 to 12 months.

Advantages. By collecting data directly from the targeted populations, this technique avoids some of the questionable assumptions that must be made when using other approaches. Techniques exist for estimating the reliability of the data. Comparisons with similar databases may establish validity.

Disadvantages. This technique tends to be expensive and time-consuming. Due to population mobility, it may be difficult to adequately sample groups within the targeted populations. Serious questions of validity must always be answered about self-reported data. These data frequently lack stand-alone validity, and planners cannot be sure of their accuracy without going to another source for verification. Planners should be cautious in presenting self-reported data as objective information.

Steps in Implementation. Eleven steps detail the community survey process:

1. *Describe the goals and objectives of the assessment.* An essential first step is to describe the goals and objectives of the community survey needs assessment. Another vital step indicates how the data will be used so it will be possible to design a study to provide relevant data.

2. *Define carefully the targeted populations.* To be able to develop an appropriate sampling design, the planner must know exactly to what community assessment issues and to what populations the findings are to be generalized.

3. *Develop criteria for sampling.* Goals and objectives of the survey assessment determine the populations to be selected for examination, the use of any special statistical techniques, and the available resources impacting upon the most appropriate sampling method. Common sampling techniques include the following:
    *   *Random sampling.* Each member of the population has an equal chance of being selected in the sample.
    *   *Stratified random sampling.* On the basis of characteristics such as age, sex, race, or socioeconomic status, the population is divided into strata assuring that subgroups are adequately represented in the survey.
    *   It is advisable to use sample areas that are consistent with census tracts and census enumerative districts. If this can be done, census data or other data collected by federal or state agencies may be available for comparison. Community demographic profiles from census data may be used to examine the validity of the needs assessment survey sample.
4. *Develop a sampling methodology.* Planners must determine how the sample is to be selected. Common approaches include:
    *   *Area sampling.* Members of the targeted populations living in a given geographic area are selected. Decisions may be made about single family dwellings to be selected, apartments in multifamily dwellings, and which individual in a family is to be surveyed.
    *   *List sampling.* Listings such as telephone directories, registered voters, high school students, or clients in treatment may be randomly sampled or with stratifications relating to individual characteristics.
5. *Select the sample.* When actually choosing the survey participants, the planner should verify that the lists and the maps are complete and up-to-date.
6. *Develop a data collection methodology.* Obviously, data collection must be responsive to the restraints imposed by the available resources, the sampling methodology, and the types of data needed. Still, the planner must select from choices of operating variables:
    *   *Methods of data collection*
        —Face-to-face interview at residence in a door-to-door survey
        —Face-to-face interview in institutional setting
        —Face-to-face interview in public setting, such as a street survey
        —Telephone interview
        —Mail survey
        —Self-administered questionnaire in a group or institutional setting.
    *   *Structure of the approach*
        —Interview with structured instrument
        —Interview structured with interviewer's guide
        —Self-administered questionnaire
        —Unstructured interview.
    *   *Type of questions to be asked* (if a structured approach is used)
        —Open-ended
        —Forced choice.
7. *Construct the instrument.* Generically, the goals and objectives of the survey determine what data will be needed. It is often advantageous to outline the type of reports and tables desired before data collection begins. Instruments should ask *only* for information that will actually be used. Questions should be asked in a logical, well-ordered manner, with difficult or sensitive questions asked last. A pretest can be done easily and is recommended for all surveys.

If automated processing is anticipated, the instrument should be designed to lend itself to easy coding and key punching. Time can be saved by printing instruments where responses filled in with lead pencils can be read directly by the computer to produce tallies and analyses.

8. *Schedule data collection.* Timetables for collecting data, especially in a relatively large effort, should be established well in advance and should take into account seasonal considerations, holidays, and days of the week.

9. *Collect the data.* While data are being collected, the process should be monitored by a logistics coordinator since scheduling flexibility is usually necessary. Validation procedures should provide for recontacting selected respondents to confirm their interviews and to thank them for participating.

10. *Reduce the data.* Depending on the sample size, it will probably be desirable to use automated computer processing and analysis of the data. To initiate this process, the data must be edited and coded, cards must be punched, and computer files must be created. A variety of existing computer packages are available for data analysis.

11. *Analyze the data.* Two types of statistical analysis may be performed for needs assessment:
    *   *Descriptive analysis.* To describe the sample, this involves percentage distributions, contingency tables, and measures of central tendency such as the computation of means, medians, and modes.
    *   *Prediction models.* Statistical techniques yield predictive statements about the sample population. A projection of the demand for prevention services. Identification of the geographic area in need. Specification of populations using specific services.

Demographic Analysis

Description. With demographic data from existing sources such as the U.S. Census Bureau, the Bureau of Labor Statistics, the Department of Health and Human Services, income and education study data, voter registration lists, and school registration records, the demographic analysis technique can be used to make projections about the target populations and about the needs of those target populations. Demographic analysis data are used as a baseline for making projections about needs. Usually, the data are used in combination with other information from national surveys, from major studies, from inferential indicators, or from community surveys. If the high-risk populations can be described demographically, the demographic analysis technique can locate the high-risk areas geographically. Demographic data should be examined carefully beforehand to make certain that the populations of interest are well represented.

In addition, data on births, death, and migration can give a picture of what the population of a given area will be like in the future. These estimates allow the development of predictions of the need and demand for health services.

Purpose. Demographic analysis attempts to identify the target populations and to project their needs. Creatively applied, these extant data sets can be extremely meaningful to the strategic planner.

Resources Required. Published public access data are widely available and usually inexpensive to use. However, computer analysis of expansive data sets and management information system files can become expensive. Nevertheless, purchasing relevant existing data is considerably less costly than generating that information anew.

Obviously, the demographic analysis technique is less expensive than primary data collection. A major factor affecting the cost is the method of access of the data. Cost estimates include the following factors:

- Personnel cost
- Cost of having the agency generate special reports,if necessary
- Cost of secondary analysis, if necessary
  —Charges for computer tapes
  —Computer time expenditures
- Cost of reports purchased, if necessary
- Reproduction charges for reports.

Staff members, consultants, or community resources are required to collect the data, analyze the data, and to write reports. Following are person-day estimates by task areas:

- Assessment, design, planning, and administration: 3 to 8 person-days
- Identification of data sets: 3 to 8 person-days
- Extraction of data from available reports: 3 to 20 person-days
- Secondary analysis of data: 10 to 30 person-days
- Report writing: 5 to 30 person-days.

Often, published data are immediately available. If special reports must be generated by the agencies, several weeks may be required. Total elapsed time may range from 10 days to 6 months.

Advantages. A prime advantage is that the data are available and relatively inexpensive to use. In addition, data files are expansive and, in some cases, data are available on the entire population. Generally, the data are objective and validity estimates are available.

Disadvantages. Because existing data are collected for general purposes, it is possible that the specific need assessment information desired may not be included.

Steps in Implementation. Five steps in the demographic analysis follow:

1. *Describe the goals and objectives of the assessment.* As usual, the essential first step is to describe the goals and objectives of the needs assessment study. Again, it is essential to determine how the data will be used so that it will be possible to structure the accumulation of appropriate data.
2. *Define the types of data needed.* To determine what data are needed, it is useful to outline the report that will be produced and even lay out dummy tables.
3. *Contact local, state, and federal agencies to determine what data are available.* A major source of demographic data will be the U.S. Census Bureau. In addition to the latest census data, information may be obtained from the income and education survey, from census bureau projections and estimates, and from additional census bureau reports. Other major sources include the Department of Labor's Bureau of Labor Statistics, state health departments, the National Institutes of Health, and the National Center for Health Statistics. Community and local groups should also look to local health departments as a source for demographic data.
4. *Access the data.* If it is necessary to have special reports produced, it will probably be most

cost effective to have the agency from which the data are requested to do the computer processing.

5. *Reduce and analyze the data.* Demographic data may be used in two ways for needs assessment:

- *Descriptive analysis.* Data are presented in a straightforward manner. Logical inferences are drawn about the meaning of the population frequency distributions.
- *Statistical models.* In combination with data from other sources, the demographic analysis allows for statistical inferences to be drawn about the problems and needs of the population. Used in either of these two ways, the data may be presented in one of two formats:
- *Table and chart format.* Percentage distributions, contingency tables, measures of central tendency, or matrices are used to describe the population.
- *Map format.* A map or a series of overlapping maps is used to visually illustrate the population distributions.

Value may be gained from ranking the geographic areas according to population densities or population characteristics that may be related to specific health needs. Those rankings may be used in combination with inferential indicators to compare the needs in various areas.

Inferential Indicators

Description. Existing data sets of direct and indirect indicators are used to make inferences about the need for health services in the target populations. Since inferences are being made, cautious and careful interpretation of the data are mandatory.

Purpose. Inferential indicators are used to draw conclusions about current and potential health care service needs in the target populations and to facilitate estimations of the need for services.

Resources Required. Reports, published and unpublished, may be available for quick, inexpensive review. Secondary analysis of data sets is usually moderately expensive and may take a few months. Observational data, which may take a relatively long time to collect, is inexpensive relative to its quantity.

Inferential indicators analysis is less expensive than techniques involving primary data collection. Major factors affecting cost are the number of data sets used and the accessibility of the data. Costs include the following:

- Personnel cost
- Cost of having an agency generate special reports, if necessary
- Cost of secondary analysis, if necessary
  —Charges for computer tapes
  —Computer time charges
- Cost of reports purchased, if necessary
- Reproduction charges for reports.

Staff members, consultants, or community resources are required to collect the data, analyze the data, and write reports. Following are person-day estimates by task areas:

- Assessment design, planning, and administration: 1 to 10 person-days
- Identification of data sets: 1 to 10 person-days
- Literature search or review of other data to identify indicators: 1 to 10 person-days
- Statistical consultation is recommended: 1 to 5 person-days
- Extraction of data from available reports: 1 to 15 person-days
- Secondary analysis of data: 5 to 25 person days
- Report writing: 5 to 20 person-days.

Published data may be immediately available. If special reports must be generated by the agencies, several weeks may be required. Total elapsed time may range from 10 days to 6 months.

Advantages. Data are available, often comprehensive, and relatively inexpensive to use.

Disadvantages. Existing data, because they are not collected for needs assessment, seldom contain all of the information desired. Access to some data sets may be limited because they contain confidential information.

Steps in Implementation. Eights steps are involved in using the inferential indicators technique:

1. *Describe the goals and objectives of the assessment.* An essential first step is to describe the goals and objectives of the needs assessment study.
2. *Identify the indicators to be used.* Indicator variables which can be correlated to the specific subject areas of the needs assessment should be identified. A list of variables found to be correlated with various aspects of health care follows. Note that the correlation is open to discussion about a causal relationship. If it is known that a direct or indirect indicator is causely related to the subject area, the indicators may be used to address the problem and allow for projections about the needs of the population.
   - *Sociodemographic characteristics.* Including sex, race, age, occupation or vocational interests, family history, and socioeconomic status.
   - *Personality characteristics.* For example, sociability, achievement orientation, independence, socialization, tough-minded versus tender-minded, breadth of interests, impulsivity, flexibility, openness to experience, social activity, and social recognition.
   - *Attitudes and opinions.* Toward authority, parents, health, fatalism, societal institutions, religiosity, school, concern for future, and social activism.
   - *Social and interperson variables.* Such as peer conformity, parental conflict, morality, social conformity, conventionality, orientation of parents toward health and socioeconomic background.
3. *Define the types of data needed.* Again, strategic planners may find it helpful to outline the report to be produced and even to lay out the tables that should be presented. This draft plan should indicate exactly how the data should be broken down, and what categories are desired for each variable.
4. *Contact local, federal, and state agencies to determine what data are available.* Inferential indicators may make available the great number and variety of existing data sets, many of which may be easily and inexpensively obtained from a variety of sources.

5. *Determine how the data may be accessed.* In some cases, reports or computerized data sets may be available. In other cases, the data may have to be extracted manually. Census data and data user instructions, for example, can be acquired through the Census Bureau's regional offices.
6. *Develop agreements regarding confidentiality.* It is necessary to consider the protection of the individual's right to privacy. Federal and state laws protect the confidentiality of case records and data sets such as those mentioned above. However, the need for social research is recognized and accommodated in these regulations. Legitimate planners should be able to negotiate access to such data, but the data may be used only in aggregate form.
7. *Access the data.* If it is necessary to have special reports produced, it will probably be most cost effective to have the agency do the computer processing.
8. *Reduce and analyze data.* Inferential indicator analysis may be used in two ways for needs assessment:
   - *Descriptive analysis.* Percentage distributions, contingency tables, and measures of central tendency are presented in a stand-alone fashion. Logical inferences are drawn about the need for health care services.
   - *Statistical models.* Statistical models, combining variables from the same or from different data sets, are used to draw statistical inferences about the need for health care services.

Programmatic Data

Description. This technique uses information from a health care provider's own files and experiences and from the files and experiences of other agency's programs to provide data for planning and decision making. Data collection may involve interviews with personnel, statistical analysis of records, management information system data, or participant observation in the program.

Purpose. Programmatic data techniques provide planning information to new or expanding programs, data for service planning and decision making, and information on available resources.

Resources Required. Access to informants and information from health care service programs is required. Expense is relative to the number of programs surveyed.

Programmatic data collection is relatively inexpensive compared to the other techniques. Elements to be considered in developing cost estimates include the following:

- Personal cost
- Travel expenses to interview personnel or extract data from files, if necessary
- Telephone costs to interview personnel, if necessary
- Computer cost to extract data from computerized management information systems, if necessary
- Reproduction costs for reports.

Staff members, consultants, and community resources are required to collect the data, analyze the data, and write reports. Following are person-day estimates by task areas:

- Assessment design, planning and administration: 3 to 8 person-days

- Identification of programs or service providers: 3 to 30 person-days: very time consuming for a state trying to identify all public and private programs and service providers
- Identification of relevant data: 3 to 8 person-days
- Interviewing staff of program or facility, if necessary: 6 to 60 person-days
- Data reduction and analysis: 6 to 15 person-days
- Report writing: 4 to 10 person-days.

Very quick turnaround is possible for local programs. Total elapsed time may range from 10 days to 4 months.

Advantages. This technique is quick and simple, and the data are often most useful.

Disadvantages. Information may sometimes be sketchy and subjective, and definitions may vary from program to program. Data are problem-oriented and are concerned only with clients using services.

Steps in Implementation of the Programmatic Data Technique. An essential first step is to describe the goals and objectives of the needs assessment study.

1. Define the types of data needed.
   Data may be needed to:
   - Identify patient populations
   - Identify areas of unmet need
   - Identify duplication of services
   - Facilitate appropriate use of available services
   - Develop directories.
   Such information may be obtained by identifying:
   - Information sources
   - Services provided
   - Staffing patterns
   - Funding
   - Client profiles
   - Patterns of use.
   Some data may be obtained from other programs and used for needs assessment planning. For instance, useful information from other assessment studies might describe:
   - Target populations
   - Needs identified
   - Indicators used
   - Needs assessment methodologies.
   Additionally, information may be gathered which might be used as models for program development, including
   - Evaluation of programs
   - Management information systems
   - Case studies of programs
   - Budgets
   - Personnel analysis
   - Analysis of available services.
2. Locate the programs from which information may be obtained.

3. Collect the information by contacting the programs with data and arrange for interviews, analysis of data sets, or program observation.
4. Analyze the data using statistical procedures, content analysis, or interviewers' and observers' reports.

Index of Well-Being

Bush, Chen, and Patrick [1974] created an index that measures changes in health status and well-being with some sensitivity. That well-being index has two dimensions: a function level [how a person performs his activity of daily living at a point in time], and a prognosis [changes that occur to his health and mental health at future times and result in shifts in his functional performance from one level to another—either higher or lower]. Bush explains function status as "conformity to society's standards of physical and mental well-being, including performance of the activities usual for the social role" [Bush et al., 1974, p. 5]. A person's malfunctioning can result from both physical and mental origins and represent degrees of deviation from well-being norms. Investigators seek to classify functional performance levels on a scale from complete well-being to death. Problems arise relative to determining the levels between the continuum of well-being and death and the calculation of valid values to each level. Health status is differentiated from functional status. Bush states that health status refers to changes in a person's well-being from one level to another while functional status refers to a person's capacity to perform his/her social activities at some specific point in time.

Three separate scales measure a person's mobility, physical activity, and social activity. Exhibit 2-4 uses a 31-level scale combining these functions with measured values assigned to each within a .00 to 1.00 continuum [Bush et al., 1974, p. 26]. Exhibit 2-5 shows these levels and assigned values [Bush et al., 1974, p. 17].

Algebraically, the index of well-being is expressed as follows:

$$F = j\frac{N_jF_j}{N},$$

where $0 < F < 1$ and
N = total number of persons in a population
N_j = number of persons in function level j,
F_j = measured weight or social preference for function level j, and
j = index for the function level—0, 1, 2, . . . 30.

Exhibit 2-6 demonstrates an application of the well-being index formula based on the 31-level scale. About 95 percent of the population functions at 30—the highest performance level. Three percent of the index includes people with various degrees of deviation from the highest level of functioning.

Advantages of the Index. Bush identifies the following advantages for the function status index:

1. A concise index of the health/mental well-being of a community.
2. Sensitive to the variations of individuals with different degrees of functional capacity.
3. Data are easily observable and can be used without knowledge of medical terms or diagnoses, or without being dependent on a person's memory.

Exhibit 2-4.   Scales and Definitions for Functional Level Classification.

Scale	Step	Definition
		Mobility Scale
5	Traveled Freely	Used public transportation or drove alone. For below six age group, traveled as usual for age.
4	Traveled with Difficulty	[a] Went outside alone, but had trouble getting around community freely, or [b] required assistance to use public transportation or automobile.
3	In House	[a] All day, because of illness or condition or [b] needed human assistance to go outside.
2	In Hospital	Not only general hospital, but also nursing home, extended care facility, sanitarium, or similar institution.
1	In Special Unit	For some part of the day in a restricted area of the hospital such as intensive care, operating room, recovery room, isolation ward, or similar unit.
0	Death	
		Physical Activity Scale
4	Walked Freely	With no limitations of any kind.
3	Walked with Limitations	[a] With cane, crutches, or mechanical aid; or [b] limited in lifting, stooping or using inclines or stairs; or [c] limited in speed or distance by general physical condition.
2	Moved Independently in Wheelchair	Propelled self alone in wheelchair.
1	In Wheelchair	For most or all of the day
0	Death	
		Social Activity Scale
5	Performing Major and Other Activities	*Major* means specifically—play for below 6, school for 6–17, and work or maintain household for adults. *Other* means all activities not classified as major, such as athetics, clubs, shopping, church, hobbies, civic projects, or games appropriate for age.
4	Performed Major But Limited in Other Activities	Played, went to school, worked, or kept house, but limited in other activities as defined above.
3	Performed Major Activities with Limitations	Limited in amount or kind of major activity performed, for instance needed special rest periods, special school, or special working aids.
2	Did Not Perform Major Activity But Performed Self-Care Activities	Did not play, go to school, work or keep house, but dressed, bathed, and fed self.
1	Required Assistance with Self-Care Activities	Required human help with one or more of the following—dressing, bathing, or eating and did not perform major or other activities. For below six age group, means assistance not usually required for age.
0	Death	

Exhibit 2-5. Function-Level Classification and Measured Values.

Level Number	Mobility [Step]	Physical Activity [Step]	Social Activity [Step]	Measured Values
L 30	Traveled freely [5]	Walked freely [4]	Performed major and other activities [no symptom/problem complex] [5]	1.000
L 29	Traveled freely [5]	Walked freely [4]	Performed major and other activities [symptom/problem complex present] [5]	.804
L 28	Traveled freely [5]	Walked freely [4]	Performed major but limited in other activities [4]	.689
L 27	Traveled freely [5]	Walked freely [4]	Performed major activity with limitations [3]	.694
L 26	Traveled freely [5]	Walked freely [4]	Did not perform major but performed self-care activities [2]	.646
L 25	Traveled with difficulty [4]	Walked freely [4]	Performed major but limited in other activities [4]	.516
L 24	Traveled with difficulty [4]	Walked freely [4]	Performed major activity with limitations [3]	.536
L 23	Traveled with difficulty [4]	Walked freely [4]	Did not perform major but performed self-care activities [2]	.495
L 22	Traveled with difficulty [4]	Walked with limitations [3]	Performed major but limited in other activities [4]	.519
L 21	Traveled with difficulty [4]	Walked with limitations [3]	Did not perform major but performed self-care activities [2]	.463
L 19	Traveled with difficulty [4]	Moved independently in wheelchair [2]	Performed major activity with limitations [3]	.503
L 18	Traveled with difficulty [4]	Moved independently in wheelchair [2]	Did not perform major but performed self-care activities [2]	.458
L 17	In house [3]	Walked freely [4]	Did not perform major but performed self-care activities [2]	.594
L 16	In house [3]	Walked freely [4]	Required assistance with self-care activities [1]	.505
L 15	In house [3]	Walked with limitations [3]	Did not perform major but performed self-care activities [2]	.519

(*continued*)

Exhibit 2-5. (Continued)

Level Number	Mobility [Step]	Physical Activity [Step]	Social Activity [Step]	Measured Values
L 14	In house [3]	Walked with limitations [3]	Required assistance with self-care activities [1]	.436
L 13	In house [3]	Moved independently in wheelchair [2]	Did not perform major but performed self-care activities [2]	.491
L 12	In house [3]	Moved independently in wheelchair [2]	Required assistance with self-care activities [1]	.444
L 11	In house [3]	In bed or chair [1]	Did not perform major but performed self-care activities [2]	.334
L 10	In house [3]	In bed or chair [1]	Required assistance with self-care activities [1]	.436
L 9	In hospital [2]	Walked freely [4]	Did not perform major but performed self-care activities [2]	.528
L 8	In hospital [2]	Walked freely [4]	Required assistance with self-care activities [1]	.440
L 7	In hospital [2]	Walked with limitations [2]	Did not perform major but performed self-care activities [2]	.440
L 6	In hospital [2]	Walked with limitations [3]	Required assistance with self-care activities [1]	.388
L 5	In hospital [2]	Moved independently in wheelchair [2]	Did not perform major but performed self-care activities [2]	.445
L 4	In hospital [2]	Moved independently in wheelchair [2]	Required assistance with self-care activities [1]	.387
L 3	In hospital [2]	In bed or chair [1]	Did not perform major but performed self-care activities [2]	.428
L 2	In hospital [2]	In bed or chair [1]	Required assistance with self-care activities [1]	.343
L 1	In special unit [1]	In bed or chair [1]	Required assistance with self-care activities [1]	.267
L 0	Death [0]			

Exhibit 2-6.   Computation of Function Status Index.

Index of Function Level [j]	Number of Persons [N_j]	Function-Level Values [F_j]	[$F_j N_j$]
30	95,000	1.00	95,000
27	3,000	.69	2,070
17	1,000	.59	590
10	700	.44	308
2	300	.34	102
Total	100,000 [=N]		98,070 [=$F_j N_j$]

$$F = \frac{F_j N_j}{N} = \frac{98,070}{100,000} = .98$$

4. Each person is exclusively assigned to only one level.
5. Flexibility permits cross-sectional comparisons among populations, disaggregation for comparison among populations within the community by nature of functioning or specific causes of dysfunction such as diabetes, schizophrenia, and so on, and the construction of longitudinal studies of the community over time.

However, the function status index is not without fault. If health status is not directly related to an individual's capabilities, the function status index overlooks changes in physical well-being or prognosis impacting upon functioning over time. Furthermore, years may pass before health status changes are reflected in the overall index. Improvements in one level of the function index may be canceled out by lower levels of functioning in other levels. While recognizing the advanced state of the index's development, critics noted additional shortcomings [Haig, Scott, & Wickett, 1986; Anderson, 1982]. As a component of illness, discomfort is not recognized as of equal importance to dysfunction. More importantly, the index does not have a ratio property. Critics claim that the index is vague in its case descriptions and inaccurate in its scaling method. Bush and his colleagues answer these and other criticisms in a detailed paper in support of the constructions, reliability, and validity of the index [Bush, Anderson, Kaplan, & Blischke, 1982].

To deal with and account for changes in a person's physical well-being or prognosis, Bush and his associates developed the "value-adjusted life expectancy" measure based on four functional levels: A—well, B—nonbed disability, C—bed disability, and D—death.

Calculating a 90-year potential life period and 10-year breakpoints, Bush computed the following "equilibrium function level expectancies:" .724 in a well state, .050 with nonbed disability, .021 with bed disability, and .205 as years of death with a longevity expectation of about 72 years. Doing the mathematics, Bush found that individuals can anticipate living in a well state for 65.2 years during their life (.724 x 90 years), with nonbed disability for 4.5 years (.050 x 90), and experience 1.9 years of bed disability (.021 x 90). Furthermore, people dying prematurely years before reaching their potential of 90 years of age, lost 18.4 years of productive life (.205490).

Multiplying function-level expectancies ($Y*j$) by FSI scale measures (F_j), yields the value-adjusted life expectancy ($Q*$): $Q* = F_j Y*j$.

This formula is applied to a community in Exhibit 2-7. Value-adjusted life expectancy is comparable to the expected dysfunction-free years of life. Evaluations can be made of all

Exhibit 2-7.   Computation of Value-Adjusted Life Expectancy.

L_j	Y^*_j	F_j	$Y^*_j F_j$
L_A Well	65.2	1.00	65.2
L_R Nonbed Disability	4.5	.59	2.7
L_C Bed Disability	1.9	.34	.6
Value-adjusted life expectancy $[Q^*]$ = 68.5 [years]			

population age groups in a community or of the health status of the same population over time. As such, Q* serves as a health indicator.

There are several advantages of Q*:

1. Combines morbidity with mortality in a single number that is independent of both age and medical diagnoses.
2. An excellent indicator to measure the health status of total populations.
3. Easy replication and serves as a longitudinal comparison of the health status of a population over time.

A disadvantage follows:

1. Causal inferences cannot be drawn from intervention procedures used to improve the health status of a population, unless a controlled experiment is designed.

Duke—UNC Health Profile

This profile was developed in the late 1970s [Parkerson, Gehlbach, & Wagner, 1981] to measure adult health status in a primary care setting. There are four components to the profile: symptom status, physical function, emotional function, and social function. With the emphasis on wellness, there are 74 items in the profile.

Symptom status is included because that generally represents the first stage of dysfunction in bodily health.

Physical status includes disability days, ability to ambulate, and use of upper extremities as the three major components These are used as measures to perform tasks.

Emotional status' key measure is self-esteem, which the researchers describe as a person's liking him/herself and/or getting along with others. This represents an indicator of a person's ego strength and emotional well-being.

Social function is measured by a person's capacity to perform his/her usual tasks in society including self-care, working and/or taking care of a home, engaging in community activity, and interacting with others.

Exhibit 2-8 displays the 74 items linked to the four components of the UNC health profile. Twenty-eight elements deal with symptom status and 26 with emotional function. Social function has only five elements.

Each item is scored individually with a zero given for the least desirable health status. For the most desirable, scores of two are given for a three-point scale, three for a four-point scale and four for a five-point scale. A person's score on an item is divided by the highest desirable score possible. For example, a person stating that he/she had some physical difficulty peeling an apple [item 11 on physical function] would receive a "1" score. That score would be divided by

Exhibit 2-8.   Duke—UNC Health Profile: A Health Status Instrument.

HERE ARE A NUMBER OF QUESTIONS ABOUT YOUR HEALTH AND YOUR FEELINGS. PLEASE READ EACH
QUESTION CAREFULLY AND GIVE YOUR BEST ANSWER. YOU SHOULD ANSWER THE QUESTIONS IN YOUR
OWN WAY. THERE ARE NO RIGHT OR WRONG ANSWERS.

[Symptom Status] *

During the <u>past week</u>: How much trouble have you had with:

		None	Some	A Lot
1.	Eyesight	____	____	____
2.	Hearing	____	____	____
3.	Talking	____	____	____
** 4.	Smelling odors	____	____	____
5.	Tasting food	____	____	____
6.	Appetite	____	____	____
7.	Chewing	____	____	____
8.	Swallowing	____	____	____
9.	Moving your bowels	____	____	____
10.	Passing water / urinating	____	____	____
11.	Breathing	____	____	____
12.	Sleeping	____	____	____
**13.	Walking	____	____	____

During the <u>past week</u>: How much trouble have you had with:

		None	Some	A Lot
14.	Headache	____	____	____
15.	Hurting or aching in any part of your body	____	____	____
16.	Itching in any part of your body	____	____	____
17.	Indigestion	____	____	____
18.	Fever	____	____	____
19.	Getting tired easily	____	____	____
20.	Fainting	____	____	____
21.	Poor memory	____	____	____
22.	Weakness in any part of your body	____	____	____
23.	Feeling depressed / sad	____	____	____
24.	Nervousness	____	____	____

During the <u>past month</u>: How much trouble have you had with:

		None	Some	A Lot
25.	Weight loss	____	____	____
26.	Weight gain	____	____	____
27.	Unusual bleeding	____	____	____
28.	Sexual performance	____	____	____

[Physical Function]*

During the <u>past week</u>:

		none	1-4 days	5-7 days	
1.	How many days were you <u>in bed</u> most of the day because of sickness, injury or health problems?	____	____	____	
2.	How many days did you stay <u>in your home</u> because of sickness, injury or health problems?	____	____	____	

		none	some	a lot	can't go outside
** 3.	How much trouble have you had <u>getting around outside your home</u> because of sickness, injury or health problems?	____	____	____	____

<u>Today</u> would you have any <u>physical</u> trouble or difficulty:

		None	Some	A Lot
4.	Running 5 miles	____	____	____
** 5.	Holding a baby	____	____	____
6.	Walking up a flight of stairs	____	____	____
** 7.	Hearing the radio or TV	____	____	____
8.	Running a mile	____	____	____
** 9.	Walking the length of a football field [100 yards]	____	____	____
10.	Walking to the bathroom	____	____	____
11.	Peeling an apple	____	____	____

(continued)

57

Exhibit 2-8. *(Continued)*

```
**12.  Reading a street sign                        ___  ___  ___
  13.  Running the length of a football field [100 yards]  ___  ___  ___
**14.  Reading a newspaper                          ___  ___  ___
  15.  Combing your hair                            ___  ___  ___
```

[Emotional Status]*

HERE ARE SOME STATEMENTS YOU COULD USE TO DESCRIBE HOW YOU FEEL ABOUT YOURSELF. PLEASE READ EACH STATEMENT
CAREFULLY AND PLACE A CHECK IN THE BLANK THAT BEST FITS HOW THE STATEMENT DESCRIBES YOU. HERE IS AN EXAMPLE:

	Describes me exactly		Somewhat describes me		Doesn't describe me at all
I like TV soap operas.	___	X	___	___	___

IF YOU PUT AN "X" WHERE WE HAVE, IT MEANS THAT LIKING TV SOAP OPERAS DESCRIBES YOU MORE THAN "SOMEWHAT"
BUT NOT "EXACTLY."

Answer each item as best you can. Remember there are no right or wrong answers.

	Exactly		Somewhat		Not At All
** 1. My body is in good shape for my age	___	___	___	___	___
2. I am a pleasant person	___	___	___	___	___
3. I don't feel useful	___	___	___	___	___
** 4. My friends look to me when they're in trouble	___	___	___	___	___
5. I get on well with members of the opposite sex	___	___	___	___	___
6. My family doesn't understand me	___	___	___	___	___
7. I like who I am	___	___	___	___	___
8. I feel hopeful about the future	___	___	___	___	___
9. I try to look my best	___	___	___	___	___
10. I am a clumsy person	___	___	___	___	___
** 11. I hate parties and social occasions	___	___	___	___	___
12. I have difficulty making decisions	___	___	___	___	___
13. I like meeting new people	___	___	___	___	___
14. I'm not an easy person to get along with	___	___	___	___	___
15. I'm a failure at everything I try to do	___	___	___	___	___
16. I'm basically a healthy person	___	___	___	___	___
17. I wish I had more sex appeal	___	___	___	___	___
18. I give up too easily	___	___	___	___	___
19. I like the way I look	___	___	___	___	___
20. I'm not as smart as most people	___	___	___	___	___
21. I have difficulty concentrating	___	___	___	___	___
22. I'm satisfied with my sexual relationships	___	___	___	___	___
23. I am happy with my family relationships	___	___	___	___	___
24. I don't treat other people well	___	___	___	___	___
25. I am comfortable being around people	___	___	___	___	___
26. I can take care of myself in most situations	___	___	___	___	___

[Social Function]*

During the past week how often did you:

	5-7 days	1-4 days	Not At All
1. Do your usual work [either inside or outside the home]	___	___	___
2. Get your work done as carefully and accurately as usual	___	___	___
3. Take part in social, religious or recreation activities [club meetings, movies, dancing, sports, parties, church]	___	___	___
4. Socialize with other people	___	___	___
5. Care for yourself [bathe, dress, feed yourself]	___	___	___

   * = Bracketed titles were not printed on instrument given to patients.
  ** = Item eliminated from instrument at time of analysis.

Source: From "The Duke–UNC profile: an adult health status instrument for primary care," by G.R. Parkerson, Jr., S.H. Gelbach, & E.H. Wagner, 1981, *Medical Care, 19*[8], 824–828. Reprinted with permission of Lippin-cott/Harper & Row.

the maximum possible score of 2, giving the person a .5 mean for that item. Each item receives equal weighting. By summing and dividing each of the item mean scores, that person receives a score on the four health components between a 1.0 for a perfect score and 0.0 for the worst score.

In a test run on fairly healthy adults attending a family health care center, the mean scores for the various profile components of 395 persons were:

Symptom status	0.84
Physical function	0.72
Emotional function	0.77
Social function	0.74

An average of 10 minutes was required for the respondents to complete the self-administered test. This profile could be used as an outcome evaluation measure of medical intervention. Or it can be used to ascertain the level of functioning of a population in a specific neighborhood or community.

Advantages of the profile are:

1.   Easily understood by respondents.
2.   Easily completed in a short period of time.
3.   Self-reporting data are both reliable and valid.
4.   Able to measure both broad measures of health and to identify small changes in health status.
5.   Oriented toward positive health.

Disadvantages are:

1.   Has not been fully tested on other populations.
2.   Clinical applicability has not been tested.
3.   Not suitable for the very sick.

Sickness Impact Profile

A Sickness Impact Profile [SIP] was developed in the 1970s with extensive testing on various populations before reaching its final form [Bergner, Bobbitt, & Carter, 1981]. SIP measures dysfunction and as such is a measurement of negative health rather than positive functioning. Designed to measure health outcomes, SIP can be utilized for evaluation, program planning, and policy formation. Furthermore, the SIP has also become an instrument against which other indices measure their own reliability and validity [Deyo & Inui, 1981; Mackensie, Charlson, DiGioia, & Kelley, 1986]. In addition, the SIP can also be used to measure changes across types and severities of illness and across demographic and cultural subgroups. That makes the SIP especially relevant in a community assessment of medical need in a population to develop targets of opportunity. This measure can also evaluate how well a health care institution is doing in dealing with the medical needs of special populations.

SIP is a 136-item test that can be self-administered in 20–30 minutes. Health-related dysfunctions are divided into 12 areas of activity. Five independent categories deal with sleep, rest, eating, work, home management and recreation, and pastimes. In addition, there are two dimensions, one for physical and the other for psychosocial functioning. Three categories [ambulation, mobility, and body care and movement] relate to the physical dimension. Four categories [social interaction, alertness behavior, emotional behavior, and communication] are linked to the psychosocial dimension. Each category has one or more items related to it. For example, in the physical dimension/ambulation category, the item states: "I walk shorter distances or stop to rest often." [See Exhibit 2-9 for a schematic illustration of the profile.]

Respondents indicate whether an item describes a dysfunction they feel currently because of their illness. Scores are produced for the profile as a whole, for each category and for the two dimensions [physical and psychosocial]. Predetermined weights are based on the severity of each dysfunction. Weighted scores are summed for all items checked in a category to produce a raw score. A percentage score is produced by dividing this raw score by the highest possible score for the category. Scoring is illustrated in Exhibit 2-10.

Exhibit 2-9.   Sickness Impact Profile Categories and Selected Items.

Dimension	Category	Items Describing Behavior Related to:	Selected Items
Independent Categories	SR	Sleep and Rest	I sit during much of the day I sleep or nap during the day
	E	Eating	I am eating no food at all, nutrition is through tubes or intravenous fluids I am eating special or different food
	W	Work	I am not working at all I often act irritable toward my work associates
	HM	Home Management	I am not doing any of the maintenance or repair work around the house that I usually do I am not doing heavy work around the house
	RP	Recreation and Pastimes	I am going out for entertainment less I am not doing any of my usual physical recreation or activities
I Physical	A	Ambulation	I walk shorter distances or stop to rest often I do not walk at all
	M	Mobility	I stay within one room I stay away from home only for brief periods of time
	BCM	Body Care and Movement	I do not bathe myself at all, but am bathed by someone else I am very clumsy in body movements
II Psychosocial	SI	Social Interaction	I am doing fewer social activities with groups of people I isolate myself as much as I can from the rest of the family
	AB	Alertness Behavior	I have difficulty reasoning and solving problems, for example, making plans, making decisions, learning new things I sometimes behave as if I were confused or disoriented in place or time, for example, where I am, who's around, what day it is
	EB	Emotional Behavior	I laugh or cry suddenly I act irritable and impatient with myself, for example, talk badly about myself, swear at myself, blame myself for things that happen
	C	Communication	I am having trouble writing or typing I do not speak clearly when I am under stress

Source: From "The sickness impact profile: development and final revision of a health status measure," by M. Bergner, R.A. Bobbit, & W.B. Carter, 1981, *Medical Care*, 19[8], 789. Reprinted with permission of Lippincott/Harper & Row.

Exhibit 2-10.   Summary of Sickness Impact Profile [SIP] Structure and Content With a Scoring Example.

Category	No. of Items in Scale	Maximum Possible Score	Hypothetical Patient's Raw Score [Sum of Item Weights for Positive Responses]	Hypothetical Patient's Percent Score [Raw Score/Maximum Possible Score]
Ambulation	12	84.2	47.4	56.3
Body Care and Movement	23	200.3	38.3	19.1
Mobility	10	71.9	25.8	35.9
Physical Dimension Total	45	356.4	111.5	31.3
Emotional Behavior	9	70.5	25.1	35.6
Social Interaction	20	145.0	71.0	49.0
Alertness Behavior	10	77.7	36.4	46.8
Communication	9	72.5	30.7	42.3
Psychosocial Dimension Total	48	365.7	163.2	44.6
Work	9	51.5	15.5	30.1
Sleep and Rest	7	49.9	16.2	32.5
Eating	9	70.5	0.0	0.0
Household Management	10	66.8	20.4	30.5
Recreational Activities	8	42.2	7.7	18.2
Total	45	280.9	59.8	
Overall SIP	136	1003.0	334.5	33.3

Source: From "Toward clinical application of health status measures, Sensitivity of scale to clinically important changes," by R.A. Deyo & T.S. Inui, 1981, *Health Services Research, 19*[3], 288. Reprinted with permission of the Hospital Research and Educational Trust, Chicago, IL.

Advantages

1. Thoroughly tested for reliability and validity.
2. Relatively easy to use by respondents without supervision as a self-administered test.
3. Sensitive to clinical changes in large groups.
4. Can be completed in a relatively short time period.
5. Can measure differences in populations over time.

Disadvantages

1. Relatively insensitive to measuring changes in individuals over time because of the difficulty in interpreting the meaning of the score changes. However, using a highly modified profile of SIP, Mackensie et al. [1986] were able to significantly improve upon this shortcoming.

Sentinel Health Events

Sentinel health events [SHE] emerged in the late 1970s from a group of Harvard University investigators [Rutstein, Berenberg, & Chambers, 1976]. An SHE signals cases of unnecessary disease, unnecessary disability, or unnecessary untimely death. There are three types of SHEs. About 90 *Single-case indexes* are conditions in which even a single death or disease should not have occurred [Carr, 1988], such as Hodgkin's disease or a malignant neoplasm of the bladder. About 25 *Indexes based on rates* are events in which a rate of occurrence of deaths or diseases above an acceptable level could have been decreased by specific medical care such as hypertension, vascular complications, malaria, viral hepatitis A, and dental caries. If such an SHE did occur, the appropriate question is, "Why did it happen?" *Medicosocial problems* such as alcoholism and schizophrenia are considered multiple etiology conditions that require intensive study and analysis relative to need indicators.

These illustrations point out that the occurrence of an SHE is not due solely to errors of omission or commission by physicians. However, Rutstein et al. do opt for initial and continuing responsibility for the physician in providing leadership and guidance in doing something about the warning SHE. These SHEs were revised by Rutstein et al. [1976, 1980].

Data for studies of SHEs can usually be obtained from a health care provider's information system or on a statewide basis from a state health information data bank such as SPARCS [Statewide Planning and Research Cooperative System of New York State]. It should be noted that SHEs only account for a small percentage of all reported deaths and diseases for those utilizing a health care facility.

In a recent New York State study [Carr, Heiniken, Charles, & Stimson, 1988, p. 12], about 12 percent of the total incidence of reported diseases and 21 percent of the total number of deaths were classified as SHEs. In a San Francisco primary care setting, only 4 percent of the diseases and 13 percent of the deaths were so classified [Heiniken et al., 1985]. Nevertheless, the 336,000 preventable diseases identified in New York State for 1983 represent a sizable number of persons who might have benefited from the proper kind of health care assistance.

Of the 62 single case indexes of preventable diseases in San Francisco that coincided with the SHEs, none of them could have been prevented by primary care treatment. All of the patients came into the clinic with long histories that predated their initial contact. This was also the case with the 14 preventable deaths. However, among the indexes based on rates, six of the 20 patients who died with hypertensive disease complication could have been prevented by proper medical care. Data collected for the New York State study were generally expressed as ratios of deaths per 1,000 hospital deaths or per 100,000 population and diseases as events per 1,000 hospital discharges or per 100,000 population. In sum, the mathematical manipulations are rather elementary. Exhibit 2-11 provides illustrations of single case indexes and indexes based on rates.

Sentinel health events can be used for several purposes: to assess the level of health and unmet needs of geographically defined populations; to identify the quality of care provided by health care institutions; and instrument versatility allows basic information to be used in evaluation, in health planning, and in setting health policy.

Advantages

1. Data are usually already available in a health care institution's information data system to provide the raw information needed.
2. Statistical manipulation is relatively simple.
3. Accuracy of the data is fairly high.
4. Health care institutions can use it for strategic planning, evaluation, and policy formation.
5. Can identify disease and death-specific changes over time by various subpopulations or geographic areas.

Disadvantages

1. Categories of indexes based on rates and medicosocial problems have not been defined or operationalized to permit proper utilization.

Exhibit 2-11. Unnecessary Disease, Disability, and Untimely Death: Indexes Based On Rates.

9th Rev. No.	Condition	Unnecessary Disease	Unnecessary Disability**	Unnecessary Untimely Death	Notes
001	Cholera	P		P,T	
002.0	Typhoid fever	P		P,T	
003.0, 003.1	Salmonella gastroenteritis & septicaemia	P		P	
005.0	Staphylococcal food poisoning	P		P,T	
005.1	Botulism	P		P	
010–018, 137	Tuberculosis (all forms)	P		P,T	P—Contact spread prevented by frequent tuberculin testing and treatment of converters
013	Tuberculosis of meninges & central nervous system	P	P,T	P,T	Sensitive index, TBC testing of maternity hospital personnel & persons from high risk groups
020	Plague	P		P,T	P—Urban—domestic rat control
021	Tularaemia			T	
022	Anthrax	P		P,T	P—Occupational exposure
026	Rat-bite fever	P		P,T	
032	Diphtheria	P		P,T	
033	Whooping cough	P		P	
034	Streptococcal sore throat & scarlatina			T	
036	Meningococcal infection: Type A & Type C	P		P	P—Limit epidemics & household outbreaks by immunization of prophylactic treatment
	Type B	P		P	P—Limit houshold outbreaks by prophylactic treatment
036.2, 038.2, 038.8M	Overwhelming septicaemia following splenectomy(s)	P,T		P,T	P—Prophylaxis against infection with pneumococcus, II, influenzae, & miningococcus
037, 771.3	Tetanus	P		P	Including neonatal tetanus
045	Acute poliomyelitis	P	P	P	
050	Smallpox	P		P	
055	Measles	P		P	
056, 771.0	Rubella	P	P	P	Congenital rubella syndrome & disability in offspring
060	Yellow fever	P		P	

(continued)

Exhibit 2-11. (Continued)

9th Rev. No.	Condition	Unnecessary Disease	Unnecessary Disability**	Unnecessary Untimely Death	Notes
070.2, 070.3	Viral hepatitis B (serum hepatitis)	P	P	P	P—Via transfusion of blood & blood components (see Table B)
071	Rabies	P		P	
072	Mumps	P	P	P	
073	Ornithosis	P		P,T	
080	Louse-borne [epidemic] typhus			T	
081.0	Murine [endemic] typhus (flea-borne)			T	
082.0	Spotted fevers			T	Age under 2 yrs.
090.0, 090.1, 090.2	Early congenital syphilis	P	P	P,T	
091	Early syphilis, symptomatic	P	P	P,T	P—Prevent disease in case contacts
093–094	Major complications of syphilis(s)	P,T	P,T	P,T	
098	Gonococcal infections	P	P,T	P,T	P—Prevent disease in case contacts
102	Yaws	P		P,T	
124	Trichinosis	P		P	
126	Ancylostomiasis & necatoriasis (hookworm disease)	P		P,T	
127.0	Ascariasis	P		P,T	
140	Malignant neoplasm of lip	P		P,T	P—Pipe smokers & sun exposure
141.1, 141.2, 141.3, 144, 145.0	Malignant neoplasm of dorsal & ventral surfaces, borders & tip (not base) of tongue, floor of mouth, or buccal mucosa	P		P,T	P—Tobacco smokers & cud & betelnut chewers
160.0	Malignant neoplasm of nasal cavities	P		P	P—Occupational—chromium industry & wood workers
161	Malignant neoplasm of larynx	P		P,T	P—Cigar & cigarette smokers
162	Malignant neoplasm of trachea, bronchus, & lung	P		P	P—Cigarette smoking, asbestos & occupational exposure
163	Malignant neoplasm of pleura	P		P	P—Asbestos exposure—"mesothelioma"
172	Malignant melanoma of skin			T	T—Diagnosis & treatment in early stages of disease
173	Other malignant neoplasm of skin	P		P,T	P—Radiation & sun exposure

Code	Condition			Remarks
180	Malignant neoplasm of cervix uteri		T	
182	Malignant neoplasm of body of uterus		T	
184.0	Malignant neoplasm of vagina	P	P	In offspring of mothers treated with diethylstilbestrol early in pregnancy
188	Malignant neoplasm of bladder	P	P	P—Aniline dyes & cigarette smoking
198.0M	Malignant neoplasm of kidney, except pelvis—Wilm's tumor (during infancy & childhood)	P	T	Early recognition & treatment
190.5	Malignant neoplasm of retina—retinoblastoma (under age 5)	T	T	Genetic—screening & treatment
NIC#	Neuroblastoma		T	Under 1 yr of age & early stage at any age
193	Malignant neoplasm of thyroid gland	P	P,T	P,T—Papillary & follicular carcinoma following radiation exposure treated early P—Medullary carcinoma diagnosed early in patient & family contacts by plasma calcitonin test
201	Hodgkin's disease	P	T	Lower stages of malignancy
205.1	Myeloid leukaemia, chronic	P	P	P—Radiation exposure or benzene
240.0	Goitre, specified as simple			Iodine deficiency
242	Thyrotoxicosis with or without goitre		T	Includes excessive thyroid material ingestion
243, 246.1	Congenital hypothyroidism (cretinism) & dyshormonogenic goitre(s)	T	T	Thyroid screening test (T4 & TSH)
244	Acquired hypothyroidism (myxedema)	T	T	Including that from drugs: early diagnosis by high TSH level
260–269	Nutritional Deficiencies (including avitaminoses)	P	P,T	Not associated with neoplasia or malabsorption
261	Nutritional marasmus	P	P,T	Under 1 yr of age
274M	Gout—tophaceous	T	T	
275.1	Hepatolenticular degeneration (Wilson's disease)	T	T	T—Early recognition by testing patient, screening siblings & treating positives with penicillamine
278.2	Hypervitaminosis A	P	P	
278.4	Hypervitaminosis D	P	P	
280	Iron deficiency anaemias	P	P,T	Good public health index for malnutrition

(continued)

Exhibit 2-11. (Continued)

9th Rev. No.	Condition	Unnecessary Disease	Unnecessary Disability**	Unnecessary Untimely Death	Notes
281.0	Pernicious anaemia		T	T	
281.1	Other Vitamin-B_{12}-deficiency anaemia		P,T	P,T	
281.2	Folate-deficiency anaemia		P,T	P,T	
284	Aplastic anaemia	P	P	P	P—Benzene exposure, drugs including chloramphenicol, & radiation
320.0	Haemophilus meningtis (II, influenzae Type B)			T	Early recognition & prompt treatment
362.2	Retrolental fibroplasia(s)	P	P		P—Excessive oxygen therapy in premature babies
365.1M	Blindness—glaucoma, chronic (simple)		T		
382, 383	Otitis media (suppurative) or mastoiditis(s)		T	T	
390–392	Acute rheumatic fever		P	P	P—Prevent recurrences
416M	Chronic pulmonary heart disease secondary to chronic pulmonary disease	P	P	P	P—Occupational & environmental exposure
460–466, 480–483, 485, 486, 490	Acute respiratory infections, pneumonia, & bronchitis			T	Deaths less than age 50 unless associated with immunologic defects or neoplasms
487	Influenza	P		P,T	P—Vaccine immunization to targeted population defined by virulence of particular strain T—Deaths less than age 50 unless associated with immunologic defects or neoplasms
492, 496	Emphysema or chronic obstructive lung disease(s)	P	P	P	P—Cigarettes & other environmental risks
493	Asthma			T	T—Self-inhalation therapy deaths under age 50
495, 500–505, 506, 507.1, 508.0, 508.1	Extrinsic allergic alveolitis, pneumoconioses, chemical fumes & vapours, lipid inhalation, & radiation effects(s)	P	P	P	

Code	Condition			Notes
531M	Ulcer, gastric (stress)	P	P	P—From severe trauma including major surgery & burns—antacid prophylaxis
550–553	Inguinal or other hernia of abdominal cavity with or without obstruction(s)		T	Deaths under age 65
574, 575.0, 575.1	Acute or chronic cholecystitis and/or cholelithiasis(s)		T	Deaths under age 65
633	Ectopic pregnancy		T	
680–686	Infections of skin & subcutaneous tissue		T	
692, 693	Dermatitis from contact & substances taken internally(s)	P	P	P—Environmental & occupational exposure to specific agents
711.0	Pyogenic arthritis	P,T	P,T	P—Secondary to pyogenic infection
714.32	Blindness—pauciarthritis(s)	T		Repeated slit-lamp examination &, if positive, local steroids
730.0	Acute osteomyelitis	P,T	P,T	P—Secondary to pyogenic infection
730.1	Chronic osteomyelitis	T	T	
630–675	All maternal deaths (including abortion)(s)	P	P	
760–772, 774–779	Infant mortality, general(s)	P	P	Plus all other deaths less than 1 yr of age regardless of cause
773.0, 773.3, 773.4	Haemolytic disease due to Rh isoimmunization	P,T	P,T	Immune globulin
NIC	Iatrogenic prematurity	P	P	P—From too early induction or Caesarian section
NIC	Neural tube defects	P	P	P—Alpha fetaprotein measurement
758.0	Down's syndrome	P	P	P—Aminocentesis—mothers over age 35, or previous baby with Down's syndrome
317M–319M	Mental retardation induced by: Maternal nutritional deficiency Tay-Sachs disease Lead intoxication	P P P		Genetic counseling & screening
NIC	Man-made (including occupational & environmental) diseases induced by (with examples): 1. Toxic agents, icluding direct chemical hazards (car-	P	P	

(continued)

Exhibit 2-11. (Continued)

9th Rev. No.	Condition	Unnecessary Disease	Unnecessary Disability**	Unnecessary Untimely Death	Notes
	bon tetrachloride); carcinogens (vinyl chloride); mutagens (lead); teratogens (thalidomide); pesticides (cholinesterase inhibitors); contact irritants (occupational dermatoses); dusts (pneuomnoconioses with and without tuberculosis); contact sensitizers (nickel); water contaminants (polychlorinated biphenyls); air pollutants (sulfur dioxide).				
2.	*Physical hazards,* including radiant energy (medical, industrial, & war); noise (rock & roll); & vibration (jack hammers).				
3.	*Artificial environments,* including space travel, airplanes, caissons, air conditioned sealed buildings, & intensive-care units.				
4.	*Accidents* (manifold varieties inducing injury).				

	5. *Biological hazards*, including laboratory accidents, antibiotic-resistant micro-organisms, & contact allergic dermatitis (plants & wood).		
780–789, 799	Symptoms & ill-defined conditions		Unless specified as "cause unknown" frequent diagnoses consisting only of symptoms or ill-defined conditions are evidence of poor quality
28.2, 28.3	Tonsillectomy with or without adenoidectomy	P	Indications for tonsillectomy are TB, tumor, post-peritonsillar abscess, recurrent infections not responsive to adequate therapy (seldom) and obstructive hypertrophy (rare)
47.0	Appendectomy for appendicitis	P	Normal appendices should be a relatively small proportion of those removed, i.e., the result of unavoidable false positive diagnoses
68.3–68.8	Hysterectomy(s)	P	Each hysterectomy must be justified by sufficient pathologic findings in the removed uterus or by extenuating circumstances documented
66.2, 66.3, 66.5, 66.63	Tubal sterilization(s)	P	
74.0–74.9	Elective Caesarian section(s)	P	A DEATH FROM TONSILLECTOMY, APPENDECTOMY FOR APPENDICITIS, HYSTERECTOMY, TUBAL STERILIZATION, OR ELECTIVE CAESARIAN SECTION IS A SENTINEL HEALTH EVENT

Source: From "Measuring the quality of medical care: A clinical method," by D.D. Rutstein, W. Berenberg, & T.C. Chalmers, 1976, *New England Journal of Medicine, 294*, 582–588. Reprinted with permission.

2. Requires periodic updating to take into account new diseases, disabilities, or causes of death.

3. A definition of "acceptable rates" has yet to be agreed upon for most of the diseases included in the indexes based on rates.

4. "A need exists for one or more select batteries of health system indicators that would include a limited number of measures that can be used together to profile aspects of the system" [Carr et al., 1988, p. 26].

5. Medical records may require more information than is now routinely collected to provide the information needed for analysis.

6. Measure is not sensitive enough to identify deficiencies in care, especially in older adult populations.

7. While the method has real potentials as a measuring tool, it has not been sufficiently tested and revised to match the purposes for which it was designed.

HSRI's Quadrant Method for Estimating Mentally Ill Population

Estimates of the chronic mentally ill population are usually based on those actually using the system on an in- or outpatient basis. Of course, this undercounts those who are actually in need as well as those failing to use the service because of lack of eligibility, reluctance to use the services, or lack of information on availability. HSRI's [Human Services Research Institute] Quadrant Method is a relatively simple three-step method for estimating total need, including those using mental health services and those not using them [Ashbaugh & Manderscheid, 1985]. Data generated by this method can be used for setting strategic planning goals and measuring unmet needs of mentally ill persons. Areas of under- and oversupply of mental health services can also be identified. Given the current problem of accurately estimating the number of mental health beds needed, this method can provide the basic population information required to make those bed methods more accurate [Goplerud, 1986].

A "Quadrant" method uses known estimates of the size of three segments [quadrants] of the chronically mentally ill population to estimate the size of the fourth unknown segment [quadrant]. Exhibit 2-12 shows the CMI quadrants divided according to Supplementary Security Income [SSI] and Social Security Disability Income [SSDI] participation and involvement in state mental health programs.

A signal feature of the method involves estimating the size of that segment of the chronically mentally ill population that is neither participating in SSI or SSDI programs nor in state mental health programs [Quadrant D]. That estimate is based on the assumption, or variation thereof, that the proportion of chronically mentally ill persons participating in the SSI and/or SSDI entitlement programs is the same, irrespective of whether they are participating in state mental health systems of services. It is assumed that the ratio of the number of those nonmental health program clients not participating in the SSI or SSDI programs [Quadrant B] is the same as the ratio of the number of mental health system clients not participating in the SSI or SSDI programs [Quadrant C] to the number of mental health program clients participating in the SSI or SSDI programs [Quadrant A] or $D/B = C/A$. The sum of quadrants A and C, the number of clients by SSI and SSDI status, must be estimated by the state. Quadrant B is then calculated by subtracting the number of mental health system clients participating in SSI or SSDI program [Quadrant A] from the total number of chronically mentally ill adults participating in SSI or SSDI programs in the state [Quadrants A and B]. SSI and SSDI estimates are calculated for each state by the Human Services Research Institute using data obtained from the Social Security Administration.

Exhibit 2-12.   Quadrant Method for Estimating the Seriously/Chronically Mentally Ill Population.

Mental Health Program Participation

	Yes	No
Yes	A	B
No	C	D

SSI and/or SSDI
Program
Participation

Source: From *Estimating the size of the seriously and chronically mentally ill population by state: the Quadrant method*, by J.W. Ashbaugh, 1986, Washington, DC: Government Printing Office, NIMH [31 March]. Reprinted by permission.

There are three stages to developing the population estimate. First, estimate the number of chronic mentally ill receiving SSI and SSDI benefits; both programs are administered by the Social Security Administration. This step requires estimating those on both grant programs nationally and disaggregating the counts to the state level with information available from the Office of Research and Statistics of the Social Security Administration. State data are adjusted by subtracting those persons receiving both SSI/MI and SSDI/MI [MI-mental illness] benefits to reduce the double count; and excluding those already institutionalized. However, this final count would still undercount those actually in need and not receiving service; those not eligible for SSI or SSDI benefits because they fail to meet work or income requirements; those unable to prove they have a psychiatric condition; and those who are eligible but fail to apply for benefits. Furthermore, data at the state level would be too small and too subject to the vagaries of each state's special circumstances to serve as a reliable indicator of the size of the mentally ill population.

Second-stage procedures aim to overcome the deficiencies identified in stage one. States must have data that "distinguish chronic patients from other patients in publicly funded community mental health programs, and to ascertain the SSI and SSDI status of the chronic patients" [Ashbaugh & Manderscheid, 1985]. Most states do not have information systems that include this data, but it is available on records. Therefore, it becomes necessary to take a sample of these individual patient records, which can be done both quickly and at low cost. This results in identifying all those receiving SSI and SSDI benefits for mental illness and those with such benefits who are also participating in mental health programs. To estimate those not part of either system, total the number of persons enrolled in the SSDI and/or SSI programs but not participating in community mental health programs, plus the number of persons not enrolled in SSI or SSDI but availing themselves of community mental health service, and divide by the estimated number participating in both SSI/SSDI and mental health programs. This gives a conservative estimate of the total chronic mentally ill population. States may desire to adjust the figure to take into account special state conditions.

Third-stage steps involve a disaggregation of state estimates to provide projections for local mental health catchment areas falling within the domain of health care institutions. First, it is necessary to obtain zip code distributions for several years of those noninstitutionalized persons receiving SSI/SSDI benefits. Then, the strategic planner must aggregate the zip code sample counts by the institution's catchment area. This is followed by computing the percentage distribution of the SSI/MI and SSDI/MI sample counts by the catchment areas. Finally, the planner estimates the number of noninstitutionalized by multiplying the number of noninstitutionalized chronically ill adults in the state by the percentages obtained in the preceding step. Because there may be variances of more or fewer persons enrolled in SSI/SSDI programs in local communities, adjustments must be made for them. For example, local communities having a high influx of former mental hospital patients, those having a high concentration of group homes for the mentally ill and those areas where many poor live tend to undercount the number of mentally ill. In spite of these limitations, this method of counting the chronic mentally ill may be more accurate than others in use.

Advantages

1. Data are readily available at both the national and state levels.
2. Collecting data for this method is inexpensive.
3. Easy to implement.
4. Counts both those receiving treatment and the untreated needy.
5. Accuracy is improved by mental health planners taking into account local conditions.
6. Strategic planners can determine service needs for their health care institution.

Disadvantages

1. Assumptions made in estimating the data counts may make the final count less reliable.
2. Where limited data exist, levels of confidence about the accuracy of the estimates go down, especially where sample data are small.
3. Does not deal with the level of functioning of the mentally ill, making it more difficult to plan services for an undifferentiated patient population.

DEMAND ASSESSMENT METHODS

While numerous demand assessment methods exist, the following examples illustrate those commonly used. Furthermore, all the techniques combine ease of mathematical formulation with easy access to readily available data. Ingram [1988] reiterates that planners must understand the various techniques as an aid to target markets as he discusses the estimation of alcoholism treatment demands.

The Formula Approach

A Hill-Burton legislative formula approach was used by most states to project the future need for medical facilities, particularly beds. This formula technique anticipates future utilization via calculations involving the use rate and an estimated population as illustrated below [LeTouze, 1984]:

$$\frac{\text{Current patient-days}}{\text{Current population}} = \text{Use rate} \quad \frac{400,000}{1,600,000} = .25$$

$$\frac{\text{Use rate} \times \text{Projected population}}{\text{annual days}} = \frac{\text{Average}}{\text{daily census}} \quad \frac{.25 \times 2,000,000}{365} = 1,370$$

$$\frac{\text{Average daily census}}{\text{Desired occupancy rate}} = \frac{\text{Projected beds}}{\text{required}} \quad \frac{1,370}{.80} = 1,713$$

If the estimated population for the region was 2 million people eight years later, future utilization results from multiplying the population by the use rate: .25 x 2,000,000 = 500,000 patient days. Average daily census computes by dividing the anticipated total annual patient days by 365, the number of days in a year: 500,000 / 365 = 1,370 average daily census.

Dividing the average daily census (1,370) by the usually desired occupancy rate, between 80 percent and 85 percent, results in the number of beds required eight years later.

$$\frac{1,370}{80} = 1,712.5, \text{ or } 1,713 \text{ beds required}$$

With adjustments, it is possible to integrate the following variables: changes in the use rate; the differential utilization of the hospital's medical/surgical, obstetric, and pediatric components; age/sex differences among those using the hospital such as child-bearing women between the ages of 15 and 44; and differences between patients living within the boundaries of the area as compared with those residing outside the area. If the use rate increased .005 per year due to an increase in the aged population, the formula could be adjusted as follows:

$$\frac{\text{Future}}{\text{use}} = \frac{\text{Current}}{\text{use rate}} \times \left[1 + (\text{rate of change}) \times \frac{(\text{number of}}{\text{projection years})} \right]$$

$$= .25 \times [1 + (.005 \times 8)]$$
$$= .25 \times (1 + .04)$$
$$= .25 \times 1.04 = .26$$

Future utilization = 2,000,000 × .26 = 520,000 patient days

$$\text{Average daily census} = \frac{520,000}{365} = 1,425$$

$$\frac{\text{Beds needed}}{\text{8 years later}} = \frac{1,425}{.80} = 1,781$$

Due to an increased aged population, the area will need 68 additional beds (1,781–1,713). Advantages of the formula approach include the following:

1. Data to compute the formula are readily available and generally reliable.
2. Formula is fairly simple to use.
3. Adjustments in the formula allow for a changing population and a realistic assessment of future bed need.
4. Reliable and valid when used in a region with a relatively stable population.

Disadvantages include the following:

1. Formula does not consider alternatives to bed use influencing the need for future beds such as health maintenance organizations, same-day surgeries, and an emphasis on preventive care.

2. Formula does not include vital cumulative factors such as diagnosis, family circumstances, or insurance coverage that influence the use rate and the need for beds.
3. Fails to discriminate between critical appropriate and inappropriate utilization of the facility, since anywhere from 10 to 60 percent of the admissions to facilities are inappropriate for the level of care required.
4. Formula does not consider persons who are not using the facility even though they have a legitimate and proper need for the services.

The Stochastic Method

Using probability theory, the stochastic method calculates a facility's bed needs [Dufour, 1974]. An assumption is made that patient admissions and discharges are random choices. These random occurrences can be matched against a normal distribution of Poisson curve by averaging the percentage of persons entering and leaving the facility during the year. Comparing the pattern of patient admissions with the Poisson and normal distribution curves allows for the use of queuing theory. Times that the average daily census will be exceeded during the year can be predicted by applying the standard deviation of the average census. Then, a facility's governing body decides how often the facility wants to have a higher-than-average daily census to calculate how many beds are needed. In contrast to the formula method linked to population changes, the stochastic method relies on fluctuations in the facility's census.

Steps in this method follow:

1. A frequency distribution is prepared of the actual census level fluxations of a health care facility showing the number of times that a census level is reached each year. A frequency pattern will probably resemble a bell-shaped curve.
2. That pattern is compared with frequency curves predicted by Poisson and normal distributions.
3. A standard deviation of the average census is calculated.
4. Facility's decision makers choose an acceptable census level to meet projected patient population needs.

Suppose the facility's average daily census is 10,000. Under the Poisson and/or normal distribution, the standard deviation is the square root of the mean and would be 100 in this case. To meet the census demand on all but nine days a year, 10,196 beds would be required [10,000 divided by 1.96 x 100]. If the facility wanted to guarantee enough beds 99 percent of the time, then 10,233 beds [2 standard deviation] would be required [Dufour, 1974]. Exhibit 2-13 illustrates the application.

Application of the stochastic method can accurately project the need for beds in a single institution while also providing the flexibility to set varying bed need levels. In a cost containment climate the method tends to reduce the number of hospital beds needed. The larger the hospital, the higher the occupancy rate; the smaller the hospital, the more excessive capacity is needed to produce a specified level of care.

However, the stochastic method does not consider the interchangeability of beds such as pediatric for surgical, or that beds in one hospital are interchangeable with another hospital. That drawback limits the technique's use in projections for an entire region. As with the formula approach, the method does not consider alternative care influencing the need for beds such as same day surgery, health maintenance organizations or the use of preventive health services. Furthermore, there is no guarantee that past utilization will continue to hold true in the future.

Exhibit 2-13.   Probabilistic Distribution of Daily Census, Pediatrics.

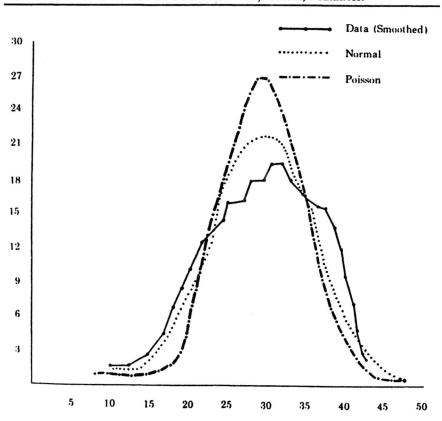

Finally, the stochastic method relies on a normal curve distribution. Unless such a distribution is present, the technique is of questionable validity.

Markov Chain Process

A Markov Chain Process can be used to predict or forecast where people starting out at one level of care will likely be three and four time periods removed [Lapin, 1988, Chap. 29]. This is an excellent method for determining the number and kind of facilities needed when there is a starting point in terms of where people are at time one. A problem could investigate how many long-term units such as nursing homes and home care services will be needed at some future date for an aging population entering the system as new patients? A Markov Chain process has no memory, and the probability of moving from one level of care to another does not depend on previous occurrences. Further, the long-run probability of being in a particular condition is constant and will hold regardless of the initial probabilities. Thus, it is possible to make fairly accurate predictions of how many aged will be in what type of long-term facility two, three, and four years or more from the time the patients first enter the system.

In using the Markov Chain, there are two important caveats that must be taken into account. First, there is an assumption that outside influences will not change the constancy of the long-run probability such as a new health regulation or the marketing of a new magic pill.

Should that occur, those influences would have to be considered and new probabilities determined. Second, a marketing research study must be undertaken to establish the transition probabilities of a series of patients moving from their initial long-term care placement level to the next. This requires developing a transition matrix and determining the probabilities of how many people will move from one level to the next. That transition is similar to asking an automobile owner what make of automobile he/she will buy as their next purchase. One can speculate that the great majority, 75 percent or more, will have been satisfied with their current automobile and purchase another one of the same make. The other 25 percent are likely to switch to several different brands. Probabilities are determined by knowing how many will switch from one automobile make to another. An example of an automobile owner transition matrix is shown below in Exhibit 2-14.

This example indicates that 70 percent of the owners of compact size automobiles will buy a compact in their next purchase. Twenty percent will buy a medium-sized care, and 10 percent will buy a full-sized luxury automobile. These become the transition probabilities that are used to determine where automobile owners will be in their successive movements. These probabilities for current compact owners will add up to 1.0 so that any probability must be between 0.0 and 1.0 for any level.

Transferring the concept to long-term care patients, the utility of the Markov Chain process becomes apparent. In this example, there are a total of nine possibilities: seven long-term care facility levels; two levels of home care; a discharged alive status; and a dead status [Lane, Uyeno, & Stark, 1985]. Exhibit 2-15 shows how many aged persons entered each level at the admission year and what actually happened to them four years from their initial admission. At admission, 759 persons entered the first level of home care and by the fourth year, 167 were still using that service. That does not mean that all of the same persons in the first year of admission were still among the 167 four years later. Patients could have transferred from other levels of long-term care service by improving enough to enter into the lowest-level home care status.

How close will the forecasting of the Markov Chain process come to the actual changes that take place from one status level to the next? As noted in the assumptions, the key to predicting future status depends on estimates of the transition matrix probabilities. Estimates for the nine status levels of the long-term care system (eight if the "dead" status is omitted) can be found by a "procedure . . . to search systematically for those elements of the P matrix that minimize the G statistic [the calculated X^2 value] over all forecast periods" [Lane et al., 1985]. Use of the computer package MARKFOR, designed for Markov Chain analysis, readily produces the minimum G-value. Exhibit 2-16 shows the outcome of applying the G-value probabilities and compares them to actual patient movement for years one through four. For example, the home care status of HPC had 759 persons at admission and 476 either remained or moved into it in year one. The Markov Chain Process forecast that 475.4 people would enter that level of care; a difference of 0.6. For year three, 212 people actually entered that level of care;

Exhibit 2-14.   Transition Matrix for Buyers of Three Types of Automobiles.

Current Automobile	To	Compact Size A	Medium Size B	Luxury Full Size C
Compact		.70	.20	.10
Medium		.05	.80	.15
Luxury		.00	.10	.90

Exhibit 2-15.   Markov Chain Forecast for Long-Term Care by Place and Level of Care.

States	Year 0	Year 1	Year 2	Year 3	Year 4
H_{pc}	759	476	307	212	167
H_{other}	482	333	270	220	179
F_{pc}	184	163	124	101	78
F_{11}	81	83	88	96	89
F_{12}	38	55	60	49	46
F_{13}	42	53	58	48	49
F_{ec}	64	34	37	47	33
Discharge alive	0	211	314	383	431
Dead	0	242	392	494	578
Total [N]	1,650	1,650	1,650	1,650	1,650

H_{pc} = Home personal care: a person requiring attention in the home.
H_{other} = Home care: three levels of care with increasing professioal assistance needed.
F_{pc} = Personal care in a facility/institution. Patient needs minimal care.
F_{11} & F_{12} & F_{13} = Three levels of intermediate care with increasing professional aid.
F_{ec} = Extended care in a facility. Most disabled patients require this highest care level.

Source: From "Forecasting demand for long term care services," by D. Lane, D. Uyeno, & A. Stark, 1985, *Health Services Research*, 20[4], 441. Reprinted with permission of the Hospital Research and Educational Trust, Chicago, IL.

Markov predicted 212.1 would still be there. Even when the largest difference occurred in year four, where 167 people actually entered and Markov forecast 155.1, there was a difference of only 4.1 percent.This is a very small difference given a forecast four years into the future.

A Markov chain can also be used to determine other types of demands for facilities, especially acute care hospital beds, mental health beds or rehabilitation beds. Such forecasts are needed by health care institutions for their environmental and community health assessments to determine requirements for a new type of service and whether the services are affordable.

Advantages of Markov Chain Analysis

1. Interdependence of all status levels of care are considered.
2. Use of a computer program allows for quick testing and sensitivity analysis.
3. Vital information for use in a health care institution's strategic health planning process is provided.
4. Unbiased forecasts that are fairly accurate can be provided.

Disadvantages

1. As the number of unknowns increase, the parameter estimates become less reliable.
2. If the number of periods of actual data is small, the assumptions may be difficult to defend.
3. Planners and analysts must have some familiarity with basic statistics and computer program use.

Exhibit 2-16. Markov Chain Results: New Clients.

	Final Results											Forecast Results		
	Year 1			Year 2			Year 3					Year 4		
States	A	F	Diff	A	F	Diff	A	F	Diff	MAD	Bias	A	F	Diff
H_{pc}	476	475.4	-0.6	307	306.5	-0.5	212	212.1	0.1	0.4	-0.3	167	155.1	-11.9
H_{other}	333	333.6	0.6	270	269.0	-1.0	220	220.6	0.6	0.7	0.1	179	176.8	-2.2
F_{pc}	163	163.2	0.2	124	123.1	-0.9	101	101.3	0.3	0.5	-0.2	78	80.8	2.8
F_{11}	83	82.9	-0.1	88	88.9	0.9	96	95.7	-0.3	0.4	0.2	89	97.7	8.7
F_{12}	55	55.8	0.8	60	57.8	-2.2	49	50.1	1.1	1.4	-0.1	46	45.9	-0.1
F_{13}	53	53.7	0.7	58	56.3	-1.7	48	49.2	1.2	1.2	0.1	49	45.3	-3.7
F_{ec}	34	34.2	0.2	37	37.4	0.4	47	46.7	-0.3	0.3	0.1	33	55.5	22.5
Disch. alive	211	210.4	-0.6	314	316.5	2.5	383	330.8	-2.2	1.8	-0.1	431	426.7	-4.3
Dead	242	241.5	-0.5	392	394.8	2.8	494	493.6	-0.4	1.2	0.6	578	566.3	-11.7
TOTALS	1,650	1,650.4	4.3	1,650	1,650.3	12.9	1,650	1,650.2	6.5			1,650	1,650.2	67.9
WAD [%]		0.3			0.8			0.4		0.5			4.12	
WB [%]		0.0			0.0			0.0		0.0			0.01	
G Stat [years 1–3]		0.29										G Stat = 11.52		
Degrees of Freedom		N/A						Degrees of Freedom = 8				Degrees of Freedom = 8		

MAD = Mean Absolute Deviation
WAD = Weighted Absolute Deviation
WB = Weighted Bias
Diff = Difference between the number of actual and forecast of new clients

G Stat = Goodness of Fit Value
A = Actual number of patients
F = Forecasted number of patients

Source: From "Forecasting demand for long-term care services," by D. Lane, D. Uyeno, & A. Stark, 1985, *Health Services Research, 20*(4) 455. Reprinted with permission of the Hospital Research and Educational Trust, chicago, IL.

Quality of Life Index

Quality of life has been defined as "the degree to which one perceives that life's quality is good, that life is satisfying, that the individual has physical and material well-being, good relations with others, and the ability to participate in social/community/civic activities, and that the individual has personal development fulfillment, and recreation" [Padilla & Grant, 1985]. It is apparent that a quality of life index [QLI] takes many facets into account.

A QLI was developed to evaluate the outcome of a nurse's impact on cancer patients. If attending nurses can fulfill the basic QLI requirements of their patients, patients may recover more rapidly and have greater satisfaction from their treatment. In turn, the QLI raises the confidence of the community to use that health care institution. Furthermore, a high QLI increases the institution's capacity to compete with other health care providers.

A 23-question QLI for colostomy patients was developed and found to be reliable and valid. Exhibit 2-17 shows the entire questionnaire. In this self-administered questionnaire, patients place a dot on a 100 mm scale that most closely approximates their feeling, behaviors, or activities. Question 10 asks:"Do you find eating a pleasure?" Somewhere between "not at all" and "a great deal," patients place a dot. A millimeter scale finds the dot and determines the score for that question. Scores are summed and means for the overall QLI and subareas within the QLI are calculated.

QLI questions are linked to six basic factors: psychological well-being; physical well-being; body image (colostomy) concerns; diagnosis/treatment responses for surgery and nutrition; and social concerns.

Psychological well-being deals with happiness, satisfaction, fun, general quality of life, pleasure in eating, and sleep. Physical well-being concerns strength, fatigue, ability to work, health and perceived usefulness. Body image is defined by ability to look at the colostomy, tendency to worry, ability to adjust, and ability to live with the odor. Surgical diagnosis/treatment looks at sexual activity and severity of pain. Nutritional diagnosis/treatment asks about weight and sufficient eating. Social concerns delve into social rejection, social contact and privacy needs. Exhibit 2-18 shows that social concerns received the highest mean scores followed by nutritional diagnosis/treatment and body image.

For colostomy patients, self-worth is considered the most important factor in promoting the individual's quality of life. This emphasis is consistent with three of the nurse's basic characteristics: promoting a caring attitude, promoting self-care, and providing the physical care patients require. These nursing qualities were correlated with the six dimensions of the QLI scale. These "nursing interventions . . . produce cognitive-emotional changes in the patient that enhance perceptions of self-worth" [Padilla & Grant, 1985]. In turn, self-worth produces psychological well-being, the central dimension of quality of life. Nurses aim to promote a patient's control over their health or illness and this has positive effects on the patient. With modification, this QLI can readily be applied to other patient conditions requiring nursing intervention.

Advantages of QLI

1. Easy to understand and score.
2. Can be scored in a short period of time.
3. Mathematics are relatively simple.
4. Reliability and validity.

Exhibit 2-17. Quality of Life Index for Colostomy Patients.

1. How much strength do you have?
   None at all _____/ A great deal

2. Is the amount of time you sleep sufficient to meet your needs?
   Not at all sufficient _____/ Completely sufficient

3. Do you tire easily?
   Not at all _____/ A great deal

4. Do you feel your present weight is a problem?
   Not at all _____/ A great deal

5. Do you feel worried [fearful or anxious] about your colostomy?
   Not at all _____/ A great deal

6. Is your sexual activity sufficient to meet your needs?
   Not at all sufficient _____/ Completely sufficient

7. How is your present state of health?
   Extremely poor _____/ Excellent

8. How easy is it to adjust to your colostomy?
   Not at all easy _____/ Extremely easy

9. How much fun do you have [hobbies, recreation, social activities]?
   None at all _____/ A great deal

10. Do you find eating a pleasure?
    Not at all _____/ A great deal

11. How much can you work at your usual tasks [housework, office work, gardening]?
    Not at all _____/ A great deal

12. Is the amount you eat sufficient to meet your needs?
    Not at all sufficient _____/ Completely sufficient

13. How useful do you feel?

Not at all ⌐_____⌐ Extremely useful

14. How much happiness do you feel?

None at all ⌐_____⌐ A great deal

15. How satisfying is your life?

Not at all ⌐_____⌐ Extremely satisfying

16. How much pain do you feel?

None ⌐_____⌐ Excruciating

17. How often do you feel pain?

Never ⌐_____⌐ All the time

18. How good is the quality of your life?

Extremely poor ⌐_____⌐ Excellent

19. How fearful are you of odor or leakage from your colostomy?

Not at all ⌐_____⌐ Extremely fearful

20. Is your level of contact with your friends and family sufficient to meet your needs?

Not at all sufficient ⌐_____⌐ Completely sufficient

21. Do you feel rejected by your family or loved ones?

Not at all ⌐_____⌐ Extremely

22. How difficult is it for you to look at your colostomy?

Not at all difficult ⌐_____⌐ Extremely

23. Is the amount of privacy you have sufficient to meet your needs?

Not at all sufficient ⌐_____⌐ Completely sufficient

Source: From "Cancer patients and quality of life," by M.M. Grant, G.V. Padilla, & C. Peasant, 1984, *Proceedings of Fourth National Conference on Cancer Nursing*. New York: American Cancer Society. Reprinted with permission.

Exhibit 2-18.   Mean Values for Overall QLI Score and Subscores.

Score	No. of Patients	Mean
Psychological well-being	132	61.0
Physical well-being	134	45.0
Body image [colostomy concerns]	126	69.5
Diagnosis/treatment [surgical] response	94	59.5
Diagnosis/treatment [nutritional] response	133	73.5
Social concerns	134	83.5
Over QLI	134	61.0

Mean scores in this table are calculated in the following manner. The overall QLI is calculated for each subject as the mean of all the 23-item scores, and the subscores representing the factors of quality of life are calculated in the same manner but include only those items pertaining to the factor. QLI scores represent a response on a 100 mm scale.

Source: From "Cancer patients and quality of life," by M.M. Grant, G.V. Padilla, & C. Peasant, 1984, *Proceedings of the Fourth National Conference on Cancer Nursing*. New York: American Cancer Society. Reprinted with permission.

Disadvantages

1. Did not correlate with all quality of life dimensions.
2. Correlated well with only three of eight basic nursing characteristics; but these were the important ones.
3. Requires further testing, but shows promise as an important QLI for nursing care.

Criteria Mapping

A criteria map "organizes criteria into a branching logic format that uses the results of tests, physical examination and historical inquiry to create subgroups of patients" [Greenfield, Cretin, & Worthman, 1981]. Criteria mapping seeks to ascertain whether medical procedures used to treat a patient results in a proper outcome. Given that end, one can assert that the quality of care process can be predictive of the outcome. This means that all patients admitted for a condition were appropriately admitted, that is, there were no false positives; and second, that once admitted they received appropriate care and were discharged with correct outcome, that is, that no patient was discharged who should not have been.

One of the major problems in evaluating the quality of care is the difficulty of correlating medical process with medical outcome. Criteria mapping overcomes that difficulty. Health care institutions could show a high correlation between their admitting and diagnostic practices as well as the treatment patients receive and their outcome on discharge from the institution. In a community health assessment, this should be reflected in a highly positive satisfaction rating by the residents using community health services.

A criteria map could be used to determine whether a person with chest pains should be admitted to a hospital from the emergency room. In a study of 485 persons who came to one of two Los Angeles hospital emergency rooms, 233 were discharged and 252 were admitted.

A criteria map for chest pains was developed for this particular situation. Each condition would have its own criteria map. Exhibit 2-19 shows that if a person had any one of four

Exhibit 2-19.   Sample Portion of Chest Pain Criteria Map.

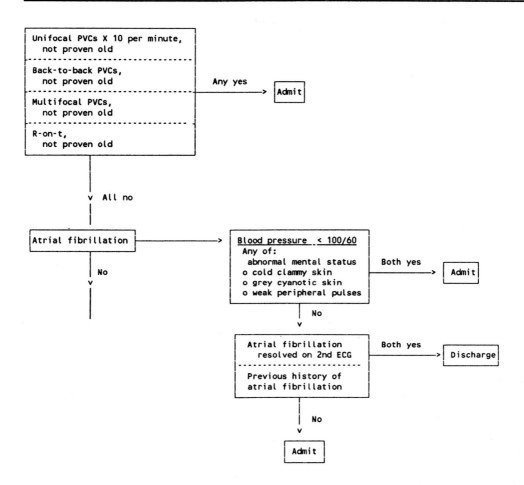

Positive responses defining a patient subgroup [left hand column] lead to the next item to the right. Negative or undocumented information responses are directed down to the next vertical item.

Source: From "Comparison of a criteria map to a criteria list in quality-of-care assessment for patients with chest pain: The relation of each to outcome," by S. Greenfield, S. Cretin, & L.G. Worthman, 1981, *Medical Care*, *19*[3], 258. Reprinted with permission of Lippincott/Harper & Row.

conditions (box in upper-left-hand corner), that person was admitted as a patient. If individuals revealed none of these symptoms, but had atrial fibrillation, those persons were admitted for follow-up if they showed any of the four symptoms noted in the larger lower-right-hand box of the exhibit, such as abnormal mental status or cold clammy skin. If not, they were still admitted if the atrial fibrillation showed a previous history and was not resolved on a second ECG. If neither condition were present, the person was discharged.

Physicians should come to a consensus in developing the key factors required for each

Exhibit 2-20.   Estimated Risk and Map Scores for Selected Patients.

Subgroup: Patients With Chest Pain and:	Consensus Estimate of Probability of Acute Serious Disease	Resultant Map Score*
Unifocal PVCs ≥ 10/min, not proven old	.60	60
Back-to-back PVCs, not proven old	.70	70
Multifocal PVCs, not proven old	.70	70
R-on-T, not proven old	.70	70
Atrial fibrillation, without shock	1.00	100
Atrial fibrillation, without shock	—	—
and no previous history of atrial fibrillation		
and atrial fibrillation unresolved on 2nd ECG	.93	
and positive previous history of atrial fibrillation		
and atrial fibrillation resolved on 2nd ECG	.05	05

*Map scores presented here are for patients with *no* other positive clinical findings.
PVC = Premature ventricular contraction   ECG = Electrocardiogram
R-on-T = Premature ventricular contraction which falls on the T-wave of the preceding beat.

Source: From "Comparison of a criteria map to a criteria list in quality-of-care assessment for patients with chest pain: The relation of each to outcome," by S. Greenfield, S. Cretin, & L.G. Worthman, 1981, *Medical Care,* 19[3], 259. Reprinted with permission of Lippincott/Harper & Row.

disease criteria map. They must consider three types of factors. First, they must identify the *signal findings*, those that contain patients' clinical findings that must be followed up. Second, they must identify the *subsequent findings*, those used to further define the clinical status of the patient with signal findings. Finally, they must establish an *appropriate disposition*: to admit or discharge.

A probability tree is developed based on the independent estimates of three physicians of the proportion of patients with signal and subsequent findings together with a final disposition.

After that, the three physicians meet together to calculate consensus estimates for each part of the probability tree. Predictive scores use the probability trees for each patient subgroup as building blocks. Map scores for signal findings are 100 times the probability of admissible disease. Exhibit 2-20 shows that a patient in shock with atrial fibrillation has a probability score of acute serious disease of 1.00 and a map score of 100. A patient with multifocal premature ventricular contraction and not proven old has a probability score of .70 and a map score of 70 [100 times .70]. Map scores consequently range from 0 for low risk of admissible disease to 100 for a high risk of admissible disease. Each patient is given a map score.

Means of these map scores are distributed on a scale of 0–100, divided into 10 unit cohorts. Exhibit 2-21 depicts the disposition of 252 patients admitted with chest pains. Those below the line were correctly admitted and those above the line should not have been admitted. As one can observe from the exhibit, almost 60 percent of those admitted were inappropriately admitted based on the criteria map factors. Almost one-fourth of the patients had very high map scores, between 91 and 100. This indicates the large percentage of false positive diagnoses for chest pain, most of which would have been reduced through the predictive power of criteria mapping. "the classification of patients based on map score alone is better both in terms of overall correct classification and, most important, is significantly better than any random rule in correctly classifying patients who do have admissible disease" [Greenfield, Cretin, & Worthman, 1981].

Criteria maps serve two important purposes in community assessment. First, since the

Exhibit 2-21.   Chest Pain Criteria Map Scores for Admitted Patients.

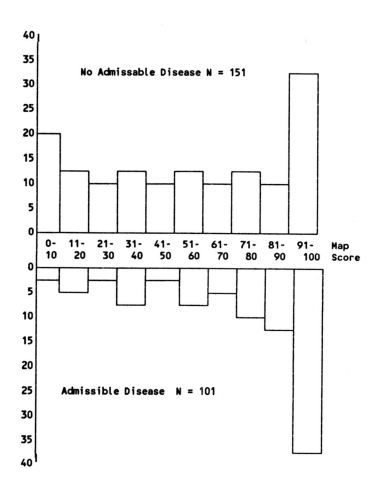

Above the horizontal axis are the scores of patients who had no admissible disease upon outcome determination. For admitted patients, this represents inappropriate disposition. The scores of patients with admissible disease are shown below the horizontal axis.

Source: From "Comparison of a criteria map to a criteria list in quality-of-care assessment for patients with chest pain: The relation of each to outcome," by S. Greenfield, S. Cretin, & L.G. Worthman, *Medical Care, 19*[3], 265. Reprinted with permission of Lippincott/Harper & Row.

maps are fairly high predictors of correct diagnosis and case disposition, community residents are assured of the high quality of the health care institution's medical competence in accurately diagnosing disease. Second, criteria maps provide an excellent method for discovering and correcting errors with improved diagnosis and treatment procedures.

Advantages

1. Once a criteria map for a specific disease is developed, most physicians specializing in that condition can use it to accurately diagnose a patient's condition.
2. While neither mathematically nor methodologically difficult to develop, criteria maps do require the expertise of medical specialists.
3. A high correlation between medical process, or treatment intervention, and outcome.

Disadvantages

1. None identified.

Functional Status Index

A Functional Status Index is a short, patient-specific instrument that measures changes in a person's physical, mental, and emotional functioning [Mackensie et al., 1986]. Exhibit 2-22 notes questions patients ask of themselves to describe their status prior to admission to a health care institution. Transition assessments allow patients to state whether they are better, the same, or worse, compared to their initial assessment one week, two weeks, four weeks, and six weeks later. By individualizing the patients' responses, changes can be identified in the patients' conditions based on their own assessment of their physical, psychological, and mental states at various points in time. Validity and reliability of the functional status index were measured and found consistent with ratings of the Sickness Impact Profile [see Exhibit 2-22].

Forty-three patients, 22 medical and 21 surgical, were followed for a period of six weeks to test the index. Exhibit 2-23 shows that among the medical patients, 26 percent were better one week after treatment, the same as for surgical patients. However, 60 percent of the surgical patients reported they were worse compared to 26 percent of the medical patients. This was to be expected because of initial reactions to surgery. By the end of the sixth week, 67 percent of the surgical patients stated they were better than they were prior to surgery compared to 39 percent of the medical patients. However, there was little difference between the two groups with respect to their mental and emotional functions. Nevertheless, this exhibit illustrates the subtle changes that affect both groups of patients over time.

Clearly, this exhibit indicates that the mathematics and the questions asked are few and simple. This index was designed for clinical evaluation of changes in patients over time as well as for clinical research. Information derived from the index can be used to determine how well patients respond to a health care providers treatment regimens.

Advantages

1. Index is very simple to understand.
2. Easily used by patients as a self-administered form.
3. Patient-specific as compared to most indexes which are either demographic or population-specific.
4. Sensitive to changes in patients over time.
5. Takes only five minutes to administer.
6. Mathematical computations are simple.

Exhibit 2-22. Functional Status Index.

We will ask you a few questions about how you have been doing before your admission [or visit] to the hospital. The questions have to do with your ability to do physically demanding things and your ability to concentrate. We also would like to know how you have been coping with stress recently and will ask about your job.

Physical Activity. My first set of questions is about things that you do that are physically strenuous. These may be things that you do around the house, activities related to work or to just getting around. Specifically, I am going to ask you what physical activity that you do requires the most physical effort.

1. Of the things that you usually do, what physical activity requires the most physical exertion or is the most physically strenuous?

2. On your good days, what would be the most [physical activity from question 1] that you could do? On your bad days, what would be the most [physical activity from question 1 that you could do?

Concentration. My next questions have to do with things that you do that require mental effort or concentration. Again, these may be activities related to work, to running the home, or to any other interest. I am going to ask you what activity that you do requires the most concentration or mental effort.

1. Of the things that you usually do, what mental activity requires the most concentration or mental effort?

2. On your good days, what would be the most [mental activity from question 1] that you could do? On your bad days, what would be the most [mental activity from question 1] that you could do?

Emotional. My next questions have to do with stressful or emotionally diffcult things that may have happened recently to you. I am going to ask you whether anything that has been going on in your life has been particularly stressful. This could include your health, family or financial worries, your job, or any other stresses you have experienced.

1. Is there anything going on in your life that has been particularly stressful or emotional difficult?

2. [If yes] What kind of problem is it?

3. How are you coping with this situation?

Physical. The last time we talked, you said that [physical activity from baseline or previous transition] was the most physically strenuous thing you could do.

1. In terms of physical activity, are you much better, slightly better, the same, slightly worse, or much worse?

2. Can you still [physical activity from the baseline or previous transition]?

3. [If yes] Is this still the most physically strenuous activity that you can do?

4. [If no] What is the most physically streunuous activity that you can do now?

Exhibit 2-22.   *(Continued)*

Concentration.   The last time we talked, you said that [mental activity from the baseline or previous transition] was the most mentally taxing thing you could do.

1.   In terms of mental activity and your ability to concentrate, are you much better, slightly better, the same, slightly worse, or much worse?

2.   Can you still [mental activity from the baseline or previous transition]?

3.   [If yes] Is this still the most mentally taxing activity that you can do?

4.   [If no] What is the most mentally taxing activity that you can do now?

Emotional

1.   I am interested in how you are not coping with the stresses in your life. Would you describe your ability to cope with stress since we last talked as much better, slightly better, the same, slightly worse, or much worse?

2.   Have you experienced anything since we last talked that you would consider stressful?

3.   [If yes] How are you coping with it?

Source: From "A Patient-specific measure of change in maximal function," by C.R. Mackensie, M.E. Charlson, D. DiGioia, & K. Kelley, 1986, *Archives of Internal Medicine, 146*[77], 1326. Copyright 1986. Reprinted with permission by the American Medical Association.

Disadvantages

1.   Not been fully tested to determine reliability with other groups of patients.
2.   Will not measure all-encompassing functional changes in patient or community populations.
3.   Index was tested on a heterogeneous population, it may perform differently on a homogeneous group.
4.   Cannot be used to distinguish levels of effectiveness between individuals or groups.
5.   Reliability of the index may be in question because it is limited to single-item scales compared to the multi-variate items on the other scales previously discussed.

SOURCES OF DATA

While it is apparent that strategic planners will be collecting and utilizing a great deal of raw data, it should be just as apparent that planners will need to know how to make sense of the data. Gathering huge quantities of statistics on every facet of a problem does not help to resolve that problem. There has to be direction and purpose in securing data. In fact, Neuman and Bonstein [1989] emphasize that strategic information systems offer a superb opportunity for the 1990s.

Planners should have some familiarity with data analysis and epidemiological methods. In a self-instruction manual on the interpretation of epidemiological data, Abramson [1988] covers basic concepts, simple measures such as rates, accuracy judgments, variable associations and cause and effect relationships. Using only simple algebra, Bland's [1987] introduction to medical statistics explains fundamental concepts of study design and the critical area of statistical inference. Illustrations and examples deal with probability, the normal distribution, significance tests, regression, correlation, cross tabulations, and statistical methods. Kahn and Sempos

[1989] discuss statistical methodology with attention to risk calculations, multivariate models, life tables, and comparative techniques. On a more sophisticated level, Jager and Ruitenberg [1988] devote their book to a statistical analysis and mathematical modeling of basic data on the spread of AIDS. Their subject matter includes statistical estimation from surveillance data, trend modeling, transmission tracing, interactive and computer simulation in decision making, prognostic analysis, and economic analysis. References such as those cited should be on the planner's bookshelf for ready access should the need arise.

Data sources are rapidly burgeoning beyond belief. At regional and state levels, information is readily available to identify needs and to analyze varying population groupings. However, information at the micro area level may be absent. Obviously, unless the huge and growing volume of data can be accessed by strategic planners, the paper, the tapes, the computer disks will merely gather dust. Since accurate and reliable data are a mainstay in need and demand determinations, a number of major sources of varying types of data are identified. This list is by no means all inclusive, but provides leads to vital data sources at the national, state, and local levels.

Exhibit 2-24 lists commonly used census data. Importantly, U.S. Census reports provide information on the general population: socioeconomic status, ethnic composition, household composition and family structure, type of housing [urbanization], condition of housing, cohabitation, and community instability. Census information is particularly useful in social area analysis and for comparisons of different subareas within a geographic boundaries. Choosing relevant characteristics as indicators allows for pertinent comparisons. High-risk populations can be identified through the use of the census data for predictions.

Additional Data Resources

Frequently, strategic planners may make decisions on insufficient data. That could occur simply because the information is unavailable. On the other hand, the planner may simply not know

Exhibit 2-23. Functional Outcomes: Response Patterns in Medical and Surgical Patients.

Study Week	Medical Patients, %			Surgical Patients, %			
	Better	Same	Worse	Better	Same	Worse	
1	26 [7]	48 [13]	26 [7]	26 [9]	14 [5]	60 [21] |	
2	7 [2]	57 [17]	37 [11]	62 [23]	21 [8]	16 [6]	} PHYSICAL
4	42 [14]	24 [8]	33 [11]	69 [22]	25 [8]	6 [2]	} FUNCTION
6	39 [15]	45 [17]	16 [6]	67 [25]	19 [7]	14 [5] |	
1	30 [8]	62 [16]	8 [2]	17 [6]	68 [28]	14 [5] |	
2	30 [9]	67 [20]	3 [1]	28 [10]	61 [22]	11 [4]	} MENTAL
4	27 [9]	58 [19]	15 [5]	44 [14]	56 [18]	0 [0]	} FUNCTION
6	26 [10]	63 [24]	11 [4]	41 [15]	54 [20]	5 [2] |	
1	29 [8]	55 [15]	15 [4]	30 [8]	55 [15]	15 [4] |	
2	33 [10]	60 [18]	7 [2]	19 [7]	70 [26]	11 [4]	} EMOTIONAL
4	24 [8]	70 [23]	6 [2]	25 [8]	72 [23]	3 [1]	} FUNCTION
6	37 [14]	53 [20]	11 [4]	21 [8]	73 [27]	5 [2] |	

Numbers in [n] are numbers of observations.
Source: From "A patient-specific measure of change in maximal function," by C.R. Mackensie, M.E. Charlson, D. DiGioia, & K. Kelley, 1986, *Archives of Internal Medicine, 14*[77], 1326. Copyright 1986. Reprinted with permission American Medical Assn.

Exhibit 2-24. Examples of Data by Type and Sources.

General Population Data

Total population by age, sex, race, marital status, etc.
Number of males and/or females [in households]
Population in group quarters
Distribution of subgroups in population

Socioeconomic Status

Income of families and unrelated individuals: median income of families and
  unrelated individuals; per capita income; unemployment rate
Families in poverty: percent of all families below poverty level; number of families receiving
  Aid to Dependent Children; number of persons receiving food stamps; number of persons
  receiving public assistance; number of persons receiving Medicaid and/or Medicare;
Low occupational status, males: percent of employed males 16 and over who are
  operatives, service workers, and laborers, including farm laborers
High occupational status, males: percent of employed males 16 and over who are
  professionals, technical and kindred workers, and managers except farm
School years completed: median school years completed by persons 25 and over
Number and percent of juvenile court referrals per 1,000 under 18 years of age

Ethnic Composition

Black: percent of household population black
Other nonwhite: percent of household population nonwhite and nonblack
Foreign origin: percent of population who are foreign born or native born of foreign
  or mixed parentage

Household Composition and Family Structure

Husband-wife households: percent of all households with husband-wife families;
  number of one parent families; household size; mobility status
Age of household heads: median age of household heads
Youth dependency ratio: persons under 18 per 100 persons 18-64 in household
  population; single parent households
Aged dependency ratio: persons 65 and over per 100 persons 18-64 in household
  population; family and/or others providing care

Type of Housing [Urbanization]

Single dwelling units: percent of all year-around housing units that are single
  detached [excluding mobile homes and trailers]; value of housing
High rise apartments: percent of all year-around housing units that are in structures
  of seven or more stories

Condition of Housing

Overcrowding: percent of persons in households in housing units with 1.01 or more persons
  per room; overcrowding index
Standard housing: percent of occupied housing units with direct access and complete
  plumbing and kitchen facilities for exclusive use

Population at Risk

Census profile from U.S. Census Bureau
Population estimates from U.S. Census Bureau, cooperative Federal/State programs for
  local population estimates, state health departments, universities, local planning
  agencies, local health and social welfare organizations

(continued)

Exhibit 2-24. *(Continued)*

Health Status

> <u>Mortality:</u> state/local death certificates; U.S. Bureau of Vital Statistics
> <u>Deaths rates:</u> state/local death certificates; National Center for Health Statistics
> <u>Natality, perinatal, infant mortality:</u> state/local birth certificates;
> <u>Marriage and divorce:</u> National Center for Health Statistics; State vital statistics
> <u>Morbidity:</u> disease registries; local surveys; school records; National Center
> <u>Disability:</u> industry records; disability claims; mental retardation registries;
>   welfare records; school records; home health agency records; local surveys; Uniform
>   Hospital Abstracts; employment commissions; Visiting Nurse Associations; vocational
>   rehabilitation administrators; American Board of Physical Medicine and Rehabilitation;
>   state and local mental health authorities
> <u>Fertility rate, live births, illegitimate births, abortions:</u> state/local birth certificates

Inpatient Facilities and Services

> <u>Characteristics of facilities:</u> Hospitals; American Hospital Association; Joint
>   Commission on the Accreditation of Healthcare Organizations; licensure boards;
>   local transportation departments; professional organizations; Chambers of Commerce;
>   National Center for Health Statistics; state/local departmental commissioners
> <u>Capacity of facilities:</u> Hospitals; state hospital association; American Hospital
>   Association; cost review commissions; National Center for Health Statistics
> <u>Staffing of facilities:</u> State directory of physicians; U.S. Department of Health and
>   Human Services Area Resource files; American Medical Association; hospital annual
>   budgets or reports; State hospital cost review commissions; Institute of Medicine
>   reports; USDHHS Health Resources and Health Manpower Bureaus
> <u>Services and utilization:</u> Boards of health; hospital records; professional
>   associations; annual reports from agencies; special studies from the literature;
>   National Center for Health Statistics; third party payers payment claims
> <u>Mental health:</u> psychiatric hospitals; mental health agencies; American Psychiatric
>   Association; agencies providing outpatient services
> <u>Payment for services:</u> Social Security Administration; Medicare and Medicaid reports;
>   Blue Cross/Blue Shield and other third party payers; hospitals; state and local
>   governments; social service agencies; VA and Defense agency payments
> <u>Quality of care:</u> Commission on Professional and Hospital Activities; Professional
>   Review Organizations; discharge abstract systems; professional activity study;
>   medical audit programs; individual facilities; hospital commissions;
>   Medicare/Medicaid investigations; National Center for Health Statistics
> <u>Ambulatory Care:</u> National Ambulatory Medical Care Surveys; data from uniform minimum
>   basic data records; National Center for Health Statistics; State and local health
>   departments; immunization program records; American Medical Association
> <u>Manpower:</u> Licensure boards; USDHHS area resource files; American Board of Medical
>   Specialists; American Dental Association; various national professional associations
>   such as nursing, osteopaths, dental hygienists, pharmacists, optometrists, etc.

Environmental Problems

> <u>Air, water, waste:</u> Environmental Protection Agencies; planning commissions; surveys

Geographic Data:

> <u>Maps, locations, transportation:</u> local planning commissions; Chambers of Commerce;
>   road maps; mass transit agencies; geography texts; parks departments

---

Sources for above data include: U.S. Census Bureau; State Labor Departments; State and local social welfare departments; U.S. Social Security Administration; local courts about available data resources. While detailing about a dozen federal and nonfederal sources, Lewis [1988] states that, "good planning requires good data." He goes on to comment that federal, state, and local data are available on tapes, diskettes, tables, or reports "commonly designated as measuring demographics, facilities, manpower, utilization services, medical economics, and measures of health."

Following are additional data resources of relevant concern to strategic planners:

Health United States series, published by the federal National Center for Health Statistics, annually updates data and past trends on numerous health indicators. Included are health status indicators on population, fertility and natality, mortality, and determinants and measures of health. There are also indicators for utilization of health services, health care resources, health care expenditures, and health prevention.

National Health Interview Survey series, published by the federal National Center for Health Statistics, provides updates on demographic data, disability days, physician visits, health conditions, long-term activity limitations, doctor visits, and number of hospitalizations. Surveys are supplemented each year with special studies on such topics as immunization, home health care, health insurance, alcohol consumption, AIDS, and health maintenance behavior. In addition, the National Center for Health Statistics (NCHS) (1988) also publishes an extensive *Catalog of Publications* at periodic intervals. This Catalog lists Vital and Health series (23 groupings), Advance Data publications, statistical notes for Health Planners, Clearinghouse on Health Indexes, Life Tables. A major economic data source, the National Medical Care Expenditure Survey, is fully explained by Cohen and Burt (1985) and Pearson (1987).

The Population of the United States in the 1980's series, published by the Social Science Research Council [New York] in collaboration with the Russell Sage Foundation [New York] and the U.S. Bureau of the Census, reports on what is happening to population subgroups and the basic issues affecting them. Some of the subjects of interest in 1987 and 1988 publications deal with women in transition, changing American income distribution, politics of numbers, color line and quality of life, Hispanic population, and housing.

Publications of the federal *Health Care Financing Administration* include discussions of marketing Medicare in a competitive environment, a data source book on Medicare and Medicaid, measuring the cost of patient care, senior citizens' access to health care, impact of prospective payment via DRGs on senior citizens, and analysis of state Medicaid program characteristics. *Health Care Financing Review* is a monthly publication published by HCFA.

Grant Formulas: A Catalog of Federal Aid to States and Localities, published by the U.S. General Accounting Office, provides a description of all formula grant programs legislated by Congress categorized by major executive departments. For strategic health planners, those relating to the Departments of Health and Human Services, Housing and Urban Development, and Labor are the most important sections.

The *Area Resource File* series, published by the federal Bureau of Health Professions, is a computerized, county-based data system of about 200 sources of the most useful data for assessing the nation's health resources. The ARF contains data on health professions, health facilities, vital statistics, health expenditures, demographic data, economic data, and health professions education. It is continually updated and is one of the few sources that provide data at the county level.

American Healthcare Systems and the Center for Health Management Research, based at the Lutheran Hospital Society of Southern California, Los Angeles, combined forces to put out a series of important health care documents in their Futures Research Program. Among those are *Health Scan*, a quarterly think piece on a variety of important topics; *Market Scan*, in-depth reports on capitation, new technologies, and other business topics; *Mini Trends*, information from non-health-related sources; *Book Digest*, reviews of books health managers should know about; and *Forecast 1988: The Economics of Change*, an annual publication on topics dealing with health professionals, leaders, governance, and regulation.

National Technical Information Service [NTIS] [Springfield, VA], a national depository maintained by the U.S. Department of Commerce, publishes thousands of research studies that are funded and sponsored by all federal agencies. Reports are available on microfilm and in paper form.

SMG Data Base, published by the SMG Marketing Groups of Chicago, Illinois, provides facility-based data on 19 providers such as nursing homes, home health agencies, and hospitals.

Microcomputer Diskette Series: State/Local Government Finance Data, published by ACIR Publications [Washington, DC], offers access to census finance data for states. Sixty-six revenue and 70 expenditure categories including population and personal income are available.

National Death Index [NDI] is a computerized central file of death record information compiled from vital statistics submitted to NCHS by the states from 1979 onward. Data items included are first and last name and middle initial, father's surname, social security number, date of birth, sex, state of birth, state of residence, marital status, race, and age at death.

Association of Public Data Users [Princeton, NJ], a national organization of users, producers, and distributors of federal, state, and local government statistical data, publishes a monthly *APDU Newsletter* aiming to enhance communications among members through electronic mail, mailing labels, a membership directory, and joint acquisition of large, once expensive data files.

The *National Infant Mortality Surveillance* monitored by the federal Centers for Disease Control [Atlanta, GA] provides a database which can be used in limited fashion for applications in evaluation and planning, that is, infant birth vs. death certificates, birthweight vs. mortality, and so on. Hogue, Buehler, Strauss, and Smith [1987] present an overview of the design, methods and results of the project.

Oryx Press [Phoenix, AZ] provides a state and city listing of licensed nursing homes with a variety of associated data about each one.

Congressional Information Service, Inc. [Bethesda, MD] publishes an *Index to Health Information* that abstracts a spectrum of publications, documents, reports, and statistics ranging from AIDS to Zoonoses.

American Hospital Association [Chicago, IL] publishes *Hospital Statistics Directory of Multihospital Systems, Multistate Alliances and Networks. A Guide to the Health Care Field* lists all US and Canadian hospitals along with additional directory type information relevant to hospital management.

Data on facilities and services are included in a directory prepared by the federal National Institute on Mental Health entitled *Mental Health, United States*.

Other organizations are developing population databases for various reasons. In Chicago, the Metro Chicago Information Center [MCIC] periodically surveys the population regarding issues such as health care, housing, race relations, education, crime, and recreation, and will make the data available to government and private institutions [*American Medical News*, 1988].

Regardless of the data source, planners need to keep in mind the strengths and weaknesses of the information. National data may be accurate but not include state- or local-level data and vice versa. Published data may be readily available but may lag in timeliness. Discovering the most accurate and useful data is no easy task. However, that is a task that must be done to achieve top-notch results.

COMPUTERS AND DATA

Microcomputers in strategic planning allow databases to be organized in a series of interactive files. A major strength of a database lies in its retrieval and reporting capabilities. As database programs gain sophistication, ease of use, and storage capacity, the files will be manipulated more easily and informatively. Software programs such as Hypertext and compact memory disks can store huge amounts of information and allow for a variety of configurations to retrieve the facts with great speed. However, Goodall [1986] does note a possible negative effect on social relationships and productivity due to the use of microcomputers and the isolation of individuals from interactions with other warm bodies.

Lemon and Toole [1987] cite the vital technological factors involved in the increased power of computer information access:

- Social factors increase the pervasiveness of computers.
- Hardware and processing speed is increasing dramatically.
- Software is becoming easier to use with an increasing use of artificial intelligence.
- Digital technology allows voice, image, data, and text to be mixed and carried at the same time.
- Local Area Networks [LANs] are allowing multi-access to single databases and interaction among computers.
- Fiber optics are increasing the speed of communications.

Peterkin and Black [1988] describe 176 online health care databases indexed by title, description and cost, producer, vendor and subject. To find medical and health care statistics, Snow [1988] elaborates on the following databases: nursing and allied health, international pharmaceutical abstracts, psycINFO, mental health abstracts, smoking and health, occupational safety and health, sport database, biosciences, embase, biosis previews, and MEDLINE. In keying into the business of medicine, Ojala [1988] suggests looking at ABI/INFORM, Promt and Nexis to find material on advertising, mergers, products, events, and geographical codes.

Management and Computer Decisions

Increasingly, artificial intelligence guides decision making and results in "medical expert systems" to assist physicians in diagnosing and treating illnesses. "Management oriented expert systems" support marketing, product planning, cost management, and financial counseling [Meyer & Boone, 1989; Norton & Neuman, 1989].

An example of an administration-oriented system would be the "case mix management" system. Case mix management can be used by strategic planners to integrate clinical, demographic, and financial data. DRGs are dependent upon six variables: age, sex, principal diagnosis, secondary diagnosis, primary procedure, and secondary procedure. To have accurate evaluation and billing, financial and medical records must be able to be integrated into a single database. A case mix system does exactly that, allowing access to a single comprehensive set of data [Rusnak, 1987].

As managers, physicians, and third-party payers depend more and more on accurate data, health care facilities are switching to use of the computer stored medical record systems. Characteristically, these systems have the ability to store clinical information from a variety of services in a common framework. That framework provides access to observations and treatment records as discrete and understandable items. Information can be retained on line for many years [McDonald & Tierney, 1988].

Use of the computer might start as soon as the patient enters the facility. Patients can have a dialogue with the computer including immediate interactions. According to the responses, the computer changes directions during the exchange. In some settings, the computer interview could increase interviewee truthfulness as well as avoid the cost and error of data entry operators [Petrovski, Olchanski, & Manoukian, 1986].

As the data are collected, it is combined with other patient data, including medical records (Korpman & Lincoln, 1988), in the format of a health surveillance database which may be on a city or county level giving information about the entire population. This data may be accessed by a strategic planner for an external audit, by a public health agency, or by any number of parties who may find it useful.

With the accumulation of data bases, strategic planners must consider a mechanism for handling and working with the information. In an extensively detailed report, McDonald and Blevins [1987] present a primer on databases. Definitions of a field, a record, attributes, and a file set the stage for a discussion of database management systems [DBMS]. Six full-featured software DBMS for microcomputers are reviewed: Paradox, R:Base 5000, dBase III+, Knowledgeman, PC/FOCUS, and Revelation. Source addresses and prices are given along with the author's recommendations. Since the computer software world changes so rapidly, the DBMS names may differ but the issues to consider will still be pertinent for planner.

Basic Software Programs for Strategic Planners

Computer software programs breed like rabbits. New and improved programs arrive on the scene every day. Now and then, it may be worthwhile for planners to review issues of computer oriented journals to catch up on what's new. Following are examples of current software programs illustrating the types of assistance that the microcomputer can provide to planners.

SUPERSTAT [Kushner, 1988], a special statistical computer software program, can assist planners requiring heavy duty analyses of significance. This program can provide means and standard deviations, frequency functions for discrete or continuous variables, graphs of frequency functions, means and variances classified by one or two variables and N-way Anova, crosstabs, plots of variables, test the differences between two or more means; individual correlations, correlation matrixes, one and two stage regressions, residuals, graphs of the regression results, and estimates of the dependent variable. At least 60 variables can be used with 15 values for each decision variable and up to 15 variables in a regression [Serendipity Systems, Valdosta, GA].

GATOR (Generalized Automatic Text Organization and Retrieval) system uses a microcomputer to index and recover data from interviews and case histories. Qualitative and quantitative data can be integrated in GATOR. Using keywords, the computer builds a master file to use in research and analysis (Giordano & Cole, 1988).

Using visual aids in a presentation or report allows a strategic planner to spend less time explaining and the audience retains more information. Computer software, such as the examples described below, can be used to create charts, diagrams, and signs to enhance planning reports and presentations. Of course, computer word processing using common programs such as Word Perfect or Word Star enhances overall report preparation abilities. Grammatik III [Williams &

Wilkins, 1989a] and RightWriter [RightSoft 1989] are software programs that correct mistakes in grammer and usage. Steadman's Medical Dictionary [Williams & Wilkins, 1989b] is also available in computer software for spelling checks.

Ashton-Tate's [1989] *Presentation-Pack* [Torrence, CA; Keil, 1988] includes three separate programs: Sign-Master, Diagram-Master, and Chart-Master. These programs can produce printed charts as well as slides. Sign-Master can make text charts that are free-form, bulleted, numbered, and columnar. Diagram-Master makes organization charts with mapped hierarchial relationships as well as text charts. Chart-Master can design pie, bar, and line charts.

Harvard Graphics [Mountain View, CA; Keil, 1988] has strong free-form capabilities. Pie and bar charts can be combined. A 3-D effect can be added to pie, bar, and line charts. Spacing, placement, and size of different elements in charts can be changes. In addition, this program allows multiple charts on one screen and provides a symbol library.

A library of public domain and user supported software for the IBM-PC exists [PC-SIG 1987]. That library lists, describes, and tells how a wide variety of useful computer software programs can be secured free or at a nominal price.

Yasnoff [1989] lists medical and health related magazines, journals, organizations, and meetings to keep you up-to-date on computer applications.

In sum, Waldrop (1987) describes how your microcomputer can be your file clerk, your secretary, your research librarian, your graphic artist, your messenger, your on-site emcee, your accountant and your pal. On the other extreme, Willbern and Walling [1989] warn that runaway computers can be hazardous to health care organizations.

CONSIDERATIONS REGARDING DATA SOURCES

Although some data sources have already been considered in the sections on need and demand assessment methods, Exhibit 2-25 lists a few additional ones. For each of the sources a few advantages and disadvantages are cited.

Representative interviews is a method similar to the key informant technique. Planners choose people they believe to be representative and interview them to collect data.

Opinion polls and surveys are familiar to most planners and to the public. Data might be available from polls and surveys that have been conducted by others and reported elsewhere such as the Harris Polls. Planners should check to see if existing opinion poll information is useful before conducting their own expensive and time consuming poll or survey.

Vital statistics in large numbers on a variety of problems are usually available from governmental agencies. Here, the problem is to select the data that can be applied to the specific problem.

An expert interview is a quick and easy information source wherein the appropriate expert is located and asked questions. Merely interviewing a few experts yields volumes of data and additional sources. Yet, considering our complex sophisticated technology, the planner has to wonder if the right expert was consulted.

Position papers submitted by vested interest parties contain information and rationales for their respective stances. Papers could be invited from experts, the lay public, concerned organizations, or individuals. Obviously, planners must judge whether the position papers present a valid viewpoint or a bias.

Public hearings are akin to the community forum approach noted under needs assessment methods. People are familiar with this technique and participate readily.

Citizen committees could take the shape of task forces, ad hoc groups, or advisory bodies

Exhibit 2-25. Considerations Regarding Sources of Data—Examples.

Data Source	Advantages	Disadvantages
Representative Interviews	Grass roots feeling Variety of viewpoints	Bias; prejudice Finding reliable source
Expert Interviews	Quick; Refer to others Mass of data rapidly	Right expert? Accurate data?
Position Papers	Quick; References Written data	Bias; prejudice May be lobbyist
Public Hearings	Community participation Legitimation	Repetitive May be controlled
Citizen Committees	Concerned participants Authoritative	Time counsuming Partisan politics
Opinion Polls	Comparative data More people covered	Expensive; expertise? Limited questions
Surveys	Population sampled Accurate collection	Expensive; expertise? Respondents' attitudes
Vital Statistics	Long term accurate data Comparative statistics	Up-to-date data? Limited to hard data
Research Studies	Authoritative Documented in literature	Expensive; expertise? Time consuming
Investigative Reports	Volume of data issued Reference materials	Expensive; takes time May be political
Literature Searches	Computerized; indexed Mass of data located	Cost; follow-up? Limited journals

appointed to secure data, to prepare an opinion and to make recommendations. Staff planners usually assist the committees. As a data source, citizen committees vary in value in direct ratio to the input of the participants.

Research studies and investigative reports generate volumes of data but both are usually expensive and time consuming. Importantly, there should be a search to assure that data does not exist before new research or investigation is imitated. A computer literature search, such as Medline, is one place to start.

In reviewing Exhibit 2-25, note that the list is representative and advantages and disadvantages are merely illustrative. For example, health diaries can record data about individual health problems ranging from absence at work to over self-medication to utilization of professional care. A diary has two advantages; as a memory aid in a retrospective interview or as a primary data source [Bentzen, Christiansen, & Pederson, 1987]. Since only about one in ten problems refers to a health care professional, diary studies are indispensable. Importantly, participants require explicit instructions, a layout with simple questions, and a simple method of collection. Respondents must be given tangible benefits to assure cooperation and the accuracy of entries. Obviously, recollective memory and incomplete notations are major difficulties with the health diaries. However, the illustration indicates that planners must consider various aspects of the sources of data.

Generally, strategic health information systems need to be managed effectively to produce desired outcomes. Neuman and Bonstein [1989], Norton and Neuman [1989], and Nolan and Grad [1989] all list a variety of guiding principles to achieve that type of management control.

OBSTACLES TO THE RECEIVING OF TECHNICAL INFORMATION

Technical and scientific data comprise much of the fodder in strategic planning, but obviously planners are not expected to be all purpose experts. There will be a need to rely on others for information and to evaluate the technical data. Difficulties arise regarding the technical information as follows:

- Although a new drug may be 99 percent effective, the one percent unlikely probability can occur. Technical and scientific data concerns probabilities with a margin for error. Physicians and scientists cannot guarantee that something will never happen. There is always a chance that some unforeseen event will occur.
- A world-famous physician creates a diet to reduce coronary artery disease. Mass media constantly interviews the physician. Just the outstanding personality of the physician involved could divert attention from the issue and overshadow efforts to secure technical data about the true value of the procedure.
- Technical differences among experts seem to have negative effects on data. When experts disagree, the public waits to see the outcome. Data from and by opposing experts get equal weight in the public's eye.
- Sensationalism in investigative areas generates mixed impacts and may attract pseudo experts with high visibility. Can such information be evaluated rationally? Weight reduction regimens are a typical example. Little can be done to blend emotion and reason.
- Unproven theories rooted in experience, myths, or visions may be be considered valid despite doubts. Testimonials from "cured" patients discount the placebo effect. Folk remedies and cures do likewise. Can intense emotional beliefs be displayed by scientific evidence? That is a serious problem.

THE VALUE OF STATISTICS

Common maxims often note that "statistics don't lie, but liars use statistics." In addition, statistics can be misinterpreted such as the hospital mortality rates released by HCFA (Chelimsky, 1988, p. 2) to assume certain hospitals are worse than others. Because statistics can readily be misused, the following guidelines provide caveats for those using statistics:

- Statistics should be interpreted with greater skill and discretion. Administrators should not be permitted to confuse them with complex, elusive realities or regard them as significant entities in their own right.
- Specious quantification of the unquantifiable can be as mischievous as ignoring subjective data. Unlike the present generation of computers, the human brain can deal with qualitative issues in their own right.
- There is a need for more and better statistics to illuminate the problems more adequately.
- There is no substitute for the intuitive feel of a problem resulting from first-hand exposure to it.

Obviously, statistics are an integral part of the required framework of strategic health planning. There can be no doubt that needs and demand assessments and analysis of resources are going to involve tons of statistics. Yet, planners should always feel a tad uncomfortable and realize that a malfunction or two *can* cause the computer to answer five when adding two and two.

REFERENCES

Abanobi, O.C. (1986). Content validity in the assessment of health status. *Health Values, 10*(4), 37–40.

Abramson, J.H. (1988). *Making sense of data. A self-instruction manual on the interpretation of epidemiological data.* New York: Oxford University Press.

American Medical News. (1988). Database seen as aid in planning health needs, *31*(4), 29.

Andersen, R., Aday, L., & Chen, M. (1986). Data watch. *Health Affairs, 5*(1), 154–172.

Anderson, G.M. (1982). A comment on the index of well-being. *Medical Care, 20*(5), 513–515.

Ashbaugh, J.W., & Manderscheid, R.W. (1988). A method for estimating the chronic mentally ill population in state and local areas. *Hospital and Community Psychiatry, 36*(4), 389–393.

Ashton-Tate [Torrance, CA]. (1989, Winter). *Update Education.*

Bentzen, N., Christiansen, T., & Pederson, K.M. (1987). Data collection using health diaries. *Scandinavian Journal of Primary Health Care, 5*(2), 67–69.

Bergner, M. (1985). Measurement of health status. *Medical Care, 23*(5), 696–704.

Bergner, M., Bobbit, R.A., & Carter, W.B. (1981). The sickness impact profile: Development and final revision of a health status measure. *Medical Care, 19*(8), 787–805.

Bland, M. (1987). *An introduction to medical statistics.* New York: Oxford University Press.

Bush, J.W., Chen, M.K., & Patrick, D.L. (1974). *Social indicators for health planning and policy analysis.* Springfield, VA: National Technical Information Service.

Bush, J.W., Anderson, J.P., Kaplan, R.M., & Blischke, W.R. (1982). "Counterintuitive" preferences in health-related quality-of-life measurement. *Medical Care, 20*(5), 516–525.

Carr, W. (1988). *Measuring avoidable deaths and disease in New York State.* New York: United Hospital Fund of New York.

Chelimsky, E. (1988). *Medicare: Improved patient outcome analyses could enhance quality assessment.* (GAO/PEMD-88-23). Washington, DC: Government Printing Office.

Cohen, S.B., & Burt, U.L. (1985). Data collection frequency effect in the National Health Care Expenditure survey. *Journal of Economic and Social Measurement, 13*(2), 125–151.

Coleman, B. (1988). Congress enacts landmark bill. *American Association of Retired Persons News Bulletin, 29*(7), 1.

Conner, D.R., & Gold, B. (1988). Hospital corporate culture and its impact on strategic change. *Dimensions in Health Care, 88*(2), 1–12.

Conner, D.R., & Newman, J.A. (1987). Managing major organizational change. *Dimensions in Health Care, 88*(1), 1–8.

De La Rosa, M. (1989). Health care needs of Hispanic Americans and the responsiveness of the health care system. *Health and Social Work, 14*(2), 104–113.

Deyo, R.A., & Inui, T.S. (1981). Toward clinical application of health status measures: Sensitivity of scale to clinically important changes. *Health Services Research, 19*(3), 275–289.

Dufour, R.G. (1974). Three case studies in planning: 1. Predicting hospital bed needs. *Health Services Research, 9*(1), 62–68.

Giordano, R., & Cole, J.R. (1988). Text retrieval on a microcomputer. *Perspectives in Computing, 8*(1), 52–60.

Goodall, R. (1986). Introducing microcomputers: Anticipating the problems. *Dimensions in Health Services, 63*(7), 22–24.

Goplerud, E.N. (1986). Assessing methods of predicting the need for psychiatric beds. *Hospital and Community Psychiatry, 37*(4), 391–395.

Gottlieb, S.R.V. (1986). Ensuring access to health care: What communities can do to make a difference through private sector coalitions. *Inquiry, 23*(3), 322–329.

Greenfield, S.S., Cretin, L.G., & Worthman, L.G. (1981). Comparison of a criteria map to a criteria list in quality-of-care assessment for patients with chest pain: The relation of each to outcome. *Medical Care, 19*(3), 255–272.

Haig, T.H.B., Scott, D.A., & Wickett, L.I. (1986). The rational zero point for an illness index with ratio properties. *Medical Care, 24*(2), 113–124.

Hawley, C. (1988). An environmental assessment is key. *Provider, 14*(4), 14–20.

Heineken, P.A., Charles, G., & Stimson, D.H. (1985). The use of negative indexes of health to evaluate quality of care in a primary-care group practice. *Medical Care, 23*(3), 198–208.

Herzlinger, R.E. (1985). How companies tackle health care costs: Part II. *Harvard Business Review, 63*(5), 108–120.

Hoque, C.J.R., Buehler, J.W., Strauss, L.T., & Smith, J.C. (1987). Overview of the National Infant Mortality Surveillance (NIMS) project—design, methods, results. *Public Health Reports, 102*(2), 126–138.

Ingram, J.J. (1988). Alcoholism treatment demand estimation. *Health Marketing Quarterly, 6*(1,2,3), 195–205.

Jager, J.C., & Ruitenberg, E.J. (1988). *Statistical analysis and mathemathical modelling of AIDS.* New York: Oxford University Press.

Kahn, H.A., & Sempos, C.T. (1989). *Statistical methods in epidemiology.* New York: Oxford University Press.

Keil, A. (1988). Presentation graphics: Two excellent packages. *Computer Center Online, 1*(2), 9–10.

Korpman, R.A., & Lincoln, T.L. (1988). The computer-stored medical record. *Journal of the American Medical Association, 259*(23), 3454–3456.

Kramon, G. (1988, June 14). "Managed Care" is top plan now. *New York Times,* p. D2.

Kushner, J.W. (1988). Personal correspondence. Serendipity Systems, P.O. Box 3293, Valdosta, GA.

Lane, D., Uyeno, D., & Stark, A. (1985). Forecasting demand for long-term care services. *Health Services Research, 20*(4), 435–460.

Lapin, L.L. (1988). *Quantitative methods for business decisions with cases* (4th ed.). New York: Harcourt Brace Jovanovich.

Lemon, R.B., & Toole, J.E. (1987). Information technology challenges the future of health care. *Healthcare Financial Management, 41*(6), 62–66.

LeTouze, D. (1984). Hospital bed planning in Canada: A survey analysis. *International Journal of Health Services, 14*(1), 105–126.

Lewis, F. (1988). Making effective use of data resources as a part of planning. *Provider, 14*(1), 16, 33.

Mackensie, C.R., Charlson, M.E., DiGioia, D., & Kelley, K. (1986). A patient-specific measure of change in maximal function. *Archives of Internal Medicine, 146*(77), 1325–1329.

McDonald, C.J., & Blevins, L. (1987). A database sampler. *MD Computing, 4*(4), 42–49.

McDonald, C.J., & Tierney, W.M. (1988). Computer-stored medical records. Their future role in medical practice. *Journal of the American Medical Association, 259*(23), 3433–3440.

Meyer, N.D., & Boone, M.E. (1989). *The information edge.* Homewood, IL: Dow Jones-Irwin.

Neuman, B., & Bonstein, R.G. (1989). Strategic information systems: Opportunities for the 1990s. *Dimensions in Health Care, 89*(3), 1–6.

Nolan, R.L., & Grad, J.H. (1989). Transforming the hospital data center into an informational utility. *Dimensions in Health Care, 89*(3), 6–12.

Norton, D.P., & Neuman, B.S. (1989). Benefits-based I/T planning for health care organizations. *Dimensions in Health Care, 89*(1), 1–4.

Ojala, M. (1988). The business of medicine. *Online, 12*(6), 88–93.

Padilla, G.V., & Grant, M.M. (1985). Quality of life as a cancer nursing outcome variable. *Advances in Nursing Science, 8*(1), 45–50.

Parkerson, G.R., Jr., Gehlbach, S.H., Wagner, E.H., James, S.A., Clapp, N.E., & Muhlbaier, L.H. (1981). The Duke-UNC profile: An adult health status instrument for primary care. *Medical Care, 19*(8), 806–823.

PC-SIG, Inc. (1987). *The PC SIG library* (4th ed.). Public domain and user supported software for the IBM-PC. Sunnyvale, CA 94086.

Pearson, C. (1987). National health expenditures, 1986–2000. *Health Care Financing Review*, 8(4), 1–36.

Peterkin, K., & Black, P.V. (1988). *The directory of online databases 1988*. Los Altos,CA: Medical Data Exchange.

Petrovski, A.M., Olchanski, V., & Manoukian, L.M. (1986). Computer aided health surveillance system—ASKIS. In R. Salamon, B. Blum, & M. Jorgensen (Eds.), *MEDINFO 86* (pp. 319–321). North-Holland, Amsterdam: Elsevier.

Pillemer, K. (1984). How do we know how much we need? Problems in determining need for long-term care. *Journal of Health Politics, Policy and Law*, 9(2), 281–290.

RightSoft, Inc. (1989). *RightWriter*. Sarasota, FL.

Rusnak, J.E. (1987). Case mix management systems: An opportunity to integrate medical records and financial management system data bases. In *Symposium on computer applications in medical care* (pp. 698–702). Washington, DC: Computer Society Press.

Rutstein, D.D., Berenberg, W., & Chalmers, T.C. (1976). Measuring the quality of medical care. A clinical method. *New England Journal of Medicine*, 294(11), 582–588.

Rutstein, D.D., Berenberg, W., & Chalmers, T.C. (1980). Measuring the quality of medical care: Second revision of tables and indexes (letter to the editor). *New England Journal of Medicine*, 302(20), 1146.

Sackett, D.L., Chambers, L.W., MacPherson., A.S., Goldsmith, C.H., & McCauley, R.G. (1977). The development and application of indices of health: General methods and a summary of results. *American Journal of Public Health*, 67(5), 423–428.

Satin, M.S., & Monetti, C.H. (1985). Census tract predictors of physical, psychological, and social functioning for needs assessment. *Health Services Research*, 20(3), 342–358.

Scotti, D.J. (1988). Cultural factors in choosing a strategic posture. In F. Simyar & J. Lloyd-Jones (Eds.), *Strategic management in the health care sector* (pp. 143–161). Englewood Cliffs, NJ: Prentice-Hall.

Snow, B. (1988). Finding medical and health care statistics online. *Online*, 12(4), 86–95.

USDHHS, National Institute on Drug Abuse. (1981). *A needs assessment workbook for prevention planning, Volume II*. (DHHS Pub. No. (ADM) 81-1061.) Washington, DC: Government Printing Office.

USDHHS, National Center for Health Statistics. (1990). *Health: United States 1989*. (DHHS Pub. No. 90-1232.) Washington, DC: Government Printing Office.

USDHHS, National Center for Health Statistics. (1988). *Health: United States 1987*. (DHHS Pub. No. 88-1232.) Washington, DC: Government Printing Office.

USDHHS, National Center for Health Statistics. [undated brochure]. *National Death Index*. Washington, DC: Government Printing Office.

Wagstaff, A. (1989). Econometric studies in health economics—A survey of the British literature. *Journal of Health Economics [Netherlands]*, 8(1), 1–51.

Waldrop, H. (1987). Make your PC your meeting-planning partner. *Successful Meetings*, 36(9), 4647.

Willbern, J.A., & Walling, M.F. (1989). Warning! Runaway computers can be hazardous to health care organizations. *Dimensions in Health Care*, 89(2), 5–8.

Williams and Wilkins. (1989a). *Grammatik III*. Baltimore, MD: Williams and Wilkins.

Williams and Wilkins. (1989b). *Stedman's Medical Dictionary*. Baltimore, MD: Williams and Wilkins.

Yasnoff, W.A. (1989). Sources can keep you informed on computers. *American Medical News*, 32(38), 15.

Young, A. (1989). There is no such thing as geriatric medicine, and it's here to stay. *Lancet*, 2, 263–265.

Zylke, J.W. (1989). Maternal, child health needs noted by two major national study groups. *Journal of the American Medical Association*, 261(12), 1687–1688.

3

Resources Mean Manpower, Materials, and Money

After problem identification and preliminary data collection, planners should take stock of the resources that are available and that will be required to achieve the institution's goals and objectives. Planners should be aware of the possibility of operating in a vacuum making these determinations. In fact, Rifkin and Walt [1988] argue that placing the decisions and resources in the hands of technicians may lead to isolation from the needs and demands of the people they are supposed to serve. A study by Farel [1988] provided "no evidence that the allocation of resources to child development reflects states' needs." She goes even further and says that "without specific federal mandates, the needs of certain populations may not be met." With or without expanded participation in the decisions, there are at least four major types of resources to account for: personnel, facilities, funding, and equipment/supplies.

Personnel includes professionals, ancillary staff, management, clerical, and even volunteers. Facilities refer to hospitals, nursing homes, satellite centers, or any other space used for an activity. Equipment/supplies include the standard and high technology apparatus as well as the usual papers and clips needed for any program. Funding relates to public and private moneys and even in terms of exchange or bartering.

In forecasting the use of health services, MacStravic [1984] enumerates five approaches to projecting the utilization of resources:

1. Using current values or standards.
2. Projections based upon past experiences.
3. Predicting resource utilization using other factors.
4. Prospective methods that use nominal group and related techniques to focus expert opinion and thus estimate future resource use.
5. Using normative standards to set factor values.

Changing utilization patterns make numbers 1 and 2 less desirable since the resource trends may not be continuous. In number 4, the expert opinion may be biased or not representative. Number 5 is essentially prospective values that have gained broader acceptance. Number 3 with additions from number 4 had advantages for MacStravic. DRGs could increase admissions, lower average lengths of stay, and modify physician practice patterns. Expert opinion could set boundaries for the related DRG factors relative to resources directly linked to each factor. Increased admissions could mean more clerical personnel, more ancillary staff; lowered length of stay could mean more alternative care resources; physician patterns could mean fewer technicians and equipment.

A critical strategic planning issue closely connected to the concepts of cost containment and scarcity of resources involves considerations of the rationing of health care services. Of course, rationing applies equally to personnel, facilities, equipment/supplies, and to funding.

RATIONING RESOURCES

Access to health care was the major cry during the 1960s and into the 1970s. Beginning in the 1970s, both cost containment and quality of care emerged as guiding themes with respect to health policy. Costs increased faster than the public or private sectors could keep pace with. By the mid–1980s, the issue shifted to the difficulty of the American people being able to afford the medical care to which they had become accustomed. Rationing, which hospitals, physicians, and other health care providers had quietly practiced, turned into a public debate in the mid–1980s. Rationing was defined in a Brookings report [Jones, 1989] as "the limiting of potentially beneficial resources." A spate of articles on the subject appeared in professional journals. Still later, a number of books came onto the market [Aaron & Schwartz, 1983; Blank, 1989; Churchill, 1987; Harris, 1987; Hiatt, 1987; Melville & Dobie, 1988; Smeeding, 1987]. No longer can the topic of health resources be discussed without taking into account the concept of rationing. There simply are fewer resources to go around to provide an equitable distribution of health care services to all who want them. A prominent health economist [Fuchs, 1984] notes that "trade-offs must be made." Individual needs must be weighed against societal needs.

One critic, who had been surprised by the crescendo of the discussion about rationing, had taken it for granted that rationing was an economic fact of life [Wilensky, 1985]. At a national conference, former Colorado Governor Richard D. Lamm spoke about America's limited health resources: "Every country and system rations health care. We pretend that we don't. . . . We find it distasteful to admit the obvious: That we can't give presidential health care to every citizen" [Perrone, 1988]. Fuchs' [1974] well-known work, *Who Shall Live?*, was a best-seller and an earlier acknowledgment that hard choices had to be made. In a like manner, Benjamin [1988] raised the same ethical question while discussing the micro-allocation of how funds are distributed. Duggan [1989] opted for sound ethical principles in resource allocation.

When there are not enough resources to go around, some groups or sectors of the population will suffer. As it turned out, low income and unemployed persons were the ones who suffered the most from implicit rationing [Gross, 1989]. This implicit and unequal rationing of health care appears even more paradoxical in light of the growing surplus of physicians and hospital beds in this country.

Making Rationing Decisions

With limited resources available, it is vital to understand how rationing decisions are made. In an economy governed by competition, the market may determine who gets what. If a person has the money to buy a Mercedes Benz automobile, that individual does so. If another individual needs a car but can't afford the upscale models, that person will have to purchase a less expensive brand. In health care, where third-party payers intervene to mask the true price of services, the consumer is not as apt to take price into account when demanding services. Consumers believe they have a right to health care as part of their employee benefit package which foregoes direct wages to pay for the health care. When sickness occurs, the consumer expects to receive whatever health care services are necessary to cure or improve their condition. There is no doubt that people consider that they have a right to obtain an equitable share of the total quantity of health resources available [Fein, 1988]. Yet, in 1982, it was estimated that about one million American families were refused needed health care for financial reasons [R.W. Johnson Foundation, 1983]. In 1984, both Bernard [1985] and Reinhardt [1985] observed that profit and nonprofit hospitals dumped critically ill, uninsured patients into municipal hospitals in unprecedented numbers. That dumping occurred despite the fact that the private hospitals recorded their highest profit margins in some 30 years. Considering the American paradox, Reinhardt [1986] concludes that "we have flattered ourselves with the pretense that ours is a one-tier health system easily accessible to all—rich and poor."

Nevertheless, when the resources are not available, they are rationed. Usually, the physician is the main gatekeeper of the health care services provided to their patients. In an intriguing study, Wetle, Cwikel, and Levkoff [1988] secured decisions about the allocation of scarce resources to geriatric patients from physicians, nurses, and social workers. Participants responded to two hypothetical situations, one to allocate resources and one to withhold treatment:

A. *Two men, a 35-year-old and a 75-year-old need treatment in an intensive care unit [ICU]. Both are similar in cognitive function, marital status, and prognosis. Who goes to ICU?*

B. *An elderly patient with acute respiratory failure and a very poor prognosis also has limited cognitive and functional ability. How strongly would you support intubation?*

Decision factors included the following with the mean level of importance for each for case A or Case B. Importance level is 1 = lowest and 5 = highest with statistical significance where * = $p.05$, ** = $p.01$ and *** = $p.001$:

	A	B
Medical factors		
Medical risk to patient	4.45	3.87***
Expected quality of life after care	4.25	4.48**
Degree of pain and suffering	4.19	4.44***
Cognitive functioning	3.58	3.54
Institutional/societal constraints and formal/informal rules	3.24	3.34*
Legal liability potential	3.14	3.33**
Patient factors		
Prior wishes of patient	4.27	4.34
Age of the patient	3.37	3.23
Family considerations	3.61	3.95***

Primarily medical factors predicted the decision relative to the allocation of scarce resources. In case A, 54 percent sent the 35-year-old to ICU; 23 percent the 75-year-old and 24 percent sent neither. A number of the 248 respondents refused to answer.

A combination of medical, societal, and situational factors predicted the decision to withhold treatment with 75 percent not supporting intubation, 11 percent in moderate support, and 14 percent in strong support of intubation.

Since the elderly population is growing rapidly, Wetle et al.'s conclusion is pointedly relevant: "No patient-related factor was significant in either decision . . . decisions of health care practitioners were strongly influenced by the medical model of decision making."

In the past, physicians generally operated on the maximalist principle: Use whatever services are necessary to obtain the best medical results for the patient. However, as national cost containment policies interacted with programs such as Certificate-of-Need, Peer Review, Appropriateness of Medical Care, and prospective payment via DRGs [Diagnosis Related Groups], the ball shifted from the hands of the physician to that of the health care institution where the physician practices. Hospitals, especially, have been forced to reconsider large financial investments in high technology equipment. In so doing, hospital management explicitly makes rationing decisions regarding the types and amounts of service to offer to the community [Wilensky, 1985; McGregor, 1989]. In turn, hospital administrators put pressure on their medical staffs to consider how individual medical service decisions affect not only the patients, but the hospital and society as a whole. In fact, Nardone [1988] comments that the use of a means test by the V.A. has been interpreted as an example of rationing. "Although the intent of the means test seemingly was to provide incentive for the V.A. to collect payments for its services, many believe it defers care and gives negative incentives for potential users of resources."

Media-Driven Humanitarianism

In July 1987, the Oregon state legislature took the unprecedented step of curtailing any further Medicaid expenditures for bone-marrow, pancreas, heart, and liver transplants [Lund, 1989a]. At that time, Oregon needed $48 million for immediate human resource needs, but only $21 million was left in the budget. Savings from the rationing of transplant procedures were transferred to provide prenatal care for 1,500 low-income mothers [Larkin, 1988].

John Kitzhaber, president of the Oregon Senate and a physician, stated that an explicit decision was made to use the state's limited funds to assist 1,500 persons rather than the 34 possibly benefiting from a transplant. At issue is whether the public will support health care rationing. When the issue was put before the public, rationing was supported. A later survey showed those favorable increasing from 37 percent to 56 percent.

In October 1987, a seven-year-old child with acute lymphocytic leukemia was denied a bone-marrow transplant. His family could not raise enough money for the procedure. There was a public outcry against the legislature's decision. Discussing how Oregon dealt with limited resources, Welch and Larsen [1988] quoted an articulate Oregonian:

> If Oregon truly has limited resources, it would make sense to allocate those resources to the individuals that would benefit the most. At the same time, perhaps we should withhold resources from those who would survive without our assistance, and we should also deny resources to those who may soon die even with our help.

In the aftermath of the negative publicity and the political backlash, Oregon's Legislative Emergency Board decided to restore the Medicaid transplant fund using private and public funds in August 1988 [Lund, 1988a]. However, private fundraising fell far short and six weeks later,

Oregon again halted the organ transplant program, except for kidney and cornea procedures [Perrone, 1988; Lund, 1988b]. Kevin Concannon, director of the state Department of Human Resources commented: "Sure, people will die because of this decision. . . . This is a striking example of the difficult health choices officials have to make with limited health resources [Lund, 1988a]. In October 1988, the boy died, a victim of health care rationing. Lamm [1988] would also label this incident a typical example of "media-driven humanitarianism." Other states—Arizona, Alaska, California, Colorado, Kentucky, and Vermont—expressed interest in following Oregon's example [Lund, 1989b, 1989c].

Rationing Guidelines

There is a strong implication that rationing is a matter of balancing benefits. How does one do this? In England, where health care services have been rationed for some time, health policy analysts developed guidelines to insure rational procedures rather than having a state legislative body respond emotionally to community sentiment. Clinicians are expected to go through a three-step process in determining the quantity and quality of medical services to be provided [Jennett, 1986]:

1. Consideration of how much benefit is likely and the probabilities of achieving that benefit.
2. Evaluation of the financial and personal costs to the patient in discomfort, hazard, or indignity.
3. Finally, clinicians weigh these two considerations against each other in making a decision.

In addition, the British physicians take into account the following five "U's" which are generally defined as inappropriate activities:

1. *Unsuccessful*—when the patient is too far gone to benefit from medical attention.
2. *Unnecessary*—when the patient's condition is not serious enough to justify evaluation and monitoring.
3. *Unkind*—when care prolongs what is a poor quality of life or imposes potential hurt such as mutilating surgery or toxic chemotherapy for an advanced cancer patient.
4. *Unwise*—when medical resources are diverted from an area where they could bring greater benefit.
5. *Unsafe*—when the risk of complications outweighs the desired benefits.

In the United States, this type of resources rationing decision making usually falls on the physician by default. Yet, hospital administrators bear the brunt of the criticism if the institution fails to balance its budget and operate in the black. Consequently, health care administrators are forced to make resources rationing decisions by adopting two principles: first, by "dumping" or transferring a poor or nonpaying patient to a public institution; and second, by allocating available resources within the institution based on the rationale of what will bring the greatest economic benefit to the hospital [Seiden, 1985]. Implementing these principles brings the administrator into direct conflict with physicians, especially those operating on the maximalist principle. Fuchs [1984] argues that it would "be a great mistake to turn each physician into an explicit maximizer of the social-benefit/social-cost ratio in his or her daily practice."

What is needed is a set of guidelines advanced and accepted by all the prime health care provider actors. This takes the burden off one set of actors of playing God with a patient's welfare. One of the major considerations in developing such guidelines is to include the benefits and costs to the community at large as well as to the individual patient. This is a role that health care administrators can logically play. In a sense, administrators should serve as the advocate of the silent, larger community. As another critic stated, without advanced planning on who gets what and how resources are allocated, it leads to the formation of God Committees to make decisions on "who shall live when not all can live" [Benjamin, 1988].

Attitudes Toward Rationing

Noting that some form of health care rationing is inevitable, a conference considered if medical care should be rationed by age [Smeeding, 1987]. That suggestion was considered an opprobrium by the participants, but none of the speakers presented a straight answer to the question. Callahan's [1987] book, *Setting Limits: Medical Goals in an Aging Society*, produced a public debate on the rationing issue. Commenting on the rash of books about rationing health care resources, Callahan [1988] summarizes the key issues involved in the subject [Blank, 1989; Hiatt, 1987; Califano, 1986]. He notes three major obstacles to rationing: the individual's belief in his/her right to unlimited medical care, the physician's maximalist approach to medical care, and the insulation of the individual from feeling the impact of the cost of treatment. Those factors produced a mass denial by society of the necessity of rationing health care services. Services have been forthcoming for so many years that the public considers it an accepted fact that medical and health resources will always be available when needed. This massive denial is a critical element in defeating efforts by Congress and organized medicine to impose solutions to bring costs under control. Without a change in the population's attitudes that acknowledges the fact that health care resources are limited, demands will continually be made to do everything possible for a patient, even in the face of the five inappropriate "U's" cited above. A full page in a popular newspaper debated the pros and cons of rationing [Cox, 1989; Kitzhaber, 1989]. In addition the paper's editorial [*USA Today*, 1989] and interviews with people on the street supported the provision of whatever care was needed.

To change these attitudes, it becomes important to modify public opinion. Churchill [1987] posits that national values are the problem in an equitable allocation of resources and America does not have the moral resources to pursue rationing as a policy. People believe that rationing can be evaded through efficiency, technological innovation, cutting the defense budget, or by outproducing our needs. As long as the majority of society believes that the system can be fine-tuned to overcome the need to ration resources, national beliefs will not change. Meanwhile, Congress and the health care sector keep trying to fine-tune the system without forcing the public to face up to the dreaded decisions involved in rationing. Ethicist Daniel Callahan [1988] commented:

> A view of reality that has optimistically declared limits to be unnecessary and even to think about them as dangerous, and that has self-righteously declared any denial of a capacity to meet some needs in an affluent society to be morally wrong, is one at war with any realistic notion of human community. That notion should encompass mutual help, mutual sacrifice and mutual limits. The present system of focusing on individual needs leaves no room for the broader needs of community as a whole. . .

From a physician provider's viewpoint, Grumet [1989] contends that health care is already rationed via the third party insurer's secret weapon—inconvenience. Rationing is achieved using eight administrative actions: procedural complexity, use of exotic terms, slowdowns, shifting of procedures, fail-safe payment systems, overlapping coverage, fragmentation of transactions, and uncertainty of coverage.

Resource allocation, as a step in the strategic health planning process, can no longer be undertaken without consideration of the serious question of the rationing of health care services. A major reason for the popularity of strategic planning is that the process operates best in a situation of scarcity or resource limits.

METHODS OF RESOURCE ALLOCATION

If the nation is operating with a scarcity of resources, there has to be methods of determining the distribution. Techniques can range from sophisticated utilization of indicators and statistics as in the RAM approach to a simple "first come first served until the supply runs out" ideology. In-between planners can use simulation games, computer modeling and mapping, survey question-naires, or creative administrative reorganizations.

Resource Allocation Methodology [RAM]

Concerned with limited resources, the Veterans Administration, the Indian Health Service, and others adopted a resource allocation method [RAM] [USDHHS, 1988]. Begun in 1985 to rationalize allocation of its resources, the VA developed RAM to overcome the disparity in allocation of its resources to its medical units. Two goals were identified by the VA: to allocate funds in accordance with the work produced and the cost to produce it, and to improve efficiency and productivity at VA medical facilities. Based on these goals, the following specific objectives were developed:

*   Allocate funds based on workload by creating standardized measures of workload.
*   Allocate funds equitably by comparing a facility's cost to produce a standard unit of work with the system average cost.
*   Support education and research.
*   Account for severity of illness by evaluating differences in degree of illness and resource consumption among similar types of patients.
*   Improve the databases to secure precise cost-per-patient information needed for an accurate assessment of a facility's cost to provide services.

To improve efficiency and productivity, the VA set three objectives:

*   Place patients appropriately.
*   Treat more patients by decreasing the average length of stay.
*   Maintain quality.

According to Roswell [1988], a VA health care administrator, the implementation of RAM "has resulted in significant improvements in the efficiency of federal health care delivery. Powerful incentives in the RAM have resulted in shortened hospital stays, greatly expanded outpatient programs and more effective utilization of limited resources."

Since 1983, the VA has seen a tremendous increase in outpatient workload, clinical complexity, and teaching responsibilities. How to respond to these changes without a commensurate increase in resources is the problem. Four major areas have been identified as targets for performance improvement: acute care, ambulatory care, long-term care, and education of physician residents.

In the VA's three-year implementation process (1985–1987), three major problems in implementing RAM were uncovered: a lack of reliable clinical data to measure workload and of financial data to measure the cost to produce it; a real question about the validity of the workload measures; and, until 1987, a lack of a monitoring system to assess the impact of RAM on the quality of care.

Major Components of RAM. There are general considerations in the RAM method. Each year the VA calculates the health care system's average cost to produce a standard measure of output called a weighted work unit [WWU]. For each of the four areas, acute, ambulatory, long-term care, and physician education, total expenditures in each area is divided by total WWUs earned in that area. Then, each facility's average cost per WWU is compared to the average for all facilities. Special salary differentials based on location of a facility in a high-cost, usually urban area, are factored into the method. For example, San Francisco personnel received a 9.3 percent salary increase beyond that of the national average. Overall, the more efficient a facility, the more resources it gains, and vice versa.

Acute care model. In three years' use of RAM, acute care's proportion of total VA funds received increased from 39 to 41 percent. DRGs are used to measure the workload. A DRG is assigned WWUs representing the expected average cost of caring for each patient in that grouping. For example, 1,000 WWUs were assigned to the most costly DRG 103 (heart transplant) in 1987. Each medical facility receives the same work unit value regardless of that unit's cost. Values are assigned only after a patient is discharged and an accurate DRG is specified. Incentives are also provided in the VA model. Psychiatric outpatient services were encouraged by overweighting the workload credit by about 44 percent. That resulted in a significant reduction in a psychiatric patient's length of stay within the facility.

Ambulatory care model. All patients are classified into one of 40 service categories, depending on their age, services provided, and number of visits. Age is an important variable in measuring workload. VA databases revealed that a patient 25 or under made 3.08 visits per year while one 85 or older made 5.95 visits. Even with multiple conditions, each patient is still placed in only one of the 40 categories with a weighted work unit value assignment. Patients are then classified into the highest cost group for which they qualify among the following five categories:

- *High psychiatry*: More than six visits to a general psychiatry clinic or more than 12 visits to a special psychiatry clinic during the year.
- *High rehabilitation*: More than six visits/year to a rehabilitation medical clinic.
- *High medicine*: More than six visits/year to a medical clinic.
- *Mid-psychiatry*: More than three visits to a general, or fewer than six to a special psychiatry, unit.
- *Standard*: Fewer than three visits/year to a general psychiatry clinic or fewer than six/year to a rehabilitation, special psychiatry, or medical clinic.

Excess visits are funded at only 50 percent of the established rate. Those using specialized clinic services such as cancer chemotherapy, radiation therapy, or computed tomography scans are credited to the medical facility on the actual cost basis.

Long-term care model. Patients are assigned to groups based on their expected use of resources rather than on a particular diagnosis. Ten resource utilization groups [RUGs] were formed by classifying patients by their degree of independence in dressing, mobility, and eating. Average nursing minutes per RUG were converted to WWUs by assigning 1,000 WWUs to the highest nursing requirement group, RUG 9; the others were weighted proportionately down to 507 work units for RUG 1. RUG 10 was given one-half the weight of RUG 1 because patients in this group were functionally independent in the three activities of daily living.

Consideration is being given to changing the weighting method by taking into account medical and behavioral characteristics in addition to functional ability. Five clinical categories are being considered:

- Heavy rehabilitation or special care (comatose or requiring nasal gastric feeding).
- Clinically complex treatments required (dialysis or chemotherapy).
- Severe behavioral problems (physical aggression or hallucinations).
- Reduced physical functioning.

Measures of functional dependence (eating, toileting, and transferring) are used to divide the clinical categories into 16 RUGs.

Education modification component. A three-tier system was adopted in 1986, indexed to the number of full-time equivalent physician residents assigned to a medical facility. A facility was categorized as:

- Fully supplemented if it had three full-time residency programs, of which two had to be in Internal Medicine and Surgery, and included 35 or more total residents or 17.5 full-time equivalents;
- Intermediately supplemented if it had 10 to 34.9 physician residents; or
- Without supplementation if it had fewer than 10 physician residents.

In 1987, this method was changed by using the reported expenditures for education and subtracting the average cost per WWU produced in unaffiliated medical centers from the similar cost in affiliated medical centers. This was used to adjust the target allowance of facilities with physician residents by $17,771/physician resident in 1987.

By taking these four component areas into account, the VA is aiming to allocate its resources in a more equitable manner.

Indian Health Service RAM. At least since 1980, the Indian Health Service [IHS] has been experimenting with various approaches to reducing the disparity in its allocation of resources to its area and subarea medical facility units. IHS finally developed a Resource Allocation Model [RAM] in the mid–1980s as shown in Exhibit 3-1. IHS's RAM is based on a different set of factors than the VA's. Exhibit 3-2 shows the four health care indices used in IHS's RAM: population, services, health status, and performance. Through an intricate weighting mechanism for each of the four indices, the RAM evolves into the formula below which ranks whether a medical facility will receive funding supplementation beyond its basic funding level and what proportion of the supplemental funds it will receive. Each component is assigned a weight, the total of which adds up to 100 percent: 50 percent for health services, 30 percent for health status, and 10 percent each for performance and population.

$$\text{Amount Allocated by each Index} = \text{Percentage Weight} \times \text{Total RAM Fund}$$

Exhibit 3-1. A Public Health Care Model: Problems; Intervention; Effects.

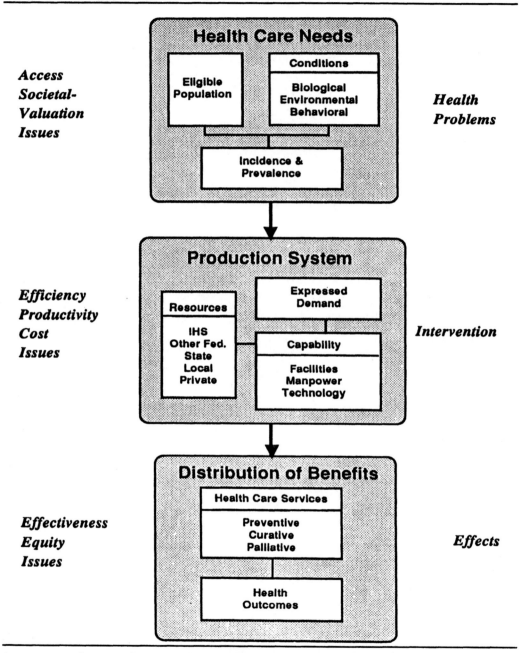

Access
Societal-
Valuation
Issues

Health
Problems

Efficiency
Productivity
Cost
Issues

Intervention

Effectiveness
Equity
Issues

Effects

Source: From *Allocation of resources*, by USDHHS, Indian Health Service, 1988, Washington, DC: Government Printing Office, p. 37. Reprinted by permission.

Exhibit 3-2.   Four Health Care Indices in Resource Allocation Method [RAM].

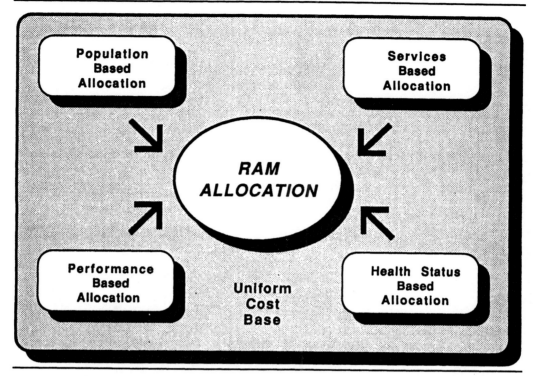

Source: From *Allocation of resources,* by USDHHS, Indian Health Service, 1988, Washington, DC: Government Printing Office, p. 56. Reprinted by permission.

Added to this basic formula is a consideration of cost which results in cost work unit workloads such as hospital admissions having 10.00 units, and primary care providers having a 1.00 unit. These are combined with the number of users to produce an expanded based formula for RAM allocation as follows:

$$\text{Allocation} = \begin{matrix}\text{Allocation}\\\text{Fraction}\\\text{for Index}\end{matrix} \times \begin{matrix}\text{Cost Index}\\\text{Adjustment}\end{matrix} \times \begin{matrix}\text{Percent}\\\text{for the}\\\text{Index}\end{matrix} \times \begin{matrix}\text{RAM}\\\text{Fund}\end{matrix}$$

This formula is expressed mathematically in Exhibit 3-3. Distribution of RAM funds is limited by applying a "qualifying hold" for each health care index. In this way, only the most needy Indian health populations and their medical facilities will be able to tap into the RAM fund.

Various factors are taken into account in computing the indices of the four components. For the RAM population index, number of users, potential user population (those who do not use Indian services because they are not available), and current Indian Health Service funding are included in the index. Health care services index includes estimation and comparison of service levels among IHS medical units, resource requirements cost projections, and level-of-need funded analysis and allocation. Health status index factors include a mortality indicator based on years of productive life lost [YPLL], a morbidity indicator, and a community income

Exhibit 3-3.   General Form of RAM Allocation Formula.

$$A_i = \sum_{j=1}^{4} F * W_j * \frac{((T_j - Q_{ji}) * X_j) * C_i}{\sum_{i=1}^{n} ((T_j - Q_{ji}) * X_j) * C_i}$$

where

A_i is the ith area RAM funding resulting from summing the individual allocations from the 4 RAM indices (j corresponds to population, services, health status, and performance indices),

F is the total amount of resources identified for the RAM fund,

W_j is the portion of the RAM fund to be distributed for the jth index,

X_j is a binary variable (0,1) which excludes areas from the RAM distribution for the jth index if their score does not exceed the threshold value T_j,

T_j is the threshold value for the jth RAM index (the score must exceed T_j in order to qualify for funding in the jth index),

Q_{ji} is the ith area raw score on the jth index and

C_i is the cost index multiplier which adjusts the allocation for area i.

Source: From *Allocation of resources*, by USDHHS, Indian Health Service, 1988, Washington, DC: Government Printing Office, p. 6. Reprinted by permission.

indicator (which serves as a proxy for the morbidity and mortality indicators for communities too small to be able to compute such an index). Finally, the RAM performance index includes manpower productivity (the average number of composite clinical work units provided per staff year), cost containment (the capacity of a medical unit to control the cost of its services based on a historical cost index), and optional performance indicators such as completeness and accuracy of patient registration data collection and initiating new programs. All of these factors are taken into account in producing the final RAM allocation for any particular community.

RAM Critics. While the methodology for the VA and Indian Health Service RAMs may be sound, critics contend that the agency's capacity to implement the method is problematical because of the difficulty obtaining reliable data or identifying valid indicators. Jemison [1988a] interviewed VA officials who commented: "The RAM is truly an Alice in Wonderland methodology . . . It is gamed to death . . . the RAM methodology has been manipulated repeatedly to protect 'flagship' VA hospitals." In fact, late in 1988, it was announced that the VA's RAM was "being sent back to the drawing board" to be partially replaced by a "patient priority" realloaction formula [Jemison, 1988b]. A General Accounting Office [GAO] study [Baine, 1989] concluded that the RAM "has had little impact on the [VA] medical centers' budgets."

Nevertheless, these resource allocation methods probably do point in the right direction. Federal government units are providing leadership in an effort at fairness, quality, and equitability in providing health care services for their patient populations.

Drug Abuse Prevention Program

Resource allocation in a drug abuse prevention program is illustrated in Exhibit 3-4. Unlike RAM, this is a much simpler, more subjective technique for determining the use and allocation of resources. In this method, a judgment is made in comparing all the resources needed in terms of personnel, skills, and financing, and their availability. If an imbalance exists between require-

Exhibit 3-4.   Resource Analysis Worksheet.

Objective: Increase number of volunteers in prevention programs by 33 percent by 8/1/91

Activities	Gather Information	Produce TV Spots	Distribute TV Spots
		Media Campaign	
Completion Date	Sept. 15, 1990	Nov. 30, 1990	Dec. 27, 1990
Resources Required			
No. of persons	1 for month	6 for 3 mos. ea.	1 for 6 weeks
Skills	Research	Advertising	Meeting people, under-standing media program
Funds	$800 car mileage, phone	$37,000	$650 mileage
Other	Photocopying	Complete production	None
Resources Available			
No. of persons	Hather available	1 for 3 months	Speedy OK
Skills	OK	No	OK
Funds	$800 OK	$37,000 OK	$650 OK
Other	OK	No	OK
Discrepancies	None	Skills and equipment for TV spot production	None
Comments	—	Subcontract to Hot Shots, Inc., for production	—
Total cost, this phase = $38,450			

ments and resource availability, the strategic planner has three options: Restructure the activity by finding alternative methods for achieving the activity or focusing the activity a little differently; reevaluate the feasibility of undertaking the activity because an indispensable resource may not be available; or request training or technical assistance, especially if deficiencies in staff skills exist.

Because this method is based on experience and subjective judgments, the technique can readily be used with representatives of an institution's trustees, staff, and service users to determine which of the three alternatives to use when resources do not match need.

Resources Allocation Simulation in Model Locality

Taking gaming seriously, Folmer [1987] describes a simulation in health resources allocation. Beginning with a model of a rural area of 500,000 residents, any type of health care delivery system can be created. Given information about the area includes a map with geographical features, population distribution, demographics, socioeconomics, morbidity causes, costs of resources, and the annual budget.

During the initial stage of the game, participants meet separately in groups of four to five. Each group considers preventive and curative coverage, quality of care, mortality prevention, and morbidity reduction. When all the groups decide on their resource allocations and place their choices on their map with plastic symbols, the first stage of the game is ended.

In the second stage of the game, each group has to plan for a sample of 200 people seeking care. Ailments range from trivial to serious and the level is indicated on each person's card. Each group is given the frequency of the illness plus the appropriate treatment modalities. This stage ends when each group categorizes all the problems of the 200 people into one of three choices: level too high, level right, or level too low. Participants in the simulation can combine the unfeeling statistics with experiencing the emotional impact of "standing in the shoes" of a parent with a sick child seeking relief.

For the final stage of the game, the outcomes and experiences of all the groups are discussed. Results can be reviewed in comparable, quantified terms using formulae and disease reduction curves.

This game can take one or two days depending upon the interest and experience of the participants. While the simulation remains constant in the basic setup, new trends and concepts can be added as events change.

Computer Simulation of Emergency Room Use

With the use of a computer and the General Purpose Simulation System [GPSS] language, a strategic planner simulates utilization in the emergency room of a pediatric hospital [Klafehn & Owens, 1987]. Administrators of the hospital are considering expansion plans and contemplating future needs of their emergency room. Using data that simulates the flow of patients through the emergency room, the planners are able to come to a tentative conclusion. They find that more patients would complete their treatment in a shorter time through using a second orthopedic group rather than only the existing one. Further analysis confirms a major drop in the length of stay for all patients. However, there are a significant number of patients for whom the length of stay in the emergency department will not decrease. These contradictions create some ambiguity in the findings requiring a longer period of simulation to determine the appropriate course of action.

This case example of computer simulation reveals both the positive possibilities of simulation as well as the limitations and ambiguities.

In a related computer simulation, Liss, Moller, and Sandblod [1986] describe a simulation-based system for regional planning of care resources in oncology in Sweden. Using the program, it is possible to plan for the long-term effects of projected variations in the care system structure, in care services, and in the incidence of the illness. Input for this technique includes program data, incidence/prognosis data, organizational data, a resource lexicon, and the simulation algorithm. This particular simulation "describes the studied care unit in enough detail to be of great use in the planning process."

Computer Mapping of Resources

Another graphic method highlights resource considerations in geographic areas. With the use of mapping overlays, correlations between needs and resources can readily be identified. In a comprehensive review, Gesler [1986] summarizes the techniques and terms used in spatial analysis along with the method's shortcomings. Spatial analytic techniques include point patterns, line patterns, area patterns, surface patterns, map comparisons, and relative spaces. Though strictly spatial and quantitative methods may be limited, the use of several together can shed light on health care resource allocation problems.

Harvard University's Laboratory for Computer Graphics is a prime resource for obtaining software to generate and plot all types of health-related maps. An example of a graphic map [Exhibit 3-5] shows the market penetration rates by zip code areas in greater Boston. Exhibit 3-6 reveals heart condition mortality rates for the elderly in Alabama. Overlaying a health resource facility map upon the computer graphic will quickly pinpoint where services are needed to lower the high area mortality rates identified by the color codes.

Poizner [1986] describes the computer mapping programs and software utilized by Strategic Locations Planning Consultants [Burbank, CA]. He states that the five following basic components are required to develop microcomputer maps:

- A computer with graphics capabilities
- An output device (monitor, printer or plotter)
- A data file
- A boundary file
- Mapping software.

In addition, Poizner points out that mapping is used for six basic functional tasks: site location analysis, target market studies, trade area analysis, sales performance monitoring and sales territory design, government resource planning, and market research data display. Obviously, a number of these mapping functions are relevant for strategic health planning.

Two simple methods of spatial analysis and their applications in location-oriented health services research are described by Kahn [1986]. Cartographic analysis uses map comparisons to detail specific spatial patterns and to propose pertinent theories based on locational relationship among the mapped phenomena. Centrographic analysis goes on to even further define the characteristics of a point distribution and also generates a graphic summary, the Standard Deviational Ellipse [SDE]. An SDE yields a handy direct comparison of multiple spatial patterns. Used in conjunction, the two methods can be particularly useful in analysis of locational characteristics of health care personnel and facilities as well as in access to health care decisions.

Exhibit 3-5.   Market Penetration Rates by Zip Code: Boston.

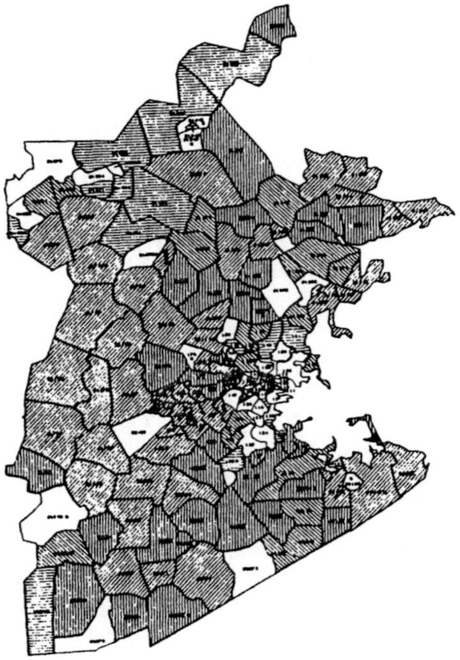

Market penetration rates by Time Magazine in Boston, using zip codes as the basis for geographic segmentation. Graphics prepared by Demographic Research Company. From **Executive Introduction to Computer Mapping,** by Allan Schmidt.

Source: From a brochure on Computer Graphics Week, by Laboratory for Computer Graphics, Harvard University, 1980. Reprinted with permission.

Thouez, Bodson, and Joseph [1988] use mapped patterns of potential accessibility and a graphic display of the delivery system's potential effectiveness to measure geographic access in rural regions of Canada. As Exhibit 3-7 indicates, only modest data information about the location of services and client populations is required for this method.

Self-Administered Questionnaires

In a study of five hospitals in Scotland to determine accessibility to rural versus urban hospitals, Parkin and Henderson [1987] used a self-administered questionnaire. Although the findings revealed that it took a shorter time for patients and their visitors to travel to rural hospitals, cost savings required that the smaller rural hospitals be closed in favor of using the larger urban ones. Closing the rural hospital would result in a savings of 500 pounds for each patient. This led to two basic issues regarding resource allocation. First, is it fair to the rural populations to save funds at their expense when they will not receive 500 pounds of alternative services such as

Exhibit 3-6.   Acute Myocardial Infarction Death Rates by County, Alabama.

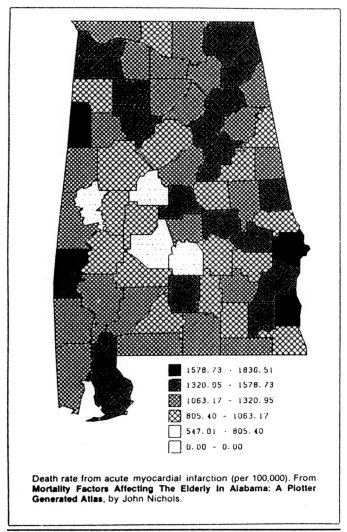

Death rate from acute myocardial infarction (per 100,000). From **Mortality Factors Affecting The Elderly In Alabama: A Plotter Generated Atlas**, by John Nichols.

Source: From a brochure on Computer Graphics Week, by Laboratory for Computer Graphics, Harvard University, 1980. Reprinted with permission.

roads or education? Secondly, should the National Health Service pursue an objective of equity in resource allocation? In sum, the study revealed how the values of cost and equity can get confused in the stated goals of a national health service. Parkin and Henderson [1987] conclude that "decision makers must decide how much weight should be given to equity, to costs falling on patients, to under-utilization, for what sort of equity the NHS should strive, and in what services health boards/authorities should be self-sufficient."

Exhibit 3-7.   Supply and Potential Spatial Accessibility of General Practitioner Services in Abitibi-Temiscamingue, Canada.

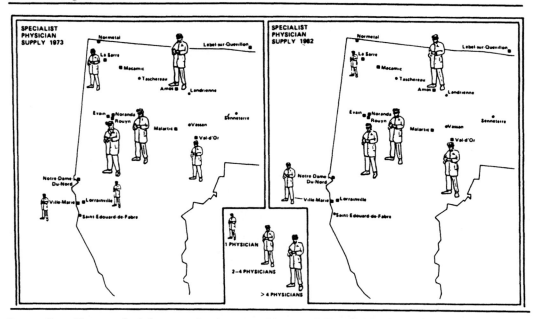

Source: From "Some methods for measuring the geographic accessibility of medical services in rural regions," by J.M. Thouez, P. Bodson, & A.E. Joseph, 1988, *Medical Care*, 26(1), 34–43. Reprinted with permission of Lippincott/Harper & Row.

Structural Method for Increasing Resources

As health care providers, particularly hospitals, find themselves under increasing pressure to maintain their viability, affiliation arrangements added operating resources [Reid, Fulcher, & Smith, 1986]. One affiliation variable involves relationships with managed health care plans such as health maintenance organizations [HMOs], preferred provider organizations [PPOs], and individual practice associations [IPAs]. Managed health care plans have grown rapidly in recent years for two reasons: their cost-containment attractiveness to employers, and the hospitals' competition for patients in an era of DRGs and reduced hospital census. Exhibit 3-8 defines the five characteristics of health care plans: contractual responsibilities; defined enrollment; voluntary membership; fixed periodic payment; and assumption of risk. The larger the enrolled membership of a health care plan in the hospital's catchment area, the stronger its negotiating leverage in obtaining better prices for its members. Furthermore, in areas where hospitals are in competition with each other, the plans will also have a stronger bargaining role. "It is imperative that hospital managers develop effective strategies for interacting with these plans and aggressively seek the establishment of productive relationships with them. Failure to act in a timely manner may erode current market share and provide an unnecessary threat to long-term survivability" [Reid, Fulcher, & Smith, 1986]. Forging contractual relationships with managed health care plans will put hospitals in a position to expand their patient population resource.

PEOPLEPOWER, MANPOWER, AND PERSONNEL

According to Fottler, Hernandez, and Joiner [1988], links exist between strategic decision making, organizational design, behavioral systems, and human resources management in health services organizations. Topics in their book include planning, recruitment, training, performance appraisal, and the impact of technology on health care personnel. In a labor-intensive industry such as health care, a critical dimension of resource allocation obviously involves the personnel employed by health care providers. In a period of limited resources, planning must consider personnel availability, situations of over- and under-supply, standardization of units of service to ensure efficient use, maintaining morale, and work station locations. Trivedi, Moscovice, Bass, and Brooks [1987] use a semi-Markov model to plan for the services of physicians, nurse practitioners, and physician assistants among different settings and geographic sites in a health care provider's system. Gallina [1989] used a Nominal Group technique to resolve a shortage of pharmacy personnel. Since physicians are dominant in the health care system, recruiting, developing, and nurturing of physicians usually has the highest priority among health care providers, followed by registered nurses and allied health staff.

Physician Hiring Process

With a projected oversupply of physicians and a limited patient potential for certain specialties, it becomes critical for health administrators to make rational decisions when physicians request medical staff privileges [Langstaff, 1987]. Credentialing in hospitals is no longer a "rubber stamp" process. According to one official: "Hospital boards are more selective about the physicians they allow to use hospital facilities, and they are holding physicians accountable for the resources they consume and for the quality of care they provide" [Cohen, 1986].

Exhibit 3-8.   Five Defining Characteristics of Health Care Plans.

Characteristics	Implications
Contractual Responsibilities	• HCP physician acts as informed purchasing agent for client, concerned with both the quality and costs of care • HCP administration addresses policy and financial matters with client • HCP hospital increases admission and collection efficiencies with potentially reduced bad debt expenses
Defined Enrollment	• Provides HCP providers with access to prescribed client groups • Provides demographic characteristics of HCP members
Voluntary Membership	• Comprehensive product must be offered at a competitive price • HCP hospital must deliver cost-efficient services and maintain favorable reputation to remain affiliated • HCP hospital may be actively involved in marketing efforts
Fixed Periodic Payment	• HCP requires minimal enrollments • HCP administration seeks provider affiliates that minimize health care costs
Assumption of Risk	• Risks assumed by HCP components reflect respective bargaining strengths • HCP hospital's risk is manifested in its negotiated payment scheme

Source: From "Hospital-health care plan affiliations: Considerations for strategy design," by R.A. Reid, J.H. Fulcher, & H.L. Smith, 1986. Reprinted from *Health Care Management Review, 11*(4), 55 with permission of Aspen Publishers Inc. Copyright Fall 1986.

Medical Planning and Impact Analysis

MPIA [Medical Manpower Planning/Impact Analysis] is a process to assist hospital officials in selecting physician appointments [Langstaff, 1987]. Exhibit 3-9 identifies the MPIA process. Key to the process is the involvement of the institution's chief executive officer [CEO]. This commitment is shown by the CEO calling for a retreat to develop a strategic mission statement and clinical role strategy for the institution. Included in the plan is an MPIA form, an administrative process for MPIA, and an ongoing evaluation and monitoring process. Information is also required related to the prospective physician's status, research, teaching and clinical interest, space and equipment requirements, and a profile of his/her past clinical practice. MPIA strategic plans are mechanisms that can assist chiefs of staff in identifying the institution's patterns of clinical practice.

GMENAC Study of Physician Resources

Even with an MPIA, the dynamics of physician mobility makes it difficult to balance out the supply with the demand for services. A major report, issued by the Graduate Medical Education National Advisory Committee [GMENAC] in 1980, attempted to establish the need for physician personnel through the year 2,000 [Tarlov, 1986]. Using a fairly sophisticated methodology to project needs, the GMENAC essentially predicted that an oversupply of physicians would begin to occur in the late 1980s and rise to 13 percent by 1990. Essentially, the GMENAC supply estimates were based on four steps:

First: Using a baseline year, the number of physicians available minus those who were expected to die, become disabled, and retire by the years 1990 and 2000 was calculated.

Second: New U.S. graduates, including those who transferred from foreign schools to complete their medical education and residencies in the United States and expected to continue to practice in the United States during the 1990–2000 year period, were added.

Third: Those graduating from foreign medical schools and expecting to continue their practice in the United States after completing their U.S. residencies were added.

Fourth: Residents in training in terms of their full-time equivalent activities, computed as 0.35 service of a full-time physician were added.

These four components added up to the supply of physicians available for 1990 and 2000. Assumptions were made about physician attrition rates and percentage of foreign-educated physicians remaining in the United States to continue their medical practice. Three models were tested in developing the projections: the demand model, the needs model, and the adjusted model. Based on current utilization of medical services, the demand model adjusts current standards of care for population growth. Critics say this model "perpetuates today's limitations and inequities into the future" [Tarlov, 1986]. On the other hand, the needs model takes into account the total incidence or prevalence of disease in the entire population. That model may overestimate illness requiring physician attention. Finally, the adjusted model used by GMENAC takes both limitations into account and includes a percentage of those with illness who seek and those who do not seek medical attention.

Physicians were divided into three components or compartments: the number of physicians employed by the federal government; those not in the federal government but in solo,

Exhibit 3-9.   Medical Manpower Planning/Impact Analysis
Flow Process.

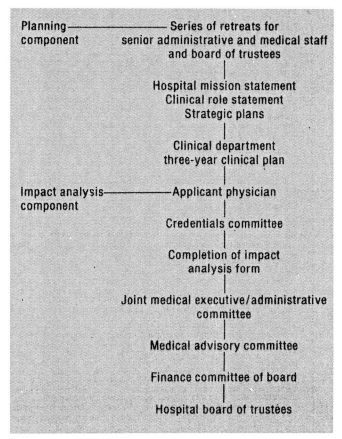

Planning————————— Series of retreats for
component   senior administrative and medical staff
                            and board of trustees

                            Hospital mission statement
                            Clinical role statement
                            Strategic plans

                            Clinical department
                            three-year clinical plan

Impact analysis—————————Applicant physician
component

                            Credentials committee

                            Completion of impact
                            analysis form

                    Joint medical executive/administrative
                                committee

                            Medical advisory committee

                            Finance committee of board

                            Hospital board of trustees

Source: From "Medical manpower planning/impact analysis, by J.H.
Langstaff, 1987, *Dimensions in Health Services*, 64, 31. Reprinted
with permission of the Canadian Hospital Association.

group, and fee-for-service practices; and those staffing health maintenance organizations. This
third component resulted in controversy over the reliability of the projections. When the study
was completed in 1980, HMO-related physicians made up a minimal percentage of all physicians. However, that percentage greatly increased. Projections to the year 2000 indicate that
HMO related physicians may number about 144,000 people serving 120 million persons, or 44
percent of the population. As the HMO physicians increase, this component can no longer be
viewed as an insignificant factor in physician supply forecasts.

Of particular importance is the fact that HMO physicians serve a far higher ratio of the
population than do federal/nonfederal physicians. While it takes 323 federal/nonfederal physicians to serve 100,000 persons, 120 HMO physicians can duplicate that feat (Tarlov, 1986).
Obviously, that fact and the sheer increase in numbers of HMO physicians will radically alter

the projections of the GMENEC for the year 2000. If the present supply continues as projected, the oversupply will be far higher than originally anticipated.

GMENAC Recommendations. Recommendations flowing from the GMENEC called for decreasing medical school enrollment by 17 percent, restricting the entry of foreign medical school educated physicians, holding the number of nonphysician health care providers steady, and making adjustments in specialties to reflect their needs for the 1990s [Iglehart, 1986]. These recommendations have met with mostly quiet and invisible resistance from the American Medical Association and key members of Congress concerned with special constituencies. "Congress wants it both ways—that is, it wants to shrink federal support for medical education but is resisting other steps that constituents might regard as limiting access to care. The AAMC [Association of American Medical Colleges] and the medical schools will remain steadfast in their opposition to paring their classes. . . " [Iglehart, 1986]. State legislators likewise prefer to maintain their medical schools and the prestige it brings to the state, even at the expense of becoming a party to the oversupply of physicians.

Validity of Resource Projections. Health analysts studying Canadian physician supply forecasts and comparing them to the GMENEC Report find the GMENEC methodology to be more sophisticated and accurate than the Canadian methods [Lomas, Stoddart, & Barer 1985]. Yet, serious flaws and limitations in all the methods cast doubt on their reliability and validity. Structurally, shortcomings result from the narrow bias of the physician-dominated membership of the committees that examined only physicians as suppliers of medical care services. Consequently, nurses, allied health practitioners, and physician assistants were ignored. Further, the reports failed to distinguish among physicians who could perform like functions such as anestheologist and general practitioner, both capable of administering anesthesia services. Double counts may occur when general practitioners are counted both in the anesthesiology specialty and in their own leading to reliability problems.

Validity questions arise over the definition of productivity. As more physicians become available, will they work longer or shorter hours and spend more or less time with their patients? Are the productivity measures used in 1980 valid for 1990 and the year 2000? Fifer (1987) addressed that question as he considered 15 attributes of the hospital medical staff of 1997. Noting a future era of "finite resources and virtually limitless demand," Fifer concludes: "Practitioners will have to decide how much health care is enough and will have to identify appropriate substitute health care methods that preserve resources without sacrificing quality."

A vital issue regarding the validity of the supply projections is the narrow lens through which the GMENEC committees viewed the future. Had they accepted the fact of limited medical resources, then the question is not "How many physicians will be needed?" but rather "What is the best mix of resources and to which health priorities should these be addressed?" This is a strategic health planning issue, not a mere forecasting one. In planning, there are tradeoffs between goals and objectives and the resources required to achieve them.

If the committees had taken a public interest perspective, they might have concluded that fewer physicians are needed and more sanitarians and housing inspectors are required to safeguard and improve the health of the population. In a like fashion, more health educators and nurse practitioners may be needed to serve the primary health care needs of the population. Taking either of these as priority objectives alters the supply of physicians required. As the health analysts concluded, "failure to place physician forecasting in this broader context can only lead to inevitable impediments to the development of more innovative approaches to the delivery of service" [Lomas, Stoddart, & Barer, 1985]. Carrying out a strategic health planning process could yield different results.

Responses to Personnel Supply Projections

Several responses can be made to medical personnel projections. Possibly, the forecasts are inaccurate and a deficit of personnel actually exists. Alternatively, existing personnel can be used more efficiently. Third, what impact, if any, will the shortage have on the health status of the population? Finally, where actual oversupply exists, alternative uses of personnel can be identified.

Shortage of Personnel Response. A July 1988 news story, one of many surfacing at that time, states that 90 percent of Massachusett's hospitals are unable to fill their staff vacancies. Specialty shortages include family practice physicians, obs/gyn specialists, neurologists, surgeons, and emergency physicians [Abraham, 1988]. As vacancies occur, those remaining on staff must work harder to take up the slack, resulting in frustration and physician burnout. That vicious cycle is further compounded by the high cost of liability insurance, state-mandated limits on physician income, and excessive state regulations. With the spread of AIDS in many large urban areas, hospital beds as well as physicians and nurses to serve those patients are frequently in short supply.

Similar reports exist regarding nurses and allied health practitioners. One study found 80 percent of the VA's 167 facilities reporting a shortage of nurses; 30 percent of the facilities stating the condition was severe [*US Medicine*, 1988a]. While there is a general shortage of registered nurses, the situation in the VA is more severe because of their noncompetitive salary and benefit packages compared to proprietary and nonprofit hospitals. Among the VA hospitals, RNs make up 67 percent of the nursing staff, with licensed practical nurses, nurses' aides, and orderlies composing the remaining 33 percent [McCormick, 1986]. Thus, any severe shortage has a serious impact on patient care. A national advisory panel estimated that up to 200,000 registered nurses were needed immediately or "the health of this nation will be at risk" [Gianelli, 1988].

In addition to nursing shortages, reports also note the increasing vacancies in allied health positions [Bradley, 1988; Page, 1988b; Institute of Medicine, 1988; Tolchin, 1988]. Openings for allied health personnel are expected to increase substantially at the same time that the American Medical Association reports a 20 percent reduction of enrollment in allied health programs. Shortages also occur in the fields of physical therapy, radiology, medical records, and occupational therapy. Reasons for this shortage include the low status accorded to the practitioners, low pay compared to other professions, repetitive work assignments, and extremely limited training funds.

A 1963–1980 retrospective study revealed that the availability of patient care physicians increased in both poverty and nonpoverty areas. Growth was greater in nonpoverty areas; office-based primary care declined by 45 percent in poverty areas and 27 percent in nonpoverty areas. Even if an oversupply occurs, there is little certainty that the physician specialty and geographic maldistribution would correct itself to provide an adequate supply of physicians in urban poverty communities [Kindig, Manassuzin, & Cross Dunham, 1987].

Innovative, Alternative Use of Existing Personnel. There is a tendency to lock health care personnel into the specialty for which they are trained. There is an assumption that a staff member in one position cannot carry out some, if not all, of the functions of another specialty. That assumption inhibits using personnel flexibly by shifting them from an area of temporary oversupply to one of shortage. Efforts to train multiskilled allied health practitioners have been stymied by some basic obstacles [Blayney, 1986]. Among the obstacles are human nature's reluctance to change, resistance of encroachment of one specialty by another, and educational institutions desiring to maintain their own identity by sticking to their own specialty and accreditation.

Registered Care Technologist [RCT]. Multiskilled personnel are especially needed in small and rural hospitals and would be welcomed by physicians seeking this type of flexibility in allied health staff. Exhibit 3-10 identifies a number of combinations of skills that can be linked together such as nurses with respiratory and laboratory testing skills or purchasing staff adding skills to become materials handlers and transportation staff. One step in this direction emanates from the American Medical Association's endorsement of a new position, the Registered Care Technologist [RCT] [Page, 1988a]. An RCT would take up the slack of RNs who have mostly given up wanting to provide bedside care and/or taking patients' requests for services. "An RCT's role is task oriented designed to focus on medical orders at the bedside" [*US Medicine*, 1988b]. This would help relieve the nursing shortage and provide a modest career ladder as RCTs demonstrate their capacity to progress into more responsible positions in the complex environment of a highly technical hospital. In addition, the RCT concept must make use of basic corporate management personnel strategies.

Not surprisingly, the national advisory panel on nursing did not endorse the RCT concept [Gianelli, 1988]. Professional nursing organizations and leaders lobbied strongly against the demonstration project viewing it as an encroachment on their functions. In fact, the Federation of Nurses and Health Professionals [FNHP] labeled the AMA's RCT "unlicensed staff" [*Healthwire*, 1989a, 1989b]. FNHP also supported U.S. Representative Wyden's position opposing RCTs [*Healthwire*, 1989c].

Within the realm of innovation, management expert Peter F. Drucker [1954] long ago expounded that hospitals must demand high performance, pile on information, and encourage development of managerial vision. Only by creating a challenging environment will hospitals be able to keep their employees.

Impact of Personnel Shortage on Health Status. A major concern about health personnel shortages relates to a potential negative impact on the population's health status. A three-year study of British Columbia's nursing shortage revealed some interesting insights [Barer, Stark, & Kinnis, 1984]. From 1980–1982, there were 1,823 difficult-to-fill nursing positions, that is, vacancies that were unfilled for 30 or more days: 4.6 months was the average period of the vacancy. Cardiothoracic nurse vacancies averaged a low of 2.8 months while surgery nurses averaged 5.8 months. Over 50 percent of the vacancies went unfilled for more than four months and 21 percent for more than six months. Most of the long-term vacancies were attributed to new positions opening rather than a continuation of existing vacancies. Further, in a three-month period toward the end of the study, the number of vacancies dropped from a high of 217 to a low of just 18. What accounts for this precipitous drop in vacancies? Of the 217 positions vacant in March, seven were eliminated [canceled or frozen]. In April, another 82 were eliminated, followed by 17 in May. Another 150 vacancies were actually filled during this period.

Key to understanding the cause of this vacancy reduction was the cost-containment policy

**Exhibit 3-10. Combination of Skills Identified by Employers
As Meeting Their Needs**

1. Nursing + limited respiratory services + radiologic skills + laboratory tests [i.e. in urgent care centers]
2. Radiographic technology generalized to a greater degree rather than the current specialization + ultrasound
3. Secretarial in laboratory area + phlebtomist duties
4. Medical technology + more microbiology skills
5. Cardiovascular laboratory + X-ray + respiratory therapy
6. Purchasing + pharmacology
7. Radiography + laboratory technology
8. Nuclear medicine + X-ray technology
9. Arterial blood gas studies + laboratory work
10. Medical records skills + risk management
11. Nursing + infection control + employee health + education and training
12. Dietetics + patient education [e.g. exercises, diet].
13. Purchasing + materials handling + transport
14. Operating room + recovery + intensive care unit

Soruce: From "Restructuring the health care labor force. The rise of the multi-skilled allied health practitioner," by K.D. Blayney, 1986, *Alabama Journal of Medical Sciences, 23*[3], 278. Reprinted with permission.

instituted by the Minister of Health in early 1982, curtailing use of funds to pay for personnel positions. Although there was no empirical evidence, policy analysts did not perceive any deterioration in the health status of the population even though news stories shrilly predicted dire consequences because of the nursing shortage. In sum, there may be no real correlation between long-term vacancies and diminished health status.

Supply and Demand Homeostasis. In a provocative article regarding homeostasis, in which an "organism behaves in a fashion which either attempts to maintain or achieve home-ostasis within a changing environment," the authors attempt to show what happens when the system or organism goes out of balance [Salmon & Culbertson, 1985]. What are the options open to physicians or nurse practitioners if the supply exceeds the demand for their services? What will or can be done to achieve a new homeostasis or balance between supply and demand?

Three options are open to the organism or system: (a) defend itself against the perceived threat [involution], (b) accommodate itself to the new environment by making adjustments within its own system or organism, or (c) take offense [innovation] by creating new opportunities for itself. Pathways open to professional organizations and their members under these three options aim their efforts at finding a new balance or integration between supply and demand forces.

Physicians have the most power, control, legal means, authority, and status to use all three options to achieve a balance between their own oversupply and creating new demands for their services [Salmon & Culbertson, 1985]. Involution strategies show that physicians are beginning to locate in rural and inner-urban areas taking over functions previously engaged in by nurse practitioners. Innovation options create new specialities or subspecialties or take on new roles in industrial, space, or wellness health care programs. Compared to nurses, physicians have a greater number of options.

Nurse practitioners and physician assistants do have some assets for dealing with any oversupply that may be created by physicians preempting their positions. Among these are social appeal, political influence because of their numbers, and pre-empting lower-level practice positions such as licensed practical nurses. However, barriers to change are also quite formidable as indicated by the dependence on physicians and institutions for positions, the limited power compared to physicians, lack of legal status, few resources, and lower status qualifications and training. Compared to physicians, the strategies of involution and accommodation are limited because of the dependence status. Their most important option for finding a new balance or homeostasis would rest on innovation [or offense]. Nursing shortages stimulate work mobility, or the ability to move into new areas of practice such as managing wellness programs, administering HMOs, and coordinating/consulting with corporations on health promotion. If nurses and other allied health personnel are aggressive they can readily move into new areas and dominate them before physicians, blinded by their concern for status, recognize the opportunities. As the health analysts note in their model, a final outcome of this struggle for achieving a new balance is extinction.

Efficient and Productive Use of Personnel

In an era of restricted resources, it is incumbent on management to use its resources in an efficient manner. Employee motivation and morale factors can be analyzed and adjusted to increase staff productivity [Gunn & Kazemek, 1986; Tabatabai, 1987]. However, Conner, Neuman, and Graham [1988] point out the complexity of the task and note that there is a "productivity fad." These authors issue a warning and tell how to avoid "productivity Nirvana" in health care. Being members of a national accounting firm, Conner et al. [1988] define optimum productivity, productivity capacity, work unit characteristics, and relate their formulae to a strategic and tactical focus.

In spite of all the data health institutions collect, information is seldom collected in a systematic manner on the behavior of their own personnel. Kelliher [1985] maintains that adequate information can assist administrators to manage productivity, performance, and the cost of services. "Labor consumption on allocation bases must be established to perform cost accounting." Aram, Salipante, and Knauf [1987] believe it is important for managers to have such information to develop indicators of human resource management effectiveness. Considering that patients may need light, moderate, or heavy levels of care, efficient personnel use is critical. Roddy, Liu, and Meiners [1987] report that heavy care patients require 2.5 times more staff effort than light care patients. Their study of 36 proprietary skilled nursing facilities over 30 months related the level of care to the time and amount of assistance with activities of daily living such as dressing, eating, bathing, toileting, and mobility.

Employee Performance Indicators. Health care managers may seldom get involved in articulating policy related to personnel conflict. By collecting data on personnel actions over time and across units within and between facilities, it is possible to spot trends and make comparisons that may call for action. Four primary indicators of potential conflict and personnel dissatisfaction are critical: withdrawal behavior, internal grievance actions initiated by employees; supervisory disciplinary actions, and individual and unit performance ratings.

Withdrawal indicators such as illness, outside activities affecting the employee, or discipline evidence an employee's degree of satisfaction with their department and/or position. Employee requests for transfers out of the unit are a particularly important indicator of dissatisfaction. A large number of grievances clearly shows dissatisfaction and employee unrest.

Supervisory disciplinary actions, on a four-point scale of severity, include a verbal warning, a written warning, suspension without pay or termination. Depending on the severity, disciplinary actions reveal how well staff members are adjusting to their work and to the organization.

Performance indicators such as merit raises, patients per staff or work produced per employee can be used to measure how well an individual or complement of employees are doing. Health care administrators should also be aware of continued on-the-job rewards such as desk accessories, theater tickets, personal jewelry, and a wide variety of meal opportunities. In addition, managers must be alert that natural rewards such as a friendly greeting, pat on the back, smile, or a verbal compliment also means a great deal to employees [Shortell & Kaluzny, 1988, p. 119]. Furthermore, salary is not everything. Bassett and Metzger [1986, p. 30] report that good wages was rated number 5 by employees in 1946 and in 1980. Number 1 in 1946 was "full appreciation of work done" and "interesting work" in 1980. Interestingly, supervisors ranked "good wages" number one in both years. However, data should be collected and analyzed on all four components of human resource indicators to enable managers to gauge the positive or negative status of the health care provider's work environment.

Efficiency can also be achieved by using lower cost personnel who are capable of performing a similar type of function as higher cost staff. Use of prospective payment reimbursement via DRGs places pressure on administrators to provide a quality service at a lower cost. Physicians, nurse practitioners, and physician assistants can all take medical histories and do physical examinations. Efficiency dictates that the lower cost personnel carry out these functions. Health care providers such as health maintenance organizations, home health agencies, and urgicenters are cost-conscious and prone to use less costly staff where possible. "As the significant cost advantages in the utilization of these practitioners [nurse practitioners and physician assistants] whenever or wherever possible is realized by health care administrators, it is likely that the ability of the medical profession to preserve their market share by exerting economic and political pressures may diminish" [Leiken & McTernan, 1985].

Standard Costs for Activities. To develop efficiency in the use of health personnel and thereby extend health resources, health care providers must know the standard costs for each unit of activity related to patient care [Bennett, 1985]. Information systems need to be able to:

- Compare the cost effect of changes in case mix.
- Measure or evaluate the cost effect of clinical management decisions.
- Compare or evaluate the cost effect of alternative treatment and operational methods.

Standards are usually developed for direct labor [hourly rates to perform a procedure and expected time to perform the task re an efficiency standard], direct material and supply standards [expected prices and amount of materials and supplies to perform the required tasks], and operational overhead standards [variables that fluctuate with changes in output volume and fixed variables that do not change with volume output]. Each of these variables can be measured using the following four potential levels:

- Basic standard—does not change over time and is seldom used.
- Theoretical or ideal standard—best possible performance under existing conditions with existing equipment.
- Currently attainable standards—allowance made for idle or down time.
- Average past performance standards—past serves as basis for standards.

"Currently attainable standards" are most often used because they permit employees to achieve goals set for them.

To implement a standard cost system, the following actions are necessary:

• Involve top management to develop and sustain the system.
• Develop a strategic action plan, showing data needs, goals, and trustee expectations.
• Carry out scientific studies of patient care departments to identify the most effective ways of achieving the most important prospective payment classifications necessary for carrying out the institution's objectives.
• Identify fixed and variable costs related to each patient care department overhead and allocation. As determined by accounting, operations, and clinical staff working together.
• Review standards for reasonableness by departments and management.
• Periodic reviews and upgrading of standards should be constant.

Exhibit 3-11 illustrates how the three categories of cost come together to produce a Patient Care Unit [PCU], a unit of service where cost information is related to a clinical application. Several of these PCUs accumulate into a resource consumption profile [RCP] for each DRG. For example, under direct variable labor costs, an RN will work 4.05 hours at $7.36 to cost $29.81 worth of resources to produce this unit of work, a physician $25.00 and a LPN $7.89. Additional indirect variable and fixed costs for other personnel are also factored into the production of this service and costs $221.90 at this health institution. Total PCU cost, direct and indirect, for this procedure is $382.23, representing the "currently attainable standard" for this procedure at this institution. Eight or more PCUs may have to be added together to produce the total cost of one DRG. Management can ask the following three test questions to determine whether a specific PCU should be developed:

• Relevance test—Does the cost of an item make a difference?
• Collectibility test—Can the data be collected in a cost-effective manner?
• Meaning test—Will knowing the cost have any impact on decision making?

If the answer is "no" to any of these questions, it is not likely the PCU will make a difference to the health care provider's management.

A standard cost-accounting system provides several advantages:

1. Budgets can be readily prepared from standard costs.
2. Accurate cost information for decision making is provided in the areas of pricing, profitability level, and performance.
3. Management and clinical staff that worked together to develop the PCUs will also be motivated to maintain them.
4. Management can measure performance and cost control by comparing PCU's to actual costs incurred.

There are also disadvantages to a standard cost-accounting system:

1. There may be too much reliance on standard costs without comparing them to actual costs.
2. Untrained staff can impair the operation of the system.
3. Failure to collect proper data will prevent development and maintenance of the system.
4. Standards may not be kept current and thus lose their effectiveness.

**Exhibit 3-11. A Patient Care Unit Example—
Portable Acute Hemodialysis.**

Category	Quantity	Unit Cost	Cost
Labor			
1. Direct [variable]			
• Physician	—	—	$25.00
• RN	4.05 hrs.	$7.36	29.81
• LPN	1.25	6.31	7.89
2. Indirect [variable]			
• Physician	—	—	—
• RN	2.66 hrs.	7.36	19.28
• LPN	1.39	6.31	8.77
3. Indirect [fixed]			
• Physician	—	—	—
• RN	6.99 hrs.	7.36	51.45
• LPN	5.04	6.31	31.80
• Clerical	4.62	4.77	22.04
4. Vacation, holiday, sickness	4.05	6.38	24.86
Subtotal			$221.90
Direct Material			
1. Artificial kidney			
• Gambro-17/13.5	1.00 ea	24.95	24.95
2. Standard supply profile	1.00	38.04	38.04
Subtotal			$62.99
Departmental Overhead Expense			
1. Equipment cost:			
• Depreciation rentals	$1.00	6.84	6.84
Subtotal			$6.84
Allocated Overhead Expense			
1. Type I	$1.00	57.21	57.21
2. Type II	0.15	221.90	33.29
Subtotal			$90.50
PCU Total Cost			$382.23

Source: From "Standard cost systems lead to efficiency and profitability," by J.P. Bennett, 1985, *Healthcare Financial Management, 39*(5), 48. Copyright 1985, Healthcare Financial Management Association. Reprinted by permission.

Obviously, strategic health planning plays an important role in determining what resources are needed, the proper mix, and methods of determining their costs. Having either an oversupply or a shortage of personnel creates an imbalance problem. Homeostasis, or the right balance, is what strategic planning strives to achieve relative to the program's objectives. However, projections of personnel needs by themselves do not constitute planning nor merit the innovative thinking required to identify and achieve objectives. Much more is required. Strategic planning is an excellent process for understanding the full implications of any resource needs.

Looking for People Power

Directories listing health care personnel are published by many professional associations geographically listing providers such as physicians, dentists, registered nurses, psychologists, social workers, physical and occupational therapists, and hospital administrators. However, these professional directories may only list members of the American Medical Association, American Dental Association, American Public Health Association, or any other professional organization. In that event, the yellow pages of the telephone book can provide locality listing for the various types of personnel. It is also possible that professionals who require State registration may be listed by the appropriate licensing body in that State.

Ancillary health care workers could include individuals with a variety of skills that may be useful in resolving a problem. People with first aid certificates may be listed by the agency that provided the training; former armed forces medical corps personnel might be located through the Department of Defense; and technicians could also be identified through licensing, or membership in a labor union or professional group.

Administrative talent most likely will come from the agency sponsoring the planning activity. However, local industries may be persuaded to loan an executive to a public interest project for a short time. In fact, the loaned executive is a common procedure in communities having a United Fund type of organization. In a strategic planning context, the highly trained industrial executive can provide particularly appropriate direction to activities that more closely resemble routine commercial administrative tasks such as marketing, product-line promotion, consumer surveys, and bottom-line evaluation. Falkenburg and Jacobson [1989] call attention to the selection and grooming of an organization's future leaders to assure management continuity planning.

Traditionally, volunteer unpaid clerical personnel have been secured from the ranks of retired persons, high school and university students, fraternal associations, and workers given released time by their employers. Those visiting hospitals are familiar with the "gray ladies," "candy stripers," and others who donate their time and energy to perform crucial tasks for the facility. Of course, a core of salaried workers is usually included in the planning of any activity since volunteers may or may not be reliable every day in every way.

Strategic planners can also advertise for professionals and lay people to volunteer their services for a specific project. Ads can be placed in newspapers, on radio and TV, on bulletin boards and anywhere in the community where people will notice the ad. Announcements can be made at parent/teacher organizations, social clubs, religious services, and union meetings. There are public-minded individuals in the community who readily participate in activities that aim to serve people in need.

In addition there are publications such as the multivolume *Encyclopedia of Associations* [Koek, 1988] that lists 25,000+ national and international trade, business and commercial organizations in classifications such as health and medical, social welfare, government, public administration, education, cultural, public affairs, ethnic, religious, and labor unions. Each organization listing gives the name, address and phone number, membership totals, staff, publications, and activities of the agency. Obviously, this type of directory is a starting point for the strategic planner looking for potential sources of personnel, facilities, equipment/supplies, and funding.

FACILITIES

Existing directories provide information about a spectrum of facilities such as alcoholism treatment facilities, agencies serving the blind, blood banks, clinical laboratories, community mental health centers, drug abuse treatment programs, facilities for exceptional children, half· way houses, HMOs, neighborhood health centers, maternal and child health centers, home health care agencies, hospitals, long-term care facilities, nursing homes, poison control centers, psychiatric clinics, inpatient facilities for the retarded, clinical programs for retarded children and suicide-prevention/crisis intervention centers, hospices, group medical/dental practices, rehabilitation facilities, and services for the aged. Many of these facility directories are published by units of the USDHHS, by the voluntary nonprofit specific disease/condition agency or by the professional association concerned with that problem such as the federal National Clearinghouse for Mental Health Information, the American Foundation for the Blind or the American Hospital Association.

Most people tend to think about "bricks and mortar" when facilities are discussed. Actually, facilities can be much broader in concept including mobile units and satellites. In all cases, however, a critical concern relates to the proprietary health care providers in a system that relegates the profit motive to a lower priority.

Issues Concerning For-Profit Hospitals

One of the phenomenal growth areas in the health care facility field is the growth and expansion of for-profit hospital chains. Previously, for-profits were small, physician-owned hospitals that maintained their viability as long as there was population expansion. When the population growth stagnated, those facilities lost their share of patients to nonprofit hospitals. In the period of the 1970s and 1980s, for-profits organized into large corporate chains developing a vertical organization of services with huge sums of capital to invest. Growth in resources resulted from buying out smaller, financially vulnerable nonprofit as well as other for-profit hospitals.

Expansion of for-profit hospitals appears to be correlated with the growth in commercial hospital insurance and the size of the Medicare population. Changes in Blue Cross coverage did not impact on their growth. Neither did certificate-of-need controls have a negative impact on hospital investment and growth. By 1977, 90 percent of all for-profit hospitals were part of several large corporate chains. As the size of the corporate chains grew, they were not very different from nonprofit hospitals in the complement of service mix and the composition of patient loads.

Since hospital corporate chains are most attuned to earning profits for stockholders, their main focus has been on identifying those factors that result in decisions to buy another hospital. Current market conditions are a key factor in whether a hospital would be purchased or not. Corporate chains would sooner buy a hospital in a dynamic growth market that was losing money because of inefficient management than buy a hospital with good management in a stagnant medical market [Alexander & Morrisey, 1988]. For-profits take advantage of existing changes rather than waiting for positive changes to occur in market conditions. Further, where investor-owned hospitals already exist in a state, new chains perceive this as a positive sign of acceptance, or at least tolerance, of for-profit health institutions. "This suggests that the political foundation for acquisition has been established earlier, thus reducing the costs of overcoming such political obstacles for the acquiring system" [Alexander & Morrisey, 1988].

In addition to weak market conditions inhibiting the purchase of hospitals, a high payroll/expense ratio also raises a "red flag." Caution prevails because the hospital may have a strong union or be located in a community of prevailing high wages. There are positive and negative factors that influence a decision to buy or not to buy a facility. Furthermore, the number of hospital facilities is finite. Ergo, there is a limit beyond which health care provider corporate chains will be able to expand through purchasing existing facilities. Instead, corporate chains are likely to turn their attention to investment opportunities that return greater profits such as insurance, long-term care, or ambulatory care centers.

As the hospital chains grow sufficiently large, organizational factors must be considered. Hospital Corporation of America [HCA] is an example of one chain that is changing its organizational structure to assure better coordination of services and to eliminate duplication [Barkholz, 1985]. HCA found that when corporate hospitals operated with fairly independent control, they even competed with each other when located in the same service area. Furthermore, HCA earnings were becoming flat, requiring greater productivity, efficiency, and control from the top. Consequently, HCA decided to structure its 400 hospitals into eight or nine fully integrated health care systems with greater centralized management in control of these clusters. This semicentralized model permits flexibility in offering an expansive range of services within each cluster such as regional laboratories, long-term care, open heart surgery, and diagnostic imaging. At the same time, HCA planned to sell inefficient hospitals to streamline services. Organizational changes will be made with the cooperation of employee physicians who are now more accepting because of their own awareness of a hospital's need to compete for patients. No doubt, other large chains will also experiment with organizational models striving to provide quality service at costs that will produce profits.

Methodology for Determining Capital Resources

It is estimated that two to three times the amount spent on capital expenditures in the 1970s will be required in the 1980s, somewhere between $50 and $193 billion [Hannan, Rouse, Barnett, & Uppal, 1987]. Obviously, that amount of resources will not be forthcoming. Therefore, it becomes necessary to determine which of the numerous capital proposals, especially facilities, should command high priority for funding. Most of these new requests will be for renovation and replacement projects and not new facilities.

Most states use an "absolute" need method in evaluating projects. If the project meets the state's Certificate-of-Need requirements, it receives automatic approval. While the criteria vary by states, most of the states use criteria such as the project's meeting a public health need, the character and competence of the provider, financial feasibility of the project, and consistency with state and regional health plans. Some analysts believe that the criteria are too flexible and fail to help decision makers to answer the question, "How great is the need and how does it compare with the need for other services?" [Hannan et al., 1987]. To answer these questions, three criteria can assess for relative need:

1. Relative public need of competing applications for capital projects.
2. Relative cost of the project compared to competing projects, including an assessment of what the applicant states the project will cost compared to what the state planners believe it should cost. These last costs are referred to as "normative costs."
3. Relative need for modernization/renovation/replacement of projects compared to each other and to the severity of the problems the projects aim to solve.

These criteria can readily be applied to the following types of projects:

1. Addition of new acute care beds.
2. Addition of new nursing home beds.
3. Modernization or construction with no change in beds.

4. Diagnostic and treatment centers.
5. Home health agencies.
6. Wide range of equipment requests such as CT and NMR scanners, open-heart surgery, and dialysis equipment.

Measurements for five health categories would have to be designed including acute care and nursing home beds, home health, ambulatory services, available equipment and emerging technologies. Each measure should identify a scale of relative need using either a continuous measure such as 0 to 100, or high, medium, low unmet need ratings. Each application would be evaluated and given a score of relative need. Similarly, cost standards would be developed. For the category of adding acute care beds, cost-per-type of acute care patient day as measured by routine costs [such as nursing cost-per-type of patient day and plant operation and maintenance cost-per-type of bed] and ancillary costs [such as diagnostic and therapeutic costs-per-type of discharge] could be used to determine the relative costs of the project compared to other proposals. In addition, incremental and capital costs would have to be taken into account.

Finally, need for modernization/renovation/replacement would have to be considered. Major concern of this criteria is on the life-safety factors as they affect the patient and the severity of the problem. Severity is measured on a 10-point scale with the highest rating given to the factor of "imminent threat to safety or continuity of operation," a middle rating to the factor of "basic treatment and diagnostic-related needs" and the lowest rating to the factor of "marketability." Exhibit 3-12 describes how this scale is set up.

Each application is rated on the three criteria, with results then summed to a final score. Qualitative factors are also taken into account before creating a priority list of proposals such as consistency with the medical facility plan, applications for poorer communities, and submission of a joint application. Additional factors in implementing a relative need system to determine a measure of unmet need would be to define a peer group against which to compare the proposal and to ascertain levels of importance for different types of capital projects. Defining these measures requires political judgments as well as technical considerations.

Such a scale has not been fully developed and tested. Obviously, that scale would have the advantage of being less arbitrary than an absolute need system. Applicants would know in advance whether their proposal would have a high priority of being found acceptable. However, unsuccessful applicants could still challenge the measures used by the decision makers to rate the proposals.

Forecasting Bed Need Methodology

Two models have been used to determine a range of mental health services for Nebraska and California [Isaacs, 1986]. Both are normative models whose standards have been determined by planners and mental health advocates. Warheit and Auth [1981] use an epidemiological model to determine psychiatric/alcohol acute care bed resources.

Nebraska Mental Health Service System Model. Beeson and Ford's [1984] model is based on estimated needs of identified service categories as shown in Exhibit 3-13. Objectively, the model aims to evaluate how well the needs of the population are being met. For 1980, the Nebraska population was 1,569,825. Unmet needs as well as the underutilized mental health services in the state that would require resource modification are identified. There is no indication of how well the services are assisting those using them, outcomes for patients in treatment, or the political implications of any effort to transfer resources from underutilized to overutilized

Exhibit 3-12.   Factors Used in Assessing the Need for Modernization / Renovation / Replacement.

Broad Rating Scale	Fine Rating Scale	Area 1: Life Safety and Structural Components	Area 2 Direct Inpatient Care and Infection Control	Area 3 Indirect Patient Care
A	1	Imminent threat to life safety or continuity of operation		
B	2	Life safety requirements		
	3		Nonwaiverable requirements	Nonwaiverable requirements
C	4		Basic needs, not code-required	
	5			Basic treatment and diagnostic-related needs
	6	Structural and mechanical nonwaiverable requirements		
	7	Routine preventive maintenance		Basic needs, other than treatment or diagnosis [not code-required]
D	8	Life safety items, not code-required	Improvement, amenities	Staff and administration amenties
	9	Marketability	Marketability	Marketability

Source: From "Methods for developing relative need criteria to accompany a health care capital expenditure limit," by E.L. Hannan, R.L. Rouse, R. Barnett, & P. Uppal, 1987, *Journal of Health Politics, Policy and Law*, *12*[1], 130. Reprinted with permission of Duke University Press.

services. Examination of these standards reveal that community mental health services have not kept pace with the large numbers of patients discharged from hospitals resulting in so many under-utilized beds. Furthermore, it is clear from this data that services have not followed patients discharged into the community.

California Community Mental Health Program Model. Crowell [1980] uses normative standards for this model as set by a consensus among a coalition of mental health providers and consumers (Exhibit 3-14). Experts also used community-based information, service utility analysis, and social indicators for the standards per 100,000 population. There is no evaluation provided of the extent to which the need is being met. Rather, the model identifies standards in terms of units of service that would be needed in this particular catchment area to meet mental health needs. These are the best judgments of experts in the community. First, these normative standards should be assessed against actual demand for services and later for need, including those needing mental health programs but not using them.

Exhibit 3-13. Nebraska Mental Health Service System Model.

Regional Level Services	Estimated ALOS*	Estimated Need per Nebraska's 1980 Pop.**	Current Resources	% of Need Met
Emergency	1 episode	60 epis/day	20 epis/day	33
Outpatient	8 hours	1,500 hrs/day	1,273 hrs/day	85
Short-term Inpatient	15 days	355 beds	682 beds	192
Community Living Services	1 year	2,156 slots	80 slots	6
Supportive/Sheltered Employment	18 mos	864 slots	6 slots	1
Multi-Regional Services				
Extended Inpatient	1 year	160 beds	320 beds	200
Specialized Children, Residential	6 mos	30 beds	10 beds	33
State-Level Services				
Security Inpatient	3 yrs	125 beds	128 beds	102
Severely Disturbed and Disruptive Adolescent Inpatient Care	2 yrs	30 beds	54 beds	180

* = Average Length of Stay
** = Nebraska's 1980 population: 1,569,825
Source: From *Acute psychiatric bed needs planning: Issues and methodologies,* by M.R. Isaacs, 1986, p. 65, Washington, DC: Government Printing Office, HRP-0906627. Reprinted by permission.

Exhibit 3-14. California Community Mental Health Program Model.

Program Function	Program/Facilities Required	Persons Served Yearly, Estimate**	Units of Service Yearly, Estimate
Short-term crisis Residential	10 beds	220	3,102
24-hour Acute Intensive Care	15 beds	310	4,654 days
Outpatient	20 beds	2,000	16,250
Acute Day Treatment	9 FTE*	160	7,000
Case Management	8.6 FTE*	400	4,800

* Full Time Employees, professional staff only
** People can receive services from several programs
Source: From *Acute psychiatric beds need planning: Issues and methodologies,* by M.R. Isaacs, 1986, p. 69, Washington, DC: Government Printing Office, HRP-0906627. Reprinted by permission.

Mental Health System for the District of Columbia

In 1982, Congress asked the General Accounting Office to evaluate the mental health system of the District of Columbia. Investigators were to pay special attention to methods of transferring the federal St. Elizabeths Hospital into an integral part of the District's mental health system [Bowskey, 1984]. GAO planners used three criteria in developing their system:

1. Provide services in the least restrictive setting.
2. Minimize the cost of operating the system while maintaining quality.
3. Utilizing existing physical plant and staff as much as possible.

Exhibit 3-15 diagrams the GAO's proposed system and Exhibit 3-16 maps locations and boundaries of various elements of the system.

Proposal of the GAO. GAO proposed a comprehensive mental health system for the District shifting the primary locus of care from St. Elizabeths to community-based programs and facilities as the clinically preferred treatment setting. The District's Mental Health Services Administration would have overall responsibility for administering the system.

Three mental health districts, corresponding to the current mental health service areas, would have budgetary and clinical responsibility for all care provided to patients living in their service areas. Each mental health district would operate: a community mental health center to provide outpatient, day treatment, and case management services; a crisis resolution unit spe-

Exhibit 3-15.   Organization of Proposed Mental Health System.

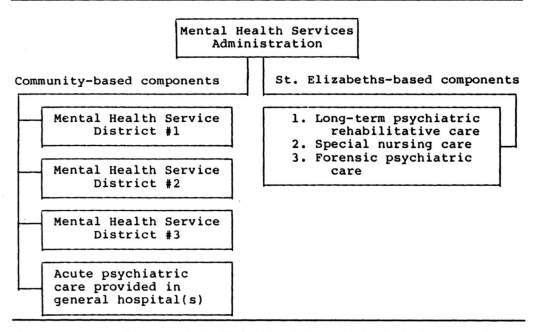

Source: From *A proposal for transferring St. Elizabeths Hospital to the District of Columbia,* by C.A. Bowskey, 1984, Washington, DC: Government Printing Office, GAO/HRD 84-48. Reprinted by permission.

Exhibit 3-16.   District Hospitals and Community Mental Health Centers.

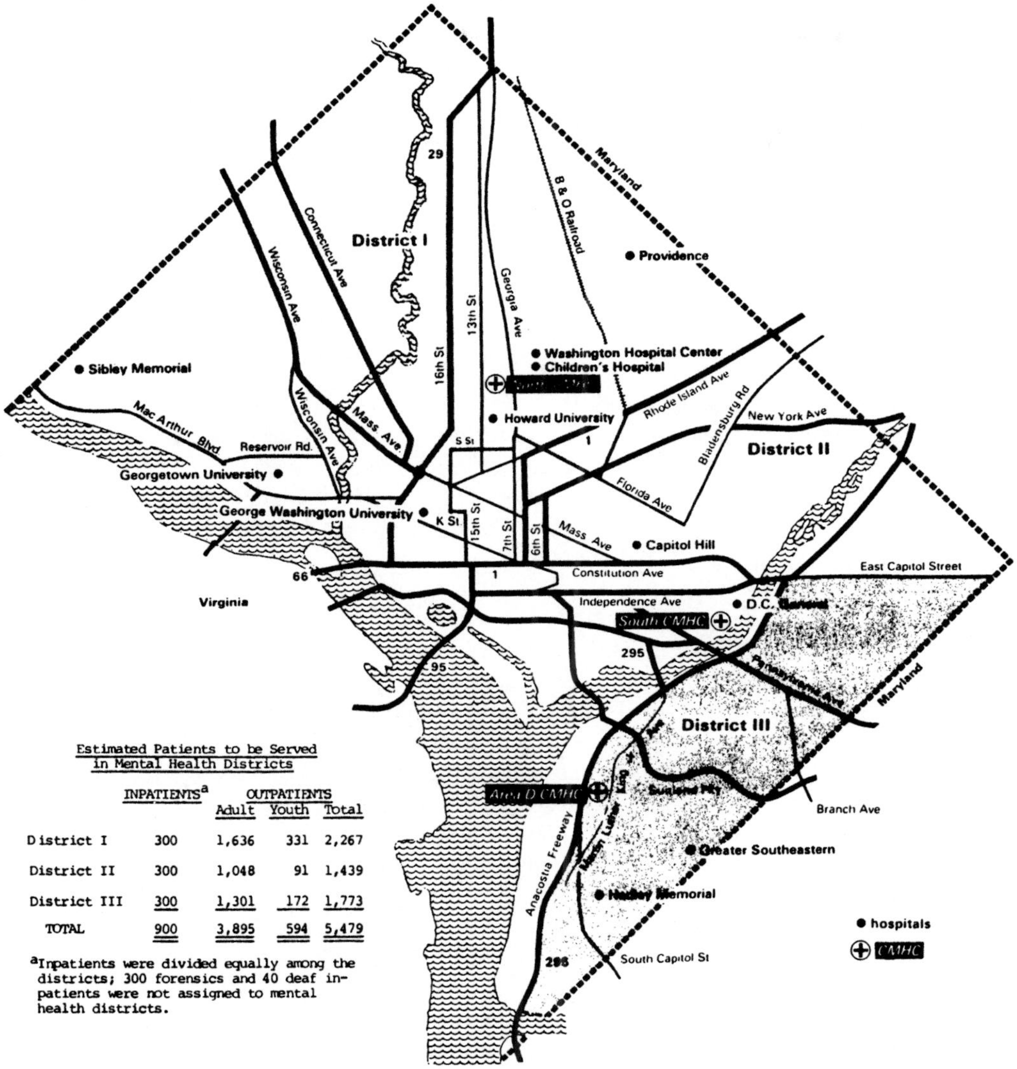

Estimated Patients to be Served
in Mental Health Districts

	INPATIENTS[a]	OUTPATIENTS		
		Adult	Youth	Total
District I	300	1,636	331	2,267
District II	300	1,048	91	1,439
District III	300	1,301	172	1,773
TOTAL	900	3,895	594	5,479

[a]Inpatients were divided equally among the
districts; 300 forensics and 40 deaf inpatients were not assigned to mental
health districts.

Source: From *A proposal for transferring St. Elizabeths Hospital to the District of Columbia*, by C.A. Bowskey, 1984, Washington, DC: Government Printing Office, GAO/HRD 84-48. Reprinted by permission.

cially trained to evaluate and treat patients experiencing a psychiatric crisis and to authorize hospitalization; and mobile treatment teams to serve difficult-to-treat patients and attempt to keep them stabilized and functioning in the community.

St. Elizabeths' role in the new system would be limited to providing long-term inpatient care; intensive and rehabilitative medical and nursing psychiatric care; and forensic psychiatric care for individuals sent to St. Elizabeths by the court system for evaluation and/or treatment. Those new roles would be accomplished in the following manner:

- Outplacing about 300 St. Elizabeths' inpatients to community treatment settings more appropriate to their needs.
- Transferring about 100 inpatients from hospital and drug abuse programs to community or institutional programs administered by the District's Alcohol and Drug Abuse Services Administration.
- Shifting about 200–250 acute, short-term patients to one or more general hospitals since federal regulations limit Medicaid reimbursements to patients under 22 and over 64 when care is provided for mental disease by institutions like St. Elizabeths. Conversion of general beds to psychiatric use would be required since District hospitals do not currently have enough excess capacity on psychiatric wards to accommodate these patients.

When these steps are completed, St. Elizabeths' inpatient population would be reduced from 1,700 to about 1,000.

Comparison of Current System With Proposed System. Exhibit 3-17 compares the fiscal year 1983 system for providing mental health services—including programs and services offered, patients served, costs, and direct patient care staffing—with GAO's proposed system. The fiscal year 1984 mental health system could be different because of budget cutbacks at St. Elizabeths and planned reductions in patients, staff, and costs. Because most of these changes have not been implemented, GAO's proposal uses fiscal year 1983 information as the current baseline.

Cost of Proposed System. GAO's proposed system estimates costs about $22 million less annually than the fiscal year 1983 system cost of about $144 million. District expenditures almost double the current payment of about $37 million. Through Medicare and Medicaid payments and payments for care provided to federal beneficiaries, the federal government's contribution would be about 38 percent of the 1983 expenditure of about $105 million. Cost savings are based on the assumption that the D.C. General Hospital would provide all acute psychiatric care. Costs of about $7.4 million would be incurred as a result of outplacing patients to community facilities and transferring substance abuse patients to District-operated programs.
At least 1,400 of the 2,300 current patient care staff would continue under the proposed mental health system. An additional 330 patient care positions would be retained if a District-run facility such as D.C. General were used for acute psychiatric care. Another 250 research and training positions would be contingent on continued federal funding.
About 80 percent of the cost reduction relates to the outplacement of current St. Elizabeths' inpatients to community facilities and the transfer of substance abuse inpatients to less costly District-operated programs. Remaining savings result from the reduced staff needed to operate the proposed system. Moving acute care to general hospitals would not result in any total cost savings but could reduce costs to the District by allowing more Medicaid reimbursements. GAO's cost estimates do not consider other economic impacts of the transfer such as unemployment costs.

Impact of Nursing Shortages on Facility Resources

In 1988, the Naval Hospital at Bethesda, Maryland experienced a severe nursing shortage so critical that 50 acute care beds were being considered for closure [Tomich, 1988]. As one of the premier facilities in the naval hospital system, that projected closure provoked outrage among the hospital's medical staff who felt their training programs were in jeopardy. Naval medical

Exhibit 3-17.   Comparison: Current Mental Health System vs. Proposed System.

	Current	Proposed
1. Programs/services:	**Responsibility/location**	**Responsibility/location**
Hospital inpatient:		
Acute psychiatric	Federal/St. Elizabeths	District/General hospital(s)
Long-term	Federal/St. Elizabeths	District/St. Elizabeths
Forensic	Federal/St. Elizabeths District/D.C. General	District/St. Elizabeths
Mental Health Program for the Deaf	Federal/St. Elizabeths	District[a]/St. Elizabeths
Outpatient	District/North Center South Center	District/ Mental Health District #1[b] Mental Health District #2[b] Mental Health District #3[b]
Crisis intervention	District/centralized crisis resolution unit	District/crisis resolution units in each mental health dis- trict
Research	Federal/St. Elizabeths	Federal/St. Elizabeths
Training	Federal/St. Elizabeths	District[a]/St. Elizabeths
2. Patients:	**Provider/number**	**Provider/number**
Inpatient	St. Elizabeths/ 1,700	St. Elizabeths/ 1,000 General Hospitals/ 200
Outpatient	St. Elizabeths/ 2,300 District centers/1,900	District centers/ 4,600
Total	5,900	5,800[c]
3. Costs [fiscal year 1983]:	**[in millions]**	**[in millions]**
District of Columbia	$ 37.0	$ 76.8
Federal	104.6	40.2[d]
Other payors	2.6	4.9
Total	$144.2	$121.9[e]
4. Direct patient care staffing:	**[No. of full-time equivalent employees]**	
Inpatient	2,006	1,088
Outpatient	286[f]	315
Total	2,292	1,403

[a]District would operate if federal funds were provided.
[b]See Exhibit 3-16 for map of Mental Health Districts.
[c]Does not include about 100 substance abuse patients who would be treated in other District programs.
[d]Includes costs of federal beneficiaries, Medicare costs, and the federal share of Medicaid.
[e]Includes costs of $7.4 million—$5.4 District, $1.8 federal, and $0.2 other] incurred as a result of patient outplacement to community facilities and transfer of patients to other District programs.
[f]Includes both District and St. Elizabeths outpatient staff.
Source: From *A proposal for transferring St. Elizabeths Hospital to the District of Columbia,* by C.A. Bowskey, 1984, Washington, DC: Government Printing Office, GAO/HRD 84-48. Reprinted by permission.

planners perceived this as an opportune time to close several small naval hospitals that were understaffed and served small populations. However, indignation on the part of elected officials in those communities prevented even that option from being exercised. Consequently, this problem was temporarily solved by "expediting a program of contracting with civilian nurses, bringing in reservists for longer than usual active duty stints, and by assigning nurses on "temporary" duty from other facilities [Tomich, 1988]. Resource allocations were also made among physicians serving the small naval hospital facilities. Having difficulty in replacing retiring naval physicians, remaining physicians had to double up on their assignments. Furthermore, the facilities were too small to permit physicians to practice their specialties. Additionally, physicians were forced to carry out more administrative duties than anticipated, further reducing their capacity to use their medical knowledge.

From this illustration it appears that severe losses and shortages of medical personnel has two significant outcomes. Larger units in the system steal personnel from the smaller units, making them even more inefficient. In turn, that tends to undermine morale and to erode medical capacity to serve naval personnel in the small facilities.

Coordination of Planning Medical Resources

In the following three examples, health planners played an important role in assisting communities to add needed resources to their areas.

In 1977, health planners in Arlington County, Virginia, found that there were no nursing home beds in spite of the fact that 25 percent of the population was composed of those 65 and over [American Health Planning Association, 1988A]. Two adjacent counties were found to have nursing home beds, with one being underbedded by 30 percent, and the others overbedded by 38 percent and 93 percent. With direct assistance from the health planners, planning studies ensued, followed by certificate-of-need recommendations to the state. Eventually, planning resulted in all the counties, including Arlington, having an appropriate number of nursing home beds equal to the needs of its elderly population.

In another example, analysis by health planners in North Central Florida [American Health Planning Association, 1988b] discovered that there was a major shortage of physicians and other medical personnel serving this small, rural, and sparsely settled population. Responding to requests by the county's citizenry, the health planners collected data and wrote an application to the Department of Health and Human Services requesting funding for a community health center. This was approved and, in addition, National Health Service Corps physicians were initially assigned to the center. Recently, the center became sufficiently fiscally sound to be able to hire two physicians and pay them out of income received from Medicare, Medicaid, private insurance, and some self-payers. With its new medical staff, the center now serves almost 3,500 patients with 12,000 visits.

In a third example, Congress gave legislative approval to the Department of Defense and the Veterans Administration to share each other's medical facilities to promote a higher quality of care and to improve efficiency [USDHHS, 1988]. While there are obstacles that prevent complete sharing of all facilities, Congress has been urged to modify laws to remove barriers. VA facilities are not penalized in their budgets when they serve DOD personnel. However, DOD facilities are not permitted to use these funds as supplements to their regular budgets. Therefore, DOD has little incentive to enter into sharing agreements. Also, DOD administers the Civilian Health and Medical Program of the Uniformed Services [CHAMPUS], which pays $2 billion annually for medical care for beneficiaries at other than their own facilities.Those funds cannot be used to reimburse the VA for services rendered to DOD personnel or their dependents, retirees and their dependents. Agreements that have been carried out are considered a success. Beneficiaries' access to certain medical services such as open-heart surgery and radiology procedures improved. In many cases, local VA or DOD hospitals provided more convenient access to the services than other federal or private providers. Since the legislation was passed in

1982, 238 of the 926 hospitals and clinics have entered into sharing agreements. Savings of over $20 million have thus far accrued as a result of this agreement.

All three examples clearly reveal that coordination and sharing of expertise and services does lead to improved medical services, quality of care, and more efficient use of resources.

EQUIPMENT AND SUPPLIES

When planners consider equipment and supply needs for a specific project, all the required resources may not be evident at first. As additional data become available, needs may change. Nevertheless, strategic planners will have to do a preliminary inventory of potential resources.

Equipment needs should be obvious relative to the problem. Is X-ray or imaging equipment needed? Do laboratory tests have to be done? Are transport vehicles required? Do the mobile clinics at night need portable lights? Are professionals bringing their own equipment to check vital signs? Taking a quantum jump from such basic equipment, planners must contend with the latest in chrome-plated hardware.

High Technology Equipment Issues

With the rapid scientific advances, an obvious planning question centers around "how to distribute the optimal quantity of high technology health care for a given population?" [Labelle, 1987]. A number of planning considerations come into play regarding the allocation of sophisticated health care technology: assurance that the technology is clinically approved and economically evaluated, identification of effective indications for use, collection of incidence and prevalence data for those indications of use, location of demographic data about the target population, derivation of a specific area forecast for the technology, assessment of the technology's output capabilities, relation of the output data to the forecasts, and calculation of the optimal technology units required for the area.

Allocation of Technology. However, a rational planning sequence may not necessarily decide who gets what in the health care delivery system. Human nature seems to motivate everyone to want to own their own piece of the "biggest and the best" technology available to cure human ailments. Gallivan [1986] reported that hospital technology planning has become increasingly sophisticated moving from an option to an imperative.

Panerai and Attinger [1986] developed a computer information system for the appropriate allocation of health care technologies and demonstrated its use evaluating 300 individual perinatal care technologies. They evaluate each technology by 10 attributes such as capital cost, recurrent costs, level of manpower, side effects and risks, service dependence, and social impact. Each attribute has subareas that are rank-ordered and/or weighted according to the effectiveness in resolution of the problem. Technologies are automatically allocated to the appropriate care level: home or mobile primary care unit, neighborhood clinic, community hospital, or teaching hospital. In addition, the computer considers the interdependence of diagnostic and therapeutic technologies as well as the grouping of technologies.

Planners have tried to establish criteria for technology such as a minimum number of procedures per magnetic resonance imaging device or minimum number of open heart surgeries per hospital. In theory, no new imaging machine could be purchased if an existing device did not meet the minimum number of procedures. Likewise, a hospital could not perform open heart surgery unless the minimum goal was surpassed. Human nature often being unpredictable, planners have to contend with competing bidding and organizations and individuals who simply cannot abide with any inhibition of their personal choices to opt for the betterment of the society.

Technology Trends Affecting Planning. High technology equipment carries with it an impact not only on physicians and nurses but also on allied health professionals. In fact, the allied health professional would probably be manning the equipment more frequently than any of the other health care workers. Bruhn and Philips [1985] list the following trends as a result of increased technology:

- Specialization of knowledge and skills with an increase in communication barriers and decreased interdisciplinary activities.
- New disciplines, professional societies, and accreditation standards with increased competition for resources, status, and prestige.
- Greater use of machines in education and patient care with higher costs for new treatment modalities.
- Increase in students in attractive high-tech disciplines.
- Ethical codes for all with malpractice coverage for all and contractual relationships with physicians re rights and responsibilities of high tech allied health workers.
- More rigorous credentialing and professional organizations requirements on keeping skills current.

Routine Equipment and Supplies

Office equipment such as desks, chairs, tables, typewriters, duplicating machinery, computers, pencil sharpeners, and staplers must also be considered. Although planners should provide some funding for purchasing, it is conceivable that much routine office equipment could be donated or loaned from a variety of sources.

Supplies provide the routine office and health care fodder that makes an activity run: pencils, pens, paper, clips, folders, lab coats, test tubes, and all the disposable material. Although most planners budget funds for the usual office supplies, there may be needs unique to the specific task that must be part of the resources. Again, potential community sources may be appealed to for assistance.

FUNDING

Regardless of whether you believe that money makes the world go around or whether you believe that money is the root of all evil, strategic planners must concern themselves with funding. Personnel may have to be paid; facilities may have to be rented or purchased; and equipment/supplies may have to be purchased. No matter how the pie is sliced, raising money is not easy. In addition, many planners are "not well-versed in the nuances of fund-raising" [Agovino, 1988].

Private funding may come from fees charged for services, insurance coverage, third party payers, or donations from individuals, businesses, or foundations. Foundation directories exist such as the 1,000 page *The Foundation Directory* [Renz & Olson, 1987] that furnish planners with details about private foundations such as the executive staff, the trustees, the officers, the donors, the typical type of award, the areas of interest, the financial holdings, and the amount of money awarded in past years. A major advantage of many private foundations is that awards can be secured within a quicker time frame that from governmental funding sources.

Public funding resources utilize tax moneys administered by local, state, and federal government agencies. Generally, funds are awarded in the form of grants or contracts with formal applications and may have peer review committees and/or professional staff evaluations. Government Printing Office publications list grant and/or contract awards and those can provide clues for planners seeking funding from specific agencies. Regional offices of the U.S. Department of Health and Human Services are often a useful starting point for planners looking to identify the appropriate bureaucratic unit to apply to for funds. It is possible for planners to be put on a mailing list to receive announcements about granting activities of the USDHHS units. In addition, local universities may have a research department that maintains computer listings and a reference library relative to funding sources. It would not be unusual for a university to allow a strategic planner to make use of their library and computer resources.

Funding need not be concerned solely with dollars and cents. Bartering, exchanging services for services, can be a vital cog in securing the resources needed for an activity. A strategic planner for a hospital could exchange an annual physical exam for the services of a carpenter who would construct an office unit. By simply allowing a business firm to have a credit line on a brochure or advertising flyer, a planner may be able to persuade a printer to produce thousands of single page advertisements.

Flexibility and Innovation

Flexibility, innovation, and creativity are key words for the strategic planner developing an inventory of resources of personnel, facilities, equipment/supplies, and funding. Narrowly pinpointing the problem eases the task of locating the relevant and alternative resources to complete the activity. However, bear in mind that a resource inventory is never really completed because a planner monitoring an activity will find Murphy's Law still active: "If anything can go wrong, it will."

Resource Classification Taxonomies

A variety of taxonomies are used to classify resources by services or by facilities. While the obvious comparative benefit of a uniform classification system is acknowledged, there does not appear to be a consistent use of any one framework.

A basic public health classification scheme combines a geographical concept with distinct levels of care to arrive at a spectrum of health care services. In a multidirectional flow system, neighborhood/local services provide entrance level primary care to the community; subregional services provide intermediate care; and regional services provide sophisticated tertiary care [USDHEW, 1977, p. A-5].

In one example, health system services are plotted against health system settings. Seven services are categorized into community health promotion and protection, prevention and detection, diagnosis and treatment, habilitation and rehabilitation, maintenance, personal health care support, and health system enabling. Seven settings include: home, mobile, ambulatory, short-stay inpatient, long-stay inpatient, free-standing support, and community. A detailed government document describes each of the services and settings with examples of each part of the classification scheme [Government Studies and Systems, 1977].

Standard categories of health care services for certificate-of-need in New Jersey comprise four classifications: 10 bed-related services, 13 nonbed-related services, 11 special services, and 13 support services [USDHEW, 1977, Appendix A].

A government health resources classification framework comes up with four categories adding a fifth with two subcategories: hospitals, nursing homes, health manpower, health manpower education institutions, and other health facilities divided into inpatient care and outpatient/nonpatient resources [Oreglia, Klein, Crandall, & Duncan, 1976, p. 7].

Collection of Inventory Data

Even after discovering all the information in the existing directories, it is possible that planners may still need to secure original data. A resource inventory provides a starting point for implementation, augments rational planning, adds primary data to discussions and also contributes to the credibility of the end product [USDHEW, 1978, p. 92].

Mail questionnaires, telephone calls, or other sources may be used to amass the information for an inventory of resources. Broad categories of data should include agency, program purpose, location[s], phone numbers, services provided, service area, eligibility policies, client capacity, legal authority, staff members, charges, hours, and accessibility [USDHEW, 1978, p. 94]. Exhibit 3-18 enumerates a step-by-step procedure with attention to the data items required, the specific listing and the periodic updating. Exhibit 3-19 illustrates an index card system for

---

Exhibit 3-18.   Step-by-Step Inventory Development Procedure.

1. **Identify resources and determine information needed about each one.**
   A. Select resources for compilation and for inventory list.
   B. Define resource to distinguish from other resources.
   C. Prepare list of data items to be collected about each resource.
   D. Define each data item.
   E. Name sources from which the data can be obtained.

2. **Develop a list of specific resources and their services using the specific resources identified in Step 1.**
   A. Compile a list of resource by name, address, phone.
   B. Check for inconsistency with those identified in Step 1.
   C. Verify the citations with other sources.

3. **Obtain data enumerated in Step 1, D.**
   A. Decide on storage mode for data; paper sheet, cards, computer, etc.
   B. Obtain the data.
   C. Check to see that data have been collected to meet needs.
   D. If data are not collected, design mechanism to obtain missing information such as phone interview, questionnaire, personal interview or combination.

4. **Update inventory.**
   A. Select appropriate time interval for updating.
   B. Update inventory as new information becomes available from existing sources.

Exhibit 3-19.   Outpatient Health Resources Collection Form and Guidelines.

[Front]   1 _____
              [Agency name]

              _____   _____
              [Agency address]   [Telephone number]

              _____   2 _____
              [City, State, Zip Code]   [Hours of operation]

           3 _____
              [Full-time personnel: number and type]

           4 _____
              [Part-time personnel: number and type]

           5 _____
              [Intake procedures, waiting list, etc.]

[Back]   6 Type of service provided: Charges, if any

              _____
              _____
              _____
              _____
              _____
              _____
              _____
              _____

           7 Date information collected: _____
              Name of respondent _____

Guidelines for Outpatient/Nonpatient Health Resources Data Collection Form

1. Full, legal name; street number and name; city, couty, state, and zip code; and area code and phone number. If another address, etc., is used for administrative offices, list both.

2. Days of week agency provides services, and hours open on each day.

3. Indicate number and type of full-time staff. Minimum categories MD, DO, dentist, RN, LPN, physical therapist, psychologist, social worker, other.

4. Indicate part-time staff as above.

5. Is there a waiting list? Is written application required in advance of treatment? Eligibility criteria?

6. List all major services provided and charges for these services.

7. Name and date person contacted.

recording data about outpatient health care resources. In some communities, this type of data may be kept by the local United Fund, Red Feather, or Community Chest organization.

Key Word Technique

Organizations vary tremendously in the appellations that are conferred upon units performing similar activities. Government agencies may use different words than voluntary nonprofit organizations and proprietary companies may use terminology different from both or all of the above. Nevertheless, from a planner's stance, they are all potential resources of peoplepower, facilities, equipment/supplies, and money. Exhibit 3-20 illustrates key words to look for in directories or

Exhibit 3-20.   Key Word List for Potential Resources.

Adolescent health	Human resources
Adult health	Immunization
Air pollution	Infant health
Alcohol abuse	Institutional care
Alcoholism	Institutions
Birth and death records	Licensing [health professionals]
Child abuse	Manpower
Child care	Maternal health
Child health	Maternal services
Child neglect	Medicaid
Clinics	Medical assistance
Colleges	Medical social services
Communicable disease	Mental health
Communicable disorders	Mental hospitals
Community health	Mental hygiene
Dental health	Narcotics treatment
Dental services	Occupational health
Drug abuse	Public assistance
Drug control	Public health
Drug treatment	Public instruction
Education	Public welfare
Emergency medical services	Radiological health
Employment security	Sanitation engineering
Employment services	Sanitation
Environmental health	Schools
Environmental protection	School health
Epidemiology	Social services
Examiners [health professions]	Social welfare
Family planning	Tuberculosis
Geriatric health	Universities
Health	Venereal disease
Health facilities	Vital statistics
Health statistics	Vocational rehabilitation
Higher education	Welfare
Home care	Youth health
Hospitals	Youth hostels

Source: Updated and modified from *Health Planning & Public Accountability Workbook* by A.D. Spiegel and H.H. Hyman, p. 98. Copyright 1976, Rockville, MD: Aspen Publishers, Inc. Reprinted by permission.

other compilations that list administrations, agencies, bureaus, departments, divisions, offices, sections, units, and the like. As more resources are identified, planners will no doubt add to the key words. Obviously, strategic planners should work up their own key words that are germane to the task or project under consideration.

A side effect of using a key word list is that planners are able at the same time to compile an inventory of agencies that may be helpful in future health planning.

Possible Resource/Potential Source Checklist

With a particular problem in mind, a strategic planner could start with a generic list of potential sources such as commercial firms, cultural groups, government agencies, hospitals, mass media, professional organizations, recreational facilities, religious organizations, schools, and voluntary health agencies. Depending upon the structural level of the planning activity, these potential sources could be considered at international, national, state, local or other organizational levels.

Exhibit 3-21 allows the planner to creatively brainstorm using a checklist of possible

Exhibit 3-21. Possible Resources and Potential Sources.

People: Leaders, Sponsors, Supporters

Clergy	Ethnic groups	Business/industry	Private practitioners
Schools	Celebrities	Govt. officials	Public health depts.
PTAs	Politicians	Medical societies	Voluntary health assns.
Unions	Social clubs	Professional assns.	Mass media
Hospitals	Mass media	Religious organs.	Retired executives

People: Health Care Providers

Clinics	First aid squads	Public health dept.	Schools [Md, RN, etc.]
Hospitals	Medical society	Professional assns.	Neighborhood health center

Staff: Consultants, Committee Members, Providers of Service

Medical:	Industry	Medical society	Voluntary health assns.
	Clinics	Public health dept.	Schools [professional]
	Hospitals	Professional assns.	Private practitioners
Clerical:	Hospital	Social clubs	Business/industry
	PTAs	Civic groups	Public health dept.
	Schools	"Y"s	Senior citizens groups
	Unions	Private citizen	Voluntary health assn.
Analytical:	Business/industry [computers]		Voluntary health assn.
	Professional assn. [statisticians]		Health planning agency
	Universities [management]		Public health dept.
Organization:	Clergy	Civic groups	Chamber of commerce
Planning:	PTAs	Medical society	Health planning agency
	Politicians	Consumer groups	Private practitioners
	Hospital	Govt. officials	Professional assns.
	Schools	Business/industry	Tenant organizations
	Unions	Public health dept.	Voluntary health assn.
	Social clubs	Retired executives	Neighborhood health ctr.
Educational:	Clinics	Consumer groups	Insurance company
	Hospital	Mass media	Professional assns.
	Schools	Medical society	Voluntary health assns.

Equipment: Office, Technical

Office:	Clinics	Business/industry	Chamber of commerce
	Hospital	Civic groups	Professional assns.
	Schools	Consumer groups	Voluntary health assns.
	Unions	Trade assns.	Neighborhood health ctrs.
	"Y"s	Public health dept.	Salvation Army
Devices:	Trade assns.	Armed forces [VAs]	Business/industry [mfgrs.]
Equipment:	Hospital	First aid squads	Professional assns.
	Schools	Govt. officials	Voluntary health assns.
	Clinics	Medical society	Advertising agencies

(continued)

Exhibit 3-21. (Continued)

Supplies: Office, Audio-visual, Laboratory, Medication			
Office Sup- plies:	Schools Unions Hospital Government	Civic groups Consumer groups Business/industry Local stores	Professional assns. Trade assns. Voluntary health assns. Rental firms
Pamphlets: Posters: A-V material:	Government Civic groups Hospital Medical society	Mass media Consumer groups Public health dept. Ad agencies	Insurance companies Union health plans Business/industry Voluntary health assns.
Lab Supplies: Medication:	Trade assns. Drug firms Government	Public health dept. Professional assns. Hospital	Business/industry Private practitioners Voluntary health assns.
How to Get Things Done in the Community Health Care System			
Current Sta- tus:	Politicians Hospital Schools	Consumer groups Medical society Public health dept.	Health planning agency Professional assns. Voluntary health assns.
Community Resources:	Clergy Clinics Hospital Schools Unions "Y"s Politicians	Fraternal societies Consumer groups Civic groups Social clubs Trade assns. Mass media Business/industry	Ethnic groups Tenants organizations Voluntary health assns. Health planning agency Public health dept. Professional assns. Senior citizen groups
Facilities: Use and/or Alteration			
Use:	Clergy Hotels Hospital Government "Y"s	Chamber of commerce Social clubs Tenant organizations Schools Unions	Business/industry Voluntary health assns. Professional assns. Neighborhood health ctrs. Civic groups
Alteration:	Business/industry [construction firms] Unions [skilled construction labor]		
Cash Money, Stocks, Bonds, Saleable Items:			
Civic groups Foundations Unions	Government Pot luck suppers Raffles	Third party payers Professional assns. Business/industry	Fraternal societies Voluntary health assns. Banks

resources plotted against potential sources. A planner needing a specific resource—people, staff, equipment, supplies, information, facilities, or cash—could go down the left-hand column and then read across to the two right-hand columns for a clue to a potential supplier of that resource item. On the other hand, if a planner knew that the agency or individual was willing to make a contribution, the two-way resource checklist could start with the right-hand columns and secure ideas about the particular resource items such an agency or individual might contribute to the effort.

This checklist uses generic listings enabling the planner to adapt the technique to the unique conditions existing in any individual community. A thrust of this method is to allow for brainstorming the actual specific sources in each particular geographic locale.

Common and Uncommon Resources

In seeking out resources, a philosophical attitude must be adopted that allows planners to move wherever the creative flow takes them. No matter how outlandish the idea, the first natural law of resource request is, "The most that anyone can do is to say no!"

Two examples illustrate the philosophical principle with an O'Henry twist. Coming to the end of a project, the planner had enough secretaries but not enough word processors to meet the deadline for the final report. Reading the daily newspaper, the planner noticed an advertisement for a new piece of equipment. Calling the local firm mentioned in the ad, the planner explained the problem to the public relations director and asked for the loan of a word processor. To the planner's surprise, the public relations director offered to loan four machines. Having the available secretarial staff at the office, the planner was able to finish the report in plenty of time. While the firm did not even ask for it, the planner mentioned the contribution in the acknowledgments of the report.

In another case, the planner arranged to borrow duplicating equipment to produce flyers advertising the location of health risk appraisal mobile units. When copies of the flyer were sent to the manufacturer who loaned the machine, the planner received a quick telephone call from the sales manager. It seems that the company did not like the quality of the reproduction of the flyer. That company sent a better machine over along with a sales representative to teach the staff how to achieve the best quality reproductions.

Exhibit 3-22 lists examples from actual experiences where planners were able to augment their own resources of personnel, facilities, materials, and money. Individual incursions into this arena can only serve to enhance these potentials. Hopefully, this list will merely be a starting point for consideration of the planner's own contacts and ideas. Simply being alert to the possibilities while reading newspapers and magazines, listening to radio or TV or perusing advertisements in professional journals will stimulate a host of resource opportunities.

Implication of Policies for Resource Allocation

A study of nursing home beds in Australia, the United States, and Canada revealed relevant implications of how admission and reimbursement policies affect utilization of resources [Howe, Phillips, & Preston, 1986]. In turn, those policies affect other parts of the health system. In the United States, each nursing home bed has almost a 100 percent turnover rate annually; while in Canada (Manitoba) only 27 percent of the beds are turned over and about 50 percent in Australia. At the same time, the United States has 64 nursing home beds per 1,000 elderly compared to Canada's 67 and Australia's between 40 and 53. When the bed ratio is multiplied by the turnover rate, an accessibility index emerges. This index shows the number of beds accessible per annum for every 1,000 elderly. In the United States, 55 of its 64 beds/1,000 elderly are available annually, while in Canada only 18 are, and in Australia around 24. In sum, accessibility appears to be directly related to turnover rate.

What causes the turnover rate to be higher in the United States than in Australia and Canada? Medicare, which pays the initial costs of nursing homes, restricts the number of reimbursement days and thereby induces patients to leave earlier than usual. In three studies, almost half the patients were discharged from United States' nursing homes within three months. In Canada, only 26 percent were discharged that soon. Around 35 percent were discharged from Australian homes within two months. Seventy-four percent of the Canadian patients stayed well over 12 months. Around 25 percent stayed that long in the United States. Canadians are heavily subsidized by their government when they enter nursing homes and only

Exhibit 3-22.   Common and Uncommon Resources.

Block associations, tenant organizations
  Volunteers cleaned the streets in sanitation effort.
Church clubs, men's and women's
  Provided clerical manpower for multiphasic screening project.
Civic associations, historical societies
  Donated funds for rodent eradication project.
Fraternities, sororities, social clubs
  Held dance marathons to raise funds for mentally retarded.
Grange, farmer's union, garden clubs
  Donated table settings for a conference of volunteers.
Health councils
  Supplied and ran off annoucements and distributed the same to
    members.
Hobby groups, photography clubs, old car collectors
  Took and prepared photos for newspapers.
Knights of Columbus, Pythian Temples
  Provided transportation for the elderly to the health center.
Labor unions
  Donated the use of their health center for diabetes screening pro-
    gram.
League of Women voters
  Supplied volunteers to work on research project on coronary care.
Lions, Kiwanis, Rotary
  Donated funds to buy volunteers awards for a tuberculosis project.
Ministerial associations
  Agreed to read messages from pulpit on AIDS education/prevention
    program.
Political clubs
  Provided consultation re community leaders and language transla-
    tors.
Professional associations
  Duplicated letters to members and mailed them on their own sta-
    tionery.
PTAs, public and parochial
  Provided personnel for community nutrition program.
Quasi-practitioners, faith healers, witch doctors
  Participated in community mental health screening project.
Radio and television stations
  Donated air time for public service announcements.
Religious charities
  Allowed the use of their computer system for research project.
Research, consultation, and management firms
  Donated funds and loaned staff to assist in planning stages.
Schools, colleges, and universities
  Graduate school class prepared promotional kits for TB screening.
Talent agencies, model agencies, and public relations firms
  Sent entertainers to blood testing program and donated popcorn
    samples.
Trade associations, merchants associations', Chambers of Commerce
  Donated 250,000 self-sticking cards for x-ray advance publicity.
Voluntary health agencies, United Funds, Community Chests
  Donated furniture, office space, and clerical help for projects.
YWCA, YWCA, YMHA, YWHA
  Supplied volunteers for training as emergency first aiders.

Source: Updated and modified from *Health Planning & Public Accountability Workbook* by A.D. Spiegel and H.H. Hyman, p. 172. Copyright 1976, Rockville, MD: Aspen Publishers, Inc. Reprinted by permission.

pay what they can afford. Thus, Canadians have little financial incentive reasons to leave as do Americans.

These findings raise vital questions for resource development which strategic planning can have a major part in answering. Basically, the question is whether nursing homes are used effectively. Is the mental health of nursing home patients affected by forcing individuals to remain institutionalized because there is no other alternative? Does an early discharge push nursing home patients to become members of the growing army of homeless because community social service alternatives are inadequate? Should reimbursement policy be used to determine a patient's length of stay or should the patient's needs be the determining factor? "Although rarely stated explicitly as such, assessment for nursing home admission is essentially a resource allocation process that determines 'who gets what.' As a gatekeeping mechanism, geriatric assessment is a principal means of implementing admission policies designed to achieve changes in use of nursing homes and in rates of turnover, and thereby bring about redistribution" [Howe et al., 1986].

In sum, there is considerable flexibility in redistributing resources within the nursing home system and between that system and other parts of the health and community social service system. Yet, it is only through some form of strategic planning that the true pattern of services required by senior citizens can be ascertained, whether for nursing homes or other services.

Resource development depends on more than methodological considerations regarding personnel, facilities, equipment/supplies, and funding. Based on reimbursement factors, political considerations, and coordination or lack of it, resources can be added or subtracted (Thompson, 1988). A comprehensive strategic health planning process would take all these and other variables into account in resource allocation decisions.

REFERENCES

Aaron, H.J., & Schwartz, W.B. (1983). *The painful prescription. Rationing hospital care.* Washington, DC: The Brookings Institute.

Abraham, L. (1988). Society's MDs find 90% of hospitals can't fill staffs. *American Medical News, 31*(28), 3.

Agovino, T. (1988). Health care planning unit hunts donors to survive. *Crain's New York Business, 4*(8), 11,14.

Alexander, J.A., & Morrisey, M.A. (1988). Hospital selection into multihospital systems. The effects of market, management, and mission. *Medical Care, 26*(2), 159–175.

American Health Planning Association (Today in Health Planning). (1988a). Health Systems Agency of Northern Virginia. *10*(5), 1–2.

American Health Planning Association (Today in Health Planning). (1988b). North Central Florida Health Planning Council. *11*(4), 1–2.

Aram, J.D., Salipante, Jr., P.F., & Knauf, J.W. (1987). Human resource indicators for hospital managers. *Health Care Management Review 12*(2), 15–22.

Baine, D.P. (1987). *VA health care: Resource allocation methodology should improve VA's financial management.* (GAO/HRD 87-123BR). Washington, DC: Government Printing Office.

Baine, D.P. (1989). *Resource allocation methodology has had little impact on medical center's budgets.* (GAO/HRD-89-93). Washington, DC: Government Printing Office.

Barer, M.L., Stark, A.L., & Kinnis, C. (1984). Manpower planning, fiscal restraint, and the "demand" for health care personnel. *Inquiry, 21*(3), 254–265.

Barkholz, D. (1985). HCA's hospital "clusters" will centralize management. *Modern Healthcare, 15*(23), 44.

Bassett, L.C., & Metzger, N. (1986). *Achieving excellence. A prescription for health care managers.* Rockville, MD: Aspen Publishers.

Beeson, P.G., & Ford, W.E. (1983). Systems planning for the 80's: The Nebraska mental health desired service system model. *Community Mental Health Journal, 19*(4), 253–264.

Benjamin, M. (1988). Medical ethics and economics of organ transplantation. *Health Progress, 69*(2), 47–53.

Bennett, J.P. (1985). Standard cost systems lead to efficiency and profitability. *Health Care Financial Management, 39*(5), 46–53.

Bernard, B. (1985). Patient dumping: A resident's first hand view. *The New Physician, 34*(7), 23.

Blank, R.H. (1989). *Rationing medicine.* New York: Columbia University Press.

Blayney, K.D. (1986). Restructuring the health care labor force. The rise of the multiskilled allied health practitioner. *Alabama Journal of Medical Sciences, 23*(3), 277–278.

Bowskey, C.A. (1984). *A proposal for transferring St. Elizabeths Hospital to the District of Columbia.* (GAO/HRD 84-48). Washington, DC: Government Printing Office.

Bradley, S. (1988). Allied care shortages addressed. *U.S. Medicine, 24*(21&22), 47.

Bruhn, J.G., & Philips, B.U. (1985). The influence of technology on the future of allied health professionals. *Journal of Allied Health, 14*(3), 289–295.

Califano, J.A. (1986). *America's health care revolution: Who lives? Who dies? Who pays?* New York: Random House.

Callahan, D. (1987). *Setting limits: Medical goals in an aging society.* New York: Simon & Schuster.

Callahan, D. (1988). Allocating health resources. *Hastings Center Report, 18*(2), 14–20.

Churchill, L.R. (1987). *Rationing health care in America: Perceptions and principles of justice.* Notre Dame, IN: University of Notre Dame Press.

Cohen, A.B. (1986). "Your papers please": Credentialing and the doctor/hospital relationship. *Health Management Quarterly, Second Quarter,* pp. 14–16.

Conner, D.R., Neuman, B.S., & Graham, R.G. (1988). The productivity fad: How to avoid Nirvana in health care. *Dimensions in Health Care, 88*(3), 6–12.

Cox, P. (1989, March 29). Government should stay out of health care. *USA Today,* p. 10.

Crowell, A. (1980). *A model for California mental health programs.* Oakland: Mental Health Associations of California.

Drucker, P.F. (1954). *The practice of management.* New York: Harper & Row.

Duggan, J.M. (1989). Resource allocation and bioethics. *Lancet, 1,* 772–773.

Falkenburger, A.J., & Jacobson, E.A. (1989). Management continuity planning: Selecting and grooming your organization's future leaders. *Dimensions in Health Care, 89*(1), 5–12.

Farel, A.M. (1988). Choice of priority area by state developmental disabilities councils: Child development as a case example. *Mental Retardation, 26*(3), 155–159.

Fein, R. (1988). Toward adequate health care. Why we need National Health Insurance. *Dissent, 35*(1), 98–104.

Fifer, W.R. (1987). The hospital medical staff of 1997. *Quality Review Bulletin, 13*(6), 194–197.

Folmer, H.R. (1987). Simulation game in health resources allocation. *Health Policy and Planning, 2*(2), 189–190.

Fottler, M.D., Hernandez, S.R., & Joiner, C.L. (1988). *Strategic management of human resources in health services organizations* New York: John Wiley & Sons.

Fuchs, V.R. (1974). *Who shall live?* New York: Basic Books.

Fuchs, V.R. (1984). The "rationing" of medical care. *New England Journal of Medicine, 311*(24), 1572–1573.

Gallina, J.N. (1989). Application of strategic planning techniques for short-term results. *Current Concepts in Hospital Pharmacy Management, 11*(1), 14–19.

Gallivan, M. (1986). Technology planning: An imperative, not an option. *Hospitals, 60*(2), 100.

Gesler, W. (1986). The uses of spatial analysis in medical geography: A review. *Social Science in Medicine, 23*(10), 963–973.

Gianelli, D.M. (1988). Shortage of nurses critical, U.S. advisory panel concludes. *American Medical News, 31*(48), 1,10.

Government Studies & Systems. (1977). *A taxonomy of the health system appropriate for plan development*. (DHEW Pub. No. (HRA) 77-14534). Washington, DC: Government Printing Office.

Gross, J. (1989, March 27). What medical care the poor can have: Lists are drawn up. *New York Times*, p. 18.

Grumet, G.W. (1989). Health care rationing through incovenience. *New England Journal of Medicine*, *321*(9), 607–611.

Gunn, R.A., & Kazemek, E.A. (1986). Employee motivation: Quality versus business concerns. *Healthcare Financial Management*, *40*(2), 76–78.

Hannan, E.L., Rouse, R.L., Barnett, R., & Uppal, P. (1987). Methods for developing relative need criteria to accompany a health care capital expenditure limit. *Journal of Health Politics, Policy and Law*, *12*(1), 113–136.

Harris, L. and Associates. (1987). *Making difficult health care decisions*. Boston, MA: The Loran Commission.

Healthwire. (1989a). Unlicensed staff: The AMA's RCT. *10*(10), 7–8.

Healthwire. (1989b). RCT resolution. *3*(3), 3.

Healthwire. (1989c). Ron Wyden: For quality care, against RCTs. *11*(4), 5.

Hiatt, H.H. (1987). *America's health in the balance: Choice or change?* New York: Harper & Row.

Howe, A.L., Phillips, C., & Preston, G. (1986). Analysing access to nursing home care. *Social Sciences and Medicine*, *23*(12), 1267–1277.

Iglehart, J.K. (1986). Health policy report. The future supply of physicians. *New England Journal of Medicine*, *314*(13), 860–864.

Institute of Medicine. (1988). *Allied health services: Avoiding crisis*. Washington, DC: National Academy Press.

Isaacs, M.R. (1986). *Acute psychiatric bed need planning: Issues and methodologies*. (HRP-0906627). Washington, DC: Government Printing Office.

Jemison, T. (1988a). RAM model unpopular in field. *U.S. Medicine*, *24*(17&18), 36–37.

Jemison, T. (1988b). RAM abandoned amidst crisis. *U.S. Medicine*, *24*(21&22), 1,46–47.

Jennett, B. (1986). Balancing benefits. *The Health Service Journal*, *96*(5005), 6–7.

Jones, L. (1989). Brookings report addresses rationing of care. *American Medical News*, *32*(9), 9.

Kahn, A.A. (1986). Two simple methods of spatial analysis and their applications in location oriented health services research. *American Journal of Public Health*, *76*(10), 1207–1209.

Kelliher, M.E. (1985). Managing productivity, performance, and the cost of services. *Healthcare Financial Management*, *39*(5), 23–28.

Kindig, D.A., Manassuzin, H., & Cross Dunham, N. (1987). Trends in physician availiabiity in 10 urban areas from 1963 to 1980. *Inquiry*, *24*(2), 136–146.

Kitzhaber, J. (1989, March 29). Ration care—but with equity. *USA Today*, p. 10.

Klafehn, K.A., & Owens, D.L. (1987). A simulation model designed to investigate resource utilization in a hospital emergency room. In *Symposium on computer applications in medical care*. Washington, DC: Computer Society Press.

Koek, K.E. (1988). *Encyclopedia of associations* (22ed ed.). Detroit, MI: Gale Research Co.

Labelle, R. (1987). Planning the provision and use of health care technology. *Dimensions in Health Service*, *64*(4), 33–35.

Lamm, R.D. (1988). An eight count indictment against America. *Medical Group Management Journal*, *35*(4), 21–24.

Langstaff, J.H. (1987). Medical manpower planning/impact analysis. *Dimensions in Health Service*, *64*(1), 31–33.

Larkin, H. (1988). Will the public support health care rationing? *Hospitals*, *62*(9), 79.

Leiken, A.M., & McTernan, E.J. (1985). Cost containment and the future utilization of health manpower. *Health Care Strategic Management*, *3*(12), 11–13.

Liss, A., Moller, T., & Sandblad, B. (1986). A simulation based system for regional planning of care resources in oncology. In R. Salamon, B. Blum, & M. Jorgensen (Eds.), *Medinfo 86* (pp. 736–740). North-Holland: Elsevier Sciences Pub.

Lomas, J., Stoddart, G.L., & Barer, M.L. (1985). Supply projections as planning: A critical review of forecasting new physician requirements in Canada. *Social Sciences and Medicine*, 20(4), 411–424.

Lund, D.S. (1988a). Oregon to fund Medicaid transplants again. *American Medical News*, 31(29), 11.

Lund, D.S. (1988b). Oregon lawmakers halt organ transplant program again. *American Medical News*, 31(36), 31.

Lund, D.S. (1989a). Oregon considers rationing Medicaid health benefits. *American Medical News*, 32(11), 1,54.

Lund, D.S. (1989b). Medicaid rationing plan gains favor in other states. *American Medical News*, 32(17), 1,36–37.

Lund, D.S. (1989c). Health care rationing plan OK'd in Oregon, stymied in California. *American Medical News*, 32(27), 1,39.

MacStravic, R. (1984). *Forecasting the use of health services*. Rockville, MD: Aspen Publishers.

McCormick, B. (1988). RNs: Two-thirds of nursing staff. *Hospitals*, 60(23), 74.

McGregor, M. (1989). Technology and the allocation of resources. *New England Journal of Medicine*, 320(2), 118–120.

Melville, K., & Dobie, J. (1988). *The public's perspective on social welfare reform*. New York: Public Agenda Foundation.

Nardone, D.A. (1988). Ambulatory care: Challenges remain. *U.S. Medicine*, 24(15&16), 19–20.

Oreglia, A., Klein, D.A., Crandall, L.A., & Duncan, P. (1976). *Guide to the development of health resources inventories*. (DHEW Pub. No. (HRA) 76-14504.) Washington, DC: Government Printing Office.

Page, L. (1988a). Controversial plan on new caregiver gets AMA support. *American Medical News*, 31(26), 1,38–39.

Page, L. (1988b). Major shortages seen in allied health; initiatives sought to gain personnel. *American Medical News*, 31(29), 10.

Panerai, R.B., & Attinger, E.O. (1986). Information system for appropriate allocation of health care technologies. In R. Salamon, B. Blum, & M. Jorgensen (Eds.), *MEDINFO 86* (pp. 253–255). North-Holland: Elsevier Science Publishers.

Parkin, D., & Henderson, J. (1987). How important is equality of access to hospital? A case study of patients' and visitors' travel costs. *Hospital and Health Services Review*, 83(1), 23–27.

Perrone, J. (1988). As needs, costs rise, states face problems of health care rationing. *American Medical News*, 31(29), 2,33.

Poizner, S.L. (1986). Micro mapping: Data imaging for information managers. *Journal of Information & Image Management*, 19(11), 35–38.

Reid, R.A., Fulcher, J.H., & Smith, H.L. (1986). Hospital-health care plan affiliations: considerations for strategy design. *Health Care Management Review*, 11(4), 53–61.

Reinhardt, U.E. (1985). Economics, ethics and the American health care system. *The New Physician*, 34(7), 20–28,42.

Reinhardt, U.E. (1986). Rationing the nation's health care surplus: An American paradox. *The Internist*, 27(2), 11–13.

Renz, L., & Olson, S. (1987). *The foundation directory 11th edition*. New York: The Foundation Center.

Rifkin, S.B., & Walt, G. (1988). Health priorities and the developing world. *The Lancet*, 2(8613), 744.

Robert Wood Johnson Foundation. (1983). *Updated report on access to health care for the American people*. Princeton, NJ.

Roddy, P.C., Liu, K., & Meiners, M.R. (1987). *Resource requirement of nursing home patients based on time and motion studies*. (DHHS Pub. No. (PHS) 87-3404). Washington, DC: Government Printing Office.

Roswell, R.H. (1988). Care patterns shift in resource model. *U.S. Medicine*, 24(15&16), 34.

Salmon, M.E., & Culbertson, R.A. (1985). Health manpower oversupply: Implications for physicians, nurse practitioners and physician assistants. A model. *Hospital & Health Services Administration*, 30(1), 100–115.

Seiden, D. (1985). Prescription for a medical ethic. Diminishing resources, critical choices. *Commonweal*, 112(5), 137–141.

Shortell, S.M., & Kaluzny, A.D. (1988). *Health care management*. New York: John Wiley & Sons.

Smeeding, T.M. (1987). *Should medical care be rationed by age?* Totowa, NJ: Rowman & Littlefield.

Tabatabai, C. (1987). Staff productivity: The other side of cost cutting. *Healthcare Financial Management*, *41*(3), 42–44.

Tarlov, A.R. (1986). HMO enrollment growth and physicians: The third compartment. *Health Affairs*, *5*(1), 23–35.

Thompson, L.H. (1988). *Further opportunities to increase the sharing of medical resources*. (GAO/HRD 88-51). Washington, DC: Government Printing Office.

Thouez, J.M., Bodson, P., & Joseph, A.E. (1988). Some methods for measuring the geographic accessibility of medical services in rural regions. *Medical Care*, *26*(1), 34–43.

Tolchin, M. (1988, April 18). Health worker shortage is worsening. *New York Times*, p. 1.

Tomich, N. (1988). Large, small hospitals in spiral. *U.S. Medicine*, *24*(13&14), 1,34,35.

Trivedi, V., Moscovice, I., Bass, R., & Brooks, J. (1987). A semi-Markov model for primary health care manpower supply prediction. *Management Science*, *33*(2), 149–160.

USA Today. (1989, March 29). Government must assure health care. p. 10.

USDHEW, Health Resources Administration. (1976). *A guide to the development of health resources inventories*. Washington, DC: Government Printing Office.

USDHEW, Health Resources Administration. (1977). *A taxonomy of the health system appropriate for plan development*. Washington, DC: Government Printing Office.

USDHEW, Alcohol, Drug Abuse and Mental Health Administration. (1978). *A manual on state mental health planning*. (Pub. No. [ADM] 77-473). Washington, DC: Government Printing Office.

USDHHS, Indian Health Service. (1988). *Allocation of resources in the IHS, a handbook on the Resource Allocation Methodology (RAM)*. Washington, DC: Government Printing Office.

U.S. Medicine. (1988a). VA showing decline in ranks of nurses. *24*(13&14), 35.

U.S. Medicine. (1988b). AMA addresses nurse shortage, pay issues, AIDS. *24*(15&16), 49,58,59.

Warheit, G.J., & Auth, J.B. (1981). *An epidemiologically based method of assessing the need for psychiatric/alcohol acute care beds*. Gainesville, FL: University of Florida.

Welch, H.G., & Larson, E.B. (1988). Dealing with limited resources. The Oregon decision to curtail funding for organ transplantation. *New England Journal of Medicine*, *319*(3), 171–173.

Wetle, T., Cwikel, J., & Levkoff, S.E. (1988). Geriatric medical decisions: Factors influencing allocation of scarce resources and the decision to withhold treatment. *The Gerontologist*, *28*(3), 336–343.

Wilensky, G.R. (1985). Making decisions on rationing. *Business and Health*, *3*(1), 36–38.

4

Generating and Considering Alternative Courses of Action

With the problem identified, with the data collected and analyzed, and with the resources inventoried, planners may consider alternative resolutions to the specific problem. However, planning does not always proceed along logical, linear lines and the methods and techniques in this chapter could also be used to identify problems, to discover sources of data, and to pinpoint available and potential resources.

Few planners will be in the position of the famous football coach who was assured of unlimited resources by the owner of the team. When questioned later, the owner remarked that the coach had even exceeded that budget. It is most likely that planners will have limited resources. Therefore, that situation requires a creative and innovative approach to make the most efficient utilization of the scarce resources.

ORIENTATION TO CREATIVITY AND INNOVATION

A slogan attributed to Alex Osborn, the inventor of brainstorming, is printed on the cover of the *Journal of Creative Behavior:* "Imagination is the Golden Key to Problem Solving." To stimulate the imagination, Osborn [1953, p. 215] suggests five devices: make a start, don't procrastinate, use checklists and make notes, set deadlines and quotas, set a time and pick a place, and think anywhere.

Psychological research clearly indicates that all aspects of creativity are within the normal abilities of the average human being. Individuals merely require practice, confidence, and encouragement to upgrade and increase their creative output. With that caveat in mind, Raudsepp [1987] delineated guideposts and "two dozen ways to turn on your organization's light bulbs." Creative problem solving to assist the average person to get into the act integrated the following admonitions:

Exhibit 4-1. Creativity Exercises.

Imagine that you are the senior planner for your hospital and each of the nine dots below represents a satellite service provided by your facility.

Your task is to coordinate all nine services using four straight lines of communication and cooperation. Federal FCC regulations mandate that your lines may cross but they must be connected. Interpreted by the hospital's legal department, that means that you can't take your pencil off the paper when starting a new line.

```
•  •  •

•  •  •

•  •  •
```

Make eight 8's equal 1,000

A longtime elected state legislator has the reputation of being competent and efficient. However, she also is noted for the fact that she always has a dour facial expression and almost never smiles. She decides to run for Governor of the state in the next election. What slogan or slogans and campaign approach can you suggest for this dour, nonsmiling but effective politician?

List as many uses as you can think of for a paper clip.

- Stretch your horizons
- Cultivate your field
- Pinpoint the problem
- Hunt for ideas
- Boost your lagging enthusiasm
- Prepare for premiere.

Obviously, these guideposts will mean different things to different people. Yet, Raudsepp [1987, p. 8] comments that the common denominator for creative people is that "the tired, the proven and the established do not have an inordinately strong hold on them."

Keeping these principles in mind, examine the four creativity exercises in Exhibit 4–1 and put this book aside while you solve the problems. Suggested solutions will be found at the end of this chapter. There are no right or wrong answers, just variations of responses. Please don't look at the possible solutions until after your own creative efforts.

Just in case you were downhearted at your results in the creativity exercises, consider the mice in council generating alternatives as related to us by Aesop in Exhibit 4–2. Creativity

Exhibit 4-2. A Dilemma for the Mice in Council.

A certain Cat that lived in a large country-house was so vigilant and active, that the Mice, finding their numbers grievously thinned, held a council, with closed doors, to consider what they had best do. Many plans had been started and dismissed, when a young Mouse, rising and catching the eye of the president, said that he had a proposal to make, that he was sure must meet with the approval of all. "If," said he, "the Cat wore around her neck a little bell, every step she took would make it tinkle; then, ever forewarned of her approach, we should have time to reach our holes. By this simple means we should live in safety, and defy her power." The speaker resumed his seat with a complacent air, and a murmur of applause arose from the audience. An old grey Mouse, with a merry twinkle in his eye, now got up, and said that the plan of the last speaker was an admirable one; but he feared it had one drawback. He had not told them who should put the bell around the Cat's neck.

[From *Aesop's Fables*, [c. 620–560 B.C.]. Revised by J.B. Rundell, 1869]

Source: From *Fragments of Heracleitus, Heracleitus, On the Universe* (English translation), by W.H.S. Jones, 1931, London: William Heinemann Ltd. Reprinted by permission.

experts should have advised the mice to produce a greater quantity of alternatives and to withhold discussion until after all of the ideas were gathered. Perhaps one of the mice would have come forward with the way to bell the cat.

GROUND RULES FOR GENERATING ALTERNATIVES

Creativity ground rules may differ considerably from the traditional scientific problem-solving method that health care providers may have learned in their respective professional schools. Generally, the scientific method proceeds from step to step beginning with a definition of the problem, data collection, appraisal of the information, formulation of a hypothesis, testing of the hypothesis, and evaluation of the results. A limitation of the applied scientific method is that people constantly evaluate as they proceed through the process. If individuals delay weighing the advantages and disadvantages of each step, there is no barrier to an outpouring of alternatives in a spontaneous and infectious fashion. Scientifically oriented persons may require practice before becoming comfortable with a freewheeling acceptance of all alternatives generated.

However, that scientific mindset need not inhibit the production of creative alternatives to a problem. Usually, individuals adjust readily to the commonality of most creative techniques that reduces inhibition, the deferring and/or postponing of judgment until all the alternatives have been generated and recorded.

In a manner not too diverse from the scientific method, Osborn [1953, p. 123] identified seven steps in the creative process:

1. *Orientation:* Pointing up the problem
2. *Preparation:* Gathering pertinent data
3. *Analysis:* Breaking down the relevant material
4. *Hypothesis:* Piling up alternatives by way of ideas
5. *Incubation:* Letting up, to invite illumination
6. *Synthesis:* Putting the pieces together
7. *Verification:* Judging the resultant ideas

Ground rules for a group problem-solving meeting must be specified and made known to the participants. As reported by J. Conlin [1987], the similarity is apparent:

1. Identify the problem and explain why it must be solved.
2. Identify the causes of the problem.
3. Rephrase the problem in "how can we" terms and use creativity techniques to produce ideas.
4. Evaluate the ideas and categorize them.
5. Reach agreement on a solution.
6. Test solution and turn into a proposal.
7. Implement the activity.

In either situation, individual or group, the well-known maxim still holds true: "A problem well defined is a problem half-solved." Equally important at a group meeting is the fact that people speak at about 120 to 180 words per minute but individuals can think at four to five times that rate. In other words, your brain can work harder and faster than your mouth.

LATERAL VS. VERTICAL THINKING—CONVERGENT OR DIVERGENT PATHS

As he comments on the virtues of zigzag lateral thinking, de Bono [1970] differentiates that mode from vertical thinking. Barrett [1978] talks about The Egnahc Makers but calls the modes divergent and convergent thinking.

Vertical [convergent] thinking is neat, orderly, and rational. There is a stepwise process with each step following the prior step in an unbroken sequence. Only relevant material is selected and dealt with at each step. In its essence, vertical thinking must be correct at every step.

Contrariwise, lateral [divergent] thinking moves sideways, zigging and zagging to apply alternatives to a problem. There is no need to be sequential and steps can be single or leap-frogged to reach a point. Deliberate use is made of random and/or unrelated data to produce creative alternatives. One can take wrong steps while still seeking the right step.

Vertical planners built a bridge with toll booths at each end. As traffic increased, long waits and hot tempers flared at both ends of the bridge. A lateral-thinking planner found that most of the drivers used the bridge to enter as well as to leave the city. His lateral solution was to double the toll, but to collect the money only one way.

Obese people are constantly told by vertical thinkers to follow a strict regimen and eat less. Reversing that thought process, a lateral thinker could recommend eating more, particularly sweets or food calculated to lessen the appetite. However, the additional food ingested would be before meals. Commercial companies have marketed that idea in "diet suppressants."

No matter what the process is called—vertical, lateral, divergent, convergent—the health planner must strive to engender an atmosphere that supports the development of creative alternatives. That task may be formidable since a large number of public and private organizations have set bureaucratic patterns that discourage innovation and reward conformity.

BREAKING AWAY FROM CONFORMITY

Addressing commercial enterprises and writing in the *Harvard Business Review,* Pearson [1988] believes that big winners marshal their resources—then they execute like the Russian hockey team. Five tough-minded ways for a company to get innovative are listed:

1. Begin with the right mindset. Create and sustain a corporate environment that values better performance above everything else.
2. One system runs the business; another one develops new ideas. This structure permits innovative ideas to rise above the demands of running the business.
3. Unsettle the organization. Define a strategic focus to realistically channel the company's innovative efforts toward a payoff in the competitive marketplace.
4. Be hardheaded about your strategy. Know where to look for good ideas and how to leverage them once they're found.
5. Look hard at what's already going on. Go after good ideas at full speed with all the company's resources brought to bear.

Pearson also commented that most good ideas look obvious—once you see how they work.

In a similar vein, Bennett and Tibbitts [1986, p. 16] listed the following seven imperatives of innovation in an organization: an enlightened culture that fosters change, a systematic view of innovation as a strategic process and a function, a credo from top management that supports innovation, a transfer of that credo from top to middle management, and so on down the line, an innovative management of human resources, an investment in money and people in innovation, and a creative work environment.

Clearly, the innovative organization accepts skepticism toward existing policies and practices, follows future-oriented decision-making directions, tolerates minor errors, and has an appetite for the unusual.

One result of creating such conditions in an organization leads to "intrapreneurship" [Pinchot, 1985, p. 20]. Employees come up with entrepreneurial ventures for their own company to undertake and therefore the change from entre to intra. Intrapreneurial ideas generated for hospitals included, in ranked order, the following: management support systems, freestanding emergency rooms, clinics, and so on, community access to in-house services, wellness programs, catering/food service management, home health care, mobile health services, occupational health programs, senior citizens programs, sports medicine programs, and hotel/hospital lodging. Goals of 137 hospital projects surveyed were identified as revenue generation [47 percent], as public relations [26 percent] and providing a needed service [23 percent] [Simyar & Lloyd-Jones, 1988, p. 236].

Pinchot [1985, p. 20], who coined the word, said, "Intrapreneurship is not just a way to increase the level of innovation and productivity in organizations, although it will do that. More importantly, it is a way of organizing vast businesses so that work again becomes a joyful expression of one's contribution to society."

Odysseum, a Boston [MA] firm, helps corporations to use tools to unlock employee creativity and innovation. An environment can be created where "whimsy, experimentation, and the introduction of the unexpected" is tolerated and even encouraged [Hancock, 1988].

ELEMENTS OF CREATIVE BEHAVIOR

In an American Management Association booklet on idea management, Clark [1980, p. 12] reported on five creative elements developed by Dr. J.P. Guilford: fluency in speech, flexibility and ability to let go of categories, originality, awareness in seeing with the mind and imagination as well as with the eyes, and the motivation of the inner drive. Expanding the positives, Bennett and Tibbitts [1986, p. 109] noted seven behavioral traits that "optimize creative potential:"

1. *Courage* to frolic in domains of activity and interest, new to most people, and in which others have feared to tread.
2. *Self-confidence* in one's own ability to change things for the better that preempts any fears of failure.
3. *Flexibility and spontaneity* that frees one from doing the same thing always in the same way, under the same conditions, accompanied with the native tendency to be unconstrained in manner or behavior.
4. *Inquisitiveness*, a state of mind that goes beyond seeing things "as they are," causing one to ask the right kinds of questions—questions that challenge one's own thinking or lead one to look for ways to reshape it.
5. *Playfulness*, in the sense of having fun at whatever one does in and out of the workplace.

6. A sense of *uncertainty*, setting one apart from the crowd that believes the way things are done is the best and only way.
7. *Discontent*, the thought that things could be better and the will to do something about it.

Writing in the *Harvard Business Review*, Quinn [1985] summed up the approach in the title of his article, "Managing Innovation: Controlled Chaos." He stated that large corporations "stay innovative by behaving like small entreprenurial ventures." Three key elements in an innovation strategy are identified: adopt an opportunity orientation; structure the firm for innovation; and use a complex portfolio planning technique to allocate resources.

Using euphemisms, Weaver [1987] capitalizes on your full creative potential with a "second wind." Kriegel and Kriegel [1988] suggest mastering the "back-burner" to let your subconscious mind take over the creativity tasks. Elliot [1987] opts for analogical thinking to spur creativity. Suggestion programs and patent systems with cash and/or intangible rewards foster creativity and innovation according to Meehan [1986].

BARRIERS TO CREATIVITY AND INNOVATION

Several quotes follow that illustrate explicitly a mindset that inhibits creativity and innovation [Albrecht, 1987, p. 142]:

- Everything that can be invented has been invented. [Charles H. Duell Head, U.S. Patent Office, 1899]
- Sensible and responsible women do not want to vote. [Grover Cleveland, 1905]
- Who the hell wants to hear actors talk? [Harry M. Warner, Warner Brothers Pictures, 1927]

Under the heading, "It Can't Be Done," Bennett and Tibbitts [1986, Figure 7C] culled additional bon mots:

- In 1797 New Jersey farmers rejected the new cast-iron plow because the cast-iron poisoned the land and stimulated the growth of weeds.
- German experts proved that if trains went at the frightful speed of 15 miles an hour, blood would spurt from the travelers' noses, and that passengers would suffocate going through tunnels.
- As the YWCA announced typing lessons for women in 1881, there were vigorous protests that the female constitution would break down under the strain.
- Baron Gottfried Wilhelm von Leibvitz, German philosopher-mathematician, expressed doubt that man would ever fly: "Here God has, so to speak, put a bar across man's path."

Taylor [1961, p. 12] identifies a rather inclusive list of 12 individualistic barriers to creative thinking:

1. Poor health—physical and/or psychological problems
2. Inadequate motivation—disinterest and lack of desire
3. Mental laziness—unwillingness to think or stupidity
4. Lack of curiosity—inability to wonder
5. Superficiality—shallowness and hastiness of thought

6. Repressive training and education via rote learning—conform! standardize! conventionalize!
7. Job degradation—regulated and stifled mental capability.
8. Emotion mindedness—feelings tend to distort thinking
9. Faulty observation—inability to see the obvious
10. Judicial mindset—reflexive criticism stops creativity
11. Labeling—thinking biased by names used
12. Conceptual blocks—stereotyped reactions

Neophobia, fear of the new, novel, or unknown, was added to the roadblocks to creativity by Raudsepp [1987b, p. 10]. In their six-point list, Hickman and Silva [1985] also included avoidance of change, reliance on rules, fear and self-doubt, overreliance on logic, black-and-white thinking, and overreliance on practicality and efficiency.

Business corporations and health care providers also develop a corporate identity that embodies attributes that may inhibit creativity. Based on research and case studies, Quinn [1985] cites seven common corporate constraints on innovation:

Top management isolation
Intolerance of fanatics
Excessive rationalism
Excessive bureaucracy
Accounting practices
Short time horizons
Inappropriate incentives

In addition to corporate-type management and structural barriers, there are verbal ripostes that tend to pop up automatically in conversations. IKE [I Kill Everything] was the acronym cited by Albrecht [1987, p. 133] among his list of "idea stoppers" while Clark [1980, p. 21] labeled his 50 or so inhibitors "killer phrases." A few of these familiar phrases that are verbalized all too frequently when a creative idea warily makes its appearance follow [Albrecht, 1987, p. 136; Clark, 1980, p. 21; Taylor, 1961, p. 176]:

That's the dumbest thing I ever heard.   Unrealistic!
We already tried that years ago.   Too idealistic!
Let's stick with what we know.   No budget for it.
That's not our job.   Are you kidding?
Boss will never go for it.   No way!
It's against company policy.   It'll never work!
Let's form a committee to look at it.   No staff on hand.

People retain a pride in their individualism and resent being told what to do, especially in their own field of expertise. In addition, people also want to partake in decisions that affect them. These combined attitudes lead to a major barrier to innovation—the NIH syndrome [Not Invented Here]. When individuals don't feel ownership or commitment, they aren't motivated to participate or to follow through.

Now that an introduction to creativity, to generating alternatives, to breaking away from conformity and to barriers inhibiting innovation has ensued, it's time to move on to specific methods and techniques that planners can employ to spur creativity.

TECHNIQUES FOR GENERATING ALTERNATIVES

In his comprehensive source book, *Techniques of Structured Problem Solving*, VanGundy [1988] describes a host of methods for producing creative ideas. He even picks out a top-40 techniques list that includes ways to redefine problems, to analyze problems, to generate ideas individually or in groups, to implement ideas and to evaluate and select ideas.

While these methods and techniques for generating alternatives are in this chapter, it should be obvious by now that the methods can be used in any phase of the planning process. Planners should not be dogmatic in using these techniques only for this or that purpose.

Since so many of the creative techniques borrow from the principles and procedures nurtured by Alex Osborn [1963], his "brainstorming" approach merits an initial look at the use of applied imagination.

Brainstorming

This technique asks participants to mentally "storm" a problem or task from all possible facets applying their aggregate brainpower. At a 1939 session, participants dubbed Osborn's efforts "Brainstorm Sessions" [1953, p. 297]. Everything is acceptable except pulling a new idea to pieces with negativism.

Specific guidelines for group sessions must be followed [Osborn, 1953, p. 300]:

1. Judicial judgment is ruled out—criticism and questions must be postponed until a later analysis
2. Freewheeling is welcomed—the wilder the better with no holds barred and caution thrown to the wind
3. Quantity is wanted—the greater the number of ideas the greater likelihood of quality winners
4. Combinations and improvements are sought—hitchhike on the ideas of others in the group

While Osborn [1963, p. 136] said that there are no real guidelines to classical brainstorming, he did list the following as typical steps in the procedure:

1. State the problem and refine and restate if necessary
2. Select 6 to 12 participants
3. Send a written memo to participants with the problem, the rules, examples and the date, place and time of the meeting
4. Have an orientation before the session—a warm-up
5. Write the problem so all participants can see it
6. Repeat the rules for the session
7. Only one idea at a time; raise hand to speak
8. Recording secretary writes down all ideas
9. Set a time limit; about 30 minutes
10. Set up an evaluation group of five people different from the participants in step 2
11. Report back to the participants and ask for more ideas
12. Present final list to the implementors

Using this technique, it would not be unusual for a group to generate 100 ideas within a five-minute brainstorming session. Even if only one usable alternative emerges, the total amount of staff time expended is minimal. Separating the activities into a creative phase and an analysis phase allows participants to focus their total energy on one task at a time. During the analysis phase, discussion will stress only the most promising alternatives.

Scientifically oriented planners and participants may find the principles and procedures of brainstorming alien to their training and experience. In a creatively controlled environment, individuals can be freed from the fear of evaluative and judgmental ridicule and/or the prospect of embarrassment or humiliation. A defensive posture is fostered when people have to be worried about negative and snide comments and they become introspective and verbally reluctant. For brainstorming to work, the health planner and/or leader must assure all the participants of psychological safety and psychosocial freedom of expression. That is a basic condition for stimulating creativity and those conditions must be apparent to all the participants.

Questioning Checklists

Since many of the techniques for generating alternatives have adapted Alex Osborn's [1963, p. 284] seminal self-interrogation questions, a complete listing is given. Principles of association via similarities, contrasts, or extensions are a major ingredient of the process as the mind is stimulated to search for ideas. As in brainstorming, planners must withhold judgment until after all the alternatives are noted. Keeping these points in mind, individuals systematically explore and probe the focused problem asking themselves the questions while maintaining the necessary spontaneity. Individual notes serve to record the alternatives.

Essentially, a self-interrogation checklist prods the planner to try out novel perspectives relative to the problem under consideration. Four types of questions usually are used: to define and uncover problems, to secure extra facts, to assist in decision making, and to generate ideas [Taylor, 1961, p. 88]. However, a comprehensive checklist of questions is only a spur to the imagination and is not a substitute for creative thinking.

Let's try using Osborn's nine category self-interrogation checklist on the problem of improving medical records.

Put to other uses?
New ways to use as is? Other uses if modified?

Adapt
What else is like this? What other idea does this suggest? Does past offer parallel? What could I copy? Whom should I imitate?

Modify?
Changing meaning, color, motion, sound, odor, form, shape? New twist? Other changes?

Magnify?
What to add? More time? Greater frequency? Stronger? Higher? Longer? Thicker? Extra value? Plus ingredient? Duplicate? Multiply? Exaggerate?

Minify?
What to subtract? Smaller? Condensed? Miniature? Lower? Shorter? Omit? Streamline? Split up? Understate?

Substitute?
What else instead? Who else instead? Other ingredient? Other material? Other purpose? Other power? Other approach? Other tone of voice?

Rearrange?

Interchange components? Other pattern? Other layout? Other sequence? Transpose cause and effect? Change pace? Change schedule?

Reverse?

Transpose advantages and disadvantages? How about opposites? Turn it backward? Turn it upside down? Reverse roles? Change shoes? Turn tables? Turn other cheek?

Combine?

How about a blend, an alloy, an assortment, an ensemble? Combine units? Combine purposes? Combine appeals? Combine ideas?

A sampling of ideas generated by using the self-questioning checklist on the problem of improving medical records follows: use different colored paper to distinguish parts of the problem-oriented record, supply disease background education on audio cassettes for attending health care providers, add larger size lettering for major problems, provide stronger binding so pages don't fall out, have records prepared by voice activated typewriters or computers, prepare records on microfiche; combine records with quality review and insurance forms, combine records with case illustrations for teaching purposes, prepare fictional simulations for training.

SCAMPER

In another version of the self-interrogation checklist, Eberle [1984, p. 16] came up with the mnemonic "SCAMPER" as a stimulus to creative imagination development. Note the similarity to Osborn's list in the questioning technique.

What can you *S*ubstitute?
What can you *C*ombine?
What can you *A*dopt? *A*dapt?
What can you *M*agnify, *M*iniaturize, or *M*ultiply?
What can you *P*ut to other uses?
What *E*lse? Who *E*lse? Where *E*lse?
Can you *R*earrange or *R*everse?

Why? Why? Why?

Bennett and Tibbitts [1986, Figure C] also derive a self-questioning checklist that encompasses the traditional newspaper reporter's "who, what, where, when and how" with five versions of the "why" [Exhibit 4–3].

Five W's and an H

Continuing to use the who, what, where, when, why, and how motif, VanGundy [1988, p. 46] zeros in on definition of the problem. Guidelines for this technique demand that judgment be deferred, an understanding that there is no such thing as a correct redefinition of the problem, adherence to using only one problem in each statement, a lack of criteria in the problem since that limits the options, and acceptance of duplication among the five Ws and the H.

Exhibit 4-3. A Self-Interrogation Checklist of W's and H's.

What is done?	*Why* is it done at all?	*Where* should it be done?
Where is it done?	*Why* is it done there?	*When* should it be done?
When is it done?	*Why* is it done then?	*Who* should do it?
Who does it?	*Why* does this person do it?	*How* should it be done?
How is it done?	*Why* is it done this way?	

Source: From *Making innovation practical*, by A.C. Bennett & S.J. Tibbitts, 1986, Chicago, IL: Pluribus Press, Inc. Reprinted with permission.

Procedures for using this method are as follows:

1. State the problem using the format: In what ways might [IWWM] . . . ?
2. Write down separate lists of who? what? where? when? why? and how? questions relevant to the general problem. Withhold all judgment during this activity.
3. Examine the responses to each question.
4. Write down any problem redefinitions.
5. Select one redefinition that best captures the problem.

Suppose the problem is to get people to come to a screening program to have their blood pressure tested. This technique could work as follows:

IWWM we motivate people to get tested?
Who are the people? Elderly? High income? Low Income? Male?
Where are those people located? Home? Work? Church? Street?
When to stimulate people? Driving car? Riding bus? Watching TV?
What is tested? Arm cuff instrument? Pressure criteria?
Why stimulate people? Better health? Increase income?
How do we stimulate? Publicity? Free speakers? Guest stars?

After answering each question and clarifying the problem each time, a redefined problem will emerge. "Who" may identify elderly white males and females. "Where" may narrow down to at home or work. "When" may focus on public transportation. "What" could specify the blood pressure criteria. "Why" may mean people who don't know their pressure is high. "How" could stress mass media actions. With those types of responses, the problem can be redefined to "IWWM mass media messages on public transportation motivate elderly white males and females at home or work to check their blood pressure?"

Charting, Mind Mapping, and Spidergram

"Is using half your brain enough?" is the question posed in a brochure offering a course on "charting." This technique uses the whole range of ways your brain works, both linear and visual. Information can be structured into a visual form or "chart." Similar to brainstorming, individuals can freewheel and write out the connections. In differing, charting is organized around a central problem expressed in a two or three words. Free associations are made and the planner draws lines to connect relevant and/or related ideas.

In a similar vein, Albrecht [1987, p. 148] labels the technique "mind mapping." Spider-

Exhibit 4-4. Free Association via Charting.

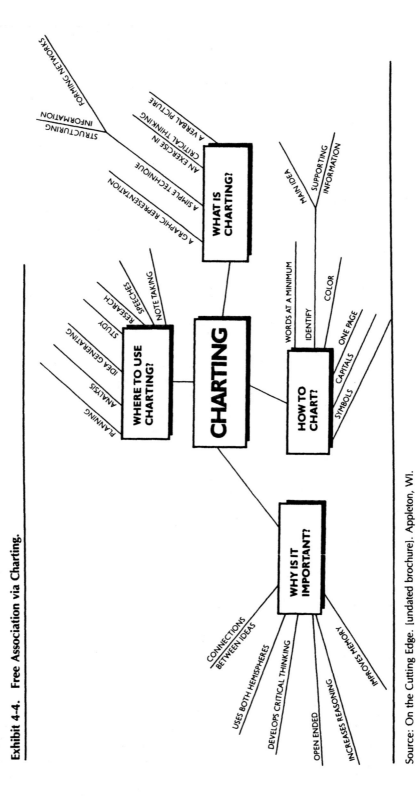

Source: On the Cutting Edge. [undated brochure]. Appleton, WI.

gram is another name for both techniques since the individual connects key words and themes with straight lines creating a spider's web effect.

Exhibit 4–4 illustrates the process using "charting" as the problem theme.

Free Association or Thought Stream

Another technique that can be used singly or in groups is "free association." Three steps were noted by Taylor [1961, p. 75] in the process:

1. Jot down a symbol—a word, sketch, picture, number—centrally related in some way to the problem.
2. Rapidly jot down another symbol suggested by the first.
3. Continue to ad lib as in step 2 until the ideas emerge.

Explain the Difficulty

Self-interrogation is given a new twist by Von Fange [1959, p. 44]. Here, the planner explains the problem to an intelligent "good listener" who doesn't understand the issue in depth. In turn, the "good listener" asks questions to clarify aspects of the alternative solution. Having the "good listener" chosen from an unrelated occupational background increases the payoff in this process.

TECHNIQUES FOR GROUPS

Moving away from individual techniques for stimulating creativity into groups working together, several points can be made. Generally speaking, most of the methods can be adapted to be used either individually or in groups. However, Sayles [1987, p. 339] comments that "it is rare for real innovations to be produced in the plans and thoughts of managers far removed from day-to-day operations . . . Innovation is inevitably the product of a small group of inspired individuals . . . " Arguing that small is better, Sayles [1987, p. 340] supports the contention that a small group creates intragroup cooperation and social solidarity, reduces the social gap between managers and workers, allows for group decisions pacing their efforts, more skills are learned and "greater productivity comes from intelligently applied group effort rather than through more fatiguing and more boring effort."

In sum, the group creative thinking process is enhanced by the interactions between the participants. Members stimulate each other to come up with solutions.

Slip Writing

In "slip writing" individual and group creativity are combined. All participants receive a pad of three-inch by five-inch slips of paper. Then the problem is presented to the group and clarified if necessary. Working individually, each person writes as many ideas as possible—each one on a separate piece of paper. Usually, there will be a time limit set for this task. Upon completion, each member of the group will present one idea, in turn, until all the ideas are exhausted. As these ideas are presented, they are written down and placed into categories on a blackboard or easel board or the slips themselves can be sorted into groupings. Participants can write down additional ideas when any of the other ideas verbalized stimulate them to do so. Up to this point, all of the participants withhold judgment about any of the ideas. With the ideas sorted into categories, the group members can the proceed to redefine and to evaluate the suggestions. "Slip writing" can be used to identify problems, to assist in fact finding, to set priorities, and to create alternatives.

Nominal Group Technique

This technique is comprehensively demonstrated in the chapter on priority determination. NGT was developed by Andre Delbecq and Andrew H. Van de Ven in 1968 [1975, p. 7]. Four steps in the process combine individual brainstorming with group interaction. In the NGT the participants know each other, meet face to face, and engage in direct verbal communication.

NGT can be used throughout the planning process to generate ideas, to set priorities, to implement a program, to evaluate an activity, to secure information, and to identify and refine a problem.

Focus Groups

A common practice in the advertising business is to convene a "focus group" of consumers to elicit opinions about a specific product. Generally, a moderator uses a prepared outline to pose questions to the group for responses. However, Schoenfeld [1988] argues that more could be learned from an unfocused group. He suggests five guidelines:

1. Throw away the prepared outline.
2. Expose the panelists to a variety of ideas and information to get the juices flowing. In this case, the material would be advertisements.
3. Never call on people directly. Ask who agrees? Who disagrees? Why?
4. Use competing data and substitute your name for theirs while separating good ideas from bad ideas.
5. Warm up the panel to practice disagreement and to relate good and bad experiences with the products. Discover who had something distasteful happen to them and find out who had good experiences with the products.

According to Schoenfeld, unfocus the group and you'll do a lot better.

In the health field, the "focus group" could be discharged hospital patients, clinic goers at a local service, parents of retarded children, or registered nurses at a facility. Patient feedback via group meetings after office hours has been a part of Dr. Marvin S. Belsky's [Belsky & Gross, 1975, p. 199] practice since 1973. Obviously, focus groups can be used to get the pulse of the public, so to speak, in an infinite variety of situations.

Phillips 66

Developed by J. Donald Phillips in the 1950s, this method transforms a meeting of 36, 66, or 666 into solution-seeking small groups [Conlin, 1987]. Steps in the process include the following:

1. Have people seated in groups of six in the meeting room.
2. Appoint a recorder for each group.
3. State the problem and display it on a blackboard or screen.
4. Allow the groups five minutes to come up with as many solutions as possible. Then, each group takes one minute to select the best ideas. [Each group of six has six minutes = Phillips 66.]
5. Each group then takes five minutes to rank-order the ideas in order of importance.
6. Completed rank-order lists are collected and the results tabulated.

Forced Association

Basically, forced association seeks to destroy habitual patterns of thinking and to establish new relationships. Examples of habitual association patterns include the following: doctor and nurse, accident and blood, dentist and drill, psychiatrist and couch. By disassociating the usual pairing, forced association looks to move participants from their conventional and orthodox thinking modes into creative approaches to generating alternative solutions. This technique may use the following steps:

1. Identify the activity or thing that needs alternatives. For this exercise, let's use the task of increasing membership in a community health organization.
2. Use free association to generate a list of words or phrases related to attributes of increasing membership: meetings, mailings, speeches, membership fee, newsletters, awards, friendship.
3. Choose an entirely different activity or stimulus such as baseball or a poem. Use free association to create another list of words or phrases with attributes of this random choice. In this example, let's use a verse:

> A Book of Verses underneath the Bough
> A Jug of Wine, a loaf of Bread—and Thou
> Beside me singing in the Wilderness—
> Oh, wilderness were Paradise enow!
>
> Omar Khayyam, *Rubaiyat*

Words from the poem include: verse; bough, wine, jug, loaf of bread, singing, paradise, book, wilderness.

4. List the words in two parallel columns:

Membership	*Poem*
meetings	verse or book
mailings	bough
speeches	wine
membership fee	jug
newsletters	loaf of bread
awards	singing
friendship	paradise or wilderness

5. Force your mind to link words from each column and then use that combination to create

alternatives to boost membership. Look for similarities, differences, analogies, similes, metaphors or causes and effects.

6. List the alternatives generated such as:
   • Mail meeting announcements in verse.
   • Invite prospective members with a singing telegram.
   • Send invitation to friendship party in a little jug.
   • Have a wine tasting party for members getting awards.
   • Meet under the bough—outdoors; at Yellowstone Park.
   • Deliver newsletters in a loaf of bread.
7. Critically analyze the ideas to choose those most useful.
8. Repeat the exercise creating new lists for step 2 [the same problem] and for step 3 [a different activity] and force relationships between the lists as in steps 5 and 6.

Once again, there should be no evaluation or negative comments while ideas are being generated by the group. In fact, Von Fange [1959, p. 54] advised participants to "use the ridiculous." In choosing the entirely different activity in step 3, participants could look at successful commercial enterprises, at hit movies, at sports attractions, travel brochures, best-selling advertisements, or theatrical events. Importantly, group members must expand their scope, free up their old thinking habits, and run wild between the two lists of key elements.

Although he called it "Focused-Object Technique," C.S. Whiting [1958] developed a similar method that forces together fixed and randomly selected attributes.

Another variation uses a random numbers table to select a specific page and a specific word on that page in a book such as a dictionary. Suppose that the 26th word on page 295 turned out to be "freezer" and the problem was "ocean dumping." Using that random stimulus, free associate and come up with alternatives. An obvious beginning is to freeze the garbage; perhaps solidify it.

Still another variation of forced association is a "word pool" where any of the words in the pool can be forced to associate with the problem as illustrated:

Visual Synetics

This forced association method originated at the Battele Institute in Frankfort, Germany {Geschka, Schwaude, & Schlicksupp, 1973]. A visual—a poster, slide, photo—provides the stimulus for the free association of forced relationships. Steps in the process follow:

1. Problem is written on the board for the group to see.
2. Visual is shown to a group of five to seven people.
3. Each persons describes what is in the visual.
4. Descriptions are written down on the board.

5. Group members relate elements from the visual picture descriptions to the problem.
6. When the group runs out of solutions, another visual is used. No more than 10 visuals used in one session.

Suppose the problem was to prevent automobile drivers from nodding off and the visual was a picture of a mountainous winter waterfall. Some ideas could include: blowing cold air on the driver automatically, create sounds when the chin drops down to the chest, a device to keep the head from going over the falls.

No matter what the technique is called—forced association, focused-object, random association, random stimulus, or free association—all these methods use a contrived method to stimulate the mind to depart from habitual thinking modes. This technique has been used in problem solving, imagination, innovation, inventions, brainstorming, and discovering new products and processes. It should be apparent that planners should enjoy similar success employing the methodology.

Synetics

By definition, synetics is a Greek word meaning the joining together of different and apparently irrelevant elements. As explained by its developer, William J.J. Gordon [1961, p. 158], there are nine phases of the synetics theory:

1. Take the problem as given—make paint adhere to smooth wall.
2. Make the strange familiar—seek elements new to the problem.
3. State problem as understood—digestion of the problem.
4. Find the operational mechanism via analogy, metaphor, or simile.
5. Make the familiar strange via a personal, direct, symbolic, or fantasy analogy.
6. Adopt psychological states such as detachment, deferment, involvement, and speculation.
7. Integrate psychological states with the problem.
8. Viewpoint from elsewhere.
9. Solution or research target.

Using the analogy of claws in reference to the adhering paint problem, one participant came up with the following [Gordon, 1961, p. 104]:

> I'm a drop of paint and I've just been put on a chalky surface . . . I'm in a panic. I'm falling, falling. I try to reach through the subsurface, but I can't. I'm slipping, slipping. I'm going to fall . . . to be killed. I'm scratching with my claws to find a decent hold . . . But I'm slipping by, faster and faster! I can't get through to the good holding stuff. . .

To make synetics, or any other "think-tank" technique work, the selection of the participants is critical. For the cross-fertilization to take hold there should be five to eight people participating. There has to be a proper meeting place away from the normal setting to enhance creativity. Obviously, the problem or goal must be clearly delineated. Group members must meet often enough for the pollinating, germinating, and flowering process to take root. Administrative tolerance for distinctively unique work habits and the flaunting of company regulations must be a given. Faith in the ability of the participants and the anticipated outcomes form the cornerstone for the acceptance of synetics or think-tanks as a productive technique for resolving problems.

Delphi Technique

Although the Delphi technique has been extensively described in the chapter on priority determination, this method can also be used to generate alternatives. Norman C. Dalkey [1967, 1972] and his associates at The Rand Corporation developed the approach in the late 1960s. Characteristically, the Delphi method has participants physically separated and anonymous to each other. This method may even be conducted by mail in a written format. Delphi can also be used for predicting future events, surveys of attitudes and views, simplified problem solving, airing controversial views, and strategy formulation.

Conceptualization

Applying this technique to the problems of campus life and to university health services, Trochim and Linton [1986] combine several methods to conceptualize for planning and evaluation. Components in the conceptualization method include process steps, perspective origins, and the representation form.

Process begins with the basic building blocks, entities—each distinguishable thought or idea expressed verbally as a word, phrase, sentence, or other text unit. Next come concepts—either individual entities or groups of entities. This leads to a conceptualization—an interpretable arrangement of concepts and/or entities. Moving from entities to conceptualization involves three steps: generation of entities via brainstorming or some other technique; structuring of the relationships between and among the entities by definition and estimation; and representation of the structured set of entities verbally [essay, outline, or lecture], pictorially [flow chart, concept map, or graph], or mathematically [written model or formula].

In their campus life example, Trochim and Linton report that 876 entities emerged from brainstorming. These were evaluated and pared down to 137 items. Using a sorting technique, 11 clusters were derived. All 137 entities were then located on a concept map using a different symbol for each cluster [Exhibit 4–5]. By grouping the plotted entities together and drawing boundary lines, the cluster map shows 11 distinct programs. With a further analysis, these 11 programs fall into one of three major categories: management, community, or programs and services [Exhibit 4–5].

These investigators make five conclusions about this methodology:

1. This process is goal-free with participants able to go in whatever direction they wish.
2. Conceptualization combines a creative opening, divergent way of thinking with a categorizing process.
3. Power over the input and output remains responsive to those involved in the process.
4. "The concept map depicts the relational data in its entirety, simultaneously showing individual entities, clusters of entities, and both of these levels in relation to each other and the whole . . . this type of data encourages synthesis across different levels of conceptual meaning."
5. Individual entities remain identifiable on the map allowing participants to retain their own personal connections—"they can see where they fit into the whole."

Innovator Computer Program

Innovator [Liberty Software, 1987] is a tool for computer-aided brainstorming and problem solving. This software uses a variety of creativity techniques to jolt the users from their

Exhibit 4-5. Concept Mapping and Cluster Grouping.

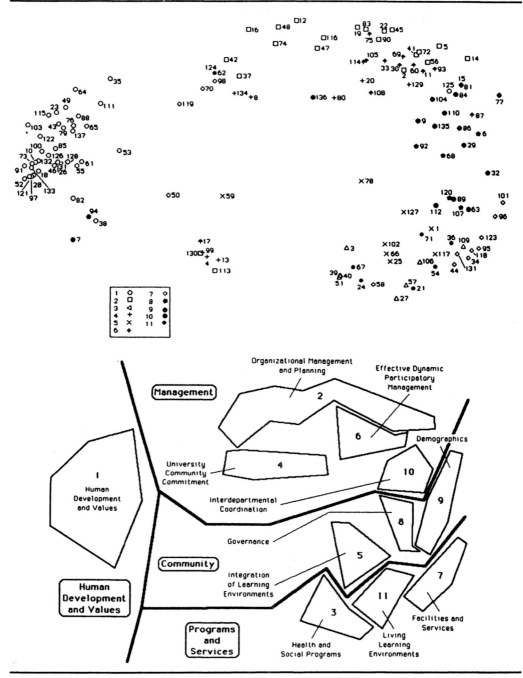

Source: From "Conceptualization for planning and evaluation," by W.M.K. Trochim & R. Linton, *Evaluation and program planning*, 9(4), 298. Copyright 1986 by Pergamon Press. Reprinted by permission.

predictable thinking ruts. Stimulators include questioning, games, words, and pictures. To get started the computer asks you to state your problem. Following that, you are asked a series of who, what, where, when, why, and how questions for clarification. After each round of questions, there is an opportunity to restate the problem. With the problem stated and refined, the computer then allows you to choose from five optional menus with pull down menu boxes: Help, Problem, Ideas, Recall, and Exit [Exhibit 4–6].

Problem menu choices lead the user to analyze the problem via a series of probing questions such as queries regarding your assumptions, the boundaries of the problem, and the pressures you face. Next you are asked to restate the problem in as many ways as possible to gain a deeper understanding of the parameters of the issue. Then, all problem statements can be listed, printed, and finally, you are asked to choose the best problem statement.

Ideas are generated through the random use of 24 different types of creativity stimulators combining fun and adventure while you are getting results. Brainstorming methods are geared to help you bypass your normal thinking strategies. Some try to knock you off balance mentally. Others depend upon your ability to make associations between old facts and new stimuli. Exhibit 4–7 illustrates the techniques. Again, the other options in this menu allow for recording, listing or printing your ideas.

Exhibit 4-6.   Innovator Computer Pull-Down Menus.

Help	Problem	Ideas	Recall	Exit
	Analyze your problem Restate your problem List your problem statements Print your problem statements Choose best problem statement Help		Recall problem file Recall idea file Help	
		Brainstorm Record your ideas List your ideas Print your ideas Help		Save your problems on disk Save your ideas on disk Exit INNOVATOR Help

INNOVATOR is set up to help you in two main areas. The first is in understanding your problem. Choosing "Problem" from the top menu bar will give you access to tools that help you analyze your problem, restate it and output the results.

Choosing "Ideas" from the top menu bar will give you access to tools that help you brainstorm for ideas, record these, and output them.

Experience shows that you should spend about one-third of your time in "Problem." This is just a rule of thumb. It will vary according to the problem, but it does help make your brainstorming more focused.

"Recall" lets you recall your work from a previous session.

"Exit" lets you save your work and return to the operating system.

[Press RETURN to continue]

Source: Reprinted with permission of Richard D. Delker, Liberty Software, PO Box 13896, Gainsville, FL 32604.

Exhibit 4-7.   Examples of Computer Brainstorming Using Innovator Software.

Help	Problem	Ideas	Recall	Exit

Problem: HOW CAN I IMPROVE THE STANDARD BRIEFCASE?
[Responses to the Innovator computer program prompts are in bold type]

Give me 3 ideas that are totally off the wall. Use your wildest imagination.
Don't prejudge any of your ideas. We're not going to use any of them directly.
   Use wild colors, patterns, texture for exterior.
   Make removable outer shells, panels, etc., that can be color coordinated.
   Have little tanks inside filled with helium to counterbalance excess weight.
Go over these wild ideas. Find 1 or 2 good practical ideas that your mind might suggest.

How would Superman handle your problems?   **X-ray vision—make a see through exterior.**
How would Perry Mason attack the problem?   **Logically, of course.**
What would Sherlock Holmes find?   **A built-in hidden compartment; a pipe holder for smokers.**

Take your problem and make it . . .
   . . . Click   . . . Transparent   . . . Concealed   . . . Reciprocate
Don't try to be a literalist on this one.
Allow the words to suggest principles or functions applicable to your problems.

Think of pizzas in light of your problem.
What are the first 5 things that come to your mind?
Stuff in briefcase
Make it easy to clean up
Carry cleaning materials—toothbrush, etc.—in compartment
Insulate the briefcase
Have built in heater
Allow your mind to make connections and suggest ideas from the best of these 5 ideas.

Find a magazine or catalog with pictures. Keep your problem in mind. Look at the pictures.
Make connections between the problem and the pictures.
What does the picture have that your problem needs?
Wheels

Select 2 words that characterize your problem.
   Looks   Function

Consider the following relationships in light of your problem.
Don't dismiss a phrase as nonsense until you think about it.

Function	below	**looks**
Looks	still	**function**
Function	if	**looks**

Give me 2 words that describe your problem.
   Carry   Briefcase

Give me 4 words similar to **Carry**
Lug   Haul   Boosts   Move
And also 4 words similar to **Briefcase**
Bag   Suitcase   Backpack   Case

Now combine these 8 similar words and look for idea suggestions.
boost . . . case
move . . . backpack
lug . . . case
haul . . . bag
haul . . . backpack

Assume that anything is possible. Not even the laws of physics need apply.
Think of some *what if* scenarios applicable to your problem.

(continued)

Exhibit 4-7. (*Continued*)

Remember, this is all fantasy. Let your imagination soar into the unknown.
    What if . . . **my briefcase would shink or grow to fit its contents?**
    What if . . . **my briefcase could disappear when not in use?**
    What if . . . **my briefcase could answer questions for me like an encyclopedia?**
Now look at the fantasies and see what kind of practical ideas that they suggest.

Pretend you are the problem. Really identify with it and put yourself into it.
           If your problem could talk, what would it say?
              I wish they would listen to me.

Think of someone who is completely outside of your field.
How would that person attack your problem?
    He'd play golf and think about it.
What principles would she apply to the problem?
      Make it fun.
Give your mind freedom to think like someone else.

Give me a 2 word phrase that sums up your problem.
    Improved carrier
What is associated with improved carrier?   **UPS**[United Parcel Service]
What else?   **Federal Express**
What else?   **Efficiency**
And one more?   **Convenience**
What does **service** suggest?   **the military—make military special briefcase**
What does **Federal Express** suggest?   **durable, able to fly, quick turnaroud**
What does **convenience** suggest to you?   **easy to open**

            [Press R to RECORD YOUR IDEA or RETURN to continue]

Source: Reprinted with permission of Richard D. Delker, Liberty Software, PO Box 13896, Gainsville, FL 32604.

By this time it should be apparent that a large number of the creativity techniques previously described in this chapter are incorporated into the Innovator program and illustrated in Exhibit 4–7.

Recall and Exit menu options are obvious from the statements in Exhibit 4–6.

Underlying the use of the Innovator program is the basic principle that you get out of it what you put into it. As your creativity skills grow, the program will become more effective as it grows with you. In addition, the Innovator program allows you to experiment in private until you are comfortable with the creative methods and techniques.

IS THERE A BEST TECHNIQUE?

Planners will find that people, including themselves, react differently to the creative techniques utilized. Common sense dictates that you use whatever works best with the individuals involved. However, there has been an effort to compare creative performance.

EXAMINING THE ALTERNATIVES

Consideration of alternative courses of action could logically be covered in the chapter on priorities. However, the subject is included at this point to directly link the methods to the generation of alternatives. Often, this process can lead to new approaches and novel ideas.

Consider a Congressional Budget Office [1984] report on planning for the future health care services of the Veterans Administration. By 1990 it is estimated that the VA will need 6,000 more hospital beds, 3,400 nursing home beds in VA facilities, and 6,500 nursing home beds in non-VA facilities. Those needs will increase costs by at least 40 percent in 1990. Three alternative actions were proposed:

- Convert underutilized hospital beds to nursing home beds.
- Recover costs from third party insurers.
- Contract for more care in non-VA nursing homes.

How would you consider the costs and benefits of each of the activities?

BASIC CRITERIA IN CEA, CBA, AND CUA

Probably the most common criteria used in the examination of alternatives relate to considerations about the costs and the benefits of each proposal [Crystal & Brewster, 1977]. Another approach considers the utility of the activity relative to costs. These concepts translate into cost-effectiveness analysis [CEA], cost-benefit analysis [CBA], and cost-utility analysis [CUA]. From the outset, the difficulty has been to avoid an underestimation of the costs and an overestimation of the effectiveness, benefits, and/or utility. Relative to decision making, Beaves, Joseph, Rohrer, and Zeitler [1988] explore the comparison of respective net benefits with special attention to the dollar value of health benefits.

Generally, costs include calculating actual dollar values for all the direct, indirect, and intangible expenditures for personnel, materials, and resources utilized for the activity. These values can usually be determined without too much difficulty and with reasonable accuracy. Bolley [1987] explains how to determine actual costs in accordance with Management Information Systems [MIS]. However, volunteer labor and/or donated materials and resources may or may not be included. Estimating those dollar values should not be a problem since there are actual comparisons available. If the intangible and indirect costs are not included, overall costs may actually be lower then if those contributions had to be purchased.

As with costs, benefits may be divided into direct, indirect, and intangible categories [Klarman, 1975; Drummond, 1987]. Commonly, benefits relate to changes in mortality, morbidity, health services changes, and improvements in the quality of life. As a benefit, health is impacted upon by a variety of factors including income, environment, nutrition, medical services, and a number of unspecified variables. Nevertheless, dollar values must be estimated for components such as the number of lives saved, the years of life added, the expenditures avoided, and the amounts that people will spend to avoid illness. When using dollar values, a difficulty arises relating to the value of the money and the need to make adjustments for future worth. In addition, the calculation of a life's worth is frequently linked to the loss of productivity. Obviously, there can be quite a bit of subjectivity in making those calculations and disagreements occur often. Unmeasureable intangibles such as lessened or absent levels of pain, discomfort, grief, rehabilitation, and emotional suffering also becloud calculating the benefits. Pieces in the benefits puzzle revolve around the data to use, the accuracy of the information, who is making the determinations, who benefits, and for whose welfare the activities were undertaken. In considering the "priceless" commodity of health, Fuchs and Zeckhauser [1987] discuss valuations in terms of wealth, time preference, risk aversion, and utility.

Utility measures are similar to effectiveness but are more comprehensive in scope such as the quality-adjusted added years of life.

Exhibit 4-8.   CEA, CBA, CUA: Costs and Benefits Formulations.

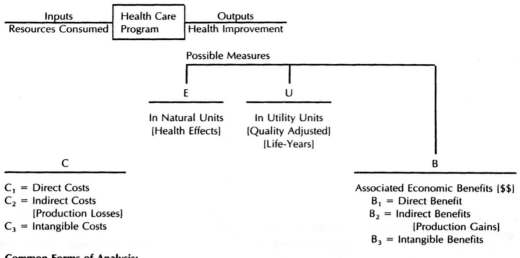

C_1 = Direct Costs
C_2 = Indirect Costs
      [Production Losses]
C_3 = Intangible Costs

Associated Economic Benefits [$$]
   B_1 = Direct Benefit
   B_2 = Indirect Benefits
           [Production Gains]
   B_3 = Intangible Benefits

Common Forms of Analysis:
1. Cost Analysis: C_1; $C_1 + C_2$
2. Cost − Effectiveness Analysis [CEA]: $[C_1 + C_2]/E$; $[C_1 − B_1]/E$; $[C_1 + C_2 − B_1 − B_2]/E$
3. Cost − Utility Analysis [CUA]: $[C_1 + C_2]/U$; $[C_1 − B_1]/U$; $[C_1 + C_2 − B_1 − B_2]/U$
4. Cost − Benefit Analysis [CBA]: $B_1 + B_2 − C_1\, C_2$; $[B_1 + B_2]/[C_1 + C_2]$
                    Also sometimes includes consideration of C_3 and B_3

Source: From "Resource allocation decision in health care: A role for quality of life assessment," by M.F. Drummond, *Journal of Chronic Diseases*, 40[6], 407. Copyright 1987 by Pergamon Press. Reprinted by permission.

Quantophrenia [Blades, Culyer, & Walker, 1987] may be a particularly relevant condition to be aware of when using direct, indirect, and intangible costs and benefits. That condition is characterized by a tendency for the quantified to assume an unwarranted status relative to the unquantified. There is a danger that the unquantifiable may be deemed "small" or "unimportant" when compared to the quantified.

Exhibit 4–8 schematically shows the relations between costs, CEA, CBA, and CUA after acknowledging the inputs and outputs of the health care program. Drummond [1987] defines the inputs as the resources consumed such as the direct costs to the health care sector and to patients/families in providing care, the indirect costs in production losses when workers are unable to perform, and the intangible costs such as pain and suffering. Outputs could include health improvement measures such as the number of cases treated, the number of years of life gained, the improvements on a quality-of-life scale, the quality-adjusted life-years, the savings in dollar terms of direct medical costs, or the value to patients/public of feeling healthier. According to Drummond: "Therefore CBA *as practiced* is often a more limited form of analysis that CEA or CUA, as seen from the formulations for each" in Exhibit 4–8 [author's emphasis].

COST MEASUREMENT TERMINOLOGY

Health planners are likely to encounter the following cost measurement terminology in a discussion of alternative considerations:

- Average costs $= \dfrac{\text{Total dollars expended on the activity}}{\text{Total end product}}$

  Examples: Cost per patient day $= \dfrac{\text{Total hospital expenditures}}{\text{Number of patient days}}$

  Cost to find cases of AIDS $= \dfrac{\text{Total screening expenditures}}{\text{Number of new AIDS cases}}$

- **Averted costs.** These refer to the future costs of health care avoided by the individual or society in general. Averted costs are particularly relevant in preventive activities [Blades, Culyer, & Walker, 1987].
- **Discounting.** This is the assignment of a value or discount rate to the present value of the programs so it is possible to compare different programs by their costs and benefits at any future time. Currency fluctuations impact upon the value of immediate and anticipated costs and benefits. Discounting is particularly important when the costs and benefits occur over varying time periods.
- **Incremental costs.** Example: If a clinic added two more service days, the incremental costs would include items such as the additional salaries and supplies. Depreciation and overhead are not included since those items were already calculated in facility costs.
- **Marginal costs.** This is essentially a law of diminished returns problem. Example: Six sequential stool guaiac tests are used to discover asymptomatic cancer of the colon. With six tests the number of cancers missed fell to a tiny fraction. If one test was done, six cancers out of 10,000 would be missed. However, "the marginal cost per cancer found by the sixth stool guaiac was more than $47 million" [Blades et al., 1987].
- **Opportunity costs.** This occurs when available resources are being used for one activity and that prohibits the resources from being used to initiate a different activity of potential value—benefits are foregone. If the value of the existing program is less than the opportunity cost of a desired alternative, planners should consider dropping the old and substituting the new.

Obviously, the material presented thus far is a general introduction to an examination of considerations related to CEA, CBA, and CUA. However, the volume of literature on these methods is voluminous and investigators have applied the techniques to diseases/conditions such as alcoholism, cancer, influenza, mental illness, ulcers, and syphilis. In the future, D.W. Conlin [1988] expects alternative health care activities such as holistic medicine, faith healing, acupuncture, and homeopathy to compliment and to be considered along with traditional medical approaches. Since future health care will emphasize self-responsibility, self-care, and prevention with a movement toward wellness and illness prevention, there will be a need to apply CEA, CBA, and CUA to those emerging programs.

COST-BENEFIT ANALYSIS

Basically, CBA allows for the comparison of alternatives wherein mathematical calculations provide a mechanism for assisting in resource allocation and decision making. Preferably, costs and benefits are stated in monetary terms and the advantages and disadvantages of competing activities are primarily weighted on economic feasibility criteria.

Purposes and Limitations

Three major reasons for using CBA follow:

1. Decision makers find CBA an excellent tool providing additional technical data for resolving management conflicts among competing interests.
2. Planning-budgeting processes achieve greater integration when CBA provides technical analysis and improves the analytical capacity required of such processes.
3. While not replacing the decision making process, CBA forces planners to prepare alternative choices and background analysis regarding the use of limited resources.

Typically, CBA provides comparative evaluation in four modes:

- Should emergency medical services transport patients by helicopters or conventional ambulances? [Intrasystem comparison]
- Should care be delivered via a curative medicine system or a preventive medicine system? [Intersystem comparison]
- What combinations of health care systems can achieve the same general objective of maximizing health during an entire life span? [Intraprogram comparison]
- Given their competing goals, should the health program or the welfare program be given additional funds? [Interprogram comparison]

There are limitations to the use of CBA. According to Higgins [1986] "the inability to monetize program benefits is the most serious limitation." Assigning a monetary figure to the human life troubles and confounds the use of CBA. In a "willingness to pay" method, the value of life depends upon the amount the individual is willing to pay to avert death or sickness. In a "human capital" method life is valued as an economic commodity having the potential to produce goods or render services. Additionally, that inability to monetize applies especially to important intangible values that are not easily quantified or measured in comparable terms.

Subjectivity is another limitation because there are numerous points at which value or ethical judgments are made. Costs and benefits mean different things to different people. Government authorities and politicians may be concerned about the allocation of budgets for competing needs. Health insurance authorities study the coverage of health care goods and services relative to reimbursement. Hospitals and medical personnel worry about the extension or restriction of therapeutic measures. Mass media and the general public stress the assessment of true or claimed therapeutic innovations. Those same groups could also have different opinions about any cause and effect conclusions regarding the activity's impact. Obviously, many variables are beyond objective unbiased control and measurement.

Controversy also takes place over which discount rate is appropriate, whether nonworkers are discriminated against in a nonequality placed on the value of human life, whether the potential consumption of goods and services ought to be deducted from future earnings, and the applicability of assumptions of future trends [Dinkel, 1985].

Despite these and other possible limitations, CBA remains a valuable tool for the planner. CBA enhances the planner's intuition, experience, and knowledge and applies the sum total to the decision-making process.

Steps in CBA

Since dollar values are vital to CBA, the steps in the analysis reflect that emphasis. Both Simyar and Lloyd-Jones [1988, p. 169] and Higgins [1986] detail the procedural process in that style as follows:

- Specify program objectives in clear and unmisinterpretable terms and describe the characteristics of your program and the alternatives.
- Identify all present and future program costs and express them in current dollar values.
- Identify all present and future program benefits and express them in current dollar values.
- Select an appropriate discount rate and apply it to future costs and benefits to determine their current dollar values.
- Express the comparison of costs and benefits as a summary measure, such as the ratio of benefits to costs.
- Conduct a sensitivity analysis to explain how benefits were identified and valued, why the particular discount rate was chosen, and other aspects of the analysis which involved subjective judgments.

Costs include personnel, equipment, and facilities committed to the program currently as well as the future costs such as interest, depreciation, and maintenance. Opportunity costs are also included here. Benefits could include increased services, improved health status, decreased absenteeism, greater worker productivity, or lower service utilization.

A benefit-cost ratio can be determined by dividing the projected savings [benefits in monetary terms] by the projected dollar costs. Priority consideration should begin with the alternative having the highest benefit-cost ratio and proceed down the ranking. However, Blades et al. [1987] point out that the ratio method loses any sense of the scale of benefits and costs. Suppose one alternative had a cost of $100 and a benefit of $500 for a B/C ratio of 5. Another option has a cost of $10,000 and a benefit of $11,000 for a B/C ratio of 1.1. Choosing the program with the B/C ratio of 5 results in a net gain of only $400 while the much lower 1.1 B/C ratio activity results in a net benefit of $1,000. These authors state that "in general, *ratios* are best avoided altogether in favor of benefit-cost *differences*" [author's emphasis].

A sensitivity analysis elaborates the reasons for specific assumptions and value choices made during the CBA. This procedure heightens the objectivity and the results by explicitly exposing the CBA assumptions to discussion.

CBA Examples

Four CBA illustrations deal with budgetary allocations for three different service options, a choice of parenteral nutrition in the hospital or in the home, a comparison of four medical information systems, and Medicaid abuse control efforts.

Comparing Three Different Services. In this hypothetical illustration, Charny and Roberts [1986] posit that there is a budget of £360,000 and a choice must be made to spend all the money on one of three options: a hip replacement, an expensive drug treatment for duodenal ulcer [DU], or screening for spina bifida by looking for neural tube defects [NTD]. Exhibit 4–9 presents the CBA data.

A hip replacement allows a 55-year-old man to continue working at full productivity until retirement at age 65. His salary for 10 years, discounted at seven percent, represents the benefit to society [£7,000 × 7% × 10 = £52,607]. That calculation yields a B/C ratio of £43.84 for each £1 invested [£52,607 − £1,200 = £43.84].

Drug treatment for 10 people with DU costs £3,000 per year. Without this treatment, those 10 patients would require £500 worth of symptomatic care yearly and one patient per year would need hospitalization for seven days at a cost of £1,000. Assuming that the hospital admission avoidance is the only benefit produced by the DU drug therapy, then £1,000 is the resultant benefit. Using those figures, a B/C ratio of £.40 for each £1 spent emerges [£1,000 − £3,000 (discounted) = £.40].

NTD screening for spina bifida costs £5,200 and produces a benefit of £19,900 per year that would have to be spent caring for each child. With discounting, that results in a B/C ratio of 3.80:1 [£19,900 − £5,200 (discounted) = £3.80].

Exhibit 4–9 also shows the gross benefit for each option derived by multiplying the number of outcomes by the benefit per outcome [hip replacement gross benefit = £52,607 × 300 = £15,782,00]. Net benefit results from multiplying the cost by the number of procedures and deducting that from the gross benefit [hip replacement net benefit = £15,782,000 − £1,200 × 300 = £15,422,000].

Clearly, the DU treatment is not worthwhile since the benefits generated are less than the costs. If the entire £360,000 budget was allocated to DU, society would have a net loss of £216,000 plus an additional loss of £17,380,000 because of the opportunity lost to earn gross benefits on the other two programs [−£0.216 − £15,782,000 − £1,378,000].

Putting all the resources into hip replacement yields a net benefit of £15,422,000 because of the high B/C ratio. That "profit" could then be used to fund additional activities such as the NTD screening. Deducting the gross benefits of £144,000 foregone by not funding the DU treatment and the £1,378,000 foregone for not funding the NTD still yields a net benefit of £13,900,000 [£15,422,000 − £1,378,000 − £144,000]. That remaining £13,900,000 could still be used to fund other activities.

In the last scenario, the entire budget could be used to fund the NTD screening and there would be a net benefit of £1,018,000 on hand to fund other programs. However, even though funding NTD screening yields a net gain, society still faces an overall loss of £14,910,000 by foregoing the gross benefits of hip replacement [£15,782,000] and DU [£144,000].

Exhibit 4-9.   CBA: Hip Replacement vs. Ulcer Drug vs. Spina Bifida Screening.

Activity Funded	Cost [$]	Benefit [$]	No. of Outcomes	Gross Benefit [$]	Net Benefit [$]
Hip replacement	1200	52,607	300	15,782,000	15,422,000
DU treatment	2500	1,000	144	144,000	−216,000
Screening for NTD	5200	19,900	69	1,378,000	1,018,000

Notes   Cost = cost per outcome whose benefit is measured in column 2.
Benefit = benefit outcome.
Number of outcomes = the number which can be obtained with the resources available to the health service, in this case 360,000 pounds.
Gross benefit = number of outcomes times benefit per outcome.
Net benefit = gross benefit minus 360,000 pounds invested in the programme.

DU = duodenal ulcer   NTD = neural tube defects $ = pound sterling [British]

Source: From "The distinction between worth and affordability: Implications of costs and benefits for the allocation of health care resources," by M.C. Charny & C.J. Roberts, 1986, *Postgraduate Medical Journal*, 62(734), 1107–1111. Reprinted with permission of The Macmillan Press, Ltd.

If society's objective is to achieve maximum benefits for a given resource input, there can be no doubt that hip replacement should be the first choice even though Exhibit 4–9 does reveal a significant net benefit for NTD screening. That decision occurs because the three services are compared with each other as well as for the fact that benefits exceed costs. In addition that decision to fund the program with the greatest B/C ratio may also mean that the other options may suffer, no matter how worthwhile. Charny and Roberts conclude that "it is unrealistic to believe that a choice *for* one activity can ever avoid being a choice *against* others" [author's emphasis].

Critics may say that the hypothetical imposition of a budget constraint of £360,000 in the above example is unrealistic. Taking on that issue, Birch and Donaldson [1987] deal with the use of CBA considering indivisible projects and fixed budgets. They start by noting that CBA is usually performed in the absence of budget constrains. Then, the researchers use sophisticated mathematical permutations of the overall budget to consider the identification and evaluation of alternative uses of the residual resources to maximize the total benefits for society. Their conclusion is that "considerable net benefits may be offset by the relatively small benefits produced by the limited use of residual resources. Greater net benefit . . . might have been produced by implementing a smaller project with lower net benefits which enabled more productive use of the residual resources. . ."

Parenteral Nutrition in Hospital or Home. Exhibit 4–10 provides a cost comparison of parenteral nutrition costs in the Federal Republic of Germany when that service is delivered in the hospital versus that service rendered in the patient's home. Costs are compared for society and for the health insurers with benefits assumed in monetary savings. Society saves about 111 DM per day [633 − 521 = 111] on care in the home while health insurers save about 72 DM per day [432 − 360 = 72] if care is delivered in the hospital. Dinkel [1985] comments that this example indicates that "CBA can no longer evaluate new therapies purely from the perspective of society as a whole." To be an effective decision-making tool, CBA must identify every interest group affected by a decision and clearly explain the cost-benefit differential to each of the concerned parties. In addition, Dinkel suggests that CBA be linked to clinical trials and be carried out prospectively rather than retrospectively; otherwise CBA may "degenerate into a mere theoretical mental exercise."

A Composite Health Care System: Four Criteria and Costs. While not exactly a CBA, the U.S. General Accounting Office reviewed the proposals of three competing vendors to supply a state-of-the-art medical information system for the Defense Department [Bowsher, 1988]. A projected monetary outlay of $1.1 billion was the cost factor while the benefits resulted from the vendor's Composite Health Care System ability in four areas in priority order: health care functions, technical approach, deployment, and management. Gradations were made in each area with scaling such as higher/lower cost, few/many weaknesses in health care functions, complete/extensive lack of integration in technical approach, acceptable/unacceptable deployment and effective/ineffective management. Exhibit 4–11 graphically compares the costs to the benefits to be derived in each of the four components from each of the three vendors.

Clearly, Science Applications is superior. "This vendor developed more health care functionality, offered the only completely integrated system, received slightly better ratings . . . in management and slightly lower ratings . . . in deployment and cost is significantly less. ، . The ranking appears appropriate because cost, health care functions and technical approach were the more critical evaluation areas" [Bowsher, 1988, p. 5].

Within the Defense Department, a three-tier CBA process involved a Source Selection

Exhibit 4-10. CBA: Parenteral Nutrition—Hospital vs. Home.

	Hospital		At Home	
I. Costs for Society [DM per day]				
Personnel costs	288.60		22.20	
Costs of medical supplies	144.10		451.40	
Costs of laboratory tests	22.10		7.70	
Other non-personnel costs	56.20		17.60	
Total: direct costs		481.00		498.90
Indirect costs	152.00		22.80	
Total costs		633.00		521.70
II. Costs for Health Insurance Scheme				
Hospital allowance [average]	360.00		—	
Personnel costs	—		0.70	
Costs of medical supplies	—		420.80	
Costs of laboratory tests	—		7.70	
Other non-personnel costs	—		2.40	
Total: direct costs		360.00		431.60
Indirect costs	—		—	
Total costs		360.00		431.60

Source: From "Cost benefit analysis: a helpful tool for decision makers?" by R.H. Dinkel, 1985, *Health Policy*, 4(4), 328. Reprinted with permission of Elsevier Science Publishers B.V.

Evaluation Board of 46 government employees who submitted their reports to the Source Selection Advisory Council of 11 Department officials who in turn sent their recommendations to the Source Selection Authority—the Assistant Secretary of Defense for Health Affairs [Bowsher, 1988, p. 4].

In sum, recommendations noted that Baxter's proposal represented an unacceptable technical risk. While the McDonnell Douglas bid was technically acceptable, there would have been increased costs without concomitant benefits because the proposal was noncompetitive. On that CBA, it was recommended that the Baxter and McDonnell Douglas systems operational test sites be removed as soon as possible. On the other hand, the "Science Application's proposal is technically superior and is significantly lower in total life cycle costs" [Bowsher, 1988, p. 28].

Medicaid Recipient Control Programs. Medicaid abuse occurs when a provider prescribes services that are not needed or are too expensive. In addition, abuse can take place when a Medicaid recipient obtains drugs or other services at a frequency or in an amount not medically necessary. States are required by law/regulation to identify and investigate cases of suspected Medicaid abuse by reviewing 0.01 percent of their recipients' and 0.5 percent of their providers' involved in Medicaid services. In 1985, state and federal costs for Medicaid Management Information Systems [MMIS] totaled about $430 million [Fogel, 1987, p. 2].

State activities to control abuse include activities such as using only specified providers, counseling recipients on proper use of services, requiring prior approval for nonemergency services, warning letters to abusing providers, review of claims and provider termination, and/or suspension from participation in the Medicaid program.

Exhibit 4-11.   CBA: Four Technical Information Components and Costs.

GAO GAO'S COMPARISON OF TECHNICAL AND COST EVALUATION RESULTS BY VENDOR

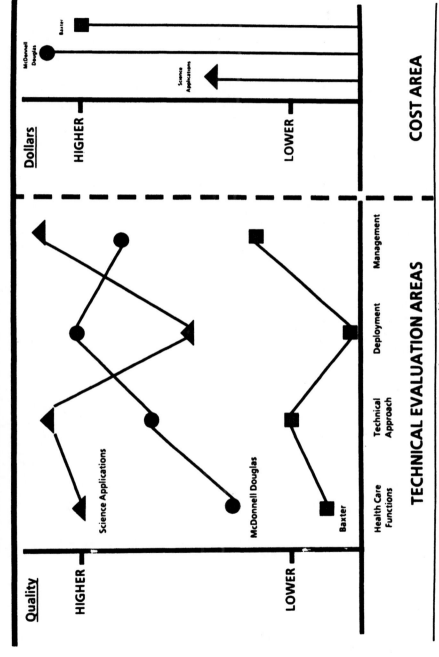

Source: From *Composite health care system acquisition—fair, reasonable, supported,* by C.A. Bowsher, 1988, Washington, DC: Government Printing Office, GAO/IMTEC 88-26. Reprinted by permission.

From a CBA viewpoint, the question is whether or not the costs expended for abuse control activities result in greater benefits than costs, a high B/C ratio. An assumption is made that the costs of the MMIS include larger start-up expenditures for equipment followed by much lower annual operating costs. Furthermore, the investment in equipment is considered wasted if it is not used at its maximum.

While not presented in usual CBA style, Exhibit 4–12 from the U.S. General Accounting Office investigation of improvements needed to prevent Medicaid abuse [Fogel, 1987] makes a strong point about costs and benefits. Four scenarios are illustrated using different variables. An assumption is made that 0.5 percent, 1.0 percent, or 1.5 percent of the nationwide Medicaid population is in a state's recipient control program. Most states have few of their Medicaid recipients in control programs. Another scenario assumption estimates the annual savings per recipient at $500, $750, $1,000, or $1,250.

Using the minimum variables of 0.5 percent of the Medicaid population in control programs and the annual cost avoidance of $500 per recipient, the total potential annual savings is about $54.5 million. That total increases to more than $400 million using the highest assumptions for the two variables, 1.5 percent and $1,250 per recipient.

In conclusion, the GAO report says that "controlling Medicaid abusers can avoid payment for millions of dollars in unnecessary Medicaid services . . . both the National Governors'

Exhibit 4-12.   Potential Savings in Medicaid Abuser Control Program.

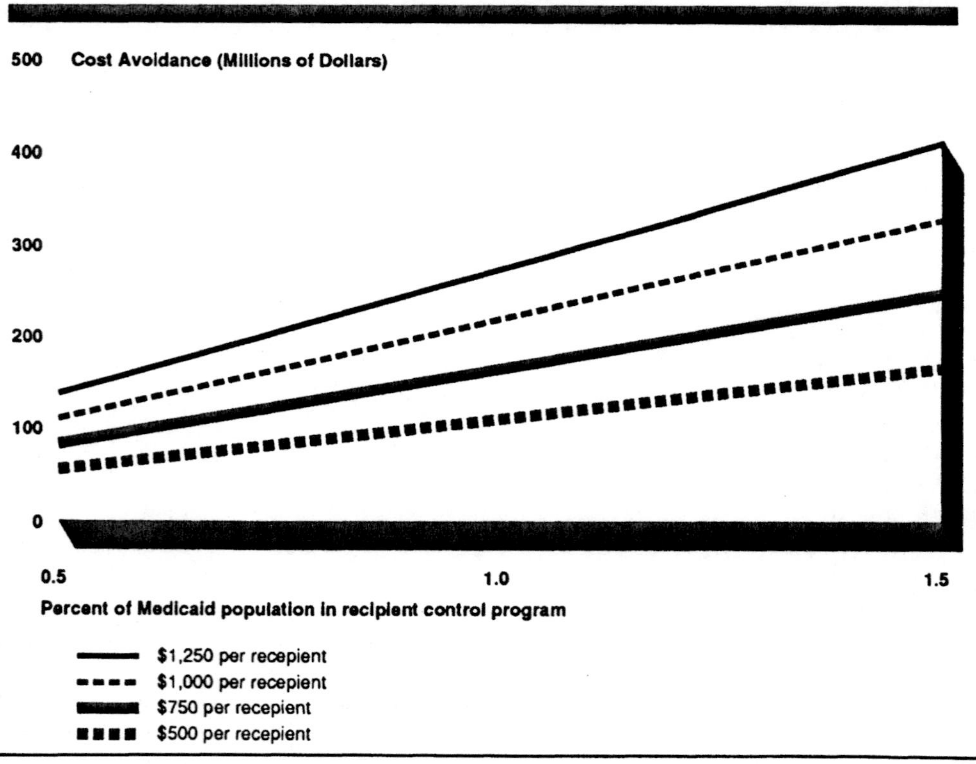

500   Cost Avoidance (Millions of Dollars)

400

300

200

100

0

0.5   1.0   1.5

Percent of Medicaid population in recipient control program

——— $1,250 per recepient
- - - - $1,000 per recepient
▅▅▅▅ $750 per recepient
■ ■ ■ ■ $500 per recepient

Source: From *Medicaid. improvements needed in programs to prevent abuse,* by R.L. Fogel, 1987, Washington, DC: Government Printing Office, GAO/HRD 87-75. Reprinted by permission.

Association and the HHS's Inspector General concluded that they [restriction programs] were cost effective and should be expanded" [Fogel, 1987, p. 26].

Whither CBA?

An Office of Technology Assessment [1980] study indicates that the high point of CBA use occurred in the 1950s and 1960s. During that period the Program Planning Budget System [PPBS] was in vogue and utilized CBA for decision making. Since that time, there appears to be a movement toward using CEA instead of CBA. Sisk [1987] guesses that the trend may be related to the distaste for assigning monetary values to health and life. As with all tools, the limitations of CBA must be kept in mind if and when that technique is utilized.

COST EFFECTIVENESS ANALYSIS

At times, CBA and CEA are not differentiated, but there does appear to be a difference that is particularly relevant when considering alternatives. CBA "addresses the problem of combining different health effects by using monetary units to express all effects" [Sisk, 1987]. Generally, CEA "seeks to identify *either* the least-cost method of achieving a given objective which is usually treated as single-dimensional [e.g., per case, per life-year gained] *or* the maximum output [usually single dimensional] attainable for a given cost" [Blades et al., 1987]. Simply put, CEA looks at the costs and effectiveness of alternate programs to reach a fixed level of output for an activity that has already been determined to be worthwhile. Both monetary and nonmonetary information is used to select the optimum alternative based on cost and effectiveness and gives CEA more flexibility than CBA.

CEA Limitations

CEA is limited by the fact that the technique shows which of the alternatives is better, not which is the best. Guidance in choosing a least-cost way to achieve a fixed goal or goals is a major end result of CEA. Importantly, CEA does little for the intertwined questions relative to the societal values of contracting, continuing, extending, or initiating a new service. In addition, this method limits quantitative comparisons to programs within the same health care system.

A Senate Appropriations Committee hearing dealt with identifying cost-effective forms of treatment. Dr. John E. Wennberg noted that physicians don't have data to compare treatment options and are forced to make treatment decisions based on that inadequate data. He testified that despite a bewildering array of treatment options, physicians receive little guidance on cost or effectiveness of medical procedures. To offset that limitation, Dr. Wennberg suggested that data on the effectiveness and cost of procedures used by hospitals in a community should be published [Fackelmann, 1985].

In a GAO study of the cost-effectiveness of home and community-based services [Zimmerman, 1987] also pinpointed the data limitation. He was quite blunt in saying that "the majority of states' reports were neither accurate or usable for assessing cost-effectiveness" [Zimmerman, 1987, p. 3].

Steps in CEA

Basically, CEA involves a series of analytical and mathematical procedures. Six steps in the process are identified by Higgins [1986]:

1. Establish program objectives.
2. Identify at least two alternatives for attaining these objectives.
3. Estimate the current dollar value of all present and future costs associated with each alternative.
4. Select a quantifiable measure of effectiveness.
5. Estimate the effectiveness of each alternative.
6. Compare alternatives with respect to costs and effectiveness.

Following through the steps, a program objective could aim to reduce automobile injuries. Alternative activities could include seat belt use, restraint devices, reduction of driver drinking, driver skill improvement, and driver licensing screening. Costs are calculated in the usual manner with direct, indirect, and intangible components. Measures of effectiveness could include a variety of indicators such as the B/C ratio, the savings, cost per death/injury averted, number of deaths/injuries averted, observed behavior changes, participation level, reported satisfaction and improved public relations. Effectiveness of each alternative for specific aspects can be compared such as which achieves the greatest reduction in mortality? In injuries? In drunken driver arrests? Finally, an overall comparison looks to find the optimal alternative that results in maximum effectiveness per dollar expended. That may not always be the least costly program. One CEA analysis showed seat belt use to be the least costly way to reduce automobile deaths—$87 per death averted. However, restraint devices at $100 per death averted may be more efficient since the human variability factor is eliminated via an automatic restraint [Drew, 1967].

Continuing with automobile accidents, Orsay, Turnbull, and Dunne [1988] studied the cost-effectiveness of safety belts on morbidity and health care costs relative to 1,364 patients at four Chicago hospitals. "We demonstrated a 60.1 percent reduction in severity of injury [51 percent after adjusting for other variables], a 64.6 percent decrease in hospital admissions, and a 66.3 percent decline in hospital charges [49 percent for adjusted means] in safety belt wearers." Only 7 percent of seat-belt users needed to be admitted as compared with 19 percent of the nonusers. Adjusted means costs differed by about $600 more for those not wearing seat belts. These authors also make a striking comment, "To our knowledge, this is the first study evaluating the efficacy of safety belt use in the U.S. based on medical data."

Regarding measurements, Zimmerman [1987, p. 4] raises the issue of choosing one alternative in lieu of another on the basis of cost-effectiveness. Are there viable alternatives to nursing home care? was the question. Home- and community-based services were the alternatives. When the costs of home and/or community care alternatives for Medicaid recipients are less that the costs of nursing home care, HCFA concludes that those options are cost-effective [Zimmerman, 1987, p. 3].

CEA Examples

Five CEA illustrations concern seven different programs to reduce infant mortality, seven screening options for genital infections, smoking cessation alternatives for pregnant women, a comparison of home health care services, cervical cancer screening for elderly women, and emergency room admissions for chest pains.

Infant Mortality Reduction Strategies. Seven different program activities were examined by Joyce, Corman, and Grossman [1988] to determine which were most cost-effective in improving birth outcomes in the United States. Program options included teen family planning, Women, Infants and Children [WIC] supplemental food program, neonatal intensive care, abortion, prenatal care, and Bureau of Community Health Services [BCHS] activities such as Maternal and Infant [M&I] and community health center [CHC] programs [Exhibit 4–13]. Two birth outcome effectiveness measurements were used: the number of additional neonatal deaths averted, and the number of additional low-birth weight births averted per 1,000 additional program and input users. Costs were calculated on the expenditures for increased utilization of each program and input per 1,000 users. Interestingly, the researchers said that "we chose a cost-effectiveness approach as opposed to a cost/benefit analysis because the estimation and information requirements of the latter were beyond the scope of our study."

Exhibit 4–13 indicates that prenatal care in the first trimester is the most cost-effective program to prevent neonatal deaths among whites, ranging from $23 to $39 per life saved. Among black populations, the WIC program is ranked first, ranging from $21 to $47 per life saved. Cost-effectiveness rankings, after the prenatal and WIC reversal, are the same: abortion, family planning, BCHS activities, and neonatal intensive care. Although the most effective way

Exhibit 4-13.   CEA: Six Strategies to Reduce Neonatal Mortality.

Program	Lives Saved per 1,000 Additional Participants		Cost per Additional 1,000 Participants [$1984 in Thousands]	Cost per Life Saved [$1984 in Thousands]**	
	High [1]	Low [2]	[3]	High [4]	Low [5]
Whites					
Teen Family Planning*	0.8	0.6	122	203	153
WIC*	3.7	1.2	145	118	39
Neonatal Intensive Care*	15.3	2.8	13,616	4,778	890
Abortion	2.1	1.9	356	191	169
Prenatal Care*	7.6	4.5	176	39	23
BCHS Project Use*	.1	0.1	146	2,281	1,123
Blacks					
Teen Family Planning*	1.1	0.9	122	130	107
WIC*	6.9	3.1	145	47	21
Neonatal Intensive Care*	10.0	4.6	13,616	2,940	1,361
Abortion	7.6	4.0	356	90	45
Prenatal Care*	11.7	3.0	187	62	16
BCHS Project Care*	0.5	0.0	146	—	270

* = A variable that is race-specific.
** = High cost per life saved obtained by dividing column [3] by column [2]
      Low cost per life saved obtained by dividing column [3] by column [1]
      Due to rounding the estimates of cost-effectiveness may differ slightly than if calculated directly from the exhibit.
Source: From "A cost-effectiveness analysis of strategies to reduce infant mortality," by T. Joyce, H. Corman, & M. Grossman, 1988, *Medical Care*, 26[4], 348–360. Reprinted with permission of Lippincott/Harper & Row.

to reduce mortality is probably neonatal intensive care [Exhibit 4–13, Columns 1 and 2], that program is one of the least cost-effective activities. "With but one exception, all the programs are more cost-effective for blacks than whites. This is a critical finding given the racial differences in adverse birth outcomes." That finding is important because the need for a vital outreach effort is directly related to the study's CEA assumptions. This cost-effectiveness analysis assumes that additional funding would increase availability as well as utilization. In addition, it is assumed that the costs of increasing services are similar to existing average expenditures.

Seven Screening Options for Genital Infections. Nettleman and Jones [1988] determined the cost-effectiveness of seven options for screening women at moderate risk for urogenital infections caused by *Chlamydia trachomatis*. Moderate risk was calculated at 7.9 percent. Strategies included the following:

1. Neither test nor treat for chlamydial infection.
2. Obtain a culture specimen from all patients and treat if positive.
3. Perform a direct antigen test on all patients and treat if the results are positive.
4. Perform a direct antigen test on all patients, obtain a a culture specimen from those with positive direct antigen test results, and treat if the culture is positive.
5. Perform IFA [indirect immunofluorescent antibody] serological testing on all patients and treat if results are positive.
6. Perform IFA serological testing on all patients, obtain a culture specimen from those patients with positive IFA results, and treat only if the culture is positive.
7. Perform IFA serological testing on all patients and a direct antigen test on those patients with positive IFA results and treat only if the direct antigen test results are positive.

Costs associated with these screening alternatives ran as follows: culture—$25; direct antigen test—$12; and IFA serological test—$8. In addition, the cost of complications of uncured chlamydial infection was estimated at $347.66 per uncured woman. This assumes that 25 percent of the uncured infections lead to symptomatic salpingitis and in turn 25 percent of those women will require hospitalization. Outpatient care can cost $150 while inpatient care can cost $2,865.

Considering these seven screening options in combination with concerns about false and positive testings, Exhibit 4–14 shows the decision tree analysis. With the authors' caveat that "cost-effectiveness is not the only measure of a strategy and may be less of a concern in some situations than the accuracy of a diagnosis," Exhibit 4–15 displays CEA values along with positive and negative predictive values.

If the direct antigen test cost was less than $11.60 per test, the authors felt that would be the most cost-effective screening option. They said: "In summary, the use of a low-cost direct antigen test as the sole basis for treatment represents the most practical approach for many clinicians and is a cost-effective alternative to neither testing nor treating." Again, returning to the issue of screening sensitivity and specificity, a word of advice was given. "It is imperative, however, that both the patient and the physician understand that treatment is based on an increased risk, and not firmly documented evidence of infection." That last statement reflects the fact that only 53 percent of patients with positive results would actually be infected.

Despite the difficulty with the determination of infection, this CEA allows planners to choose an alternative still calculated to provide a most effective return for the output.

Smoking Cessation for Pregnant Women. Three alternative methods were tested in activities designed to stop pregnant women from smoking. One group received standard clinic

Exhibit 4-14. CEA: Decision Tree Outcomes for Direct Antigen Testing

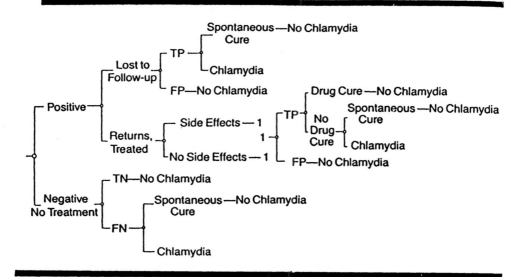

—Decision tree describing outcomes associated with strategy of employing direct antigen test in all n. TP indicates true-positive; FP, false-positive; TN, true-negative; and FN, false-negative.

Source: From "Cost-effectiveness of screening women at moderate risk for genital infections caused by Chlamydia trachomatis," by M.D. Nettleman & R.B. Jones, 1988, *Journal of the American Medical Association*, 260(2), 207–213. Reprinted with permission. Copyright 1988 by American Medical Association.

advice to quit the habit. Another group was given the standard clinic advice plus a manual "Freedom from Smoking in 20 Days." Lastly, the third group received the advice, the manual, and a stop smoking guidebook that was specific for pregnant woman. Quit rates were 2 percent,

Exhibit 4-15. CEA Values and Sensitivity of Predictive Testing.

Strategy	Cost-Effectiveness Value, $	Positive Predictive Value	Negative Predictive Value
Neither test nor treat	26.74	—	—
Obtain culture specimen from all	34.41	.99	.98
Perform direct antigen test on all	27.11	.53	.96
Perform direct antigen test on all; if positive, obtain culture specimen	34.33	.99	.95
Perform IFA* on all	16.88	.17	.98
Perform IFA; if positive, obtain culture specimen	32.28	.99	.97
Perform IFA; if positive, perform direct antigen test	32.10	.73	.95

*IFA indicates indirect immunofluorescent assay for serum antichlamydial antibodies. Prevalence of infection = 7.94%
Source: From "Cost-effectiveness of screening women for genital infections caused by Chlamydia trachomatis," by M.D. Nettleman & R.B. Jones, 1988, *Journal of the American Medical Association*, 260[2], 207–213. Reprinted with permission. Copyright 1988 by the American Medical Association.

6 percent, and 14 percent respectively. Alternative three, clinic advice plus Freedom manual plus specific guidebook, proved to be the most cost-effective. That higher quit-smoking rate was achieved at one-half the cost of the other two groups [Windsor, Warner, & Cutter, 1988].

Home Health Care CEA. Assuming that patients can receive quality care in their own homes, a number of investigators conducted CEA comparisons. Cabin [1985] reported on 26 examples such as $270,830 per year for a ventilator-dependent person in a hospital as compared to $21,192 per year at home; spinal cord injury with quadriplegia costing $23,862 per month in the hospital as against $13,931 per month at home; and nursing home care cost at $482 per month as compared to $222 per month at home. Spiegel [1987, p. 211] devotes an entire chapter to the question of the cost-effectiveness of home health care. Numerous studies are cited that compare home health care to hospital care, to nursing home care and to hospice care.

Cervical Cancer Screening. Elderly women in the United States account for 25 percent of the incidence of gynecologic cancer and 40 percent of the deaths. Therefore, Mandelblatt and Fahs [1988] conducted a CEA of a screening program designed to prevent cervical cancer in a targeted population of elderly women. Their CEA model calculations follow:

$$CEA = \frac{\text{net costs}}{\text{net effects}} = Crx + Cse + Cmorb + \frac{(Cxle)}{LYS}$$

Crx = direct medical costs
Cse = costs of adverse side effects of performing a Pap smear
Cmorb = savings in health care costs due to early detection
Cxle = added costs of treating illness during life years saved
LYS = life years saved

Overall, the cancer screening program saves money and extends the life of the patients. Early detection of cervical neoplasia saved $5,907 and 3.7 years of life per saved. Using a 5 percent discount rate, the favorable B/C ratio yields the total of $1,589 saved per year of life saved. Based on their results the authors' recommend the implementation of similar screening programs.

Emergency Room CEA via Computer. In an interview, Gildea [1986, 1987] reports on a project that allows emergency physicians to ascertain the most cost-effective way to deal with a patient arriving with chest pains. Attending physicians punch the patient's symptoms into a computer. After that, the computer determines the probable outcomes of three scenarios: if the patient is admitted to intensive care; if the patient is hospitalized, but not placed in intensive care; and if the patient is sent home. CEA is demonstrated in savings when people are sent home who do not have to be hospitalized and when lives are saved through an appropriate hospitalization instead of a patient being sent home [*Health Cost Management,* 1984].

COST UTILITY ANALYSIS

In essence, CUA emerged because of a dissatisfaction with CEA. Investigators believed that CEA's limited view of *outputs* "seriously failed to capture some important dimensions of benefit that ought to be taken into account [Blades et al., 1987]. In CUA, the approach is similar to CEA with the exception of the consideration of a more comprehensive sets of *outcomes.*

Additional questions are raised regarding the measurement of outputs, "how far superior performance in one outcome dimension may compensate for less good performance in another, in a comparison between options, and other related issues" [Blades et al., 1987]. In fact, Drummond [1987] discusses CUA as a subset of CEA [Sisk, 1987]. "Outputs of health care programs can be measured in quality-adjusted life-years [QALYs], where the life extension gained is adjusted by a series of 'utility' weights reflecting the relative value of one health state compared to another. Utility, therefore, is a specific kind of quality of life measure which has gained prominence in economic evaluation in health care. An evaluation having utilities in the denominator would be called a *cost-utility analysis.*

Obviously, there are critical questions arising about the use of quality of life assessments in economic evaluations. Firstly, there is the matter of who assesses the quality of life. Should it be the health care provider? Should it be the patient? Directly related to the "who" is the "how" to obtain the quality of life measures. Should the assessments be made during the activity? Should there be a consensus at the conclusion? Should the measurement be made in conjunction with a clinical trial?

Secondly, is a generalizable quality of life measure needed? Here, the issue is whether a measurement can be used for a range of differing population groups. In economic terms, the quality-adjusted life-year provides an index allowing for comparisons across programs. However, it is possible that small clinical differences may be undetected although those differences are medically important.

Finally, is it right to construct comparative tables of alternatives in terms of their cost per quality-adjusted life-year? That could lead to "caps" on expenditures for specific procedures and de facto rationing by dollar amount, by age, and so on.

Basically, there are a number of subjective edges to the use of a quality of life assessment as used in CUA. Nevertheless, Drummond [1987] still makes a strong pitch: "Of the various forms of economic evaluation, CUA, where the consequences of interventions are expressed in terms of the quality-adjusted life-years gained, is the most promising approach for all but the most limited choices."

VALUE DISTINCTIONS AND CHOICES

Whether a planner uses CBA, CEA, CUA, or any other technique to assist in the decision making, choices may be profoundly impacted upon by differences in values. These include the values of individuals, the values of specific groups, and the values of the larger society. Putting it another way, Charny and Roberts [1986] pointedly state that "little attention has been paid to the important distinction between the affordability and the worth of health services, perhaps because the implications are unpalatable."

An example of the values influencing choices arises in the case of an individual who requires an expensive transplant operation but cannot afford the procedure. If that person happens to be older than 55 and lives in a country where the national policy prohibits "unaffordable and unworthwhile" kidney transplants at that age, societal choices prevail. However, if that individual happens to be a young child who was denied the transplant due to budget restrictions, another scenario could unfold to change the value choices about worth and affordability. Pleas could be made by the child's parents using the mass media to appeal for funds. Societal values would be bypassed, waiting lines would be bypassed, and the choice would be made on an emotional basis. Rational value choices based on worth and affordability disappear. It is apparent that a single identified patient with a name and a visible face attracts more attention than a statistical anonymous case who joins large numbers of other anonymous patients. Furthermore, the decision maker who attributes the value choice to the saving of a life also enjoys the commendations of the mass media and the public for making the "right choice."

In a different scenario, a planner might consider air pollution control and kidney transplant alternatives (USDHHS, 1977). In the same time period, air pollution is expected to cause 1,000 deaths and 100 people will need transplants. Statistically, it will cost less and benefit society more to save those 1,000 air pollution victims than the 100 kidney transplant patients. Yet, the individual visibility factor could influence the choice to a severely reduced B/C ratio for society.

Often, recognizable identified individuals who are known to be dying attract a great deal of public attention. With the attention comes an outpouring and mobilization of resources to try to save that person's life. Such expensive intervention might reduce the risk slightly and extend life for a short period. To use those same resources to reduce the mortality risk of another group of patients from 25 percent to 23 percent would hardly motivate an equal mobilization of resources. Again, the B/C ratio would be favorable for the nondying population group.

Some would contend that ethical, physical, and emotional concerns constitute a rightful part of the decision-making process. On the other hand, some would say that those concerns are not a rational part of the health planning procedure. Charny and Roberts [1986] put it in monetary terms: "It is ironic that economics, which explicitly attempts to explore the consequences of scarcity, has been used to cloud the distinction between affordability and worth."

At times, planners will be unable to influence the sociopolitical value choices that have to be made. However, planners will still have to arrive at some conclusion about the relative weight to give to the varying individual, group, and societal concerns.

CREATIVITY EXERCISES—POSSIBLE SOLUTIONS

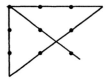

Some have connected all nine dots with three straight lines. Someone has even been able to connect all nine dots with *one* straight line by folding the paper. (See puzzle on page 160.)

---

888 + 88 + 8 + 8 + 8 = 1000   (See puzzle on page 160.)

Campaign strategists decided to play up the candidate's unsmiling visage using a picture of her grim look in connection with a related slogan: *What does she have to smile about?* Responses to the question stress the negative aspects of the past administration. *High taxes! Crime in the streets! Corruption in government! Congested highways!*

Partial listing of uses of a paper clip.

necklace	chain	picture hanger	lock pick
tie clip	belt	art sculpture	sign holder
money clip	wedge	checkers	clothes pin
earrings	missle	advertising	ring
key ring	ruler	book marker	pen holder

etc., etc., etc., etc., and etc.

REFERENCES

Albrecht, K. (1987). *The creative corporation*. Hubbard Woods, IL: Dow Jones-Irwin.

Barrett, F.D. (1978). Creativity techniques: Yesterday, today, and tommorrow. *SAM Advanced Management Journal 43*(1), 25–35.

Beaves, R.G., Joseph, H., Rohrer, J.E., & Zeitler, R.R. (1988). Cost-effectiveness. How should it be determined? *Evaluation & the Health Professions, 11*(2), 213–230.

Belsky, M.S., & Gross, L. (1975). *How to choose and use your Doctor*. New York: Arbor House.

Bennett, A.C., & Tibbitts, S.J. (1986). *Making innovation practical*. Chicago, IL: Pluribus Press.

Birch, S., & Donaldson, C. (1987). Cost-benefit analysis: Dealing with the problems of indivisible projects and fixed budgets. *Health Policy, 71*, 61–72.

Blades, C.A., Culyer, A.J., & Walker, A. (1987). Health service efficiency: Appraising the appraiser—a critical review of economic appraisal in practice. *Social Science in Medicine, 25*(5), 461–472.

Bolley, H. (1987). Determination of actual cost in accordance with MIS Guidelines. Part 1. *Dimensions in Health Service, 64*(8), 55–57.

Bowsher, C.A. (1988). *Composite health care system acquisition—fair, reasonable, supported*. (GAO/IMTEC 88–26.) Washington, DC: Government Printing Office.

Buyer, L.S. (1988). Creative problem solving: A comparison of performance under different instructions. *Journal of Creative Behavior, 22*(1), 55–61.

Cabin, W. (1985). Some evidence of the cost-effectiveness of home care. *Caring, 4*(10), 62–67, 70.

Charny, M.C., & Roberts, C.J. (1986). The distinction between worth and affordability: Implications of costs and benefits for the allocation of health care resources. *Postgraduate Medical Journal, 62*(734), 1107–1111.

Clark, H. (1980). *Idea management: How to motivate creativity and innovation*. New York: American Management Association.

Congressional Budget Office. (1984). *VA health care: planning for future years*. Washington, DC.

Conlin, D.W. (1988). Future health care: Increasing the alternatives. *The Futurist, 22*(3), 13–15.

Conlin, J. (1987). Who's running this show anyway? Managing meeting dynamics. *Successful Meetings, 36*(13), 38–46.

Crystal, R.A., & Brewster, A.W. (1977). Cost benefit and cost effectiveness analyses in the health field: An introduction. In L.E. Weeks & H.J. Berman (Eds.), *Economics in health care*. Rockville, MD: Aspen Systems Corporation.

Dalkey, N.C. (1967). *Delphi*. Santa Monica, CA: The RAND Corporation.

de Bono, E. (1970). *Lateral thinking: Creativity step by step*. New York: Harper & Row.

Delbecq, A.L., Van De Ven, A.H., & Gustafson, D.H. (1975). *Group techniques for program planning. A guide to nominal groups and Delphi processes*. Glenview, IL: Scott, Foresman & Co.

Dinkel, R.H. (1985). Cost-benefit analysis: A helpful tool for decision makers? *Health Policy, 4*(4), 321–330.

Drew, E.B. (1967). HEW grapples with PPBS. *The Public Interest, 7*, 10.

Drummond, M.F. (1987). Resource allocation decisions in health care: A role for quality of life assessments? *Journal of Chronic Diseases, 40*(6), 605–616.

Eberle, R. (1971). *Scamper on (for creative imagination development)*. Buffalo, NY: DOK Publications.

Elliot, L.B. (1987). Creativity management and analogical thinking. *Data Management, 25*(2), 20–21.

Fackelmann, K.A. (1985). Experts ask for research to locate treatments that are cost-effective. *Modern Healthcare, 15*(1), 28.

Fogel, R.L. (1987). *Medicaid. Improvements needed in programs to prevent abuse*. (GAO/HRD 87–75). Washington, DC: Government Printing Office.

Fuchs, V.R., & Zeckhauser, R. (1987). Valuing health—a "priceless" commodity. *American Economic Review, 77*(6), 263–268.

Geschka, H., Schlicksupp, H., & Schwaude, G.R. (1973). Modern techniques for solving problems. *Chemical Engineering, 80*(18), 91–97.

Gildea, J. (1986). Forecasters of a more cost-effective future. *Health Cost Management, 3*(5), 13–16.

Gildea, J. (1987). Forecasters of a more cost-effective future. Part two. *Health Cost Management, 4*(1), 10–17.

Gordon, W.J.J. (1961). *Synectics. The development of creative capacity.* New York: Harper & Row Publishers.

Hancock, S.H. (1988). Unleash creativity. *Sucessful Meetings, 37*(12), 30.

Health Cost Management. (1984, July/August).

Hickman, C.R., & Silva. (1985). How to tap your creative powers. *Working Woman, 10*(4), 26, 28–30.

Higgins, C.W. (1986). Evaluating wellness programs. *Health Values, 10*(6), 44–51.

Joyce, T., Corman, H.E., Grossman, M. (1988). A cost-effectiveness analysis of strategies to reduce infant mortality. *Medical Care, 26*(4), 348–360.

Klarman, H.E. (1975). Application of cost benefit analysis to health services and the special case of technologic innovation. *International Journal of Health Services, 4*(2), 325–352.

Kriegel, M.H., & Kriegel, R. (1988). How to master back-burner thinking. *Working Woman, 13*(1), 46.

Liberty Software. (1987). *Innovator.* Gainesville, FL.

Mandelblatt, J.S., & Fahs, M.C. (1988). The cost-effectiveness of cervical cancer screening for low-income elderly women. *Journal of the American Medical Association, 259*(16), 2409–2413.

Meehan, R.H. (1986). Programs that foster creativity and innovation. *Personnel, 63*(5), 31–35.

Nettleman, M.D., & Jones, R.B. (1988). Cost-effectiveness of screening women at moderate risk for genital infections caused by Chlamydia trachomatis. *Journal of the American Medical Association, 260*(2), 207–213.

Office of Technology Assessment, U.S. Congress. (1980). *The implications of cost-effectiveness analysis of medical technology, background paper: Methodological issues and literature review.* Washington, DC: Government Printing Office.

On The Cutting Edge. [undated brochure]. Appleton, WI.

Orsay, E.M., Turnbull, T.L., & Dunne, M. (1988). Prospective study of the effect of safety belts on morbidity and health care costs in motor vehicle accidents. *Journal of the American Medical Association, 260*(24), 3598–3603.

Osborn, A.F. (1953). *Applied imagination: Principles and procedures of creative thinking.* New York: Charles Scribner's Sons.

Osborn, A.F. (1963). *Applied imagination* (3rd ed.). New York: Charles Scribner's Sons.

Pearson, A.E. (1988). Tough-minded ways to get innovative. *Harvard Business Review, 88*(3), 99–106.

Pinchot, G., III (1985). *Intrapreneuring.* New York: Harper & Row.

Quinn, J.B. (1985). Managing innovation: Controlled chaos. *Harvard Business Review, 63*(1), 73–84.

Raudsepp, E. (1987a). Establishing a creative climate. *Training and Development Journal, 40*(2), 50–53.

Raudsepp, E. (1987b). *Growth games for the creative manager.* New York: Perigee Books.

Sayles, L.R. (1987). Organization size, effectiveness, and human values. *Administration & Society, 19*(3), 339.

Schoenfeld, G. (1988). Unfocus and learn more. *Advertising Age, 59*(22), 20.

Sisk, J.E. (1987). Discussion of Drummond's article. *Journal of Chronic Disease, 40*(6), 617–619.

Simyar, F., & Lloyd-Jones, J. (1988). *Strategic management in the health care sector. Toward the year 2000.* Englewood Cliffs, NJ: Prentice-Hall.

Spiegel, A.D. (1987). *Home health care* (2nd Ed.). Owings Mills, MD: National Health Publishers.

Taylor, J.W. (1961). *How to create new ideas more than a book—a comprehensive course in the art and science of creative thinking.* Englewood Cliffs, NJ: Prentice-Hall.

Trochim, W.M.K., & Linton, R. (1986). Conceptualization for planning and evaluation. *Evaluation and Program Planning, 9*(4), 289–308.

USDHHS, Health Care Financing Administration. (1987). *Findings from the National Dialysis and Kidney Transplantation study. Comparative analyses of four treatment modalities.* (HCFA Pub. No. 03230). Washington, DC: Government Printing Office.

VanGundy, A.B. (1988). *Techniques of structured problem solving* (2nd ed.). New York: Van Nostrand Reinhold Co.

Von Fange, E.K. (1959). *Professional creativity.* Englewood Cliffs, NJ: Prentice-Hall.

Weaver, R.L. (1987). Second wind. Capitalizing on your full creative potential. *Vital speeches of the day*, *53*(1), 235–237.

Windsor, R.A., Warner, K.E., & Cutter, G.R. (1988). A cost-effectiveness analyses of self-smoking cessation methods for pregnant women. *Public Health Reports*, *103*(1), 83–88.

Whiting, C.S. (1958). *Creative thinking* New York: Van Nostrand Reinhold.

Zimmerman, M. (1987). *Medicaid. Determing cost-effectiveness of home and community-based services.* (GAO/HRD 87–61). Washington, DC: Government Printing Office.

5
Limiting and Ranking Options: Selecting Priorities

Currently, and for the foreseeable future, scarce resources and increased competition will dictate that health care providers set priorities from among all the available alternative objectives. Planners must be able to use methods and techniques to provide rationales for the difficult choices. As Williams [1988] bluntly states: "Priority setting means deciding *who* is to get *what* at *whose expense* [author's emphasis].

PRIORITY SETTING EXAMPLES

Beginning with a global determination of priorities by the World Health Organization, illustrative examples move to U.S. national choices by a volunteer coalition and governmental agencies to governing boards, health care executives, and consumers.

WHO Plan for Health

With respect to international health goals, the World Health Organization [1981] and the Pan American Health Organization [1988] developed a Health for All plan listing the following priorities as most important [Patel, 1986]:

- A commitment by heads of state to guarantee health for everyone within their population.
- Mobilization of community and interest groups in the implementation of this comprehensive goal.

Those broad goals were followed by 12 yardsticks for specific priorities [*World Health*, 1986] that included:

1. A minimum of five percent of the gross national product should be spent on health.
2. A fair share of this should be allocated for primary health care, excluding hospital care, at the local level.
3. Equitable distribution of health resources should be available to all groups in the population.
4. Wealthier nations should assist poorer ones which are making good-faith efforts toward achieving these goals.

Five research areas for the Health for All program targeted the following: health policy and organizational behavior, inequities, community participation and collaboration, information systems, and collaborative studies [*International Nursing Review*, 1989].

In addition, the World Health Organization's plan set measurable specific objectives that should be achieved such as increasing life expectancy for all nations at birth to 60 or more years, spending at least $500 per capita of the nation's gross national product on health care and achieving an adult literacy rate of at least 70 percent. Mason, Katz, and Lord [1985] set 10 global goals, including reduction of infant mortality to less than 50 per 1,000 live births and elimination of vaccine preventable diseases in children. Of course, more advanced nations have already achieved most of these goals.

In keeping with current trends, Stroot [1989] notes that the WHO promotes healthy lifestyles stressing exercise, sport, nutrition, and personal responsibility.

Health Policy Agenda for the American People

In 1987, an ad hoc organization called the "Health Policy Agenda for the American People" [HPA] composed of 172 leading organizations in the United States, issued its priority health reforms for the American people [Cherskov, 1987]. Among their recommendations are:

1. Assist consumers in comparing costs and services among competing providers.
2. Develop a basic health care benefits package to serve as a benchmark for consumers and governmental bodies to assess the adequacy of their current benefit package.
3. A guaranteed 10 percent annual increase in federal funds for basic and applied biomedical research.
4. Guarantee that all persons who are below the poverty line receive Medicaid benefits.
5. Reform the Medicare program to assure its continued solvency.

While there are other health priorities, these suffice to show the direction in which this particular body is heading. These priorities aim to foster the consumer's self-direction in using medical care while guaranteeing access to the best medical care available, especially for those on government assisted programs.

Healthy People Priorities

In 1979, the United States Surgeon General issued a report, Healthy People, in which 15 detailed priorities were identified for health promotion, health protection, and personal preventive services to improve the health of Americans [USDHEW, 1979]. These were promulgated as specific, measurable objectives to be achieved by 1990. Achievement of those objectives was expected to improve the population's health status.

In his discussion on setting the 1990 objectives for public health, Breslow [1987] reiterated examples of the priorities in each of the designated areas:

Personal Preventive Health Services
- At least 90 percent of all children should have completed their basic immunization series by age 2—measles, mumps, rubella, polio, diphtheria, pertussis, and tetanus.
- The fertility rate for 16-year-old girls should be reduced to 25 per 1,000.
- At least 60 percent of the estimated population having definite high blood pressure [160/95] should have attained successful long-term control at or below 140/90 for two or more years.

Health Protection
- The annual estimated incidence of hepatitis B should be reduced to 20 per 100,000 population.
- At least 95 percent of the population should be served by community water systems that meet federal and state standards for safe drinking water.
- At least 25 percent of workers should be able, prior to employment, to state the nature of their occupational health and safety risks and their potential consequences, as well as be informed of changes in these risks while employed.

Health Promotion
- The rate of suicide among people 15 to 24 should be below 11 per 100,000.
- The proportion of adults 18 to 65 participating regularly in vigorous physical exercise should be greater than 60 percent.
- Laws should exist in all 50 states and all jurisdictions prohibiting smoking in enclosed public places, and establishing separate smoking areas at work and in dining establishments.

Both Millar and Myers [1983] and Rall [1988] reported on progress toward *Healthy People* 1990 objectives in the area of occupational and environmental health. Significant progress was noted regarding priorities concerning environmental levels of lead, reduction in pelvic radiation exposure, toxic waste dump testing, chemical exposure to dioxin in soil, and accumulation of information on 4,100 compounds with potential health risks. With respect to infant mortality, teen-age birth rates, homicides, and cigarette smoking, Breslow [1987] noted substantial improvement toward meeting the 1990 objectives. In totality, progress in meeting the specified health priorities would indeed herald a major advance in the health status of the American population.

Moving forward from the 1990 objectives, the current emphasis is on the *Year 2000 National Health Objectives* [*Federal Register, 1989*; USDHHS, CDC, 1989; Windom, 1989].

Priorities in Public Health

A former Assistant Secretary for Health, Dr. Edward N. Brandt, Jr. [1988], delineated several major problems inherent in the priority setting process in public health programs. His observations noted that the national process of priority setting may be unduly influenced "by the vector sum of forces operating on decision makers, leading more and more into a 'disease-a-month' approach to public health." Those vector sum of forces include the mass media, the legislative process, and an army of vested interests lobbyists. In addition, Brandt mentioned the undefined responsibilities of public health organizations and the inconsistency of the priorities even after the choices are made. In conclusion, Brandt states: "There are hard choices to be made because our predecessors have already solved the simple ones."

AIDS Priorities. One of the hard choices must be related to the AIDS epidemic. In a discussion of the setting of priorities regarding the AIDS outbreak, Henry [1988] calls for a closer alliance of public health and clinical approaches toward the control of AIDS. He offers the following three priority actions to facilitate efforts to limit HIV transmission:

- Provide resources to study basic questions about the biology of the principal infective unit of HIV in the genital tract.
- Give priority to developing drugs which have clinical efficacy in HIV infection and simultaneously decrease infectivity.
- Institutions and physicians involved in studies and care of people with AIDS should study and implement educational and counseling programs that minimize further HIV transmission.

These priorities do appear to be reflected in the funding of specific projects in those three areas.

Shifting Federal Priorities. Stating that priorities in the U.S. "are at best askew and at worst wrong," Holloman [1986] argues that it is time to reorder our priorities. Addressing subtle factors or barriers that may be completely ignored in the priority-setting process, Holloman discusses the absence of a national health policy, access to care, physician and hospital maldistribution, and attitudinal prejudices against the poor. With particular attention to the economic factors influencing decisions, Holloman ponders: "If our great nation is to survive and reach its potential, it must reorder its priorities so that the materialism of the few will not destroy the humanity of the many."

To back up Holloman's point, an earlier article headlined the fact that the federal government's health care priorities had shifted [Kosterlitz, 1985]. In a review of the major divisions of the Health and Human Services Department, Kosterlitz came to a jolting conclusion: "HHS has presided over a drastic shift in priorities driven by a philosophy that the federal government should not be the frontline of defense against social problems and poverty, that a strong economy is the best guarantor of the general welfare and that the operations of the free market will ultimately be in the best interest of consumers of health care goods and services."

A Congressional Commission, an Institute of Medicine study group, and the Children's Defense Fund all are urging that the health of mothers and children should become a national priority [Zylke, 1989; Ries, 1989]. While Garfunkel [1989] comments that "the life of a child is priceless," he also tempers that remark with the observation that "hard choices may need to be made."

President Bush's Secretary of HHS [Sullivan, 1989] identified five priority areas of immediate concern: addressing HIV infection, stopping the use of illicit drugs, improving the quality of care for the poor and minorities, restraining the escalating costs of health care, and providing more affordable long-term care for the elderly.

Technology and Priorities. Public health priorities must also keep pace with technological advancements such as organ transplants and artificial organs. Governmental policy decisions toward technology fall into four basic areas: research and development, evaluation and assessment, regulation of efficacy and safety, and controls on investment and use [Banta, 1986]. After an analysis of vaccination against pneumococcal pneumonia by the Congressional Office of

Technology Assessment [OTA], the legislators amended the Medicare law to cover that preventive intervention [OTA, 1984]. On the other hand, Congress did not act after an OTA study showing the cost-effectiveness of influenza vaccine [OTA, 1981]. These and other examples lead Banta [1986], a former OTA physician administrator, to conclude that the U.S. Congress lags behind European nations in realization of the links between technology assessment and setting specific public health priorities.

State Health Priorities. A survey of 46 state crippled children's agencies by Ireys and Eichler [1988] revealed considerable unanimity among administrators. In order of priority, the following activities were judged very important: coordinating patient case activities [73 percent], team conferencing on individual cases [69 percent], developing standards of care [64 percent], eligibility criteria [60 percent], collecting payments [60 percent], advocating with state legislators [58 percent], linkages with other government agencies [58 percent], prospective payment plans [52 percent], and continuing education for staff [47 percent].

In a similar fashion, the then-president of the American Psychiatric Association, Dr. John A. Talbott [1985], commented on the national priorities identified by state mental health commissioners and published in the same journal. However, Talbott said that the specification of the priorities was only a halfway step in the right direction. He commented that "decisions seem to be made by legislators, businessmen, and third-party payers . . . propelled more by outside forces—economics, legal advocacy, and the social zeitgeist—than by philosophical and therapeutic principles."

Adding to Talbott's emphasis on outside forces, Sleet [1987] contends that "public health priorities arise from the convergence of a disease threat, public awareness of the threat, demand for proper protection from the threat, and a body of scientific literature to support the effectiveness of prevention/protection measures." Nelson [1989] agrees and talks about shared values and priorities in public mental health systems.

Strategic Directions for Governing Boards

Trustees of health organizations gave serious thought to restructuring board composition and reorienting the role such a board would play [Delbecq & Gill, 1988]. Considering that strategic planning for growth, and sometimes survival, is more important than maintaining and conserving a health organization's resources, a special study recommended the following priority changes:

1. Board size should be reduced to an ideal number of seven board members as compared to the usual existing 11 to 15 board members.
2. Board membership should be composed of technical and strategic experts rather than representatives of specified groups in the community.
3. Lay volunteer members of the board should be replaced, largely by compensated experts whose special knowledge is required to make policy decisions in a fast-changing economic environment.
4. Of possible internal directors, only the health institution's chief executive officer should serve on the board with powers and influence equal to that of the board's president.

If these organizational priorities were instituted in health organizations, there could be a radical shift from the "traditional, conservative, risk-aversive lay trustee model" [Delbecq & Gill, 1988], to a strategic, corporate model of governance.

CEO Priorities

Priorities can be determined by experts simply stating their opinions. A sample of hospital chief executive officers [CEOs] were asked to identify the activities requiring their most urgent attention. As early as 1984, more than 430 hospital CEOs were asked to rank their five most critical concerns from a list of 22 choices. Strategic planning was number one [66 percent], followed by medical staff relations [61 percent], cost containment [61 percent], marketing [51 percent], and alternative revenue sources [38 percent] [Moore, 1984]. Furthermore, CEOs ranked the following areas of expertise extremely or very important: strategic planning [91 percent], finance and accounting [89 percent], marketing [83 percent], human resources [82 percent], and management information systems [75 percent] [Moore, 1984]. Strategic planning was still rated the most important activity in 1986, followed by medical staff relations, financial planning, and communications with staff and consumers [*Hospitals*, 1986].

In terms of power shifts within health organizations, the executives predicted that chief executive officers would gain the most influence followed by market specialists and financial officers. This power shift would come at the expense of physicians, policy analysts, and nurses.

Consumer Priorities

In a survey conducted by the National Research Corporation in 1984, consumers recommended their top priorities for alternative health care services [Jackson & Jensen, 1984]. First priority was the consumer's desire for more home health care services. This was followed by adult day care, longer physician office hours, wellness centers, alcohol treatment, more family physicians, emergency facilities, and finally nursing homes. With the recognition that there are more two-family workers and more elderly who need care in the home, it is not surprising that home health care services was the number one priority.

In an opinion poll of 1,000 adults commissioned by the American Federation for Clinical Research, 53 percent chose improving health care as the top national priority [Hsueh, 1989].

A poll of 529 homeless adults, perhaps surprisingly, chose good health as the top priority need over a steady income, a permanent job, a permanent home, and regular meals [Linn & Gelberg, 1989].

Patients, local health board members, and health care professionals in Finland were asked to rank priorities in primary care from six statements expressing essential qualities about continuity of care, availability, empathy and humanity, comprehensiveness, and knowledge. Treatment without delay [availability] received highest priority from patients and board members; continuity of care was ranked highest by health care professionals [Hagman & Rehnstrom, 1985].

INDIVIDUAL AND IRRATIONAL PRIORITIES

Individuals and organizations do have their own distinct personalities and perspectives. There really is not one set of priorities to which all are likely to subscribe. Each entity must decide for itself what is in its own best interests and/or those of its client population. Essentially, strategic planning starts from the premise that each institution has its own mission, cultural environment, and set of values to guide it in selecting priorities from among a number of options. Values that may be rational for one institution may appear to be irrational when seen through the eyes of another. Dr. Theodore Cooper [1987], a prominent health care administrator, teacher, and policy analyst, contrasted how the priorities of macro-level health policy makers viewed the spending of so much money on dying people as irrational. While at the micro-level, a dying person's family and friends rationally opted to spend the funds. Cooper stated: "People by nature are given to doing irrational things. In the United States, that includes spending huge sums of money for a small gain—a few months of life, a slim hope of a cure, an off chance that one might start feeling better." Most people believe that a cure or a breakthrough may be just around the corner. They have faith that science and biomedical progress will ultimately result in finding the causes and cures of all our diseases. Ergo, why shouldn't we spend large sums of money to keep dying people alive if a cure may be coming at any moment? As with fine art, rationality is in the eyes of the beholder.

CHANGING PRIORITIES OVER TIME

Even as priorities are set for one decade, they are open to change in the next. Witness the demise of the 10 priorities of the National Health Planning and Resources Development Act [PL 93–641], promulgated in 1974 by Congress. Selected priorities dealt with strategic issues such as primary care services, coordination of institutional health services, improvement in quality of care, health education, and uniform cost-accounting procedures. For almost 10 years, these priorities played a strong role in guiding the creation and later implementation of regional health plans developed by the nationwide 200 or so Health Systems Agencies [HSAs]. Now, these HSAs and their goal priorities have almost vanished. Isolated county and/or state governments or individual health institutions may still use these goals as their priorities. For the most part, the objectives are no longer a part of the mainstream priorities. Only when those specific priorities are part of an institution's strategic plan will they have the importance they once had for the whole nation.

Obviously, health priorities are not meant to last forever. Priorities articulate the beliefs and values of a people at some point in time and are subject to modification or elimination as circumstances and conditions change. Seeking to effect change while reacting to the commercialization and privatization of health care in this era, Mahaffey [1986] exhorts mental health professionals "to make use of the political process to re-establish health and mental health care as a national priority."

GOALS AND PRIORITY DETERMINATION

A close relationship exists between goals, objectives, and priorities. In choosing priorities, planners make decisions selecting rank orders and deciding which priorities require more funding and/or support from the community. Within that environment, four elements of the process can be identified: determination of priorities, criteria for determinations, uses of the process, and component of the process.

Determination of Priorities

A vital step in the determination of priorities integrates community values and judgments into the raw data. However, that step could be taken by an elite authority figure acting on behalf of the public's best interests. There is no doubt that priorities are frequently set just that way. In recent years, the process has expanded greatly. Legislation and changing times spurred the inclusion of an array of consumers, a variety of providers and public officials in the deliberations about the priority needs of the community. A greater emphasis upon egalitarianism in determination of priorities resulted. However, Rada [1986] comments that the patient per se is not gaining any more input into the priority setting process. It is the patient shifting from the medical chart to the active consumer who is receiving greater control over health care decisions by voting with his/her dollars.

Representation from this wider population spectrum makes it more difficult to arrive at a consensus on health priorities. Differing values and vested interests are certain to arise in setting priorities as patients, community organization representatives, business people, labor representatives, physicians, institutional trustees, and various subgroups participate in the process [Carlyn & Hicks, 1986]. That distinction in values and vested concerns can be critical. Weiner, Boyer, and Farber [1986] point out the differing attitudes of administrators and physicians making priority choices regarding patients in life-threatening scenarios. When individuals need cardiopulmonary resuscitation, physicians think in terms of "future worth or quality" of a patient's life. On the other hand, administrators tend to focus more on existing "worthiness." This small philosophic and/or moral difference in values may have profound implications on priorities as the balance of power shifts to administrators.

However, given that all these groups must be taken into account, who determines priorities? Cynics believe that in the end it is the institutional priorities of health care organizations that influence the final decision based on self-interest and the concerns of the various community trustees and/or stakeholders [Fuchs & Deber, 1987].

In the glare of public priority determinations, value juxtapositions do cause difficulties. Should AIDS care be funded in preference to care for the elderly? Is acute care more pressing than long-term care services? Are prevention programs worth more energy and funding than disease alleviation activities? It is obvious that people are going to feel differently about different issues. Data may set the stage for a discussion, but on the final vote the attitudes and values may be the major factor in decisions. Until agreement can be reached on which statistics really represent true priority needs, decision makers will be troubled translating data into priorities.

An oft-quoted maxim states: "Statistics don't lie but liars use statistics." Numbers alone, assuming their validity, may not reveal the total picture. One community may have twice as many services as another. On the face of it, there may be no reason for the disparity. However, closer examination reveals that the first community has four times the need of the second; that cultural habits inhibit access to services; and that residents can't use the streets at night. Statistics do not illuminate the environmental, social, and psychological factors impacting on the health care services.

In the strategic planning process, the community and environmental health surveys can provide the data and insights to permit decision makers to comprehend priorities of various segments of the population.

Criteria for Priority Determination

At least three criteria should be used to set priorities: fairness, community participation, and a mixture of data and values.

Fairness includes a selection of representatives from all concerned groups affected by the forthcoming decisions. Both individuals involved in decision making and the general public should be guaranteed participation opportunities. In addition, fairness means that choices can be made impartial. Methods and procedures should assure everyone an equal opportunity to make decisions without undue influence or pressure.

Community participation in the priority determination process involves more than the neighborhood leaders and board members. People actually using the health care services should be involved since locality-wide priorities may not be harmonious with subarea needs or organizational priorities. Specific differences must be brought to light and discussed before priorities are set.

A priority-setting process must be able to link quantifiable data with community values. Both factors should be taken into account with neither ranking higher in the fairness deliberations.

In addition to these fairness criteria, additional specific criteria are usually linked to the priority options being considered. When a health care institution considers expansion or addition of new services, criteria such as cost, accessibility, quality, continuity, and effectiveness guide strategic planners and decision makers to ranking choices. When the federal Food and Drug Administration considered consolidating laboratories, criteria included condition and suitability of the facility, age of the facility, recent renovation work, and ownership prior to consolidation determinations [Fogel, 1987]. When the Toronto [Canada] Department of Public Health evaluated existing and proposed health protection program priorities, four criteria were used: whether the department had legal responsibility; whether it had the expertise; whether it had the capability of carrying out the programs; and whether any new priority options would be coordinated with existing ones [Hancock, 1986].

A final example concerns the development of long-stay services. Henderson [1985] reported that the following criteria were used in determining priorities:

- Improve the integration of patients with the community.
- Raise the quality of the patients' environment.
- Increase access for patients' families and visitors.
- Facilitate communications between staff.

Components of the Process

A priority determination process can set priorities among issues evolving from a needs assessment and a ranking of alternative resolutions of identified problems. In this way, general and specific criteria can assist in setting goals and objectives. Furthermore, priority determination can select specific program activities to achieve the stated goals and objectives.

Three vital components are involved in the priority-setting process: the inputs, the process itself, and the outputs.

Input refers to the information or data given to the decision-making group, the identification of decision elements, a complete list of decision criteria, and a format for recording decisions. Information or data could be mortality data, number of people living in an area, or the rate of admissions to hospitals. At this stage of the planning process, information is mainly linked to the group or agency's goals and program objectives under consideration for priority ranking.

Decision elements refer to all the goals and program objectives to be prioritized. These should be specifically identified in writing so everyone accepts the list and has no additions to make to it. It is essential to have a consensus on what should be included in the list before any decisions are made. Adding new items after the process is fairly well along results in confusion and raises questions about the fairness of the process.

Decision criteria are those measures used by each participant to judge the importance or value of the decision elements, the goals, and/or objectives. Criteria could relate to "percentage of people affected by the goal," "costs of achieving the goal," or "availability of service to special target populations, such as the elderly." Obviously, these decision criteria should have some relevance to the goals and program objectives under consideration.

Format details the procedure of recording the choices made by the decision-making body. A chart, a table, or a simple tabulation of "yes" and "no" votes could be used, but the format should be applicable to the methods and process involved.

A priority-setting process usually includes the rules to follow to have an orderly decision-making process as well as procedures for mathematical calculations to score the decision. Rules should cover factors such as the group's size, who should make decisions, how voting takes place, and the selection of a leader or chairperson for the meeting. Procedural rules generally follow prior experience. To make some changes, it may be necessary to adapt to different priority-setting methods. Computational rules determine how the group arrives at a consensus. Complex statistical procedures are inappropriate, and simple addition, multiplication, or averaging usually can serve the purpose. Individual preferences to rank goals and objectives can accurately reflect the group's thinking.

Output results in a list ranking goals and program objectives encapsulating the thinking of the decision makers. Potentially as crucial, outputs indicate the relevance of the criteria used by the decision makers to judge objectives. If the list is too long or the objectives vaguely written, it will be difficult to separate one priority ranking from the other. Ideally, a priority-setting process identifies data of benefit the next time decision makers engage in the priority planning process. Ancillary outputs can lead to sophisticated and valid decision making in future cycles of the planning process.

These major components of the process—inputs, the process itself, and the outputs—are generic to all the priority-setting techniques to be discussed. This rational, systematic approach is consistent with the strategic planning process adopted as the general framework for linking the illustrative methods to the components of the planning process.

PRIORITY-SETTING METHODOLOGIES

These baker's dozen of priority-setting techniques range from simple to complex and from preference to statistical analysis. All have been used in strategic planning and the techniques are not confined solely to priority setting.

The Simplex Method

In the Simplex method [Drake, McCann, Adams, & Isaacs, 1977, pp. IV:1–40], individual perceptions are garnered using questionnaires. Members of a decision-making body can work effectively responding to a variety of structured questions that analyze each proposal. Responses to the questions are scored and the results totaled. Top priority is given to the proposal with the highest total and the others follow in numerical order.

Structured Questions for Considering Solutions. A set of structured questions are used in the Simplex method. Structured questions concerning the solutions might fall into the following four categories:

1. Questions regarding the impact on the community's health (Exhibit 5–1).
2. Questions about general social concerns (Exhibit 5–2).
3. Questions of a strategic health planning nature (Exhibit 5–3).
4. Questions dealing with political factors (Exhibit 5–4).

Each set of structured questions may be expanded or modified to meet specific situations.

A Step-by-Step Example of Simplex. Either problems or solutions can be rank-ordered using the Simplex method. A group may be confronted with a situation in which one of several proposals must be chosen to deal with an identified problem. After the group answers all the

Exhibit 5-1.   Simplex Questions on Community Health.

1. This solution will benefit:
    1. few people
    2. some people
    3. half the people
    4. a majority
    5. everyone

2. This solution would make manpower, facilities, and money available to:
    1. very few
    2. a minority
    3. half the people
    4. a majority
    5. everyone

3. The effect of this solution on premature deaths [those deaths before the end of the normal life span] will be:
    1. none
    2. a slight reduction
    3. a reduction
    4. a great reduction
    5. elimination

4. This solution's effect on the community health environment will be:
    1. very harmful
    2. harmful
    3. without effect
    4. improvement
    5. great improvement

5. This solution will probably solve the problem:
    1. never
    2. eventually
    3. in good time
    4. soon
    5. immediately

6. The effect of this solution on pain, discomfort, and/or inconvenience will be:
    1. an increase
    2. no change
    3. moderate reduction
    4. substantial reduction
    5. great reduction

Exhibit 5-2. Simplex Questions on General Social Concerns.

1. The effect on lost work time by this solution will be:	1. an increase 2. no effect 3. a reduction 4. a great reduction 5. elimination
2. The distress or danger to others caused by this solution will be:	1. increased 2. not affected 3. moderate 4. reduced 5. eliminated
3. This solution will:	1. create many other problems 2. create few other problems 3. create no other problems 4. solve a few other problems 5. solve many other problems
4. This solution's impact on a patient's employability will be:	1. a substantial reduction 2. a moderate reduction 3. no change 4. a moderate increase 5. a substantial increase
5. The aesthetic effect of this solution will be:	1. bad 2. poor 3. fair 4. good 5. excellent
6. Public attitudes toward this solution are:	1. antagonistic 2. disapproving 3. tolerant 4. sympathetic 5. whole-hearted support
7. Public opinion toward financing this solution will be:	1. antagonistic 2. negative 3. indifferent 4. favorable 5. highly favorable

questions bearing on the selection of proposed solutions, the following steps result in a priority choice:

Step 1: Develop A Simplex Questionnaire. Sample questions listed in Exhibits 5–1 to 5–4 may be generically useful in a priority selection process. Obviously, unique conditions may dictate that certain questions be added and others deleted. In fact, members of the decision-making group may have knowledge about the immediate area certainly unknown to the developers of the illustrative questions.

A list of questions should be developed, approved by the entire decision-making group, and classified appropriately. A two-thirds or greater approval vote is suggested to consolidate the consensus. Any disagreements regarding the list of questions should be completely resolved prior to starting the Simplex process.

Structured questionnaires can be as lengthy or as specific as the group desires. However, given limitations on time, available information, and related extremities, the greater the number

**Exhibit 5-3.   Simplex Questions on Strategic Health
Planning Concerns.**

1. In practice this solution would be:
   1. difficult to change
   2. inflexible
   3. somewhat rigid
   4. fairly easy to change
   5. highly flexible

2. This solution will benefit:
   1. few at high costs
   2. few at moderate costs
   3. many at moderate costs
   4. a majority at low costs
   5. everyone at low costs

3. The return for the dollar spent on this solution will be:
   1. a losing proposition
   2. break-even
   3. moderate
   4. substantial
   5. very high

4. This solution's effect on manpower requirements will be:
   1. a great increase
   2. an increase
   3. no effect
   4. a reduction
   5. a substantial reduction

5. The phases of the problem attacked by this solution will be:
   1. one
   2. a few
   3. many
   4. a majority
   5. all

6. The amount of beneficial side effects produced by solution will be:
   1. none
   2. a few
   3. some
   4. many
   5. very many

7. The amount of health care manpower, facilities, and money used by this solution will be:
   1. unacceptable
   2. excessive
   3. acceptable
   4. minimal
   5. negligible

8. Necessary technology for this solution is:
   1. unavailable
   2. difficult to find
   3. accessible
   4. largely available
   5. completely available

9. There are many other solutions to this problem 1
   There are several other solutions to this problem 2
   There are a few other solutions to this problem 3
   There is another solution to this problem 4
   This is the only solution to this problem 5

of questions, the increased possibility that responses overlap or distortions occur. In addition, if the group uses complex techniques to evaluate the responses, the larger number of questions could compound the difficulties.

Exhibit 5-4.   Simplex Question on Political Concerns.

1. The political attitude toward this solution is:	1. antagonistic 2. indifferent 3. complacent 4. concerned 5. very interested
2. This solution will affect public opinion:	1. very adversely 2. adversely 3. not at all 4. favorably 5. very favorably
3. Because of this solution, coordination among official agencies will be:	1. greatly discouraged 2. slightly discouraged 3. unaffected 4. slightly encouraged 5. greatly encouraged
4. Because of this solution, coordination among public and private agencies will be:	1. greatly discouraged 2. slightly discouraged 3. unaffected 4. slightly encouraged 5. greatly encouraged
5. Community participation and support for this solution will be:	1. negligible 2. slight 3. moderate 4. high 5. very high

Step 2: Familiarization with Proposal Background Information. Before answering the structured questionnaire, group members should discuss all the proposed solutions. Any additional information should be made available to all about the purpose, scope, probable effectiveness, and overall value of each proposal. Openness and honest exchange should be encouraged.

Step 3: Complete the Simplex Questionnaire. Simplex questionnaire(s) on the solution(s) is/are distributed to all group members and completed for each proposal. Group members complete the questionnaires independently and answer each question with one of the structured responses. All questionnaires are collected by the staff for tabulation.

Step 4: Tabulation of "Solution(s) Questionnaire" Results. Tabulation involves averaging the numbers corresponding with each selected answer from each member of the group. Multiple-choice questions guarantee that the higher the number selected [1–5], the better the solution. As all the answers for one question are totaled and averaged, the resulting number presents the group's assessment of the value of that proposal. That value judgment can be numerically compared with the assessments of the other proposals.

In the second tabulation step, all the averages for all the questions are totaled. Resulting totals for each proposal can then be compared with the other proposals, which in this case ranged on a scale from 28–140. The proposal with the highest total number would be considered the priority choice.

Optional Weighting Techniques. Each of the structured questions in all questionnaires is implicitly given equal weight. However, the overall importance of each question may vary.

"Return for dollars spent" [Exhibit 5–3, Number 3] may be seen as significantly more important than "aesthetic value" [Exhibit 5–2, Number 5]. If the group decides that specific questions should express relative impacts, there are several weighting mechanisms. An easy weighting method assigns each structured question a value based upon comparative importance. "Relative importance" can be determined through a polling process. Using a specified numerical range such as 1 to 3, each member assigns a value to each question and the values are averaged. That average score is used as that given question's weight.

Suppose the group rates the relative importance of each question on the Solution Being Considered [Exhibits 5–1 to 5–4] on a scale of 1 [low importance] to 10 [high importance]. For the first question, "This solution will benefit" [Exhibit 5–1, Number 1], the average rating turns out to be seven, indicating relatively great importance. If a group member judged the proposed solution to affect "half the people," that response [#3] would be multiplied by the weight [7] to result in a weighted response of 21. Each of these weighted scores would be totaled and then divided by the number of members, resulting in a weighted score for that specific question as related to a particular proposal.

All question responses are weighed in the same fashion. Sums of all questions for each proposal are still comparative and the highest weighted score is still the most desirable.

The Nominal Group Process Model

A Nominal Group Planning method developed by Delbecq, Van de Ven, and Gustafson [1975; Van de Ven & Delbecq, 1972] explores problems and issue dimensions. In 1968, the developers noted that the technique could be used for the following applications: problem exploration, knowledge exploration, priority development, program development, and program evaluation.

In each application, the mechanics of the process are essentially the same. Although a variety of data can be integrated into this method, the process generally utilizes consensus opinions and values to arrive at systematic choices.

A basic foundation of the nominal group process lies in the composition of a decision-making group to include individuals with diverse backgrounds, expertise, and perceptions. This method achieves planning goals by cross-fertilization of the differing inputs of the participants to reach a consensus.

As a method of establishing priorities, the Nominal Group involves fewer statistical manipulations. Instead, group discussion and information exchange constitute the key phases.

Nominal group methods begin with the group members specifying details re the specific topics to be discussed. If the topic was program activities, specific details could include a listing of all the health care problem solutions perceived by the participants. If the issue was the creation of decision guidelines, a list of specific criteria to evaluate health care options could evolve. After lists are developed, participants exchange information and reach consensus on the question by a simple voting process.

Step-by-Step Example. After developing all perceived options, the Nominal Group members must choose among solutions. Within funding limits, that chosen solution should receive priority in the allocation of efforts and resources. How to arrive at the priority choice is detailed in the following step-by-step example.

Step 1: Set Up the Structure of the Decision-Making Group. Two immediate questions at this point are: "How large should the group be?" and "Should the group be broken down into subgroups?"

Answers to these two questions relate to the breadth and complexity of the subject matter. In addition, the existence of subtopics may lend itself to the formation of different smaller decision-making groups. Each subgroup can tackle specific components of broad-ranging decisions.

After each subgroup reaches a consensus, the full group begins a nominal group process based on the collected decisions of each subgroup. Normally, the nominal group process is improved by first achieving subtopic consensus.

Subgroup members can be recruited from specific existing committees corresponding to the topic in question. However, the inclusion of noncommittee members exposes the subgroup to a wider range of perspectives. If a topic-oriented committee structure does not exist, subgroup members may be randomly selected or assigned according to background or expertise. Maximum success occurs when participants apply broad-ranging perspectives and knowledge to a given problem.

A minimum size for a nominal group process is six to 10, but the decision group can be larger. As the number of participants increases, the outcomes will be improved, but the time requirements and complexity of the process also increases. Even a group of 15 to 20 participants can reach a consensus in a single session as the nominal group process still remains very workable.

Step 2: Define the Dimensions of the Problem. Each nominal planning session is led by a coordinator who explains the process and outlines the problem. After this explanation, each participant receives a "Nominal Group Task Statement Form" which specifies an exploratory question seeking group consensus. Multiple forms and questions may be used to arrive at an overall consensus on the problem.

In addition to the overall problem, each form states the type of input sought from the participants. Exhibit 5–5 illustrates two Nominal Group Task Statement Forms to elicit input:

- List all the problems/solutions, whether subjective or objective, which you perceive as affecting the delivery of health care in your area.
- List the criteria by which you would judge the seriousness of a solution affecting the institution's health care delivery system.

Independently, each participant completes the Task Statement Form[s] within a predetermined time limit. On Task Statement Form I, each participant lists as many criteria as possible to be considered while reviewing the institution's health care delivery solutions. Criteria might be drawn from the participant's personal knowledge and experience, staff suggestions, federal, state or local regulations or from public opinion.

For the second form, each participant lists all the subjective or objective problems/solutions perceived to impact upon the delivery of health care. Objective problems/solutions may relate to the organization, resources, or environmental barriers to meeting the areas needs. Subjective problems may result from emotions, feelings, and undefined reactions. A person may presume that treatment is unavailable without money when in fact services are free.

When the allotted time period concludes, the coordinator compiles a master list of all the problems/solutions and criteria. In a round-robin fashion, each participant contributes one problem/solution [criterion] aloud from their nominal group task statement form to be recorded on a large flip-chart or blackboard. There is no discussion while the list is recorded. One after the other each person reads an item from their list until all the items from all the lists are recorded. Participants can add to their list if ideas are suggested by any of the noted items.

Exhibit 5-5.   Nominal Group Task Statement Forms.

```
NOMINAL GROUP TASK STATEMENT FORM 1

To identify health care solutions that should receive priority
    with regard to the allocation of effort and resources

    List the criteria you would use to judge the seriousness of
a solution affecting the institution's health care delivery system.

1.
2.
3.
4.
--
--
--
--
--
--
--
N
```

```
NOMINAL GROUP TASK STATEMENT FORM  2

To identify those health care solutions that should receive priority
    with regard to the allocation of effort and resources.

    List all the problems, whether subjective or objective, which you
    perceive as effecting the delivery of health care in your area.


1.
2.
3.
4.
--
--
--
--
--
N
```

Step 3: Discussion of the Statement Items. After all items are recorded, the coordinator leads the discussion of the listed problems, criteria, and solutions. This discussion aims to clarify, to elaborate, to defend, or to dispute existing items. While items may be added at this time, items are deleted at this point. Discussion progresses item by item until all listings are clarified to the satisfaction of the group. A specific time limit can be set.

Step 4: Solutions and Evaluation. At this step, the group has separate lists of problems/solutions and criteria. Since each list has been discussed, each participant is asked to evaluate the problems/solutions in light of the predetermined criteria. Based on individual preferences and the discussions, the participants can choose any of the criteria to evaluate the problems/solutions. Another option allows the group to first select a certain number of the criteria using a voting or ranking procedure. Selected criteria would then be used by the participants to evaluate the problems/solutions.

Whichever method is used, each member comes to an individual decision relative to the importance of each of the problems and the solutions.

Step 5: Rank Ordering of Problems/Solutions. At this stage, each participant lists their 10 most important solutions in rank order. Each solution is recorded on a separate index card by solution name, and ranking number. Top choices rate a 10, next choice a 9 and so on through all 10 solutions.

When participants finish their rank ordering, the votes are individually marked on a tally sheet on the flip-chart or blackboard (Exhibit 5–6). Relative importance of each solution is reflected in the right hand total column that sums up the votes for each solution.

Step 6: Discussion of Ranking. Once the votes are recorded and summed on the tally sheet, the coordinator initiates a discussion of the results. In this session, participants can reclarify, elaborate, defend, or dispute these preliminary outcomes.

Step 7: Final Ranking. After the discussion of the rankings, the coordinator allows participants the opportunity to change any of the 10 priority items on their index cards. Then,

Exhibit 5-6.   Nominal Group Vote Tally Sheet Example.

Master List of Solutions	Rank Ordering of Solutions on Master List [Ranks Assigned to Solutions by Each Participant]							
	Participants							
	1	2	3	4	5	6	7	Total
A	10	9	8	8	7	9	7	58
B	—	2	—	4	—	—	—	6
C	9	10	7	6	5	7	5	49
D	6	—	—	5	4	—	6	21
E	8	7	6	7	6	6	4	44
F	5	8	5	9	—	5	—	32
G	7	—	—	—	—	4	3	14
H	—	3	—	—	2	3	1	9
I	4	4	3	2	—	—	2	15
* * * * *	[2,3]	[1,5,6]	[1,2,4,9,10]	[1,10]	[3,8,9,10]	[1,8,10]	[8,9,10]	
[N]	1	—	—	3	1	2	—	7

Exhibit 5-7.   Nominal Group Final Rank Tally Sheet Example.

Master List of Solutions	Rank Ordering of Solutions on Master List [Ranks Assigned to Solutions by Each Participant]							
	Participants							
	1	2	3	4	5	6	7	Total
A	90	100	85	88	76	78	92	609
B	—	85	—	70	—	42	—	197
C	83	65	55	100	100	100	72	575
D	100	—	—	48	59	—	95	302
E	95	92	86	82	70	64	100	589
F	85	90	100	80	—	45	—	400
G	81	—	—	—	56	42	30	209
H	—	32	21	10	—	91	15	169
I	65	78	41	30	—	—	22	236
J	32	65	27	—	29	—	61	214
K	—	51	91	82	73	60	87	444
L	22	10	—	51	18	45	1	146
M	—	—	31	—	57	—	—	88
N	15	—	16	42	22	45	—	140

participants rate their priority items giving a value of 100 to the most important priority card and values between 0 and 99 to the other nine cards. This revised rating of priorities is collected by the coordinator.

Final ratings are recorded on a tally sheet (Exhibit 5–7) and the individual ratings are totaled. Solutions with the highest scores delineate group consensus on the priority solution to achieve the agency's goal and objectives.

Caveat on this Technique. A Nominal Group process relies heavily on the subjective analysis of the subject matter by each participant. In fact, the process itself can be modified to adapt to specific issues, to the preferences of the governing body and to the vested interests of all concerned parties. Even though the process may take different forms, the basic procedural steps should be retained in the suggested order.

Criteria Weighting Method

A Criteria Weighting Method [Blum, 1974, chap. 6] applies simple mathematics to a number of decision options criteria to achieve a significance level for each alternative under consideration. Basic steps in this process are:

- Assignment of weights to the criteria selected as appropriate to the issue.
- Rating of each proposal according to each criterion.
- Multiplication of the weighting value by the rating yields the significance level.
- Review and comparison of each alternative in light of the significance level values.

It is possible that the final value ordering may not reflect the final decision. Yet, higher rank-ordered alternatives indicate a belief in their superior merit and the nature of the process demonstrates a consensus of the group.

A Step-by-Step Example of the Method. In this illustration, the group is required to choose from among three alternative proposals for the use of resources to improve health care in the area: A: Alcoholism Clinic; B: Mental Health Clinic; and C: Hypertension Clinic. All three proposals are known to the group and there is agreement on the criteria applicable to priority determination. If the proposals or the criteria are not known or agreed to, the initial step should resolve that situation. A useful method to do so is a simplified Nominal Group process as described earlier.

Step 1: Development of Criteria. Criteria can be grouped into topical generic categories such as technological issues, community health issues, general social issues, or financial issues.

Decision criteria under each of these categories should be agreed upon and listed. Methods to develop specific criteria could use group process techniques that have been described in earlier sections.

Step 2: Weighting the Criteria. Importantly, each criterion is discussed thoroughly to assure that each participant comprehends them. Of course, the validity and appropriateness of each criterion must also be supported. A criteria weighting proceeds as follows:

- Each participant places a value of one [low] through five [high] on all criteria in each category.
- Members privately assign their own values to each criterion.
- Averaging of the scores for each criterion reflects the relative weight of each criterion as shown below:

Criteria	JBC	ISH	TOL	Weighting
A	5	4	3	12/3 = 4
B	4	3	3	9/3 = 3
C	2	2	4	8/3 = 2.6

These weighted criteria values indicate that the participants believe that criterion A is more important in making the final decision than criteria B and C.

Step 3: Rating Solutions by Criteria. To rate the three proposals, a subjective process is used similar to the assignment of weights to the criteria. Each member independently reviews each proposal successively according to each criterion. For each criterion, the participant values each proposal by scoring the activity between -10 and $+10$. Use of negative numbers allows for accurate distinctions between alternatives.

After rating each proposal, scores for each criterion are averaged resulting in single positive or negative numbers that reflect consensus on relative importance. Each combination of one proposal and one criterion should have a numerical rating.

Exhibit 5–8 displays the results of this process in columns 1 and 2 with column 2 divided into the three proposed activities—A, B, C.

Step 4: Obtaining Criterion Significance Levels. Multiplying the proposal rating by the criterion weight produces a "significance level." Adding all the positive and negative criterion significance levels results in the total significance for each proposal. Seven specific criteria on "community health issues" are weighted and rated in Exhibit 5–8. "Accessibility to health services," has a high weight of five. Average rating for activity A and for that criterion is +2 [2 + 3 + 1/3]. By multiplying the weight five by the rate of two, the significance level of accessibility for activity A is ten. That same process for each criterion/activity combination is shown in Exhibit 5–8.

Step 5: Standardization of Significance Levels. All criteria significance levels are totaled for each proposal. Standardization occurs by dividing the total significance level by the number of criteria used to rate each proposal. However, the total is divided only by the number of criteria actually used. Significance level is intentionally skewed by dividing by the number of criteria applied rather than by the sum of the weights. Proposals can be arranged in a priority sequence according to the average standardized significance levels; the higher the average standardized significance level, the higher the priority.

Column 3 in Exhibit 5–8 demonstrates this step. Note that the criterion for "morbidity impact" was not used to evaluate activity C and that column C is divided by six rather than by seven criteria.

Step 6: Determine Priorities. Results of the criteria weighting process for all three activities are shown in Exhibit 5–9. Each cell applies to one proposal and one group of criteria. Each number value reflects the group's consensus as to the importance or the effectiveness of the

Exhibit 5-8. Criteria Weighting: Determining Significance Levels for Community Health Issues Criteria.

Example Criteria	Example Weights	Average Rating			Significance Level		
		A	B	C	A	B	C
Accessibility to Health Services	5	2	3	1	10	15	5
Health Manpower Requirements	4	4	3	2	16	12	8
Public Education about Topic	2	−1	0	−2	−2	0	−4
Probable Duration if Left Unattended	2	3	3	1	6	6	2
Mortality Impact	2	2	1	3	4	2	6
Morbidity Impact	2	−1	−4	—	−2	−8	—
Prevalence or Attack Rate	3	−3	−3	−2	−9	−9	−6
Total Health Planning Significance Levels					23	18	11
Divided by the number of criteria applied to each proposal					7	7	6
Average Standardized Significance Level					3.29	2.57	1.83

Note: The criteria and weights used are merely examples and are not intended in any way to represent any particular real-life situation. They are solely for the purpose of presenting how the criteria weighting methodology operates.

A = Alcoholic Clinic   B = Mental Health   C = Hypertension

Exhibit 5-9.   Criteria Weighting: Significance Level Rating of Importance of Three Proposals.

Category of Example Criteria:	Proposal A	Proposal B	Proposal C
Group of Criteria on Technological Issues	+4	+2.1	+2
Group of Criteria on Financial Issues	+3	+2.5	+2.1
Group of Criteria on General Social Issues	+3.4	+2.3	+2.4
Group of Criteria on Community Health Issues	+3.29	+2.57	+1.83
Total Significance Level	17.69	9.47	8.33

proposed solution. Criteria group values for each proposal are totaled yielding the final proposal weighting. That number can be compared to any of the other proposal values. A total significance level yields a priority among the three activities. Obviously, the consensus is that proposal A [17.69] exhibits greater significance and should be addressed first. Given constraints on resources, proposals would most likely be considered in rank order. In the final analysis, the process makes no conclusions about implementation. However, the process does reveal, using the selected criteria and the alternatives, that the number "one" proposal is considered to be most serious and most in need of resolution.

A rationale for this process builds on the assumption that the use of this analytical tool persuades participants to more readily agree on complex issues. Considering proposals using relevant weighted criteria and rating each proposal for significance levels, allows decision-making groups to arrive at reasonably acceptable choices.

The Hanlon Method

Hanlon and Pickett [1984, chap. 11] list three major objectives for their method of choosing priorities:

- To permit decision makers to identify explicit major factors to be included in the priority-setting process.
- To organize the factors into groups that are weighted relative to each other.
- To allow the factors to be modified as needed and scored individually.

Based on repeated demonstrations in various health care contexts a consistent pattern evolved and is reflected in the following four components used in the Hanlon Method:

- *Component A* = the size of the problem.
- *Component B* = the seriousness of the problem.
- *Component C* = estimated effectiveness of solution [solubility of the problem].
- *Component D* = PEARL factors relating to administrative practicality.

These components are a collection of one or more criteria that may be appropriate to the question at hand.

Scores expressing these four components are inserted into the following two formulas:

- Basic Priority Rating [BPR] = [A + B] C.
- Overall Priority Rating [OPR] = [A + B] C × D.

The difference between the two formulas is the presence of component D in the OPR formula. This distinction will become apparent as component D [PEARL] is explained in the step-by-step process.

Hanlon Method: Step-by-Step Example. This example intersperses explanation in a hypothetical situation along with the mechanics of the Hanlon Method.

Hypothetical Situation. For the past two years, the Able Medical Center has been losing patients. Occupancy fell below the 80 percent break-even point in the past year. Employing a strategic planning consultant, a community needs survey revealed that the area's population had been changing for some time. Residents were more affluent and more concerned with self-responsibility in caring for their own health and the use of nonhospital-based health services. An internal audit by the strategic planner found that the Able Medical Center's trustees were concerned with conserving resources rather than entering into new opportunities. Recommendations to improve the medical center's image and financial base focused on streamlining the Board of Trustees from 18 to 7 members, reorienting the Board to a strategic policy-making corporate board, and vesting more power and authority in the chief executive officer. Consequences of the Board doing nothing would eventually result in bankrupting the Able Medical Center. Changes would be necessary for the medical center to meet the needs of the new population's interest in health promotion and concerns with home health services, especially for the growing elderly population. Furthermore, many new residents would welcome extended physician hours to cater to the growing number of two employed spouses. With the transition in population to a more affluent and older one, the number of persons in the catchment are decreased from 55,000 to about 50,000 over the last 10 years.

To forestall a change in the Board's composition, representation, and role, the current trustees agreed to use the Hanlon method to rank the community needs spelled out in the consultant's report. While still maintaining a conservative orientation, the Board was willing to invest in one new strategic program opportunity if it would help improve the Center's community image and cash flow problems.

This component may deal with only one factor, but the choice remains with the group. In any event, that factor[s] must be spelled out carefully to avoid misinterpretations such as which population group and how to corner the population.

Step 1: Determine Component A—Size of Problem. Faced with dealing with the three community needs expressed in the consultant's report, the only criterion considered in component A was the size of the population affected. "I" refers to the community's health promotions needs; "II," to home health care needs; and "III," to extended physician hours.

A community survey revealed that 10 percent of the population wanted health promotion services; 15 percent desired home health services; and 30 percent wanted extended physician hours. A table correlated percentage of population with community needs and weighted scores as follows:

Percentage of Population	Community Need	Score
30%	III	10
25%		8
20%		6
15%	II	4
10%	I	2

On component "A," size of problem, the Board collectively gave a 10 score to extended physician hours, a 4 to home health care needs, and a 2 to health promotion needs in this procedure. Group decisions define the factors in all four components of the formulas and also the relative weights for the components. In the evaluation of programs and activities, individual rater judgments are applied in the formulas. However, scientific control may be instituted using a representative sample of qualified raters, a precise definition of terms, the delineating of exact rating procedures, and the utilization of available statistical data to guide ratings.

Step 2: Determine Component B—Seriousness. At this point, the group lists the elements determining the seriousness of the problem. Using a group process, each participant prepares their own list of relevant factors.

A composite list is compiled from the individual lists. Participants vote to choose the factors critical to the assessment of the seriousness of the problem. Less than 10 factors would be considered a "reasonable" list. Factors might include the following areas:

1. Urgency
   - Public concern
   - Public health concern
2. Severity
   - Mortality rates
   - Morbidity—degree and duration
   - Disability—degree and duration
   - Accessibility—average distance to care
3. Medical Costs
   - To individuals directly affected
   - To third-party payers
4. Trends in Health Care Needs [forecasts]
   - Potential number of persons who may acquire problem or be affected by the problem, and relative degree of involvement.

In the Able Medical Center example, three factors were selected to measure seriousness: degree of severity, cost per person, and urgency of need. It is also possible for the group to weigh factors if one element is considered more important. Scoring ranged from zero [least serious] to 10 [most serious]. Factor breakpoints can be in dollars, percent or a rating score as determined by the group. Breakpoints should be kept to about five or six and compromise the total range of scoring as noted below:

Degree of Severity	Cost/Person	Urgency Score	
Very Severe	0–$150	Very Urgent	10
Severe	151– 300	Urgent	8
Moderate	301– 450	Some Urgency	6
Minimal	451– 600	Little Urgency	4
None	601– 750	No Urgency	2
—	over 750	—	1

On these three seriousness criteria, the collective average score of the Able Medical Center Board is shown for each community need:

	Community Need	Severity	Cost	Urgency	Total	Score Average
I	Health Promotion	4	6	4	14	4.7
II	Home health care	7	1	6	14	4.7
III	Extending MD hours	6	4	6	16	5.3

On the component of seriousness, extending physician hours has the highest average score with 5.3. Home health care and health promotion are tied with 4.7 average seriousness scores.

Step 3: Determine Component C—Solubility. Taking into account the resources of the Able Medical Center, the Board must determine the effectiveness of resolving each of the three identified needs. In many cases, measurements of effectiveness are estimates since the task is difficult and the instruments leave much to be desired in terms of validity. If the Center dealt with problems rather than needs, Board members might be asking, "How effectively can this problem be solved, if at all?" Individual estimates may again be a major part of the response.

Keeping in mind the current resources and technology of the Able Medical Center, each Board member ranks the three needs between .5 and 1.5 based on an individual estimate of realistic solubility. A .5 indicates that the need is not likely to be solved by the medical center; a 1.0 value indicates no likely change; and a 1.5 suggests that the need can be resolved. Importantly, both the Basic Priority Rating formula and the Overall Priority Rating formula receive a multiplier effect from the value of component C: a .5 reduces the priority and a 1.5 increases the priority.

Regarding the need for health promotion services, the consultant's report estimates that 10 to 20 percent of those desiring the service will use it: about 500–1,000 persons. There were serious questions whether a greater number of people would utilize the services of a new health promotion program. While such a program might improve Able Medical Center's community image, the activity would not do much to increase occupancy rates or to improve the cash flow problem. On the effectiveness scale, the Board rated community need I a 1.04.

With respect to home health services, the community needs survey indicated an estimated 5,000 to 7,500 persons requiring such a service. Board members estimated that available resources would permit an initial program to serve about 3,000 persons, but realistically expected only 1,500 clients. That number would not exceed current informal arrangements with family and friends. Consequently, it was estimated that starting such a program would not add more services. Starting such a service might not add anything to the medical center's image but could add to the cash flow losses. Collectively, the Board gave community need II a score of 0.95.

On extending physician hours an estimated 15,000 persons expressed a need for this service. With the number of two-worker families, single-parent families, and reduced availability of parents and grandparents to assist, there is a real and growing need to extend physician hours. Board discussion led to the realistic conclusion that 50 percent of those 15,000 already have their own physicians and would not change. Another 25 percent would probably go to the new urgicenters that recently opened in the medical center's catchment area. However, the remaining 25 percent [3,700 persons] might utilize a physician satellite center or clinic with extended hours. That could mean an estimated 3,700–4,000 new medical center visits per year—an increase of 15 percent over current clinic utilization. In turn, if 10 percent of those seen required hospitalization, that would increase the occupancy rate about 2 percent. Community need III received a score of 1.15 on the scale.

All three community needs are placed on the continuum rating and the Basic Priority Rated calculated below:

$$\text{not likely to solve need} \quad \underline{\quad \overset{II}{0.5} \quad \overset{}{0.75} \quad \overset{I}{1.0} \quad \overset{III}{1.25} \quad 150 \quad} \quad \text{likely to solve community need}$$

Basic Priority Rating   = [A + B] × C]

Health promotion   I = [2 + 4.7] × 1.04 = 6.97

Home health care   II = [4 + 4.7] × 0.95 = 8.27

Extending MD hours   III = [10 + 5.3 × 1.15] = 17.6

Obviously, the Board gave III the highest Basic Priority Rating followed by II and I.

Step 4: Determine Component D—PEARL. Each of the community needs must be appraised in terms of PEARL: *P*ropriety, *E*conomic Feasibility, *A*cceptability, *R*esource availability, and *L*egality. Do any of the PEARL factors preclude pursuing solutions to the problem? For each element of PEARL, Board members vote using the number one for a "yes" vote and a zero for a "no" vote. A zero could mean that the proposal may be improper, illegal, unfeasible, or unacceptable. However, since component D is a multiplier and not a sum, any one zero makes the Overall Priority Rating also zero even if the proposal received a high Basic Priority rating.

Votes for each element of PEARL are tabulated and the results discussed. Members may change their votes if they wish. As a unit, the Board comes to a decision as to the one or zero value to assign to each element of PEARL. Remember that a zero vote on any PEARL element negates that proposal. Results of the medical center's Board overall priority rating [OPR] is shown below:

Community Need	Component D P E A R L	D × BPR = OPR	Final Rank
I	1 1 1 1 1	= 1 × 6.97 = 6.97	2nd
II	1 0 1 1 1	= 0 × 8.27 = 0.00	0 = no rank
III	1 1 1 1 1	= 1 × 17.6 = 17.6	1st

Computations for PEARL indicate that I [health promotion] and III [extending physician hours] meet all the implementation requirements. On the other hand, community need II [home health care services] get a zero or no vote by the Board for economic feasibility. Because the use of medical center resources may result in further losses, the implementation of home health care services is not feasible at this point in time. Consequently, Board members clearly believed that extending physician hours would be in the medical center's best interests and voted to implement this priority.

Step 5: Evaluate Other Factors. Before making a final decision, Able Medical Center Board members evaluated several additional factors. Resources existed to extend hours of existing outpatient clinics or to establish a free-standing medical satellite. However, it was not clear whether sufficient physicians, especially the specialists with admitting privileges to the medical center, would be willing to change their hours of practice to evenings and weekends to meet community needs. Possibly, the combination of a growing surplus of physicians and the flexibility of new physicians moving into the area might induce the existing physicians to accept the medical center's request to cooperate with this program.

A second factor was that one of the two urgicenters was staffed by several physicians having admitting privileges at Able Medical Center. A new satellite medical office would be in direct competition. It was considered essential to discuss the Board's decision with that urgicenter regarding a feasible means of cooperating or coordinating the new satellite center. At any rate, the Board reaffirmed the necessity to strike out in a new direction. Here was an opportunity to utilize the consultant's report to stem the financial losses and to improve the Able Medical Center's image in the community. At the same time, depending on the response to the new satellite center, the Board could keep the second priority on the back burner. Possibly, many of the new persons using the satellite center might also be interested in health promotion. If so, there might be a direct link and built-in incentive to open such a program either within the satellite center or as a separate program at a later date.

Delphi Forecasting

Delphi is a method for forecasting social and organizational changes. This method was predominantly used for technological forecasting. Determining the needs, priorities, organizational structure, and program objectives for hospitals and other health care provider services are some of the current uses of Delphi.

In another Delphi application Yang, Yu, and Cho [1987] used the technique to determine priorities for research fields in South Korea. About 30 panelists used three Delphi rounds to select 20 priority research fields from among 85 choices. Population, family planning, and environmental pollution emerged as the top three research priority areas.

Basically, Delphi obtains consensus from a panel of experts on the probability that future events will occur. Panel members do not interact with each other, but through an intermediary. This permits the experts to present their best estimates without being biased by the presence of strong-willed persons of high status or prestige, as in a face-to-face situation. Panelists do not know each other's identity during the proceedings, except that all are experts in specific fields. This process takes three to four rounds before the differences among the panelists can be narrowed to form a consensus about the future. In each round, the respective panelist's descriptions and predictions of the future are circulated among the other panelists, leading to anonymous comparisons and contrasts among them. In time, through refinement and clarification of each panelist's positions, a consensus is reached.

Panelists should have heterogeneous backgrounds to ensure that a range of values is offered to the subjects under discussion. Each panelist must be an expert in their own right to avoid a situation where someone else's point of view is summarily accepted without question. Criteria should be developed to guide the panelists in their evaluations.

One set of criteria was devised for a dental Delphi [Whittle, Grant, Sarll, & Worthington, 1987]. Panelists used four-point scales to rate criteria related to importance [priority or relevance], confidence [validity of argument or premise], desirability [effectiveness or benefit], probability [likelihood], and feasibility [practicality]. Other criteria, such as accessibility, affordability, satisfaction, and personal counseling, might have been used. On the criteria of importance, the panel of 10 might have rated the particular question as follows:

Criteria of Importance	Number	Percent
Very important	4	40%
Important	3	30%
Slightly important	1	10%
Unimportant	2	20%

This result shows that four of the 10 panelists considered the issue very important and three, important. Since the combined ratings of seven of the 10 panelists were in the highest two categories, the issue must be considered significant. Had only 50 percent considered it important or very important, a second Delphi round would have been necessary to try to reach consensus. Each panelist would receive the scores of the other panelists and any rationale provided for their answer. By the third or fourth round, a consensus usually develops as panelists are influenced by each other's answers and change their own minds to favor or reject a program objective.

Where there are two or more panels such as private physicians, hospital administrators, and health policy experts responding to the same question, a method referred to as the Polarization Index [PI] is used to evaluate the range of differences among the panels. This PI is the sum of the differences between the ratings of pairs of the groups. Where three groups are used, the PI is twice the range. On the criteria of desirability for a particular program option, the rating for the three groups might have been 81, 63, and 49. Then, the PI = 2 × range = 2 × [81 − 49] = 64.

Each of the criteria for the statement are treated in the same way and the polarization indices summed to provide an overall score. The larger the score, the more disagreement among the groups.

Three groups were asked to respond to a series of policy practice questions. Public health dentists, private practice dentists, and a community health advocacy group for senior citizens agreed to participate in a Delphi process regarding dental care for the elderly [Whittle et al., 1987].

Three of the 15 statements illustrate the Delphi process:

Statement 1: Senior citizens should receive dental examinations at low or no cost at least annually.

Statement 2: Dentists should be given the responsibility of informing their senior citizen patients when their annual, routine examinations are due with a notice of a specific appointment time.

Ratings for the three statements are shown below.

Rating criteria	Statement Number 1	2	3
Importance	90	54	77
Confidence	80	41	61
Desirability	93	58	74
Probability	74	35	58
Feasibility	90	61	67
Polarization Index	312	356	136

Based on these evaluations, statement 1 can be considered significant because the overall criteria scores for the three panels range above the 70 percent level. However, it is evident that the high PI for both statements 1 and 2 reflects much disagreement among the three Delphi panel groups. An examination of the scores for each panel on question 2 reflects this difference.

Criteria	PI	Private Dentists	Public Dentists	Community Advocates	Overall Score
Importance	124	87	54	25	54
Confidence	74	62	45	25	41
Desirability	76	75	72	37	58
Probability	40	37	45	25	35
Feasibility	44	62	72	50	61

These scores show a wide disagreement existing between private dentists and consumer health advocates regarding the taking of a senior citizen's blood pressure during routine dental examinations. Consumers are opposed and private dentists are in favor. Public health dentists take an intermediate position. These differences are responsible for the low-significance scores on the five criteria and would require several iterations of the Delphi process to determine whether a consensus could be achieved.

Using statement 3 as an illustration, the findings show how the Delphi process can bring closure and significant agreement from one round to the next.

Criteria	First Round	Second Round
Importance	77	96
Confidence	61	92
Desirability	74	96
Probability	58	85
Feasibility	67	88

All criteria demonstrate a major increase in agreement and the formation of a consensus. A 31 percent increase in the significance of the "confidence" criterion indicates agreement that dentists should take the responsibility of keeping their senior citizen patients informed when their routine examinations are due.

A Delphi process method can predict the significance of policy and program objectives and rank the alternative options as to their priority. However, there are strengths and weakness in using this method.

Advantages

1. An excellent method to use where quantitative data are not available and the subject is complex.
2. A fairly inexpensive method to use.
3. Democratic in that each person makes their own decision without being biased by a dominant expert and results in a maximum of options.
4. Forecasts of future changes in programs can be monitored so additional changes can be made by a further iteration of Delphi as needed.

Disadvantages

1. Selection of panel members must be done carefully to avoid bias.
2. Panel fatigue, usually by the third round, may lead to premature closure.

3. Can be used for unintended purposes such as assuming that the results are based upon available date and are statistically significant.
4. Because assessments are subjective in nature, they are neither valid nor reliable and another panel could come to different conclusion.

ADDITIONAL METHODS FOR SETTING PRIORITIES

Size of Need Gap

Data are collected for the subject under discussion and compared to agreed upon predetermined standards. Differences between the desired goal, the standard, and the current level of attainment are calculated. Those objectives with the greatest size of need gap between the current level and the future level are ranked a higher priority that those with a lower need gap.

Officials of the Indian Reservation Public Health Clinic in South Dakota completed a strategic planning community health analysis of the clinic's Indian population, alcoholism, cirrhosis, highway fatalities, and suicides [Morrow, 1987]. These goals were based on the state's mortality rates for these four conditions. Exhibit 5–10 reveals that South Dakota has lower mortality rate for three of these four conditions than the United States. Public health strategic planners reasoned that conditions in South Dakota were more amenable to lower death rates than in the United States as a whole. Consequently, the planners preferred using the South Dakota rates as the standard to be achieved.

Exhibit 5–10 reveals the following:

1. Mortality rates for cirrhosis are 76 percent higher in the Indian Reservation population than for South Dakota.
2. Mortality rates for alcohol-caused deaths are 29 percent higher for the Reservation population than for South Dakota.
3. Mortality rates for fatal highway accidents are 20 percent higher for the Reservation than for South Dakota.
4. Mortality rates for suicide are 6 percent higher for the Reservation than for the state of South Dakota.

Exhibit 5-10.   Mortality Rates for Four Disease Conditions: Indian Reservation, South Dakota and the U.S.

Region	Mortality Rate per 100,000 Population			
	Cirrhosis	Alcoholism	Highway Accident Fatalities	Suicide
Reservation*	28.7	3.6	53.9	15.1
South Dakota	16.3	2.8	44.8	14.3
United States	20.9	3.1	30.8	17.4

* Indian reservation data are partially ficitious and illustrate the method.
Source: Wilson, R., H. Malin, and C. Lowman. 1983. Uses of mortality rates and mortality indexes in planning alcohol programs. *Alcohol Health and Research World*, 8[1], 41–53. Reprinted with permission.

On the basis of these findings, the size of need gap between the existing rates and the state standard results in the following priority rankings:

First priority: reduction of cirrhosis-induced deaths
Second priority: reduction in alcohol-caused deaths
Third priority: reduction in highway fatal accidents
Fourth priority: reduction in suicides.

Advantages of Method

1. Simplicity permits easy use by almost any planning group.
2. Use of a simple criterion as size of gap avoids the value issues that often arise when persons with different orientations try to find a consensus.

Disadvantages

1. In reality, this method is an oversimplification of complex issues.
2. This method does not indicate the degree to which the gap can be reduced or whether the reduction is dependent on achieving a related goal. Are alcohol deaths related to the lack of job opportunities for the Indian population resulting in a sense of anomie?
3. There is no indication that the goals can be achieved within the time frame set by the strategic planning process.
4. If the program objectives are of different types, there is questionable validity in comparisons.

Increasing medical personnel affects the performance of the health institution while reducing cirrhosis affects the health status of the population.

Cluster Method of Prioritizing

Starting with the size of need gap a cluster method of prioritizing adds a new dimension. Planners become concerned with the relative importance of the problems. Participants know the facts and identify the size of the need gap. Then, the issues are compared to each other to judge significance.

Using a simple three-step continuum, group members assign each problem a high, medium, or low value. High-priority issues are identified from the rankings and priority clusters can be created.

Exhibit 5–11 notes 30 major diseases from a larger list of preventable conditions that occurred in New York State. Rates for various groups were measured: whites, blacks, and hispanics; those discharged from hospitals with Medicaid benefits; and those discharged with Blue Cross benefits. Six disease entities—anemia, bladder cancer, emphysema, iron deficiency, lung cancer, TB—comprised almost 80 percent of all diseases that could have been avoided with either proper early treatment, modified lifestyles, or healthier environmental conditions. Initial priority rank is based on size-of-need gap. With the introduction of the criterion of "importance," each of the 10 members on the strategic planning committee voted on the degree of importance on a scale of 1 to 10 with 10 rated most important. Raw scores in the second column are attached to the group suffering from a specific illness.

Exhibit 5-11.   Single Health Event Disease Ocurrences by Major Diagnoses and Selected Groups: New York State Residents.

Major Disease	Size of Need* Gap Rank	Raw Score Criterion: Importance	Rank Based on Importance Criterion	
1. Cancer of lung, Black	1	98	1	
2. TB, Black	2	84	6	
3. TB, Medicaid	3	83	7	
4. Emphysema, Medicaid	4	52	22	First
5. Iron deficiency, Black	5	48	23	Priority
6. TB, Hispanic	6	82	8	Cluster
7. Iron deficiency, Medicaid	7	63	19	
8. Lung cancer, Blue Cross	8	78	14	
9. Emphysema, White	9	43	25	
10. Bladder cancer, White	10	79	13	
12. Lung cancer, White	12	94	2	
13. Anemia, White	13	42	26	
14. Anemia, Blue Cross	14	38	29	
15. Iron deficiency, White	15	28	30	Second
16. Lung cancer, Hispanic	16	81	10	Priority
17. Iron deficiency, Hispanic	17	40	27	Cluster
18. Emphysema, Black	18	63	18	
19. Lung cancer, Medicaid	19	87	4	
20. Iron deficiency, Blue Cross	20	38	28	
21. Anemia, Medicaid	21	53	21	
22. Bladder cancer, Medicaid	22	80	11	
23. Bladder cancer, Hispanic	23	82	9	
24. Anemia, Black	24	44	24	Third
25. Emphysema, Blue Cross	25	79	12	Priority
26. TB, Blue Cross	26	66	19	Cluster
27. Anemia, Hispanic	27	54	20	
28. TB, White	28	75	15	
29. Bladder cancer, Black	29	85	5	
30. Lung cancer, Hispanic	30	90	3	

* Size of need gap based on New York State as a standard on cases per 1,000 discharges.
Source: Carr, W. 1988. *Measuring avoidable deaths and diseases in New York State.* NY: United Hospital Fund, Paper Series 8, Table B-4, p. 48 [January]. Reprinted with permission.

Lung cancer for blacks is still rated the number one priority in Exhibit 5–11. However. only four of the first 10 priorities measured by the size-of-need gap still remained in the first 10 high-priority items ranked by the "importance" criterion. Three fell to the second cluster of medium priorities, and three to the third cluster of low priorities. At the other extreme, two of the lowest ranked diseases on the size-of-need gap ranking shifted into the first 10 high priorities when the "importance" criterion was used. By dividing the 30 items into three clusters of 10 each, the committee is in a better position to determine high-priority goals for the five-year, long-range strategic plan.

Committee members could also have clustered the 30 items into groups of 10 without ranking them as was done in Exhibit 5–11. Each item could have been treated as equally important and other criteria or circumstances could determine which would be implemented in what order.

A combination of differing human values and technical expertise is represented in the final high-, medium-, or low-priority clustering of issues. Final decisions are also placed on the community participants rather than on the planners. This is important because the data base may be weak and technical planners tend to use quantitative statistical analysis techniques to create rankings that take on an aura of authority. However, there is little validity to attach such importance to manufactured rankings. As much, if not more, validity accrues from arriving at a group consensus, even if the choice relies on the subjective opinions and personal experiences of the members.

Clustering results in an advantageous double-ranking process tending to narrow the highest priorities by weeding out the less desirable options. Participants have an opportunity to reconsider new dimensions that may not have been included in the initial priority rankings.

Weaknesses similar to the size-of-gap method pertain to the clustering method. However, clustering adds a second criterion to set priorities and there is some consideration of the complexities of the issues missing in the size-of-gap method. In addition, participants may vote for priorities based on their own biases. Members with the most influence or who comprise a block of common interests may easily secure a high ranking for their programs.

Preference Surveys

Essentially, each group member declares their personal preference for any of the options relying on individual attitudes and experiences. Typically, 15 to 20 persons review the alternatives and vote "one" or "zero" for each.

Exhibit 5–12 is an example of four alternative options open to a Board of Trustees considering the fate of their deficit-ridden health institution. Among the options considered by the 15-member board are affiliation with another institution, an outright merger with a stronger organization, closing the facility, or selling it outright to another organization. Each board member ranks the four choices from 1, first choice to 4, last choice. This illustration shows that the trustees prefer affiliation over any of the three options. Merger was preferred only over closure; selling out was preferred over the options of merging or closing. The sum of the scores for each of the participants is added to determine the total group score and the final ranking.

A preference survey method is relatively simple to use only requiring a list of alternative and tallying as in Exhibit 5–12. Since subjective choices are made, the technique does not use weighting or predetermined criteria. In all probability, preferences will cluster to form a consensus negating the extremes. In as each individual indicates preferences privately, the influence of other group members on voting is minimal. If the participants are representative of the popula-

Exhibit 5-12. Priority Alternative Options for a Deficit-Ridden Facility.

	Alternative Options				
	Affiliation	**Merger**	**Closure**	**Sell-Out**	**Total**
Affiliation	—	1	1	1	3
Merger	0	—	1	0	1
Closure	0	0	—	0	0
Sell-Out	0	1	1	—	2

Priority Ranking of Options: #1 = Affiliation   #3 = Merger
                                 #2 = Sell-Out   #4 = Closure

tion at large, the preferences will reflect appropriate concerns. However, there should be no more than 10 alternatives in the preference survey otherwise the matrix turns unwieldy.

Shortcomings of the preference survey reside in the fact that the consensus choices are a limited reflection of the larger differences normally existing in a community. Even though the preference survey has some validity as an expression of priorities re issues or goals, the method has poor reliability. It is doubtful that the same participants would reconvene at a second meeting to choose preferences and subsequently the priorities would change at the second meeting. Since a strategic plan typically deals with more than 10 issues, a preference survey is usually not recommended. Subcommittees or task forces can use a preference survey to deal with six or seven alternatives related to a specific subset of the total range of problems such as ambulatory care, utilization of inpatient services, or environmental control.

Timing of Implementation and Priorities

Forces hindering or promoting the implementation of each option are usually determined by the planning staff. An estimate is made of the time required to implement each alternative. Variables regarding time factors are reviewed by the entire strategic planning group examining additional elements either overlooked or given too much emphasis by the planners. As a result of this collaborative effort, adjustments can be made relative to the length of time estimated to reach the goals. Tangible and intangible considerations such as available funding, legislative cooperation, appropriate scientific and technical knowledge applicable to the problem, and social acceptability by the target populations impact upon the length of time required to initiate each alternative. With the staff input and consideration of the other influences, a consensus emerges on the priority timing of the implementation.

A health institution's strategic planning committee concludes that it would like to add five new physicians to its staff, four paraprofessionals to work with women in reducing the percent who smoke, and to reduce lung cancer in men. Each of these will take estimated time periods to implement. Although physicians are being graduated in greater numbers, the specialists the institution is seeking will require an estimated two years to recruit and hire. Paraprofessionals are in greater supply and it is estimated they could be recruited and hired in about a year. As a service to the community and to improve its public image, the institution wants to engage in an extensive health education program to stimulate women to stop smoking. A goal of a 10 percent reduction has been advanced by the strategic planning committee. Finally, studies indicate that lung cancer in men is almost 50 percent higher than the state average. Since there are an unusual number of industrial and chemical plants in the area, the committee reasoned that work place conditions are probably a major factor in the high incidence of lung cancer. However, the committee also recognized that affecting the economic interests of major producers of income and tax dollars in the community may require a fairly long time span to produce positive results in the health of the male workers in the community.

Criteria helps to set priorities. Should importance of the problem be critical? Is curing cancer more important than additional physicians, regardless of time factors? Should easily achievable objectives automatically be ranked higher than those requiring more time? If both physicians and paraprofessionals are needed, which should be recruited first? In a like manner, the etiology of cancer is still a mystery, so an undefined time factor is linked to that goal. If cigarette smoking and air pollution are deemed to be related causes of cancer, time estimates could be made regarding the implementation of air pollution emission controls and the time needed to change personal habits about cigarette smoking.

As a result of this style of reasoning, time alone can be used as the basis for setting priorities as indicated below:

Alternative	*Time for Implementation*	*Rank*
More physicians	2 years	2nd
More paraprofessionals	1 year	1st
Cigarette smoking reduction	2–5 years	3rd
Air pollution control	4–10 years	4th

Using time required for implementation as the sole criterion, the obvious conclusion is that training paraprofessionals is the top priority followed by reducing the deficit of physicians. However, most planning groups would likely consider other variables in addition to the time required for implementation. If lung cancer mortality and morbidity due to air pollution is unusually high in the area, it would not be unreasonable to weigh that factor and assign air pollution control a higher ranking while decreasing the priority of paraprofessionals. If cost of expensive factory emission controls became a barrier, that option may be priced out of consideration and cause a shift in alternatives. However, as the least expensive and quickest achievable goal, more paraprofessionals still retains first place.

Time needed for implementation is infrequently used as the only criteria to choose priorities. Often the method is used as an initial indicator, but other critical considerations usually adjust the priority deliberations. Individuals may be yearning to achieve visibility and credibility with rapid results. Legislators may desire to establish a track record for re-election after a two- or four-year term in office. However, timing alone is a very limited priority choice.

Social Area Analysis Method

Federal government mental health officials [Goldsmith, Unger, & Rosen, 1977; Rosen, 1977] developed a social area analysis method using U.S. Census data for needs assessment and to set priorities. Census characteristics are correlated with mental disorders in addition to pathology rates that relate directly or indirectly to treatment modalities. Particular census groups, service utilization rates, and pathology factors are placed into clusters. Each cluster is assigned a weight and a rank. Totaling the ranks of the clusters results in a priority of need. Resources available in the area to serve individuals with mental disorders are also ranked. A cross-correlation between overall needs and available resources yields the final priorities.

Over the years, variations of social area analysis emerged. Efforts sought to identify the irreducible minimum number of census, utilization, and pathology characteristics on which to base decisions regarding which areas should receive what share of the scarce mental health dollar.

One social area analysis paradigm pinpoints four clusters deemed to be related to mental disorders: socioeconomic indicators, social pathology, welfare indices, and mental and physical illness indices. Each cluster has a subset of indicators as follows:

Socioeconomic Indicators

Median annual income per family
Number families having annual income less than $$,$$$
Unemployment in civilian labor force

Median value one-unit housing
Percentage total housing units considered deteriorating or dilapidated
Median education completed by people over 25
Percentage of people over 25 with less than five years education

Social Pathology

Total number of arrests by local and state police
Number of commitments to youth service facilities
Number of arrests for drunkenness
Number of arrests for violation of narcotics laws

Welfare Indices

Old age assistance recipients
Medical aid to the aged
Disability assistance
Aid to dependent children
General relief

Mental and Physical Illness Indices

Number of admissions to mental hospitals
Number of mentally retarded children in special classes
Number of physically handicapped children in special classes.

Statistical data related to each cluster are classified by each indicator in the grouping. "Median annual income per family" for each geographic area is comparatively ranked among all the areas. Likewise, each indicator in each of the four clusters is ranked. Ranks for each indicator are summed to produce the total ranking for each of the four clusters.

As the four clusters may not have equal programmatic significance, weights are usually assigned as follows:

Category	Weight
Socioeconomic Indicators	2
Mental and Physical Illness Indices	4
Social Pathology	4
Welfare Indices	3

Actual social pathology and mental and physical illness is awarded a higher weight than the specific socioeconomic factors that may contribute to pathology such as low income, poor housing, or unemployment. Weights are applied to the geographic area rankings for each respective cluster. New rankings are summed and averaged to produce the final ranking of need for the areas. Exhibit 5–13 is a hypothetical illustration of how indicators produce a priority list of need. From the 15 geographic areas in Exhibit 5–13, area C has the greatest need for mental health services based on the combined four indicator clusters, while area D has the least need for mental health programs.

Then the 15 areas are divided into thirds with the five localities with the highest needs grouped together; the next five are part of the medium class priorities, and the final five have the lowest priorities. Next, an analysis inventories the resources currently available to provide services to each of the 15 geographic areas. Resources are also divided into three levels: limited

Exhibit 5-13.   Priority Rank on Each Need Category and Total Need for 15 Mental Health Areas.

Area	Socioeconomic [Weight 2]	Illness [Wt. 4]	Social Pathology [Wt. 4]	Welfare [Wt. 3]	Total Need Rank
A	3	3	4	2	2
B	7	11	6	9	4
C	4	1	1	1	1
D	12	12	14	13	15
—	—	—	—	—	—
—	—	—	—	—	—
—	—	—	—	—	—
0	11	9	12	8	12

resources, average resources, and major resources. A cross-correlation of available resources with the overall need identifies those areas requiring the most urgent attention [Exhibit 5–14]. Area L, which ranked fifth in terms of overall "need," became part of the highest priority grouping because of severely limited available resources. On the other hand, area C fell to a lower rank because the area has major resources to serve the overall needs of its high priority population. This cross-correlation clearly demonstrates how priorities change as differing criteria are considered.

In another priority determination model, Exhibit 5–15 identifies seven indicators related to alcohol deaths [Wilson, Malin, & Lowman, 1983]: cirrhosis rate, alcohol psychosis rate, alcoholism rate, alcohol poisoning rate, fatal highway accident rate, suicide rate, and homicide rate. Indicators are given for each of the 32 counties in New Mexico. Based on the rates, indicators are ranked from 1 [highest need] to 32 [lowest need]. In turn, the ranks are summed. McKinley County has the highest alcohol mortality rate and is ranked first while Los Alomas has the lowest and is ranked 32nd. Because the precise number of deaths for the various indicators is not known, a low and high range [columns I and J] is provided. McKinley County ranges from a low of 199.7 to a high of 280.4 on death rates associated with alcohol. A comparative rank for the United States is also shown. Unlike the mental health model, this priority determination does not correlate the resources currently available to deal with the problem. However, that could be readily added by strategic planning officials.

Social area analysis has several strengths. Utilization of clusters and specific indicators

Exhibit 5-14.   Program Development Priorities by Need and Resources for 15 Mental Health Areas.

		Limited [5]	Resources Average [6]	Major [4]
O V E R A L L	High [5]	L A	J B	C
	Medium [5]	M	F H	I N
N E E D	Low [5]	E G	K D	O

Exhibit 5-15. Seven Indicators of Alcohol-Related Mortality.

County	Population 15–74, 1975 (A)	Cirrhosis Rate (B)	Alcohol Psychosis Rate (C)	Alcoholism Rate (D)	Alcohol Poisoning Rate (E)	Fatal Highway Accident Rate (F)	Suicide Rate (G)	Homicide Rate (H)	Range of Death Rates Associated with Alcohol (I) (J)	Rank in State (K)	Rank in U.S.
Bernalillo	255,959	19.4	0.3	14.8	0.4	49.6	26.4	15.9	52.7– 79.6	24	326
Catron	1,686	19.8	0.0	0.0	0.0	276.8	19.8	0.0	96.1– 164.5	5	27
Chaves	33,611	31.7	0.0	4.0	0.0	53.6	20.8	21.8	48.9– 83.9	23	320
Colfax	8,908	52.4	0.0	7.5	0.0	56.1	26.2	18.7	61.5– 108.1	20	131
Curry	28,808	26.6	0.0	5.8	0.0	28.9	13.9	17.4	37.4– 62.8	26	861
DeBaca	1,801	18.5	18.5	0.0	0.0	203.6	18.5	18.5	100.9– 157.7	6	28
Dona Ana	54,747	12.2	0.0	8.5	0.0	34.1	9.7	6.7	29.5– 45.4	30	1,729
Eddy	30,476	24.1	1.1	5.5	0.0	29.5	17.5	13.1	36.1– 59.8	27	968
Grant	16,543	26.2	0.0	12.1	0.0	46.3	22.2	18.1	51.2– 81.0	25	328
Guadalupe	3,233	51.6	0.0	10.3	10.3	165.0	61.9	51.6	132.0– 211.1	2	13
Harding	891	0.0	0.0	0.0	0.0	37.4	37.4	0.0	20.6– 32.5	31	2,602
Hidalgo	3,738	8.9	0.0	8.9	0.0	205.1	35.7	0.0	83.0– 133.1	12	58
Lea	35,980	18.5	0.0	3.7	0.0	37.1	18.5	17.6	35.7– 59.0	28	1,001
Lincoln	7,068	28.3	0.0	14.1	0.0	198.1	14.1	4.7	91.0– 148.6	9	35
Los Alamos	11,403	0.0	0.0	0.0	0.0	17.5	17.5	0.0	9.6– 15.3	32	3,031
Luna	9,673	37.9	0.0	17.2	0.0	113.7	17.2	3.4	72.9– 118.9	16	86
McKinley	31,662	51.6	1.1	58.4	1.1	204.2	41.1	33.7	199.7– 280.4	1	2
Mora	3,247	61.6	0.0	20.5	0.0	112.9	41.1	10.3	95.0– 157.9	7	32
Otero	28,427	24.6	1.2	19.9	0.0	65.7	29.3	12.9	64.6– 97.2	21	154
Quay	7,834	8.5	0.0	25.5	0.0	140.4	42.6	38.3	100.5– 146.4	8	34
Rio Arriba	17,906	63.3	0.0	29.8	3.7	130.3	41.0	31.6	124.3– 196.1	3	18
Roosevelt	11,884	14.0	0.0	8.4	0.0	25.2	25.2	5.6	30.8– 47.6	29	1,579
Sandoval	14,790	42.8	0.0	36.1	0.0	121.7	54.1	18.0	112.5– 170.2	4	22
San Juan	42,039	22.2	0.8	17.4	0.0	147.5	21.4	30.1	91.7– 142.1	10	38
San Miguel	16,208	41.1	0.0	22.6	4.1	76.1	22.6	28.8	86.2– 132.4	11	53
Santa Fe	43,231	33.9	0.0	17.7	0.0	76.3	33.2	10.0	67.7– 107.4	18	115
Sierra	5,800	34.5	0.0	0.0	0.0	97.7	23.0	5.7	52.0– 94.1	22	231
Socorro	6,547	14.6	4.9	19.5	0.0	112.0	53.6	14.6	84.5– 124.2	14	66
Taos	12,768	41.8	0.0	13.1	0.0	99.2	23.5	20.9	76.0– 125.7	15	75
Torrance	4,756	35.0	0.0	21.0	0.0	91.1	28.0	0.0	69.7– 110.2	17	109
Union	3,262	30.7	0.0	20.4	0.0	81.7	20.4	10.2	67.6– 105.1	19	122
Valencia	30,155	23.2	0.0	18.8	1.1	128.2	31.0	13.3	82.1– 126.8	13	65

Source: From "Uses of mortality rates and mortality indexes in planning alcohol programs," by R. Wilson, H. Malin, & C. Lowman, 1983, *Alcohol Health and Research World*, 8(1), 41–53. Reprinted by permission.

provide immediate scientific credibility and authority for decision makers merely perusing the methodology before making a choice. Outcomes are believable, have the ring of authenticity, and appear valid. Furthermore, social area analysis uses readily available data that are usually highly reliable. Another plus is that social area analysis relies on technical, quantitative methods that are easily understood and accepted rather than on the problematic subjective attitudes and values of planning participants. Finally, the cross-correlation technique of the mental health model of social area analysis priority determination creates rankings that reflect interactions between needs and resources as opposed to a single criterion.

Importantly, strategic planners must be aware that there is no consensus on what cluster or subset specific indicators correlates better than any other cluster or subset indicators with any particular disease or condition. Critics may contend that poverty or unemployment rates alone correlate just as well with mental illness as all the other indicators combined. Wagstaff [1987] questioned the validity of social indicators, whether individually or in clusters, as a basis for program choices. In addition, the statistics may not be reliable. But trained personnel using computers to enter the raw numbers accurately and precisely does much to increase confidence in the level of reliability. At this time, validity is more of a concern than reliability.

As impressive as the social area analysis technique appears, basic implementation considerations such as cost, personnel, space, available ancillary services, and community awareness of local responsibilities to provide assistance are not part of the decision-making process.

Another negative in social area analysis centers around the fact that the specific indicators and each cluster are usually generated by technical experts on the strategic planning staff in conjunction with key administrators and governing board members. Participants may be high-status elites who do not normally use the services under discussion. For the most part, real consumers of the service are excluded from the process of selecting clusters and specific indicators to use to determine priorities. Studies in strategic health planning [Fontana, 1986; Madan, 1987] reveal that consumers and providers seem to differ in emphasis in determining priorities. In social area analysis, the providers' voice is usually added in the final priority determination.

Potentially Productive Years of Life Lost [PPYLL]

Traditionally, mortality rates for specific diseases are used to determine priorities in terms of resources. Diseases of the heart, malignant neoplasms, and cerebrovascular diseases account for the majority of deaths in the United States. Consequently, resources and research funds are a priority expenditure to identify causes and means of treating these life-threatening diseases. However, since the legislative actions in health planning in the mid–1970s, emphasis shifted to viewing death from a positive point of view, that is, the potentially productive years of a person's life lost [PPYLL] due to death. Examination of mortality rates from this perspective results in a different configuration of the leading causes of death.

Productive years are defined as the ages 15 to 70 and readily measured by the equation:

$$\text{Years of Life Lost} = p_i \times d_i$$

where d_i equals the number of deaths in the ith age category. p_i equals the difference between endpoint and the midpoint of the ith age category [Perloff, LeBailly, & Kletke, 1984; Dever, 1980, pp. 85–87].

Regular reports on years of life lost appear in the Centers for Disease Control's [CDC] publication, *Morbidity and Mortality Weekly Report*. Exhibit 5–16 reveals how the priorities

Exhibit 5-16.   Ten Leading Causes of Death and Rank by Potentially Productive Years of Life Lost [PPYLL].

	Rank	
Cause of Death	Deaths	PPYLL
Diseases of heart	1	3
Malignant neoplasms	2	2
Cerebrovascular diseases	3	8
Accidents	4	1
Chronic obstructive pulmonary disease and allied conditions	5	—*
Pneumonia and influenza	6	10
Diabetes mellitus	7	—*
Chronic liver disease and cirrhosis	8	9
Atherosclerosis	9	—*
Suicide	10	6
Certain conditions in perinatal period	—*	4
Homicide and legal intervention	—*	5
Congenital abnormalities	—*	7

* Not ranked among top ten causes for this measure
Sources: USDHHS, National Center for Health Statistics: Advance Report Final Mortality Statistics, 1979. *Monthly Vital Statistics Report,* 31 (6) Supplement, 1982. National Center for Health Statistics: Table 210A: Deaths from 27 Selected Causes, 5-Year Age Groups, Race and Sex, U.S., 1979, unpublished data, 1982.

based on death rates change when PPYLL is used as a measure of death. Among the 10 highest-ranked causes of death are heart diseases, cancers, and strokes, with accidents ranked fourth. Perinatal conditions, homicide, and congenital abnormalities are not ranked among the top causes of death. When the leading causes of PPYLL are calculated, major changes occur. Accidents become the leading cause of potentially productive years lost, while pulmonary diseases, diabetes, and atherosclerosis drop out of the top ten. PPYLL analysis causes cerebrovascular diseases to fall to the eighth rank, and pneumonias and influenza to fall to tenth place. Moving high up on the PPYLL priority scale are perinatal conditions [fourth], homicides [fifth], and congenital abnormalities[seventh]. Accidents account for 20.1 percent of PPYLL, followed by cancers [17 percent], heart diseases [16.9 percent], perinatal conditions [8.3 percent], homicides [5.1 percent], and suicides [4.7 percent]. Obviously, these differences relate to the age at which the disease-related death occurs. Cerebrovascular disease has a lower death rate among younger age groups, while accidents is a major killer among those aged 15 to 44.

A study of PPYLL can lead to insights about resources allocation. Motor vehicle accidents claim 61 percent of PPYLL with drownings [8 percent] and poisonings [6 percent] the next highest accident causes of PPYLL. Further, males are involved in far more accidents than females. For white males, motor vehicle accidents and firearm deaths are leading causes of accidental PPYLL. For nonwhite males, homicides and firearms are the leading causes.

Given these statistical findings, Perloff et al. [1984] advise strategic planners to emphasize environmental, socio-economic, and behavioral program objectives to reduce PPYLL:

First, the analysis shows the preventable nature of much premature death and the importance of improving both medical and nonmedical preventive interventions. Second, the analysis draws attention to the importance of lifestyle or environment rather than disease alone as a key factor in premature death. Finally, the analysis enables us to highlight vulnerable populations, target scarce resources more efficiently, and monitor trends in prolonging life.

As a technique, PPYLL has much going for its utilization as a priority ranking measure. Statistical simplicity and the general availability of data, especially from federal information sources, permit ready manipulation of the data to arrive at priority rankings. Further, there is an emphasis on prevention rather than on disease control. Sleet [1987] argues for priorities to promote the use of automobile safety belts, child restraints, and automatic protection to prevent PPYLL due to motor vehicle trauma. Given the increasing number of skilled employees needed in our expanding economy, our nation cannot afford to lose scarce and valuable professional and skilled employees in their most productive years of life. Disadvantages of this method are similar to the drawbacks of the social area analysis technique.

Computer Graphic Mapping Method to Identify Priorities

Computer mapping is increasingly used by strategic health planners to identify trends, to evaluate outcomes, to plan, and to make decisions. Dever [1980, chap. 9] cites the following advantages:

- Fast, efficient, simple, and economical.
- Provides information in a clear, eye-catching manner.
- Data trends can be shown in a series of maps.
- Trial computer maps can be developed before a final printed version, cutting costs and reducing errors.

Business health coalitions are concerned with how their activities impact on health policies at the state level. A computer-generated graphic map, Exhibit 5–17, shows three levels of business participation in state health policy [Bergthold, 1987]. Clearly, the greatest participation takes place in states with the largest population and industrial activity such as New York, California, and Michigan. A tier of six northern mountain states—Idaho, Montana, Nebraska, North and South Dakota, and Wyoming, had low participation. This graphic presentation highlights the degree of penetration and influence of business health coalition in determining health policy at the state and local levels.

High participation states access vital information about the health care system, engage in a partnership with state health officials to identify and collaborate in containing costs, and place pressure on traditional services by championing alternatives such as HMOs. Given this capacity to influence health policy in high activity states, business health coalition leaders should stimulate low participation states into greater activity.

Exhibits 5–18 and 5–19 show computer-mapped geographic areas with high-priority concerns related to alcohol-related chronic health problems and casualties in New Mexico [Wilson, Malin, & Lowman, 1983]. In this case, the two maps show that a high level of alcohol-related problems do not necessarily result in a high casualty index. Only one county in the northern tier of counties overlapped a high level of alcohol-related problems with casualties. Visual evidence strongly implies that the particular county requires high priority attention from state and county alcohol service agencies and strategic health planners to reduce the high rates to

Exhibit 5-17. Business Participation in Health Care Politics by State

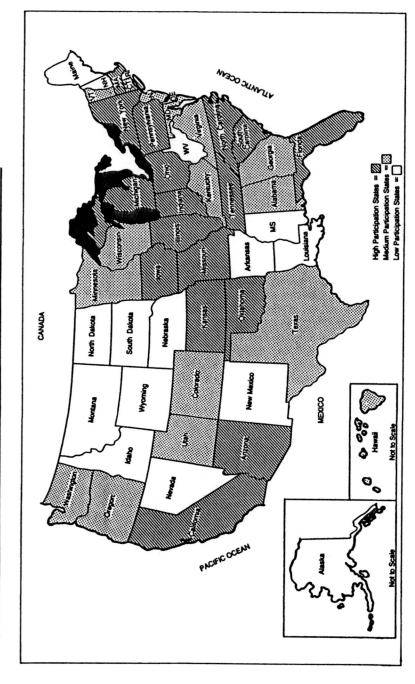

Source: From "Business and the pushcart vendors in an age of supermarkets," by L. Bergthold, 1987, *International Journal of Health Services, 17*(1), 18. Copyright 1987. Reprinted with permission of Baywood Publishing Co. Inc.

Exhibit 5-18.   Alcohol-Related Chronic Health Problems Index, New Mexico.

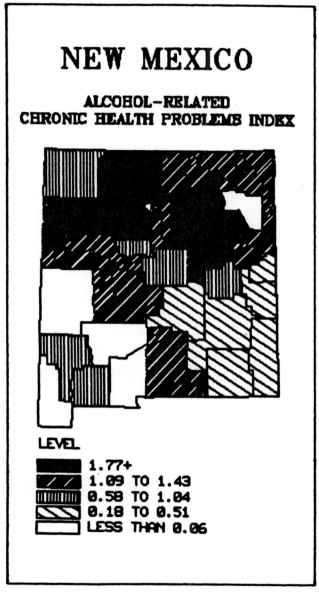

Source: From "Uses of mortality rates and mortality indexes in planning alcohol programs," by R. Wilson, H. Malin, & C. Lowman, 1983, *Alcohol Health and Research World, 8*(1), 41–53. Reprinted by permission.

acceptable average state levels. However, this conclusion may be tempered by determining whether these geographic areas are also areas of high or low population. A high mortality rate does not signify a large number of deaths in sparsely populated areas. A high casualty index

Exhibit 5-19. Alcohol-Related Casualties Index, New Mexico.

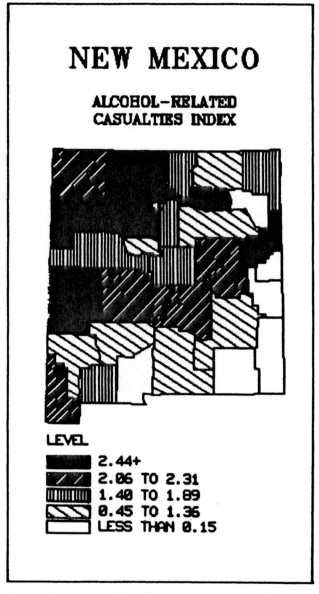

Source: From "Uses of mortality rates and mortality indexes in planning alcohol programs," by R. Wilson, H. Malin, & C. Lowman, 1983, *Alcohol Health and Research World, 8*(1), 41–53. Reprinted by permission.

could indicate a deficit of alcohol resources or other program emphases such as health education, legislative changes, or regulations.

Exhibit 5–20 maps mortality rates from cancer of the trachea, bronchus, and lung in

Exhibit 5-20.   Cancer of the Trachea, Bronchus, and Lung, Georgia.

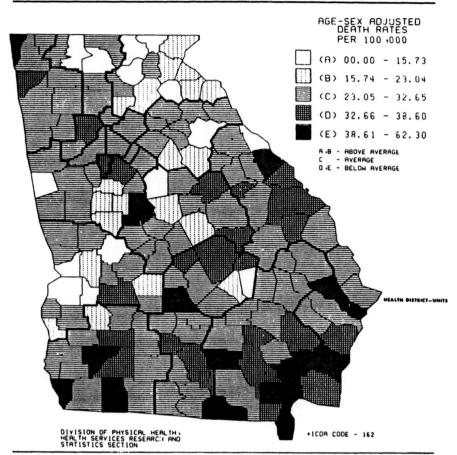

AGE-SEX ADJUSTED
DEATH RATES
PER 100,000

(A) 00.00 - 15.73

(B) 15.74 - 23.04

(C) 23.05 - 32.65

(D) 32.66 - 38.60

(E) 38.61 - 62.30

A,B - ABOVE AVERAGE
C   - AVERAGE
D,E - BELOW AVERAGE

HEALTH DISTRICT-UNITS

DIVISION OF PHYSICAL HEALTH,
HEALTH SERVICES RESEARCH AND
STATISTICS SECTION

•ICDA CODE - 162

Source: From *Disease patterns of the 70s*, by Office of Health Services Research and Statistics, 1976, Atlanta, GA: Department of Human Resources, Div. of Physical Health.

Georgia identifying five mortality groupings. Almost all of the highest rate areas are located in the lower third of the state whereas the lowest rate areas are found in the upper third. While the computer maps pinpoints high mortality rates for cancer, planners still need data such as the resources that are available, the probable causes of high rates in these areas, the demographics of those affected and transportation accessibility to existing services. This type of computer graphic map provides a visual first cut in the analysis required to set program priorities.

While computer graphic mapping has obvious advantages, there are disadvantages.

- Can be time-consuming to code and enter the data.
- Must have expertise to determine the scale and type of map and the level of measurement to use.
- User of graphic mapping often has little knowledge or awareness of the usefulness or quality of the maps produced.

PRIORITIES NOW COMPARED TO THEN

No doubt, there are additional methods and techniques to use to choose priorities and other techniques described in other chapters could be used. Nevertheless, the examples cited here are relevant and easy to apply. In tandem with other aspects of the strategic health planning process, priority setting is still developing. In any event, priority determination almost always includes a blending of technical expertise and subjective values and feelings. Illustrative methods embraced both elements. As in many other situations, there is no one perfect priority-setting method. These examples reflect the spectrum that exists for appropriate use by participants such as administrators, planning staffs, boards, trustees, and consumers.

In regard to priorities in the new medical-industrial-economic complex of DRGs, HMOs, and PPOs, Zoghlin [1987] argues that the "pendulum has swung too far, too fast." He calls for a stop to short-sighted health planning and a gradual revamping of medical-industrial-economic priorities. In concluding, Zoghlin says that, "as things are now, we're punishing institutions that reacted in good faith to other priorities in other times." In prior times, the priority objective tended to provide whatever the patient needed and damn the cost. Now, perhaps cost containment prevails as the top priority.

REFERENCES

Banta, H.D. (1986). Dutch committee assess the future of health technology. *Dimensions in Health Service, 63*(7), 17–20.

Bergthold, L.A. (1987). Business and the pushcart vendors in an age of supermarkets. *International Journal of Health Services, 17*(1), 7–25.

Blum, H.L. (1974). *Planning for health development and application of social change theory*. New York: Human Sciences Press.

Brandt, E.N., Jr. (1988). Hard choices in public health. *Public Health Reports, 103*(4), 339–341.

Breslow, L. (1987). Setting objectives for public health. *Annual Reviews for Public Health, 8,* 289–307.

Carlyn, M., & Hicks, R.S. (1986). On the designation of transplant centers in Michigan. *Michigan Medicine, 85*(6), 291–292.

Cherskov, M. (1987). Health policy agenda seeks approval. *Hospitals, 61*(8), 125.

Cooper, T. (1987). How high a priority will society accord to health care? *Vital Speeches of the Day, 53*(8), 242–245.

Delbecq, A.L., & Gill, S.L. (1988). Developing strategic directions for governing boards. *Hospital and Health Services Administration, 33*(1), 25–35.

Delbecq, A.L., Van de Ven, A.H., & Gustafson, D.H. (1975). *Group techniques for program planning: A guide to nominal group and delphi processes*. Glenview, IL: Scott Foresman.

Dever, G.E. (1980). *Community health analysis*. Rockville, MD: Aspen Systems Corporation.

Drake, J., McCann, P., Adams, S., & Isaacs, J. (1977). *Methods for priority setting in area-wide health planning*. Washington, DC: Arthur Young and Co.

Federal Register. (1989). Announcement of year 2000 health promotion and disease prevention objectives. [FR doc 89–21974]. *54,* 38453.

Fogel, R.L. (1987). *Insufficient planning for field laboratory consolidation decisions* (GAO/HRD 88–21). Washington, DC: Government Printing Office.

Fontana, L. (1986). Political ideology and local health planning in the United States. *Human Relations, 39*(6), 541–556.

Fuchs, M., & Deber, R.B. (1987). Technology acquisition in a selected sample of Ontario hospitals. *Dimensions in Health Service, 64*(6), 17–20.

Garfunkel, J.M. (1989). Priorities for the use of finite resources: Now may be the time to choose. *Journal of Pediatrics, 115*(3), 410–411.

Goldsmith, H.F., Unger, E.L., & Rosen, B.M. (1977). *A typological approach to doing social area analysis.* (DHEW Pub. No. (ADM) 77–262). Washington, DC: Government Printing Office.

Hagman, E., & Rehnstrom, T. (1985). Priorities in primary health care. *Scandinavian Journal of Primary Health Care, 3*(4), 197–200.

Hancock, T. (1986). Public health planning in the city of Toronto—Part I: Conceptual planning. *Canadian Journal of Public Health, 77*(3), 180–184.

Hanlon, J.J., & Pickett, G.E. (1984). *Public health: Administration and practice.* St. Louis, MO: Times Mirror/Mosby College Publishing.

Henderson, J. (1985). Appraising options: A practical guide. *Hospital & Health Services Review, 81*(5), 286–290.

Henry, K. (1988). Setting AIDS priorities: The need for a closer alliance of public health and clinical approaches toward the control of AIDS. *American Journal of Public Health, 78*(9), 1210–1212.

Holloman, J.L.S., Jr. (1986). It's time to reorder our priorities. *The Internist, 27*(2), 14–15.

Hospitals. (1986). Meet health care's leaders for the 21st century. *60*(5), 78.

Hsueh, W.A. (1989). Making biomedical research a national priority. *Clinical Research, 37*(3), 481–486.

International Nursing Review. (1989). Priority research for health for all. *36*(1), 30–31.

Ireys, H.T., & Eichler, R.J. (1988). Program priorities of crippled children's agencies: A survey. *Public Health Reports, 103*(1), 77–83.

Jackson, B., & Jensen, J. (1984). Home care tops consumer's lists. *Modern Healthcare, 14*(6), 88, 90.

Kosterlitz, J. (1985). The priorities have shifted. *National Journal, 17*(20), 1128–1131.

Linn, L.S., & Gelberg, L. (1989). Priority of basic need among homeless adults. *Social Psychiatry and Psychiatric Epidemiology, 24*(1), 123–129.

Madan, T.N. (1987). Community involvement in health policy: Socio-structural and dynamic aspects of health beliefs. *Social Science and Medicine, 25*(6), 615–620.

Mahaffey, M. (1986). Planning for mental health: The immediate agenda. *American Journal of Orthopsychiatry, 56*(1), 4–13.

Mason, G.O., Katz, M., & Lord, K.S. (1985). Visions of the year 2000. *American Journal of Preventive Medicine, 1*(1), 4–10.

Millar, J.D., & Myers, M.L. (1983). Occupational safety and health: Progress toward the 1990 objectives for the nation. *Public Health Reports, 98*(4), 327–328.

Moore, W.B. (1984). Survey shows CEOs' priorities are changing. *Hospitals, 58*(24), 71–77.

Morrow, R.C. (1987). Using staff input to set priorities in an Indian health service clinic. *Public Health Reports, 102*(4), 369–372.

Nelson, S.H. (1989). Values and priorities: Their effect on knowledge utilization in public mental health programs. *Journal of Mental Health Administration, 16*(1), 44–49.

Office of Technology Assessment. (1984). *Update of federal activities regarding the use of pneumococcal vaccine.* Washington, DC: Government Printing Office.

Office of Technology Assessment. (1981). *Cost-effectiveness of influenza vaccination.* Washington, DC: Government Printing Office.

Pan American Health Organization. (1988). *Health for all by the year 2000. Annual report of the Director.* Washington, DC.

Patel, M. (1986). An economic evaluation of health for all. *Health Policy and Planning, 1*(1), 37–47.

Perloff, J.D., LeBailly, S.A., & Kletke, P.R. (1984). Premature death in the United States: Years of life lost and health priorities. *Journal of Public Health Policy, 5*(2), 167–184.

Rada, R.T. (1986). The health care revolution: From patient to client to customer. *Psychosomatics, 27*(4), 276–279.

Rall, D.P. (1988). Toxic agent and radiation control: Progress toward objectives for the nation for the year 1990. *Public Health Reports, 103*(4), 342–347.

Ries, D.A. (1989). Suffer the little children. *Hospital Progress, 70*(7), 36–43.

Rosen, B.M. (1977). *A model for estimating mental health needs using 1970 census socioeconomic data.* (DHEW Pub No. (ADM) 77–63). Washington, DC: Government Printing Office.

Sleet, D.A. (1987). Motor vehicle trauma and safety belt use in the context of public health priorities. *Journal of Trauma, 27*(7), 695–702.

Stroot, P. (1989). A priority for the World Health Organization: Promoting healthy ways of life. *American Journal of Clinical Nutrition, 49,* 1063–1064.

Sullivan, L.W. (1989). The health care priorities of the Bush administration. *New England Journal of Medicine, 321*(2), 125–128.

Talbott, J.A. (1985). National priorities: Halfway there. *Hospital & Community Psychiatry, 36*(1), 5.

USDHHS, CDC, *Morbidity and Mortality Weekly Report.* (1989). Year 2000 national health objectives. *38*(37), 629–633.

U.S. Department of Health, Education, and Welfare (USDHEW). (1979). *The Surgeon General's report on health promotion and disease prevention for healthy people.* (Pub. No. 79–55071). Washington, DC: U.S. Government Printing Office.

Van de Ven, A.H., & Delbecq, A.L. (1972). The nominal group as a research instrument for exploratory health studies. *American Journal of Public Health, 62*(3), 337–342.

Wagstaff, A. (1987). Government prevention policy and the relevance of social cost estimates. *British Journal of Addiction, 82*(5), 461–467.

Weiner, J.L., Boyer, E.G., & Farber, N.J. (1986). A changing health care decision-making environment. *Human Relations, 39*(7), 647–659.

Whittle, J.W., Grant, A.A., Sarll, D.W., & Worthington, H.V. (1987). The Delphi Technique: Its use in dental health services research. *Community Dental Health, 4*(3), 205–214.

Williams, A. (1988). Priority setting in public and private health care. *Journal of Health Economics, 7*(2), 173–183.

Wilson, R., Malin, H., & Lowman, C. (1983). Uses of mortality rates and mortality indexes in planning alcohol programs. *Alcohol Health and Research World, 8*(1), 41–53.

Windom, R.E. (1989). New Year and still on course—developing goals for the year 2000. *Public Health Reports, 104*(1), 1.

World Health. (1986). Twelve yardsticks for health. 2(10), 8–9.

World Health Organization. (1981, September 3). *Global strategy for health for all by the year 2000. Health for all.* Geneva: WHO.

Yang, J.M., Yu, S.M., & Cho, W.H. (1987). Research fields and priority setting for health sciences in Korea. *Yonsei Medical Journal, 28*(1), 60–70.

Zoghlin, G.G. (1987). Stop shortsighted health planning. *Modern Healthcare, 17*(1), 81.

Zylke, J.W. (1989). Maternal, child health needs noted by two major national study groups. *Journal of the American Medical Association, 261*(12), 1687–1688.

6

Implementation

Planners may have been thinking about when action is going to replace the painstaking details of identifying the problem, unearthing the data, finding the resources, generating ideas, considering alternatives, and determining priorities. In a logical planning process, implementation time is now. However, in some instances, planners may jump into implementation quite early. If the policy has already been decided and the activity approved by the chief executive, it is conceivable that the task could be undertaken rapidly without going through the arduous procedures detailed in preceding chapters. Nevertheless, it should be pointed out that all the energy and time expended on problem identification, data collection, inventorying resources, seeking alternatives, and selecting priorities generally makes the ensuing implementation and the evaluation much more precise and targeted.

Simply stated, implementation means that planners are now about to use materials, methods, and resources to do what they have been saying they were going to do about a particular problem. In a bottom-line sense, implementation means detailing who is going to do what, when, where, why, and how. However, there has to be an explicit examination of how to change behavior with the least amount of resistance. Additionally, with the overlay of cost containment priorities, the issue of the changing marketplace of health care requires special attention.

A HUMBLING OBSERVATION

Of course, implementation requires that people do what they are supposed to do to make the program succeed. In a study of the politics of leadership and presidential power, Neustadt [1980, p. 9] reported an anecdote that surely tends to make all planners realize the pitfalls of implementing a program:

> In the early summer of 1952, before the heat of the campaign, President Truman used to contemplate the problems of the General-become-President should Eisenhower win the forthcoming election. "He'll sit there," Truman would remark [tapping his desk for emphasis], "and he'll say, 'Do this! Do that!'" *And nothing will happen.* Poor Ike—it won't be a bit like the Army. He'll find it very frustrating."

In his current perspectives on implementation, Gummer [1987] paraphrased the quote commenting that "there's many a slip 'twixt cup and lip.'"

In a discussion of marketing implementation, Bonoma and Crittenden [1988] take the bottom line approach: "It is not enough to have a science of making plans; it is also necessary to understand how they are translated into actions and into marketplace results."

IMPLEMENTATION STRATEGIES

Based on a survey of 91 service organizations such as hospitals, government agencies, social service providers and professional societies, Nutt [1986] identified the following four types of management strategies to implement programs or to initiate policy changes:

- *Implementation by intervention* has the manager/planner creating rationales for the action in the minds of key people. Task forces may be used for evaluating procedures, commenting on plans, suggesting changes, and making recommendations. Managers/planners act as change agents more or less in charge of what happens or doesn't happen.
- *Implementation by participation* starts with the manger/planner stimulating the activity and seeking decisions from the participants. Nutt classified participants by their roles in the process:

Participation	Solution Role	Involvement
• Token	solution-framing	partial
• Delegated	solution-specifying	partial
• Complete	solution-framing	full
• Comprehensive	solution-specifying	full

Task Forces are given the authority to arrive at a consensus and to make recommendations with minute probability of being vetoed by the manager/planner.
- *Implementation by persuasion* may find managers/planners relying on experts or their own expertise to initiate needed activities. Essentially, this is a selling job, or educational process, using documented benefits accruing to the organization as the foundation for making the changes.
- *Implementation by edict* relies upon personal power and control and bypasses any form of participation. Compliance with directives is expected and rationales for the changes are not needed.

In his study, Nutt also noted the success rate of each implementation strategy as well as the percentage of organizations using each type as follows:

Strategy	Success Rate	Companies Using
Intervention	100%	19%
Participation	84%	17%
Persuasion	73%	42%
Edict	43%	23%

Clearly, higher success rates are directly linked to participation in the implementation planning process. That fact has been stated many times. As an example, Erez, Earley, and

Hinton [1985] conclude that "if one participates in establishing a goal, then the perceived control over the goal may be considerably higher than when goals are externally assigned . . . behavior may be enhanced in the former compared to the latter condition." While not exactly contradicting that conclusion, Callahan and Wall [1987] stated that "absolute participation is neither realistic nor desirable for all decisions."

These four implementation strategies can be used separately or in combination. Calling them decision procedures, Yuki [1981, p. 203] describes them as autocratic, consultation, joint and delegation decisions. There is an obvious resemblance to Nutt's classifications.

Often implementation involves developing a new service or modifying an existing one. In addition to selecting an implementation strategy, there are other factors to consider. A director of strategic planning [Emery, 1986] found five critical implementation areas for management analysis in those situations:

1. *Service Description and Need* looks at compatibility with existing services, rationales, benefits, need determination, and alternatives.
2. *Market Information* examined the demographics of the community to be served, patient awareness of service, access, location, hours or operation, competitors, competitive price structure, and who will provide service.
3. *Operational Information* relates to the nuts and bolts of the activity identifying management responsibility, job descriptions, contracts required, insurance, coordination, regulations, support resources, and legal ramifications.
4. *Success Indicators* describe the strengths and weaknesses of the service, promotion of the service, acceptance of providers and the community, and scheduling.
5. *Financial Plan and Information Verification* calls for a complete multiyear financial plan, a multiyear projected return on investment, and assurance that all information is reviewed and verified.

RISK FACTORS AND IMPLEMENTATION

An important variable in implementing a program is the risk factor concept. Basically, the risk factors are determined by a risk assessment that "quantifies the relationship between environmental or personal characteristics and the probability of the occurrence of some outcome" [Kannel & McGee, 1987]. Based on the Framingham, Massachusetts classic epidemiological study that began in 1948, the intertwined connection between heart disease and risk factors such as hypertension, cholesterol level, diabetes, and cigarette smoking has been well established [Kannel & McGee, 1987]. In turn, those risk factors have led to the implementation of a wide variety of activities including screening for early detection of hypertension and high cholesterol levels, smoking cessation programs, and lifestyle modification activities.

Directly linked to implementation and to risk factors is an understanding of how the subjective decision to seek care evolves. In a health-belief model [Andren & Rosenqvist, 1987], individuals may first consider whether or not they believe that they are susceptible to the disease or condition, Next, there could be a consideration of the seriousness of the disease/condition. Thirdly, people subjectively decide whether or not securing medical care will be helpful. Finally, there is a individual review of the selectively specific barriers that inhibit seeking care.

Going through the process you realize that you are susceptible to influenza; and it could be a serious illness; and that medical care could be helpful; and that you had the money and the physician could see you immediately. Mass media notices about the flu could provide the "trigger" for you to take the action.

Planners who are aware of the factors influencing the decision to seek care can improve the targeting of their implementation activities.

IMPLEMENTATION IN ACTION

Taking into account the humbling experience, the strategies, and the risk factors, several examples of implementation activities illustrate the use of the combined knowledge.

Smoking Cessation

Reporting in the *Harvard Business Review,* Hammond, DeCenzo, and Bowers [1987] told how one company went smokeless. Blue Cross/Blue Shield of Maryland decided that the nature of the company's business demanded a smoke-free workplace. In addition, the 36 percent of the 900 employees who were smokers cost the company about $185,000 per year in sick days and diminished productivity.

A three-phase program began in January 1986 with smoking banned at meetings, conferences, and training sessions. If meetings lasted more than one hour, there would be a break for smokers. In September 1986, all work areas were made smoke-free, vending machines were removed, and there were designated smoking areas. By January 1987, there was to be no smoking on company premises. Deviations were punishable by disciplinary measures ranging from warnings to termination.

Not a single employee left or was fired. While 20 percent of the employees still smoke, they don't do so on company premises.

Why did the smoke-free edict succeed in being implemented? Five reasons were given: Top management gave unswerving support; implementation was phased in over one year; the plan's importance to the image of the company and to the health of employees was communicated; there was room for feedback and dissent; and the company offered as many kinds of medical programs to help cure the addiction as could be found.

Freestanding Ambulatory Surgery Center

Goodspeed and Earnhart [1986] label ambulatory surgery as "an excellent market opportunity" as they present their approach to planning, developing, and implementing such a center. Four implementation strategies are noted in the early stages: Pre-empt the competition to secure a greater share of the market; package prices competitively for marketing; operate as a separate product line stressing consumer satisfaction, scheduling ease, and efficient patient flow; and be conducive to wellness rather than the institutional concept of sickness.

In the work plan for the center, special attention is given to tasks that need to be accomplished in areas such as legal, financial, equipment, personnel, marketing, regulations, and facility/space/construction aspects. Since physical environment is extremely critical in a surgery center, several suggestions emerge: a light blue mood pleasing color for the operating room; plants and pictures to create a homelike atmosphere; stereo headsets for patients as a diversion; and an aquarium providing a tranquil mood in the waiting room instead of a television. During this implementation phase, pinpointing *who* does *what* and *when* is vital.

What made their implementation effort achieve its goal? "The key to success is organization, particularly before scheduling the first patient."

SETTING GOALS IN IMPLEMENTATION

Returning to the beginning of this chapter, the point was made that some planners may have wondered if and when any activity would ever be implemented. Mowll [1987] reinforces the vital nature of all the preliminary effort by commenting that most people don't reach their goals because they don't define them. He stresses the use of results-oriented management [ROM] and management by objectives [MBO] as two techniques to define and reach goals. Regardless of the technique used, implementation will flounder unless the goals and objectives are specifically delineated.

FROM A TO B TO C: IMPLEMENTING CHANGE

When any activity is undertaken, a certain amount of change takes place. There has to be an accommodation for the new or modified program. No matter who is involved in the implementation effort, those people can be agents of change. Bassett and Metzer [1987] advise the manager to constantly question changes by asking why this is being done? Is it necessary? What is its purpose? And how can it be done better?

In discussing the management of the health care professional, McConnell [1984] lists six steps to enjoy the greatest chance of successfully managing change:

1. *Inform* employees as early as possible of future events.
2. *Plan* thoroughly.
3. *Communicate* fully.
4. *Convince* employees as necessary.
5. *Involve* employees whenever the circumstances permit
6. *Monitor* implementation and assure that decisions are adjusted and plans are fine-tuned as necessary.

Changing Behavior

Generic to implementation is the truism that behavior must change. Tuomilehto and Puska [1987] discuss four theoretical models for behavioral change. Although they overlap somewhat, in combination the following models constitute the foundation for implementing a community based health program:

1. *Behavior change approach* is linked to learning theory and helps people to identify risk factors; educates people re their behavior and health; persuades and motivates to action; trains the target population; provides social support; creates favorable environment for change; and mobilizes the community support.
2. *Communication behavior approach* uses mass communication and interpersonal communication to get messages across. Community leaders are the particular target of the one-to-one communications.

3. *Innovation diffusion approach* claims that the new changes are considered innovations which then diffuse throughout the community. Innovation occurs in four stages: knowledge, persuasion, decision, and confirmation. Decisions may be made individually, by collective consensus or by an authority figure.
4. *Community organization approach* relates to the complex network of mass media representatives, health care providers, business leaders, key people in voluntary organization and political leaders that exercises influence over individual behavior and lifestyle.

Overcoming Resistance to Change

In essence, fear or uneasiness about the unknown incubates an aversion for the new or untried. People prefer to maintain the status quo that they have been comfortable with over the years. Resistance is enhanced and almost assured when the change is a surprise. Different managerial styles generate varying degrees of resistance to change as noted by McConnell [1984] in his gradations:

- *Telling* them what to do engenders the greatest degree of resistance to change. Direct orders present a major threat and require blind obedience.
- *Convincing* them of what must be done makes employees less resistant. Since regulations and mandates put the choice out of the hands of the governing bodies, health care organizations may face this task frequently in implementing changes.
- *Involving* individuals in changes that may affect them is the best way to keep the resistance at a minimum.

There are a number of options that can be used to deal with resistance to change including: education and communication, participation and involvement, facilitation and support, negotiation and agreement, manipulation and co-option, and explicit and implicit coercion. While the last two named methods are undoubtedly quicker than the other four, Jaffe [1985] points out that their use could create the same lack of trust exhibited as a major barrier to change in the first place.

To survive in the highly competitive health care market, Jaffe [1985] recommends specific implementation strategies that react to external trends and reflect internal organizational and individual philosophies:

- Develop cost-effective programs.
- Participate in health policy decisions.
- Create innovative nontraditional roles for people.
- Market the services and the people.
- Engage in studies to assess quality of care of services.

Changing Three Hospitals Into One

What change could be more threatening and create more resistance than an hospital merger? Possibly a merger of three hospitals? Fyke [1987] reports on his personal experience as a hospital administrator intimately involved in just such a process.

This merger into the Greater Victoria Hospital Society in British Columbia, Canada linked three hospitals located on four sites. There were about 1,218 acute care, 100 rehabilitation, and

448 long-term care beds with an operating budget of $160 million. There were 450 physicians on staff and 5,500 employees represented by 17 unions.

In this complex hospital merger with all the ingredients for a disaster of momentous proportions, Fyke did come away with certain beliefs relative to implementation:

- With a great deal of opportunity for discussion and persuasion, a courtship approach to unifying medical staffs works better to secure the advantages of amalgamation.
- Minimize uncertainty with open and timely communication with all levels of the organization during the merger. This is critical.
- Management skills different from day-to-day operations are required during a merger. Required negotiating skills help to recognize when people resist because of insecurity or inability to accept change. Political sensitivity recognizes a fast or a slow pace and the changes that can realistically be made and those that cannot or must be delayed.
- Chief executive officers must be sensitive to the impact of a major merger on the community and the need to be seen as working to improve services.
- Although the type of emergent organization is different, the question remains as to which is better.
- From a cost and quality viewpoint, research is needed about the advantages and disadvantages of a merger.

From a management consultant's viewpoint, O'Brien and Roemer [1989] list 11 key issues to consider when evaluating or pursuing a merger or acquistion such as alternative concepts, governance, dollar valuation, communication, legal aspects, and post-transaction activities.

CONSTRAINTS/BARRIERS/PRESSURES TOWARD CHANGE

Top-level administrators quickly learn through experience that are things you can control and those that you cannot. Furthermore, the good administrator is able to distinguish between the two and to "avoid spending undue time, energy and resources attempting to control the uncontrollable" [Seay, Vladeck, & Kramer, 1986].

Which of the following implementation and change constraints barriers and pressures fall into the controllable or uncontrollable categories in regard to hospitals?

- Less money for health care
- Shifts in population demographics
- Patients lack of insurance
- Rapid diffusion of high technology services
- Competition between hospitals and physicians
- Financing of graduate medical education
- Resource allocations for new diseases
- Great expectations of health care by the public

According to Seay et al. [1986], "except for demographic and epidemiological phenomena, hospitals potentially have far more capacity to shape their futures than they may now recognize."

Importantly, that optimistic mindset can be illustrated by past history. On May 7, 1889, John Shaw Billings spoke at the opening day ceremonies for Johns Hopkins Hospital, a facility that he had designed:

> A hospital is a living organism. . . Its work is never done; its equipment is never complete; it is always in need of new means of diagnosis, of new instruments and medicines; it is to try all things and hold fast to that which is good.

In a discussion of the health planning predicament in four nations, Rodwin [1984, chap. 9] asks three questions about the barriers to implementation:

- Are health policy instruments adapted to medical practice?
- Do structural interests in the health sector result in "dynamics" without change?
- Are there structural constraints to state intervention?

Reflect upon who determines health policy? What is the role of lobbyists? Is there a "spinning of wheels?" Why hasn't the U.S. enacted a national health service or insurance scheme? Answers, or even a discussion of the questions, should reveal insights into effecting change via the implementation of new and/or modified programs. Why did the U.S. take more than 20 years to enact the Medicare program? History has another lesson for those who wish to implement change. As with the Medicare battle, the implementation of the current cost-containment activities also raises the powerful pressures associated with the struggle for "turf" [Gibbons, 1985].

In a discussion of effective policy implementation in inner city health departments, Jones and Loe [1988] identify national and local constraints. On a national level, there may be legislative constraints as well as inhibiting factors in resource allocation and service distribution. On a local level, constraints can concern the characteristics of the agency, personnel and resources and the commitment to the policy. For the local health department to effectively implement a national policy, Jones and Loe consider six elements: the agency's suitability as an implementor, the agency's ability to achieve results, level of support from official auspices, maintenance of community support, administrative and technical competence of the agency, and the ability to acquire adequate resources.

Sometimes the hospital has the data and knows the problem, but the community implements the solutions. Major causes of hospitalization resulted from dog bites, auto accidents and respiratory infections in this Chicago area. Asking the questions, the community discovered the solutions. They implemented programs to round up stray dogs; to alter traffic flow and speeds to improve road safety; and to build rooftop greenhouses to combat the respiratory disease presumed secondary to poor nutrition. Hancock [1986] commented that the hospital must develop a community conscience rather than an institutional loyalty while pondering which implementation activity produces the "biggest bang for the health care buck."

Survival appears to be the basic issue resulting from the pressures existent in the health care industry based on a survey of 1,419 hospital executives by Touche Ross [1988, p. 5]. A flexibility to become "department stores" for health care services, providing in one location a full range of integrated services, emerged as a most probable solution for survival [Touche Ross, 1988, p. 15].

If the department store concept is feasible, implementation of marketing activities is a logical next step.

IMPLEMENTING HEALTH CARE MARKETING ACTIVITIES

In the medical-industrial complex of the health care delivery system, the corporate culture has taken steadfast hold. Marketing concerns surged forward, providers learned marketing basics, governing boards, and CEOs adopted business ethics and pondered marketing problems.

Health Marketing Surges

Between 1980 and 1984, more than 600 articles on health care marketing appeared in about 150 journals. Approximately 25 percent of the articles discussed marketing research [Cooper, Jones, & Wong, 1984]. An updated bibliography [National Technical Information Service, 1988] contains 134 pages of citations on hospital and health care marketing. This publication gives "examples of time tested corporate management functions and their new application to all types of hospitals, health care agencies and profit and nonprofit organizations in view of the recent U.S. health care industry's struggle for economic survival."

Health care marketing emerged as a discipline in the 1970s with the initial publication arriving in 1978, *The Health Care Marketing Newsletter.* In 1980, the Academy for Health Services Marketing was formed and Eisenberg [1988] reported 3,500 members by the end of 1988. Soon after, the first publication appeared, *Journal of Health Care Marketing* [Cooper & Hisrich, 1987]. In addition, a step-by-step guidebook, *The Complete Medical Marketing Handbook* [Ricardo, 1988] leads providers in developing their own plans for advertising and marketing. For physicians, there is a quarterly portfolio of practice and promotion tips including newspaper and other advertisements critiqued by a marketing specialist [Brown, 1988]. A $25,000 five-step marketing plan suitable for any physician follows [Clark, 1989]: Start with gathering basic data; distinguish yourself from competitors; reach your captive audience; time media and advertisements effectively; and offer a "freebie."

In late 1988 and early 1989, the National League for Nursing [1988] offered seven programs on "Successful Marketing Strategies for Home Care: A How-To Management Seminar." Their hard-sell brochure highlighted the key words related to learning about implementing marketing activities: survival and growth strategies, the best marketing approach for your company, targeted nurse marketing, winning joint ventures, specific strategies that will increase *your* market share, and communications that sell.

Hospitals spent $1.18 billion on marketing and advertising in 1987 with the average hospital budgeting about $200,000 for that purpose. More than 90 percent of the 7,000 U.S. hospitals advertised in 1986—up 64 percent from 1985 [Erickson, 1989]. In this competitive climate, most health care facilities and services now have a staff member assigned responsibility for marketing health care [Steiber & Boscarino, 1985, p. 92].

Marketing Basics

"Health care marketing management is the process of understanding the needs and wants of a target market. The purpose is to provide a viewpoint from which to integrate the organization, analysis, planning, implementation, and control of the health care delivery system" [Triolo, 1987]. Another, probably more commonly agreed upon definition says that marketing "is the means by which organizations identify unfulfilled human needs, convert them into business opportunities, and create satisfaction for others and profit for themselves" [Kotler, 1980, p. 4].

Distinctions are made between selling and marketing. Manassero [1988a] states that selling involves first creating a product or services and then persuading people that they need the product or service. On the other hand, marketing means discovering what people need and then creating the product or service. This distintion appeared in a printed debate. Pros said that marketing by hospitals was tailored to the needs. Cons felt that marketing filled the beds with nonmedical needs [*Pharmacy Practice News*, 1989].

Basic elements in industrial marketing are referred to as the four P's: product, place, price, and promotion. Specifically modified for health care, Cooper [1985a, p. 3] suggests the following changes:

- Product to Service—shift to emphasis on services of health care marketers
- Place to Access—reflecting consumer's concern for services and availability
- Price to Consideration—anything of value exchanged for health care services
- Promotion—shift to emphasis on public relations and health education

Though it is only one part of the marketing process, promotion is a critical element since the product [health care] is sold to potential customers [patients]. Similar to advertising campaigns, promotion activities in health care marketing seek to inform and educate people about services, to let people know where to buy, to persuade customers to buy, and to keep the company's name in the public eye. It is doubtful that a health care service can achieve continued success without an effective promotional marketing effort [Cooper, 1985a, p. 3].

To gain superiority in the health care marketplace, Grenell and Studin [1988] tell administrators that they must have a "strategy paradigm." That coined word refers to core strategic consideration at two levels: an analytic level and a tactical level. At the analytic level, the strategy paradigm includes typical corporate types of analyses: an industry analysis, a local market analysis, and a competitive analysis. At the tactical level, the model utilizes corporate marketing principles such as targeting specific market segments, adding capacity and reducing prices, and by avoiding confrontation with market leaders by selling their own competitive advantage. "Executives who resist using their strategy paradigm to promote new directions may manage, but they will not lead" [Grenell & Studin, 1988].

In a book containing 46 articles on health care marketing and trends, Cooper [1985b, p. 130] develops a marketing planning model. His model begins with consumer-oriented situational analysis marketing research. Data from that step yields segment-specific strategies and goes on to produce the mission, goals, and objectives. Implementation takes place then followed by evaluation. Data from the evaluation are fed back to each prior step as appropriate.

While Manassero [1988b] says that the marketing plan need not be elaborate, complex, or involved, he does identify four key elements to a successful plan: a goal, objectives, strategies, and resource assessment.

Although talking about marketing in home health care, Freitag [1988] outlines the following seven steps in the marketing planning process that combine the four Ps and the "strategy paradigm:"

1. *Establishing the Mission.* Goals and objectives are set by the governing body and are consistent with organizational philosophy and policies.
2. *Environmental Assessment.* Looks at opportunities and threats in the environment and the strengths and weakness evidenced in the organization's capabilities.
3. *External Forces.* Reviews forces that impact upon health care marketing such as legisla-

tive/regulatory mandates, referral sources, insurance coverage, demographics, competition, disease/condition trends, new services, and vital statistics.

4. *Referral Source Analysis and Potential Markets.* Current and potential markets are analyzed including attention to identifying specific population targets. Similarly, current and potential referral sources are examined.

5. *Decision Maker, Purchaser, and User.* A wide variety of needs and wants are involved in health care decisions. Marketing requires discovery of the way decisions are made. For example, a decision maker [physician] may look for a high quality hassle-free provider; a purchaser may search for the best value for the money; and the user wants compassionate care.

6. *Competitive Analysis.* Competitors and their marketing strategies are analyzed by asking questions such as Who are the competitors? What is their market share? What services do they provide? How are they different? What are their prices? and Where do they get referrals?

7. *Internal Assessment.* Operational trends in the organization's services are examined with attention to routine corporate details such as annual volume of business, visits by payor, services by program and by discipline, profitability by service, uncompensated care, cost per visit, visits per case, and prices of services.

As an example of its customer service philosophy [Establishing the Mission], Freitag [1988] reproduces a poster used by the Visiting Nurse Association of Boston. "Sometimes the best medicine is a home remedy" is the bold headline followed in smaller type with "There are some things you can't write a prescription for. Like the sympathetic ear of a caring professional treating you in your own home." A picture shows a happy baby in a woman's lap with another woman talking and playing with the baby.

Obviously, these health care marketing basics have dipped strongly into the existing well of corporate America.

Culture of Corporate Business

Health care providers are being advised to adopt the culture of corporate America in their approach to serving consumers. Behrman's [1987] extensive laundry list gleans the advice to managers from the business media and clearly makes the case of the impact upon health care providers:

Determine new product lines	Develop market niches
Increase market shares	Obtain capital funds
Learn to be competitive	Reorganize
Raise capacity utilization	Raise revenues and cut costs
Improve technology	Seek mergers and acquisitions
Form joint ventures	Develop/buy more modern equipment

Learn planning and strategic management
Seek vertical and horizontal integration
Research consumer attitudes toward health care

Behrman [1987] also makes several other notable points: "All these ideas are the lifeblood of business schools. . . These ideas also raise ethical issues. . . All these imperatives are techniques."

Vertical integration is akin to the "department store" concept mentioned by Touche Ross [1988, pp. 5, 15] as they spoke about survival in the health care market. Brown and McCool [1986] comprehensively explain the strategic concept. They note that vertical integration allows health care organizations to provide all levels and intensities of care under a single umbrella— one-stop shopping, so to speak. Barriers to vertical integration, as well as some of the other business imperatives, could reside with issues such as physician autonomy, our pluralistic system, support for multiple delivery sites, and a desire to maintain the status quo.

Joint ventures are popular in the health care field. Simply put, a joint venture is a cooperative agreement between two or more firms seeking similar objectives. However there are quite a few venture variations: equal equity and ownership, contractual nonequity coopera- tion, shared management, dominant management by one party, and percentage distributions. Schillaci [1987] enumerates six resources critical in a joint venture: marketing, technology, raw materials and components, financial, managerial, and political.

Apparently, not everyone believes that the adoption of the American corporate business culture is the direction health care providers should take. Dr. Arnold S. Relman [1980] has been a frequent dissenter in the pages of the *New England Journal of Medicine*. He attacked the "new medical industrial complex" and said that for-profit health care organizations had no place in medical care. Relman and others argue that the "profit motive" is inappropriate and corrupts the entire system.

If health care is a business, then the adoption of a business orientation is justified. However, Behrman [1987] strongly illustrates the differences: "But business is primarily deal- ing, not caring; business is competitive, and caring is cooperative. Business is done at arm's length; caring is done with arms linked, or with an arm around someone's shoulder. . . The conclusion that health care is a business is wrong. Health care is provided by members of a profession, which is not a business." Behrman contends that a confusion exists elevating the value of corporate business techniques over the purpose and demand for health.

Obviously, the battle over the adoption of the corporate American business culture still has to be resolved. Until that time, it is apparent that health care marketing strategies will continue to be implemented in profusion.

Governing Board and CEO Directions

Governing boards of health care organizations can decide to engage in any of the business activities listed earlier. Gone are the days when "hospital trustees leave their brains at the office when they come to board meetings" [Coddington & Moore, 1987a]. Now, members of govern- ing boards are "business strategists" who have to make the "hard decisions." With the chief executive officer carrying out their wishes, the governing board wields control over strategic planning and marketing implementation.

Nauert [1985] presents the case for the role of the chief financial officer of health care organizations in the strategic business planning process. Involvement in strategic planning includes areas such as environmental analysis, analytical research, goal setting, program for- mulation, implementation, goal achievement, and evaluation.

There can be no doubt that attention to the marketing planning model of doing business is a prime concern of the both the voluntary governing board members as well as the salaried executive employees. However, the transition to the business of marketing does create problems.

Problems in Marketing

In a telling example of "Murphy's Law," M. Campbell [1989] narrates her woeful tale of marketing gone wrong. Using tasteful newspaper advertisements, Dr. Campbell placed her OB/GYN ads in several targeted papers. She attracted drug abusers, non-English speaking immigrants, gays, and fervent anti-male physician females.

Clarke and Shyavitz [1987] report that there are few trained health care marketers. Furthermore, few health care organizations have developed marketing plans containing defined goals, objectives, strategies and tactics. If the organization has the plans, Kotler and Clarke [1987, p. 82] report there is usually a growing time lag between plan and implementation.

On top of those two limitations, marketing is usually allocated a low level of resources. Part of the difficulty may lie with the ambivalence felt by voluntary nonprofit health care organizations with the concept of "selling their services" and their interpretation of their public and social responsibilities as stated in their charters. However, Clarke and Shyavitz [1987] say that "the marketing concept is as appropriate for not-for-profit organizations as it is for for-profit organizations" and "market segmentation is not contrary to the not-for-profit responsibilities . . . the health care organization that does not compete effectively probably will not survive."

Five serious execution problems in marketing are identified by Bonoma and Crittenden [1988]:

1. Management by assumption—There is an assumption that someone somewhere is handling pricing, promotion, and assorted vital tasks.
2. Global mediocrity—Many things are done adequately, but nothing is done extremely well.
3. Empty promises marketing—Programs are created without the capability to execute at the line level.
4. Program ambiguity—Clever programs without strong leadership and a shared understanding of the unifying theme and/or identity will flounder.
5. Ritualization, politicization, and unavailability—Ritual is encased in "things have always been done that way" rhetoric. Office politics can alter facts and a lack of data or resources can effectively stall any activity.

Additional difficulties in implementing marketing tactics relate to the following considerations:

*   Providers, rather than consumers, stimulate, and demand services.
*   All activities exist solely to support the medical staff in their medical endeavors
*   Isolating specific markets begs the question of serving the poor and other undesirable groups.
*   Political consequences, such as medical staff opposition, could be hazardous to implementation of programs.
*   Marketing resources needs usually can not compete effectively against clinical needs.

Because hospitalization is falling, "hospitals must adapt more aggressive marketplace strategies" with "competitive strategies based on price and quality" [*American Medical News*, 1988]. Obviously, those comments are not restricted to hospitals but apply equally as well to all health care providers. Implementation of significant and sophisticated marketing action in health care is on the increase for the following reasons according to Clarke and Shyavitz [1987]:

- "Most importantly, competition among health care providers is fierce."
- More sophisticated management methods and techniques are being adapted by health care organizations.
- High costs and scarce resources force providers to consider potential demand and to defer new services.
- Reimbursement mechanisms, mainly prospective payment systems, focus efforts on profitable diagnoses.
- In the benefits area, consumerism is gaining momentum as a significant force.

These rationales for the potential surge in marketing by health care organizations points out the need to discuss the corporate concepts of product line management, market segmentation, and marketing research.

PRODUCT LINES, MARKET SEGMENTATION, AND MARKET RESEARCH

Beginning with the product line [health care or each DRG], the typical industrial firm selects its target audience, learns about the population, and tailors its promotion to that group.

Product Line Management

Product line management is the development, management, and marketing of distinct services to specific groups of users [Super, 1987]. There is no one planner creating one implementation model which aligns the company to be more in tune with market needs [Lutz, 1987]. A product could be a current consumer interest such as a "sports medicine center" or "wellness centers" or could be a "specialty product line" such as cardiac care, geriatrics, substance abuse, surgery, or medicine. There could be autonomous product line centers with their own budget, their own personnel, and their own autonomous product line manager. A survey of 73 California hospitals with more than 200 beds revealed that 82 percent have implemented, will implement, or are considering implementing product line management techniques [Super, 1987].

Radical change may occur within the health care organization when a product line concept is introduced. Key decisions may be shifted away from physicians and into the hands of the governing board and management personnel. Therefore, in implementing a product line strategy, the following four points should be considered:

1. Communication of clear objectives and operational policies that specifically detail authority and responsibility to all concerned, particularly to the medical staff.
2. Dedicated management professionals to implement actions.
3. Comprehensive management training programs.
4. Gradually introducing the practice with an emphasis on services most in need of marketing support.

Van Pelt [1985] notes the distinction between the historical organizational structures based on function [specific tasks for specific purposes] or division [grouped functions]. On the other hand, hybrid product line management combines functional responsibilities with focused market products. Administratively, product line management could shift organizational structures from the traditional pyramid to concentric, overlapping, coordinated rings.

Cardiovascular Product Line. After studying the marketplace and their own resources, the 450-bed University Hospital in Denver set up a modified form of product line management. Reporting to a Coordinating Committee, a Cardiovascular Care Center manages a children's cardiac unit, expanded the electrophysiology laboratory, began a heart transplant program, and set prices for five cardiovascular products. Marketing activities included the following: a Heart-line telephone number with different recorded messages daily, a Healthy Heart Cookbook, Heart-to-Heart Week when the public could get free cardiac risk assessments, and weekly radio spot announcements cosponsored with the American Heart Association.

New Product Lines. "Developing new or modified services requires considerable planning and cost analysis—including revenue projections and interfunctional cooperation and coordination" [Emery, 1986]. Specific market information needed relates to day-to-day operations such as demographics, competition, price comparisons, hours of services, location of service, and parking. Triolo [1987] outlines the seven Cs to consider when planning new product lines: quality of *C*are [technical capability], *C*aring [compassion and warmth], *C*omfort [amenities and decoration], *C*onvenience [hours and parking], *C*urative [aids to recovery], *C*oping [emotional and educational support], and *C*ost [alternatives to high cost services].

As competition intensifies for new health care markets, White [1985] reported a surge in demand for demographic data. Donnelley Marketing Information Services [Stamford, CT] saw their health care business more than double in one year. For example, data available include more than 300,000 physicians sorted by specialty and zipcode; all hospitals by number of beds, occupancy rates, bed specialty, utilization and length of stay; and integrated demographic data with patient history records. Using this type of information, health care providers could pinpoint the market for a specific service and determine the market share.

Also in the area of information marketing, St. Peters Medical Center [New Brunswick, NJ] tested the Smart-Card, a credit card-sized identification repository embedded with a 8K bit memory and/or microprocessor of the individual's demographic and medical history [Bermar, 1988]. Using a smart card reader, the hospital can call up on the screen the patient's medical history, insurance data, and personal information. Smart cards speed admissions and data can be added as events occur. "As a sales ploy, the wallet-sized IDs wed patients to the clinic whose name they now carry in their back pocket."

In one instance, a hospital tracked recent real estate transactions in its locality. Using that market intelligence, the hospital planned to implement walk-in centers to serve single adults and childless couples where condominiums were to be constructed. In single-family housing areas, the hospital scheduled a primary care physicians' office building as a referral conduit when hospitalization was required [White, 1985].

Market Segmentation

Even though you may adopt a product line management stance, the health care provider still has to specifically delineate the intended audience. While a community can certainly be seen as a whole, it also consists of a variety of different groupings. A targeted approach to marketing is vital. As testimony to the critical nature of targeting, the average American hospitals spent $236,000 on marketing in 1987 [Wager, 1988].

A marketing segmentation approach embodies three tenets related to targeting a market:

- Consumers are different.
- Different consumers have different marketing behaviors.
- Consumer segments can be isolated from the overall market.

Through market segmentation, health care providers can attempt to gain one or both basic types of competitive advantage: cost leadership and/or differentiation in services [Porter, 1985]. In his basic five-step approach to segmentation, Wager [1988] sets up a logical common-sense sequence: set specific goals; study the target; define the message; develop the strategy; and choose the tools to accomplish the task.

Through its Market Area Profile [MAP], the American Medical Association helped about 2,000 physicians to locate their practices beginning in June 1985 [Holden, 1988]. Now, the AMA sells MAP Graphics starting at $75 each for AMA members and $125 for nonmembers. Color-coded maps illustrate specific locations in up to 10 zip codes in the target area using two sets of up to 20 demographic variables such as population, median and average household income, household size, age, race, and sex. Profiles can be for the current year, the last U.S. Census year and five years into the future. In addition, MAP Graphics can show the concentration of 21 different physician specialities in any one area. Most frequent users are physicians already in practice seeking data about their target areas, particularly in highly competitive specialties such as ophthalmology, internal medicine, family practice, obstetrics, and orthopedics. Phyllis Kopriva, a product manager for the AMA's Department of Practice Development Resources, says that "the best thing about MAP is that it is personalized and can be tailored to a very specific area."

Segmentation Messages. In defining the message, the provider must clearly explain what makes your particular service better, special, and different. Messages must be created to avoid the "SW²C" reaction from the public: So What? Who cares? In addition, the message must be repeated using a combination of communication approaches. Of course, the exchange element must be mentioned wherein each party exchanges something of value: The provider gets revenue for services rendered and the patient receives care in return. While implementing marketing, MacStravic [1987] also cautions about not losing sight of retaining the loyalty of current patients. He notes that it is six times more costly to attract a new customer.

Paying attention to the average health care provider, Eisenberg [1988] notes that advertising works for the little guy, too. With a modest budget, an effective promotion campaign can get the message across. Topics covered include finding an agency, creating a strategy, where and how often to advertise, what to say and how much the marketing will cost. In marketing promotions, providers are urged to stress benefits such as short waits, friendly staff, evening hours, 24-hour coverage, convenient location, free parking, and house calls. Choose positive phrases such as "specializing in" rather than "practice limited to." Choose your words carefully aiming for a conversational tone and don't be cute since health is a serious business. Additionally, in print material, experts advise using a little bold type, lots of white space, unusual borders to attract the eye and avoid using illegible script lettering.

Depending upon the marketing program and the geographic location, providers could be charged $25 to $75 per hour with campaigns running anywhere from $500 to $6,000 for the average physician. There may be free lance advertising people who will moonlight for individual or group providers. Incidentally, Saundra Atwood of the American Academy for Health Services Marketing says that "practice development is a growing part of the hospital's strategy" and the physician's hospital may be happy to share the cost of the marketing promotion.

Exhibit 6–1 shows a marketing segmentation action plan aimed at neighborhood clergy with a target of increasing referrals to a nursing home by 200 percent per year. Note the various methods and techniques for messages and communications.

For the child-bearing female target group, Triolo [1987] appeals to a message that puts "women in charge" or by saying "Have your baby your own way."

Pointing out that claims shouldn't guarantee success, shouldn't be misleading and should be topical, MacStravic [1988] illustrates messages that communicate benefits directly or indirectly:

- We'll have you feeling human again fast.
- Take off your glasses—forever.
- Lose 15 pounds in six weeks.
- We've fixed up some of the worst joints in town [sports medicine center]
- Count sheep, toss and turn, read a book or call us [sleep disorder center].

From a health care point of view, there may be an ethical objection to promising specific outcomes due to treatment of any nature. Therefore, the advertising tends to be product oriented rather than "a money back guarantee if not satisfied."

Segmentation Samples. Noting that the nation's hospitals are likely to adopt market segmentation techniques, Super [1986] reported that there may be as many as 20 different subsets of a single grouping. Importantly, each subset, or segment, may have distinct service needs and distinct exposure patterns to a variety of communication media.

Four affiliated nonprofit San Francisco hospitals, the California Healthcare System, spent $200,000 for a print media marketing campaign promoting a physician referral service. People can phone "Physician Finder" at 800–433-My-MD and the free service will recommend one or more of their medical staff to be the family physician or to resolve that person's health care problem. Aiming at the California persona, their newspaper ad shows a slightly overweight woman in an exhaustive workout out on a pedal wheel and pull weights with a bold headline: "Maybe the best way to stay healthy is to see a Doctor."

Even highly respected providers will be marketing their "brand name" high-cost, high-quality services. The Mayo Clinic [Rochester, MN] opened outpatient facilities in Jacksonville, Florida and Scottsdale, Arizona [Super, 1986]. In New York City, the Mt. Sinai Medical Center has extensive advertising campaigns on television extolling the technical capabilities of physicians at their institution. Both of these well known and highly respected providers are engaged in marketing and seeking new patients.

In marketing women's health care, Powills [1987] keys in on the diversity of the group while Harrell and Fors [1985] concentrates on segmenting ambulatory care. Five major primary market segments among women have been isolated along with their characteristics [Harrell & Fors, 1985; Triolo, 1987]:

- *Traditional:* Medium concern about health care—occasional service users—follow organized system to get care—generally compliant with medical regimen.
- *Family-centered:* Highest health concern level—frequent contact with variety of specialists—family health care decision maker—support and promote family well being—provider "shopping" occurs in low risk situations
- *Sports-oriented:* Concerned about body performance—occasional service users—seek treatment when health interferes with performance—self-confident in decision making—high degree of experimentation—most likely to explore new health care alternatives.
- *Wellness/wholeness:* High health consciousness—frequent service users—tend to prefer alternatives to traditional medical treatment when possible—moderate confidence level and

Exhibit 6-1. Marketing Segmentation Nursing Home Action Plan.

EXHIBIT B

Target
Area Clergy—20 churches/synagogues

Goals
1. Create high level of awareness
2. Create close ongoing relationship with major churches
3. Increase referrals to 30 per year (200 percent increase)

ACTION PLAN

January
► Identify all churches and synagogues, including name, address, and phone number of clergy.
► Identify the leadership and other details of the Ministerial Association.
► Place all clergy on newsletter mailing list.

February–April
► Administrator and social worker individually to attend church functions and meet ministers and church members.

May
► Administrator meets individually with a few of the key Ministerial Association leaders to discuss meeting spiritual needs of residents. Bring up the idea of a volunteer chaplain program (VCP); garner their support for the idea.

June
► Family council meeting—discuss the desire to more fully meet residents' spiritual needs. Ask for ideas and introduce the VCP concept.
► Include suggestions from the family council meeting and the key clergy members into a written VCP.
► Present the written VCP to the same key area ministers. Ask for advice on the program and support from the Ministerial Association.

► Make arrangements to attend a meeting of the Ministerial Association to present the program.

July
► Present the program to the association with the support of the key leadership. Set up a kick-off and training meeting to be held at the center.

August
► Kick-off to be held at the center involving all area clergy. Provide written VCP, center brochures, and other promotional items. Teach them all about the center.
► Implement the VCP which will provide 24-hour (via a beeper) coverage seven days a week and regular visits to the center.
► Other promotional efforts: sign by front door indicating that a volunteer chaplain is available; name tags for volunteer chaplains; newsletter to introduce the program and to indicate who the chaplain will be each week of the month; promotional materials to include this new service; letters to hospital social workers and physicians outlining the new program; asking leaders of the Ministerial Association if a news release may be sent to local news media.

September
► Family council meeting—new program will be introduced.
► Thank-you letters to all ministers for their support. Indicate positive comments from families.
► Send news release to local media regarding the new VCP.

October–December
► Social service director to continue ongoing weekly contacts with VCP ministers.
► Continue monthly mailing of newsletter.
► Ask various ministers if they would like to contribute articles to the newsletter.
► Ask volunteer chaplains to rotate responsibility for co-chairing the monthly program for new families, along with the administrator and social service director.
► Activity director to work with all area churches on holiday season activities.
► Send a thank-you letter to the area ministry for its continuing support, signed by administrator and president of the residents' council. Send along a holiday gift.

Source: From "Approach the community as more than one public," by R.J. Wager, 1988, *Provider, 14*(6), 10. Reprinted with permission of American Health Care Association.

moderate in experimentation—holistic approach—interested in nutrition, longevity and enhancing health.

- *Avoiders:* Low health consciousness—infrequent service users—do not rely on established providers—delay seeking care—tend to be self-prescribers—behavior may be due to distrust, fear, disinterest, or lack of funds.

While these characteristics may also apply to men, and may even be generic for populations, it is apparent that specific market messages can be directed at each subset of each distinct market segment. Obviously, it is important to engage in market research.

Coddington and Moore [1987b] illustrate a number of market segments in their discussion of health care diversification. A mobile breast diagnostic center could aim for women 40 and over with their own primary care physicians. An HMO could solicit firms of more than 25 employees in the area served. An outpatient surgery center could work from data about the proportion of surgeries that could be shifted from a facility plus new business potential.

These authors were "shocked at the number of important decisions made in hospitals without the benefit of rigorous marketing and economic analysis." These missing analyses lead directly into the use of market research in implementing activities.

Market Research

In implementing market research, the eternal questions arise regarding how much information is needed to make a decision and how good is the data being used. Keckley's [1988] market research handbook covers areas such as determining market share, measuring consumer satisfaction, identifying physician needs, assessing community and professional opinions, developing new products, and effectiveness of promotional activities.

In a humorous fashion, Collins [1986] cites three important maxims relative to establishing a market research information database:

- *Get it from the horse's mouth.* Use primary data or actual comprehensive source information rather than extrapolations.
- *Pick the low apples first.* Build data in increments beginning with the most relevant and then adding additional information.
- *Pin it down.* Or will the real John Doe stand up? Use data with accurate and consistent classifications regardless of the source or integration and comparison will be invalid.

To collect data, numerous methods and techniques can be utilized. Cooper and Hisrich [1987] list the following three market research techniques with subgroupings:

1. *Observational methods* provide valid nonsubjective data if there is no bias on the part of the observer recording the information.
   - *Mechanical observation* may use a simple traffic counting device to record the number of cars passing a potential health service location or a sophisticated eye movement device to measure the attention given to competing ads for health care services.
   - *Nonmechanical observation* relies on one or more human observers. Obviously, each observer may see events in a different light. Market researchers must specify as clearly as possible exactly what is to be observed to avoid ambiguity in recorded data. A

wellness center could observe visitors to an open house and display of equipment to record potential customers' interest in using such equipment. Without guidelines, one observer could record interest only if the visitor tried the equipment for more than one minute while another could record interest regardless of the time involved.

2. *Survey methods* are most commonly used in market research and are also most useful. Choice of a particular survey method depends upon expense, response rate, speed of completion, versatility of the method, amount of information obtainable and the clarity/reliability of the data secured. Several basic ways to gather data include mail questionnaires, telephone interviews, personal interviews and focus groups. Exhibit 6–2 gives the advantages and disadvantages for each technique.
   - *Mail questionnaires* may be least costly but the response rate could be low. Due to the lack of respondent interaction, both versatility and clarity may also be low. Generally, mail questionnaires should be relatively short, easy to complete, and request non-threatening data.
   - *Telephone interviews* secure a limited amount of information in a short time with a high response rate. Computerized phone surveys appear to be less successful than personal calls. Additionally, the popularity of the telephone survey may be reducing the response rate. Costs are a function of interviewer training and the expense of business phone lines. A major attraction of a telephone survey is the ability to gather data almost overnight.
   - *Personal interviews* are quite expensive but do have a high response rate with the gathering of a volume of detailed information. Again, with the increasing popularity of personal interviews, the public may become jaded and the response rate reduced. Additionally, the data may take longer to complete and analyze.
   - *Focus groups* have been explained in detail in Chapter 4. Since there is a captive group for a moderator to discuss the issue with, the response is high and the information generated is voluminous. Versatility is a plus along with a short completion time. Costs involved include the moderator's fee, group member payments, and rental of a meeting place.

3. *Experimentation* is most commonly associated with medical and not market research because of the costs and complexity. If used in market research, variables could be manipulated to measure cause and effect reactions. Obviously, when human beings are involved, experimentation is not a simple technique. Drug companies, on the other hand, could use a controlled laboratory experiment to regulate dosage levels for treatment purposes and then use the results for marketing.

Market research techniques of observation, surveys, and experimentation directly link to implementation activities in general planning as well as specific functional areas such as pricing, promotion, availability and service development. Exhibit 6–3 ranks the utility of each technique and subset for a variety of implementation variables. Note the high degree of benefit attributed to the focus group technique for all of the factors.

Borrowing from scientific approaches, Pastides and Moore-Pastides [1986] explain and discuss the use of probability sampling, standardization, randomized controlled trial, and statistical modeling for objective decision making in marketing.

Exhibit 6-2.   Advantages and Disadvantages of Survey Methods.

Characteristics Criteria	Mail Questionnaire	Telephone Survey	Personal Interview	Focus Group
Expense	Low	Medium/Low	High	Medium
Response Rate	Low	High/Medium	High	High
Completion Time	Medium	Low [shortest]	High [longest]	Low/Medium
Versatility	Low	Medium	High	High
Amount of Information	Medium	Low	High	Medium
Clarity for Respondent	Low	Medium	High	High

Source: From "Commentary on . . . marketing research for health services: Understanding and applying various techniques," by P. Cooper & R.D. Hisrich, 1987, *Journal of Health Care Marketing,* 7[1], 56. Published by the American Marketing Association. Reprinted by permission.

Probability sampling selects the target audience for market research. Cluster sampling is suggested as the choice to bypass the need of a universe and a random stratified sample of that universe. If all residents of one or more housing complex for the elderly were surveyed, data could be secured about their knowledge, attitudes and practices regarding a wellness center to be initiated on the premises or in the neighborhood.

Standardization techniques allow for an adjustment to eliminate extraneous factors such as age or socioeconomic status that could be the cause of differences. Direct standardization could use statewide averages to compare the staff-to-bed ratio department by department or hospital wide.

Exhibit 6-3.   Health Care Marketing Techniques by Implementation Variables.

Market Research Techniques	General Planning	Functional Areas			
		Cost Consideration [Pricing]	Access/ Availability	Promotion [Communication]	Service Development
Observation					
Mechanical	Low/Medium	Low	Medium/High	Low	Medium/High
Nonmechanical	Medium	Medium	Low/Medium	Low	Low
Survey					
Mail Questionnaire	Medium/High	Medium	Medium/High	Medium/Low	High
Telephone	High	Medium	High	Low	Medium/High
Personal Interview	Low	Medium	Low	Medium/Low	Medium
Focus Groups	High	High	High	High	High
Experimentation					
Controlled Lab	Low	Low	Low	Medium	Low

Source: From "Commentary on marketing research for health services: understanding and applying various techniques," by P. Cooper & R.D. Hisrich, 1987, *Journal of Health Care Marketing,* 7[1], 58, published by the American Marketing Association.

A randomized clinical trial involves selecting two or more similar population groups from a targeted audience. One group is the control and does not receive the marketing exposure while the other groups can be exposed to one or more approaches. Suppose a mobile foot care van is proposed as a service to the elderly. Implementation activities suggested are a printed packed of information and/or a group tour with refreshments. Responses could be calculated for the control group getting nothing, a group getting only the information packet, a group getting only the tour invitation, or a group getting both the information packet and the tour.

Statistical modeling or profiling utilizes multivariable statistical techniques to simultaneously predict probabilities. If a hospital wanted to establish a kidney transplant center, data could be secured from areawide physicians as to various needs such as beds, equipment, staffing, follow-up, and organ donations. Governmental criteria and professional society guidelines could be added into the variables. Statistical computer programs could analyze the input paying attention to preferences and weighted choices. Output from the computer program would determine the probabilities of use by the physicians with statistical probabilities for each of the variables, for the composite or for selected variables.

Applications of Market Research. Noting that "complicated data sets and sophisticated analyses are *not* the rule," Collins [1986] details several market research applications.

Hospital A's bed census dropped 10 percent in the last three years. An explanation was requested of the administrator by his Governing Board. Analysis was made of the hospital's market share by each zip code area by discharge over the last three years and also by each service area. Comparisons were made to the overall discharge rate for the area and between services. Results indicated that the hospital loss was average but there was a disproportionate loss in pediatrics. Actions were taken to attract more people to that specific service.

Hospital B did a large number of "balloon catherizations" in the past few years. Now, a few drugs, such as streptokinase, can be used and eliminate the need for the balloon procedures. Did the use of the new drugs affect the hospital's services? Data was collected on numbers of patients treated, length of stay, and reimbursement coverage for a period when the balloon procedures were routine and for a period when the drugs were used. Comparisons showed that the patients were predominantly covered by Medicare and Medicaid and their length of stay was cut in half. Hospital B decided to switch to drugs and implemented an educational program for physicians still using the balloon catheterizations.

Both Ambry [1988] and Waldrop [1987] use market research forecasting techniques to predict the need for ongoing services by the turn of the century. In relation to breast cancer, Ambry correlates data on documented risk factors with age-specific incidence rates and the number of people in each age group. Data sources could include the American Cancer Society, the National Cancer Institute's Surveillance, Epidemiology and End Results [SEER] program, and the Bureau of the Census population projections. Her analysis reveals that "two million women will develop breast cancer" by the year 2000 with 30,000 new patients per year. Ambry concludes that "despite shortcomings, these figures can guide businesses in preparing for growth in the health care and specialty services market for breast cancer victims."

Using similar data sources such as the American Diabetes Association, the National Institutes of Health and the National Center for Health Statistics, Waldrop declares that "age appears to be the most important risk factor " in the demographics of diabetes. Since people with diabetes are living longer and the American population is graying, the market implications are evident. In addition, the per capita health care expenditures of diabetics are about three times higher than average. Forecasting the number of known diabetics to be about 6.4 million by 1990 with a growth rate of 31 percent in the 45 to 64 age group, the market for products and services is apparent.

LINKING MARKETING, CHANGING BEHAVIOR, AND IMPLEMENTATION

By looking at activities in emerging new or modified services, planners can examine the links between the factors involved in changing behavior, the health care marketing objectives and the actual implementation of services and programs. Ambulatory care, home health care, long-term care, wellness centers and nurse entrepreneuring provide the settings to review marketing, changing behavior and implementation.

Ambulatory Care

Choosing "convenience medicine" as a "product line" Haley [1984] describes how to position the product by "balancing a company's capabilities with the consumer's needs." Convenience medicine includes services variously labeled as satellite centers, Urgicenters, Doc-in-the-Box centers, emergency services, and Medistops. Haley reports that random surveys in Dallas, Spokane, Tucson, and Nashville showed strong support for episodic, minor emergency, and acute care walk-in convenient services. Pricing analysis aimed for a figure at a lower cost than a hospital emergency room and more accessible and available than a private doctor's office. "Advertising is essential" to promote awareness of the care available at competitive prices. In addition, the convenient "medical stores" attract walk-ins as well as scheduled visits providing a referral network to corporate related services/facilities. In combining marketing techniques with theories about changing behavior and implementation action "ultimately, the success of retailing convenience medicine depends on the physician, since his/her service is the product" [Haley, 1984].

In Detroit, Klegon and Slubowski [1985] distributed a self-administered questionnaire to almost 300 residents in the area surrounding an ambulatory care center. Respondents indicated that ambulatory care centers fared poorly in comparison to the private physician's office as the consumer's choice for care. Based on that survey, existing services in the ambulatory care center were modified regarding physician availability, patient information booklets, walk-in services, and fees. Following the modifications, two community focus groups discussed the new products and the new promotional materials. These consumers affirmed the importance of stressing the patient/physician relationship and the personal attention in the facility. In addition, the focus groups came up with major revisions in advertising such as explaining the difference between the 24 hour walk-in services and a hospital emergency room service.

Using the focus group input, the ambulatory care center developed a series of newspaper ads and a direct mail brochure. Implementing the program, Klegon and Slubowski [1985] reported 44 percent more visits in the first three months of the promotional campaign. After probing, 45 percent of the new patients recalled the mailed brochure and 33 percent saw the newspaper ads. Following the promotion campaign, a consumer telephone survey of 400 random households found 22 percent who could name the ambulatory care center. That percentage was double the recognizability of a competitive center that had been in operation 15 years longer. However, of the 22 percent who identified the new center, only six percent had tried it. Apparently, there was still plenty of room for growth. Klegon and Slubowski [1985] conclude that "appropriately designed and executed promotional strategies are likely to meet intended objectives."

In a study of the demand for ambulatory mental health services, Horgan [1986] looked at the price factor. She found that "it does appear that the demand for ambulatory mental health services is fairly price-responsive, certainly more so than the demand for ambulatory medical services." Other considerations in implementing ambulatory mental health services relate to why people do or do not use the services, the skewed nature of the users and the zero out-of-pocket expenditures of many of the users.

Using a microcomputer, Winter [1986] analyzes macrodemographic data from the Bureau of the Census and vital statistics from the National Center for Health Statistics to determine the potential utilization of an ambulatory "convenience medicine" center. Then, using a Law of Retail Gravitation [Converse, 1949; Schwartz, 1963] that is linked to distance, Winter's computer program attacks the microproblem of actually locating a prime geographic site for the ambulatory center using a 24 × 17 map grid with about 408 × 204 point combinations. There is a possibility that the proper location selection can produce market shares three to four times higher than otherwise. An American Medical Association service, MAP Graphics, offers physicians similar location selection assistance [Holden, 1988].

With a related technique, Day, DeSarbo, and Terence [1987] uses strategy maps to illustrate the spatial relations of intra-industry competition. A completed map plots items such as sales, customers, market share, cash flow, growth, and profitability.

Home Health Care

Discussing the issues of implementation and marketing in home health organizations, Ingram and Hensel [1985] noted the top priority given to marketing. Dek Hagenburger, a national corporate president of Beverly Enterprises Home Health Services Division, stated: "Home health will be *the* domain and those that will be pre-eminent in that arena will be the companies that have a solid background in understanding and creating a sensitivity to what is involved in delivering health care services" [*Home Health Line*, 1984, p. 65].

Basic marketing issues for home health agencies were identified as involving the expectations of marketing, the level of organizational commitment to marketing, definition of the market and the plans, strategies and tactics of implementation. In turn, the resolution of the basic issues leads to the consideration of the elements in the marketing mix such as channel management, product management, and pricing. Within those three elements, the topics arise of political economy, dyadic relationships, patient loyalty, product breadth versus depth, product quality, product deletion, price and quality, competition, and reimbursement risks.

Interestingly, Ingram and Hensel [1985] and L. Campbell [1989] caution that too much promotion and/or borrowed marketing strategies may have adverse effects, particularly if the promotion is not done well. Many people still feel that health care advertising is unethical, manipulative, irrelevant, insulting, and degrading. Choices of "pull" or "push" advertising/selling are related to consumer/market analysis. A "pull" advertising campaign is designed to attract people with a grassroots approach. A "push" promotion uses personal salesmanship to sway referral agencies, physicians, and other "gatekeepers" and assures them that the home health agency can meet the needs of *their* clients. Ingram and Hensel predict that "successful home health organizations of the future will have a marketing orientation that is deeply integrated within the structure of the organization." Campbell advises concentrating on client relationships, marketing the family, communicating a new image, and demonstrating superiority.

While noting the special problems and opportunities, Freitag's [1988] practical approach to marketing in home health care also relies on the traditional mix of product, price, promotion, and place. "Sometimes the best remedy is a home remedy" is the slogan theme of the Visiting Nurse Association of Boston.

Long-Term Care

Stewart [1988] proposes a niche strategy as the mechanism for implementing a long-term care program. A niche strategy offers two benefits: improved refinement of message, and a narrower target audience seeing and hearing the message frequently ["reach"]. This is similar to a market segmentation methodology. Selecting the correct target niche depends upon the application of the Profitability Impact of Marketing Strategies [PIMS] rule. PIMS posits that low or high cash generation [relative market share] plotted against low or high cash use [market growth rate] results in product "Stars," "Cash Cows," "Question Marks," or "Dogs."

A niche strategy includes a narrowly defined audience, provision of a full range of services, differentiated services for the target audience and a market growth opportunity. In Exhibit 6–4, Stewart [1988] illustrates some 16 examples of parameters, available niches and differentiators for long-term care providers. Parameters may be combined such as geographical and demographic variables to pinpoint a niche. Retirement community providers could look for states with a high percent of the population over 65 to match up with states having an affluent population over age 65.

Lar [1986] lists inexpensive do-it-yourself marketing ideas for long-term care administrators. She explains 16 activities for $200 or less; 6 for up to $1,000; and 3 that cost more than $1,000.

Surveys continue to show that long-term care coverage is a "hot" new product (McIlrath, 1989).

Wellness Centers

Vital to the implementation of any activity is a clear understanding of terminology and perceived conceptions of what the terms mean to the public and to the provider. In considering adult health promotion programs, Mullen [1986] distinguishes between three terms: disease prevention, wellness, and health promotion.

Disease prevention aims to reduce the occurrence and severity of illness utilizing risk factors and behavioral change data. People are motivated to prevention activities to avoid the pain and suffering attendant with the illness.

Exhibit 6-4.   Niches, Parameters, and Differentiators for Long-Term Care Providers.

Parameter	Niches Available	Differentiators
Geography	High elderly population High growth area	Regional lifestyles Familiarity of environment Accessibility for visitors
Income Demographics	Retirement community Home care	Quality of life Social well-being Preventive medicine Familiarity of surroundings Emergency response time
Level of Care	Transitional	Intensity of services Emergency response time
Time Divided	Day care or shift care Episodic, short-stay Episodic, long-stay	Convenience to commute Administrative burden Comfort Adequacy of services Emergency response time
Disease-Specific	Vascular Coronary Alzheimer's Rheumatoid	Emergency response time Cardiac conditioning Accountability Close supervision Advanced technologies Ease of manual tasks/locomotion Specialized facilities services
Ethnic	Hispanic Old World Asian	Menu Language Traditional medicine Religion
Business Relationships	Third party payers Hospitals	Contract services Cost Relief from fixed costs Profit contribution

Source: From "Finding the right niche for service," by J.M. Stewart, 1988, *Provider, 14*[6], 7. Reprinted with permission of the American Health Care Association.

"Wellness is described as attitudes and activities which improve the quality of life and expand the potential for higher levels of functioning." Contrary to disease prevention, people engage in wellness programs to enhance their successful existence.

Health promotion is considered to be a combination of disease prevention and wellness programs.

Mullen's point is that activities labeled as wellness programs aim solely at the prevention of disease. Even though the marketing strategies highlight the word "wellness," Mullen feels that wellness, as defined, is a missing component of many health promotion campaigns. Specific examples of wellness goals could include minimizing the tensions of urban living, strengthening the family unit, encouraging fellowship in community life, and fostering human dignity. As Dunn [1961] and others have suggested, communities and society need to promote lifestyles conducive to high-level wellness.

If Mullen's definition is accepted, wellness centers need to redefine their market segment, their rationale for changing behavior and their implementation techniques.

Nurse Entrepreneuring

Starting with changing behavior, the National League for Nursing's marketing group promoted a new book, *Entrepreneuring: A Nurse's Guide to Starting a Business* [Vogel & Doleysh, 1988]. Advertising called attention to the opportunities for independent nursing health care practitioners, a radical behavior change for people traditionally employed by institutions. After that hurdle, the promotion links marketing and implementation with "down-to-earth step-by-step instructions" in a nurse's guide to starting a business. Personal experiences, extensive research, sample contracts, marketing tools, and self-assessment exercises shows the nurse "how to survive and thrive in your own business."

Continuing in that vein, planners can now return to considering implementation techniques such as the newspaper reporter's basic who, what, where, when, why, and how. However, the planner will have the benefit of an understanding of how to change behavior, product lines, market segmentation, and market research.

IMPLEMENTATION TECHNIQUES AND METHODS

Implementation Worksheet

In its simplest form, an implementation worksheet answers the basic questions. Rudyard Kipling spelled it out in verse in "The Elephant's Child:"

> I keep six honest serving men
> (they taught me all I Know);
> Their names are WHAT and WHY and WHEN
> And HOW and WHERE and WHO.

For each implementation task/activity, the following questions must be answered in detail:

- Who does what for whom?
- In what order and when?
- With what resources?

Exhibit 6–5 lists the typical steps in the development of an implementation strategy. Note that the steps include a logical determination of dates [Step #6,7] and responsible persons [Steps # 1,2,11].

Translating the steps in the development of an implementation strategy into actuality, Exhibit 6–6 illustrates plans for a generic countywide detection and treatment center. This worksheet could be for diabetes detection and treatment or for TB, cancer, glaucoma, or a host of other diseases/conditions. Targeted to a specific audience, this generic model takes place within the governmental agency and is solely administered for county resources and services. If the program was linked to local physician participation, there would have to be steps to

Exhibit 6-5. Steps in the Development of Implementation Strategy.

1. Specify clearly who does what for whom.
2. Select one person to be responsible for the overall program and for coordination with all others carrying out specified tasks.
3. Identify all prerequisite steps before initiating the program such as written promotional materials, equipment acquisition, volunteer training, written operational manuals and treatment protocols.
4. List the steps in their sequential order.
5. Integrate missing steps into #4 as they are discovered.
6. Determine the date when each step should begin and end.
7. Check the dates to assure that enough time has been allowed for the completion of each step in the sequential order.
8. Where possible, consult and communicate with all organizations and individuals affected by the program to identify potential problems, opportunities or misunderstandings.
9. Specify what resources will be needed and their source.
10. Identify any constraints and how they will be addressed.
11. Affirm that all individuals and organizations know exactly what is expected of them and by whom.

Exhibit 6-6.   Generic Implementation Worksheet for A Countywide Detection and Treatment Center.

Activity: Develop a county detection and treatment center
Constraints: Residents of the county have to be stimulated to come in and to undertake follow-up. Deadline 1/1 of next year.

Implementation Strategy: [Who Does What]	[When]
1. Director of Ambulatory Services develops proposal for detection/treatment center	1/1
2. County Board funds proposal	3/1
3. County renovates facilities	6/1
4. Director hires staff, including administrator and medical director	6/15
5. Administrator and medical director develop protocols and procedures, including special effort to motivate residents to participate and to follow-up	8/15
6. Administrator acquires equipment and supplies	8/15
7. Data specialist develops patient record forms	9/15
8. Health educator develop education materials	9/15
9. Staff and volunteers are trained by medical director, health educator and head nurse	10/1
10. Administrator test methods and materials with county residents	10/15
11. Staff begins detection and treatment services to county residents	11/15
12. Administrator evaluates detection and treatment services	11/15

Exhibit 6-7.   Strategic Health Planning Activity Worksheet.

Objective: Increase the number of volunteers by 33 percent by August 1, 1991

1 Task or acitivity	2 Person responsibile	3 Completion date	4 Approved?	5 Comments/Constraints
Media campaign	W. Hather	January 4, 1991	Yes—vital to work of agency.	Work with educational TV stations and public service directors at others.
1. Gather information on what types of volunteers are needed where.	S. Sallace	September 9, 1990		Use initial questionnaire as a starting point.
2. Produce TV spots	Subcontract to Hot Shots, Inc.	November 30, 1990		
3. Distribute TV spots to appropriate TV stations.	B. Speedy	December 27, 1990		Match volunteer TV spots with areas where people are needed as noted in Step #1.

coordinate the detection and treatment with the local doctors and their patients. That would mean coordination steps, referral procedure steps, and follow-up steps.

Exhibit 6–7 is another example of an activity worksheet. This media campaign activity seeks to increase the number of volunteers in a health program by 33 percent by a specific date. Note the specific identification of responsible persons, the completion dates and the comments/constraints column. In addition, this activity worksheet also confirms the fact that the Social Security Agency has the appropriate authority to undertake the task.

Action Plan for AIDS Education

In a seven-step approach to educating people at risk for AIDS, four components are linked to seven steps [actions] and the options to consider within each step [Chelimsky, 1988] [Exhibit 6–8]. Note that this action plan could be enhanced with specifics such as who will be responsible for each step and details about the methods and techniques. In addition, legislative and regulatory policies regarding confidentiality and antidiscrimination must be integrated into the strategic planning choices [Gostin, 1989]. Of course, a timetable can fix responsibilities and allow for monitoring the actions.

In considering the target group, planners need to decide exactly who will be targeted. Do you want to disseminate a broad message for all adolescents or a relevant message for teenage runaways? Do you want to reach all minority adults or mainly those at high risk for drug use? Experience indicates that the more precisely the target group is defined, the more effective the implementation campaign is likely to be.

Group characteristics aid to determine exactly why the segmented audience needs AIDS education. Attributes to evaluate and weigh for their implications for access and acceptance could include urgency due to risk behaviors, capabilities related to educational background or

Exhibit 6-8.   Seven-Step Approach in AIDS Education.

Component		Step	Options to Consider
TARGET GROUP		Decide exactly who will be targeted	Race / ethnicity Community Age bracket Drug-user friendship network
GROUP CHARACTERISTICS		Decide exactly why the targeted group needs AIDS education	Risk behavior Capabilities Attitudes Cultural values AIDS awareness
MESSAGE	*Medium*	Decide which media are more likely to reach the target group	Mass Personal
	Information	Decide which facts on AIDS should be	Transmission Nontransmission Risk reduction methods Effectiveness of methods
	Skills	Provide the skills for behavior change	Interpersonal Practical
	Motivators	Offer persuasive reasons for reducing risk	Negative Positive
INTENDED OUTCOMES		Specify the intended outcomes of the effort	Knowledge Behavior change

Source: From *Educating people at risk for AIDS,* by E. Chelimsky, 1988, Washington, DC: Government Printing Office, GAO/T-PEMD-88-8.

understanding of English, attitudes and values, or level of AIDS awareness [Dawson, 1988]. Sharing of drug use paraphernalia could lead to an exchange of contaminated blood. "Survival sex," in which teenagers trade sex for food, money, or a place to sleep could expose them to high risk. Recent immigrants and illegal drug users may tend to avoid government-sponsored activities. All of these attributes must be contemplated in planning the action steps.

Message Content. Planning for the message component of the action plan requires informed decisions about the media most likely to reach the target group. Mass media can be chosen singly or in combination from among media such as radio, television, newspapers, magazines, brochures, bus or subway posters, and billboards in English and/or foreign languages. Communications research also guides the choice by noting that radio is especially effective for reaching teenagers while television appears to be a prime information source for blacks and Hispanics. Personal or face-to-face communication may be most effective if the message is delivered to the segmented target group by community leaders, celebrities, health experts, actors, classroom teachers, or trained peer group members.

With the large body of information available, planners must decide which facts on AIDS should be included in the message. Intravenous drug users should know about the modes of transmission and options available for treatment. Young school-age children and adults in general could be told about modes of nontransmission to dispel unfounded fears. People can be given information about AIDS risk reduction methods such as total abstinence from sex and illegal drugs, use of a condom, or the use of bleach to clean their drug paraphernalia. Importantly, the risk reduction message must also tell people how effective these measures are likely to be. This point is particularly relevant for those who fall into the high-risk target groups. Regardless of the message, the information must be presented in terms that are readily understandable. Obviously, sexual activity must be discussed. "Bodily fluids" need to be defined exactly since concerns about sweat and saliva cause confusion. There are three Spanish words for prophylactic: *condon, ule,* and *preservativo.* In addition, planners must decide on whether to use graphic language to achieve simple clarity. Some target groups may be distracted by the colorful words while for others the message will be the one sure way to make the facts understandable.

Changing Behavior. Skills needed to change behavior are vital to the implementation of an AIDS education program. Interpersonal skills teach high-risk groups to resist pressures to do illegal drugs or to have unprotected sex. "Just saying no" requires constructive bolstering by an individual's interpersonal skills. In addition, high-risk group members need to practice the practical skills to reduce the possibility of transmission such as how and when to clean drug paraphernalia, and how and when to use condoms. Effective mastery of these interpersonal and practical skills gives "empowerment" to high-risk individuals, especially those whose self-confidence or related experience is limited.

Both positive and negative motivators can be included in messages that offer persuasive reasons for reducing the risk of AIDS. Positive motivation could include prizes for scoring well on AIDS knowledge tests, vouchers to get into drug treatment programs, social approval for risk reduction, and "eroticizing" safe sex practices making them more attractive than riskier sex. Negative motivators could emphasize the degenerative and fatal nature of AIDS. However, communications research indicates that the effectiveness of fear is limited. Fear may effect short-term changes but may not be a factor in sustaining longer-term risk reduction. If the fear level is too high, the message may be counterproductive since people may become too frightened to think about AIDS at all.

Finally, planners need to specify the intended outcomes of the action plan. Implementation of an AIDS education program could aim to increase knowledge about AIDS, could seek to inculcate attitudes toward AIDS risk reduction, and ultimately look to change behavior. For at-risk people, behavior change is paramount while for people not at risk, prevention of the risk behavior in the first place is crucial.

Elements of Effective Messages. In summary, this proposed AIDS action plan requires a note of caution. Experience in related health areas reveals that the implementation techniques and methods still require refinement. People still smoke too much, still drink too much, and still eat too much. Research indicates [Chelimsky, 1988, p. 12] that the educational message is more likely to be effective if it is:

- *Credible*—Delivered through sources trusted by the target group and in the group's own words.
- *Clear*—Covers information, skills, and motivators neither more nor less explicit than they need to be.
- *Accessible*—Combines the mass and personal media that will reach the group.
- *Appropriate*—Designed with due attention to group values that are relevant and appealing to a well-defined group.

Flow Diagrams

If a planner is dealing with services to clients in a hospital, health center, or other type of facility, a diagram showing the flow of people through the system may be useful in implementation. Examine Exhibit 6–9 which details a flow diagram for new outpatients. Logically, the flow diagram directs attention to the manpower, materials, and funding required for each step in the process of moving through the outpatient service. Questions can be raised that fill in blanks in the implementation process. Start with the direct travel arrows and answer the following illustrative questions:

- Is there enough parking space for new patients?
- Do we need a shuttle bus from the distant parking area?
- Are there enough lights for night parking?
- Is a parking attendant needed?
- Do we need signs to direct patients?
- Is there an information desk in the vestibule?
- Does the control officer check for insurance coverage?
- How many interview cubicles are needed?
- Who does intake screening using what forms?
- Can we use physician assistants in clinic service?
- Where are laboratory specimens taken?
- Is medical social service available to all patients?
- Is there a discharge officer at check out?
- How do we decorate and equip the waiting room?
- Does the pharmacy have generic or brand drugs for sale?

These are only a few of the implementation questions that are triggered by using a flow diagram.

Another mode of working with the flow diagram entails listing the steps in the flow process and filling in the manpower, materials, and funding requirements:

Step	Manpower	Materials	Funding
Parking	Attendant	Minibus	Hospital budget
		Lights	Parking fees
Vestibule	Information	Signs	Hospital budget
	clerk	Phone	Volunteers
Control	Nurse	Phone	Hospital budget
	Messenger	Files	Volunteers
		Forms	

As each step is plotted, planners can add or delete activities and requirements as ideas occur. When all the arrows in the flow diagram are tracked through the process, the implementation effort should emerge fully documented answering the who, what, where, why, when, and how specifics for the total new outpatient program.

A computer system for hospital management developed by Klimek-Grzesiak and Stakowski [1986] in Poland has a patient traffic subsystem that gives data about free beds, length of stay, admissions, transfers, discharges, deaths, and patient identification information.

Exhibit 6-9.   Flow Diagram for New Outpatients.

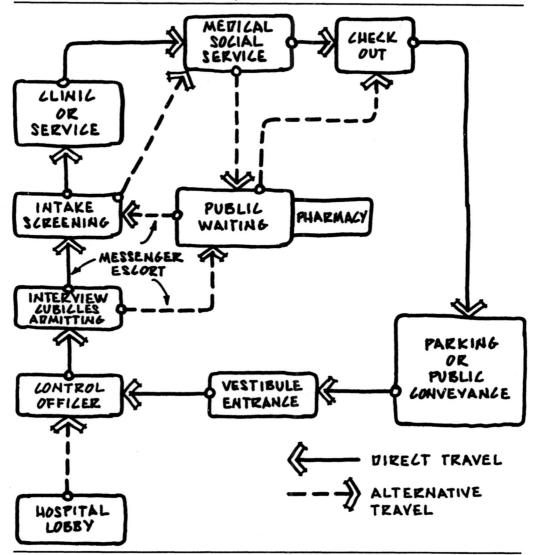

In addition, there are data subsystems for the pharmacy, dispensary, laboratories, archives, and hospital management staff.

In diagramming improvements in the Veteran's Administration patient incident investigation process, Exhibit 6–10 shows the flow with branching for the yes and no responses. Planners can determine the manpower, materials, and money needs by beginning with the incident report and considering the requirements at each step. Among the manpower needs could be a clerk to file incident reports, investigative and secretarial staff for the Board of Investigation, the Medical Center Director, the Regional Director and the Medical Inspector. Materials relate to the incident report form, the request for an investigation, report forms, review forms, recommendation forms, and the usual office supplies. Funds may be needed for

Exhibit 6-10. Patient Incident Investigative Process: Veterans Administration

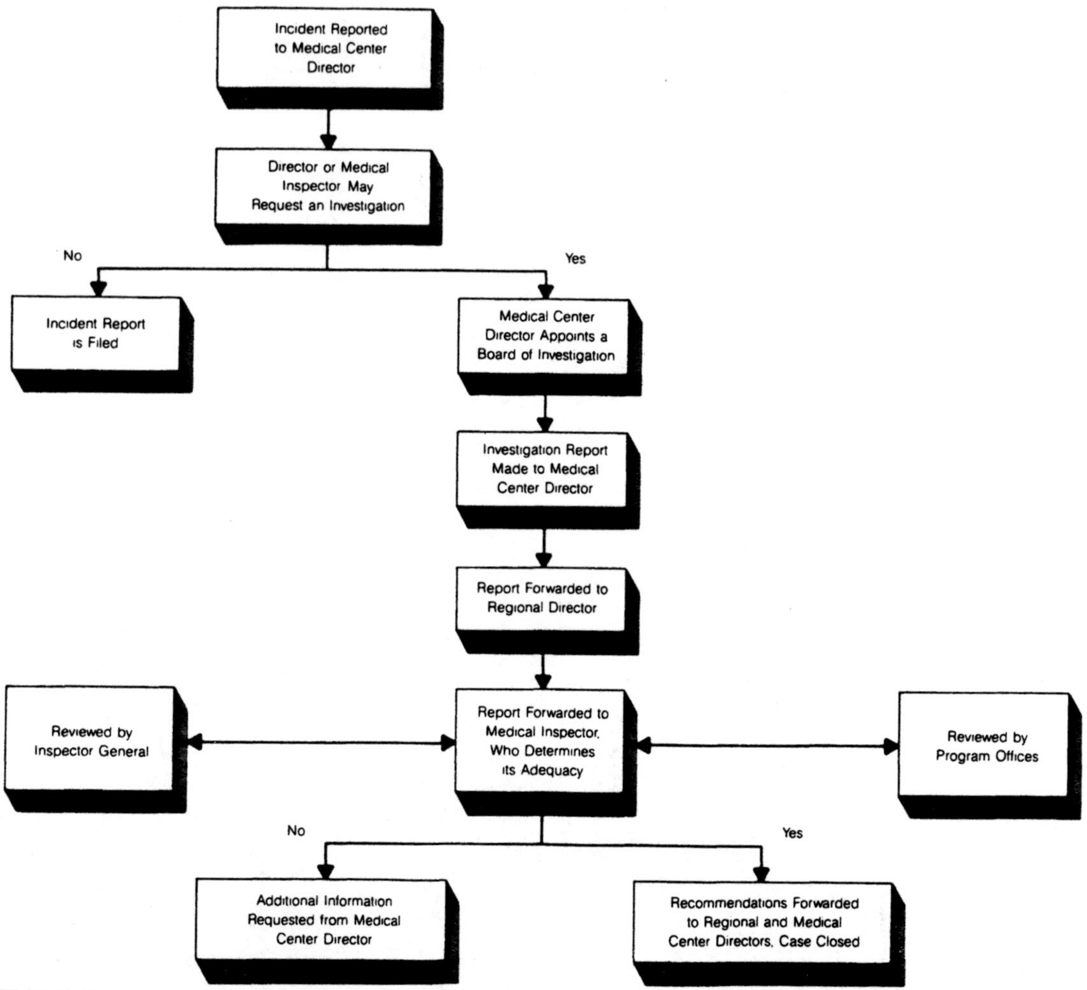

Flowchart of the Patient Incident Investigative Process:

Incident Reported to Medical Center Director → Director or Medical Inspector May Request an Investigation

- No → Incident Report is Filed
- Yes → Medical Center Director Appoints a Board of Investigation → Investigation Report Made to Medical Center Director → Report Forwarded to Regional Director → Report Forwarded to Medical Inspector, Who Determines its Adequacy
  - → Reviewed by Program Offices
  - Yes → Recommendations Forwarded to Regional and Medical Center Directors. Case Closed
  - No → Additional Information Requested from Medical Center Director
  - ↔ Reviewed by Inspector General

Source: From *VA health care. VA's patient injury control program not effective*, by R.L. Fogel, 1987, p. 36, Washington, DC: Government Printing Office, GAO/HRD 87-49. Reprinted by permission.

the additional staff, the additional printing, the postage, telephones, and office furniture. In this particular situation, existing VA staff may be used as well as existing forms and office furniture. Nevertheless, planners should still consider all the elements until there are decisions about who will supply what when.

Five steps are shown in the problem solving technique flow chart in Exhibit 6–11: problem specification, fact finding, goals and criteria evaluated for solutions, evaluation of solutions, and implementation. Note the use of the yes/no branching decisions, the dead end flow when rejection takes place and the feedback loop when data is incomplete or when redefinition is needed.

Referral Network Diagram

Similar to a flow chart, another type of implementation tool is a referral network diagram. This diagram identifies all the organizations involved with a specific problem and shows the referral relations between all the agencies and/or individuals. In addition, the services provided by each of the organizations are specified. Furthermore, the diagram can identify the various patient/client entry and exit points in the system. Since all the agencies and their services must be coordinated to implement a successful program, a referral network diagram aids considerably in defining operational aspects.

Exhibit 6–12 displays a referral network for unwed teenage pregnant girls. Note the two-way referrals in this system and the fact that some agencies appear to have more interaction than others such as the welfare department, the private family agency, the health department, and the adoption agency. There are also many client entry points into the system such as the school, the welfare department, the clergy, and private physicians. Possible services that could be provided by each of the referral agencies are also listed in Exhibit 6–12. It is also possible that the teenager may be directed into criminal or illegal channels. Obviously, the planner does not have to deal with the criminal/illegal element. However, the planner should be aware of its existence and the possible impact upon any implementation program being considered.

With the referral network diagram plotting the points of entry into the system, the services of each agency and the two-way referrals, planners can now ponder the components of a program to improve health care for the teenager during and after pregnancy and the newborn illegitimate child after delivery. Schools could implement an educational campaign. Private physicians could be provided with information to make appropriate referrals. Welfare and health departments could provide financial support and free well baby care if the teenager elects to keep the child. Hospitals may see the teenager who doesn't get into the system at the time of delivery and coordinate the services needed quickly as well as adoption activities if desired. Implementation of a program for the unwed pregnant teenager will obviously necessitate an intensive coordinative effort between all the involved parties.

Referral and Decision Network

Beginning with 1,000 hypothetical disabled beneficiaries, Exhibit 6–13 illustrates what happens to those individuals when they enter the vocational rehabilitation [VR] system. Note the flow through the various stages of the process along with the branching decisions. Organizational units and specific employees are indicated in addition to the decisions made at each level of the system. Reasons for the decisions are given along with the number of clients affected by that decision.

Exhibit 6-11.   Problem-Solving Technique Via a Flow Chart.

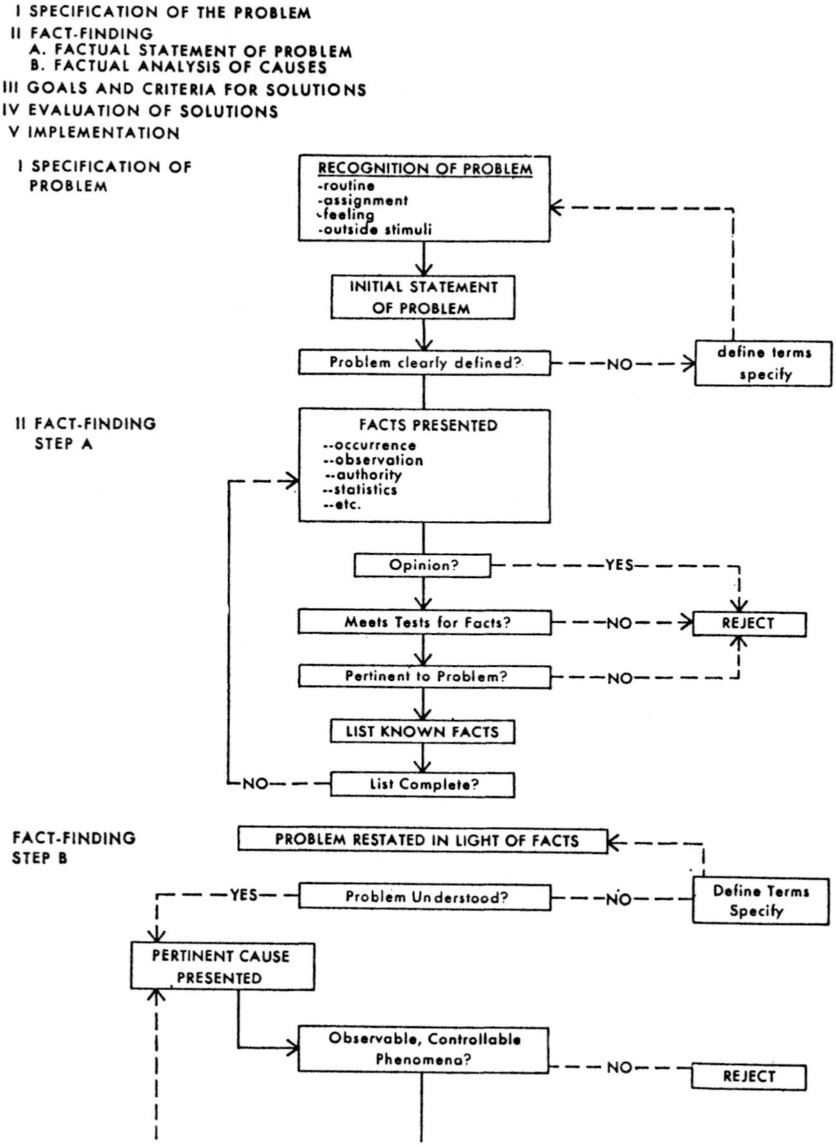

I SPECIFICATION OF THE PROBLEM
II FACT-FINDING
   A. FACTUAL STATEMENT OF PROBLEM
   B. FACTUAL ANALYSIS OF CAUSES
III GOALS AND CRITERIA FOR SOLUTIONS
IV EVALUATION OF SOLUTIONS
 V IMPLEMENTATION

I SPECIFICATION OF PROBLEM

RECOGNITION OF PROBLEM
-routine
-assignment
-feeling
-outside stimuli

INITIAL STATEMENT OF PROBLEM

Problem clearly defined? — NO — define terms specify

II FACT-FINDING STEP A

FACTS PRESENTED
--occurrence
--observation
--authority
--statistics
--etc.

Opinion? — — — YES — — —

Meets Tests for Facts? — — NO — → REJECT

Pertinent to Problem? — — NO — — —

LIST KNOWN FACTS

List Complete? — NO —

FACT-FINDING STEP B

PROBLEM RESTATED IN LIGHT OF FACTS

Problem Understood? — YES — — NO — Define Terms Specify

PERTINENT CAUSE PRESENTED

Observable, Controllable Phenomena? — — NO — — REJECT

286

Exhibit 6-11. *(Continued)*

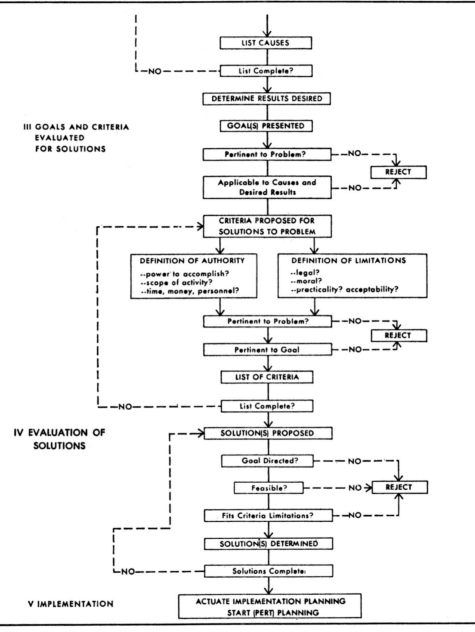

Source: From *Health program implementation through PERT,* edited by M.F. Arnold, 1966, pp. 28–29, San Francisco, CA: American Public Health Association. Reprinted with permission.

Exhibit 6-12.   Referral Network: Unwed Teenage Pregnant Girls.

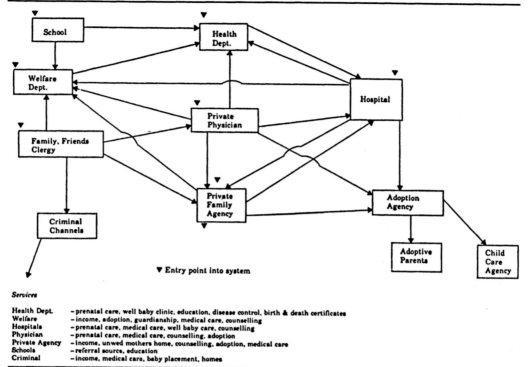

▼ Entry point into system

Services

Health Dept.	–prenatal care, well baby clinic, education, disease control, birth & death certificates
Welfare	–income, adoption, guardianship, medical care, counselling
Hospitals	–prenatal care, medical care, well baby care, counselling
Physician	–prenatal care, medical care, counselling, adoption
Private Agency	–income, unwed mothers home, counselling, adoption, medical care
Schools	–referral source, education
Criminal	–income, medical care, baby placement, homes

Source: Reprinted from *Health Planning and Public Accountability Workbook* by A.D. Spiegel and H.H. Hyman, p. 270, Aspen Publishers, Inc., Copyright 1976.

Concentrating on the points at which decisions are made, planners can determine appropriate implementation tasks that must be adequately resolved such as the following:

- Classification of problems at each decision point.
- Identification of questions and answers for employees.
- Isolation of possible actions to be taken.
- Stress when employee should seek assistance.
- Discover steps where training and supervision are needed.

When the VR counselor checks whether the client is an existing or prior case, there are three decisions to make: screen out as not promising [45 people]; a prior case not worth reopening [17 people]; or already an active client [14 people]. Planners could consider the guidelines needed for the VR counselor to arrive at any of those decisions. Do the counselors need training relative to what cases are promising or not worth reopening? When should supervisors be consulted? Even though contact is not attempted for 76 people, is there communication to those individuals?

After that initial decision by the VR counselor, there are a number of additional decision points involving the VR counselor and the claimant. Similar type questioning results in planners being able to arrange for the required personnel, materials, and funding at each decision point.

Utilizing a referral/decision network forces planners to develop a logical flow that is internally consistent, completely unambiguous, with decision points diagrammed and brought to a rational conclusion. With all the alternatives plotted as well, a comprehensive program emerges in the schematic. Once the referral/decision network is worked out, the planner can proceed to secure the resources, personnel, and funding to accomplish the implementation.

Timeline [Gantt Chart]

Graphing a timeline [Gantt chart] can help planners to place all the tasks within an operational framework. A single visual shows the overlap among the activities as well as the movement toward the end. With the years and months indicated, planners can monitor events and keep track of progress. Exhibit 6–14 illustrates 12 distinct tasks occurring during a nine-year time-frame plotted against a years/months timeline. Note that the exact month is indicated for each task and that years are included even when no tasks are concluded.

Who/What/When Computer Software Program

Chronos Software, Inc. [San Francisco, CA] created a computer program for people who manage people, projects, and time every day. Tasks can be categorized with the computer maintaining "To-Do lists" with four levels of priority. Priorities "A" and "B" carry forward each day until they are marked complete. Priority "C" is for one day only. Priority "D" is for delegated tasks and includes an automatic follow-up date reminder.

A people management view allows the computer to display the personnel involved, their projects and schedules [Exhibit 6–15]. Note that personnel are cross-referenced with co-workers, a company or unit can be identified, a phone number is listed and that there is a when, what, and description of the task. Planners will always know who is working on what and when it is due.

In a project management view, the computer displays the projects, the people involved, the milestones, and the deadlines [Exhibit 6–16]. Note that the task [brochure] is listed on top, the project manager is identified, the current and future days remaining for the task is given, a May through August calendar plots the timeline for the project with milestones marked, when and who and tasks are specified and milestones are described.

Project timecharts [Gantt] can be automatically created from daily calendar entries [Exhibit 6–17]. Tasks are listed on the left side and the May through July daily calendar shows milestones and expectations for each task.

In addition, the Who/What/When computer program has a "Meeting Maker" that allows planners to book group meetings for up to nine people at a time while checking and flagging any conflicting activities. Furthermore a "Daily Calendar" screen displays meetings, single time events, alarm reminders, and prioritized To-Do's. All the daily calendar entries are automatically cross-referenced into the people, project, and time management data banks.

Who/What/When computer software incorporates a number of the implementation tools already noted. This program is just one example of the type of advanced, but relatively simple-to-use, technology available to planners.

Exhibit 6-13. What Happens to Vocational Rehabilitation Disability Referrals?

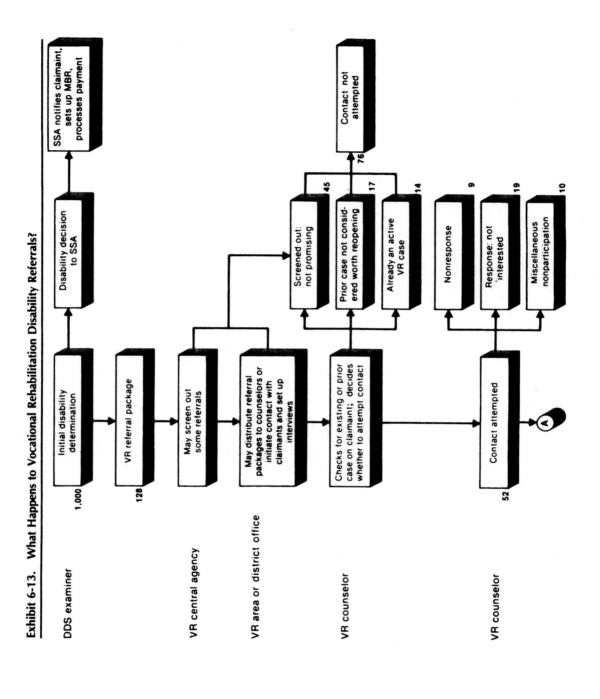

290

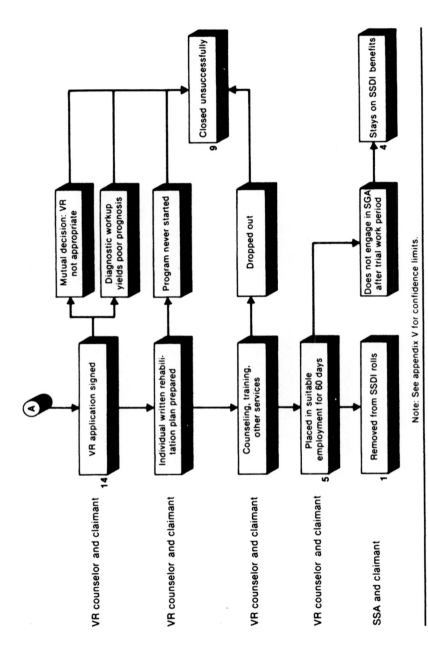

VR counselor and claimant

VR counselor and claimant

VR counselor and claimant

VR counselor and claimant

SSA and claimant

Note: See appendix V for confidence limits.

Source: From *Social security: Little success achieved in rehabilitating disabled beneficiaries,* by R.L. Fogel, 1987, pp. 36–37. Washington, DC: Government Printing Office, GAO/HRD 88-11. Reprinted by permission.

Exhibit 6-14.   Modernization Time Schedule: Veterans Benefits Department.

CALENDAR YEAR	1986	1987		1988		1989		1990		1991	1992	1993	1994
MONTH	8 9 10 11 12	8 9 10 11 12		2 3 4 5 6 7 8 9 10 11 12		3 4 5 6 7 8		5 6 7 8 9 10		12	1 2	9	9 11

1.   Define Goals and Objectives

2.   Identify Constraints

3.   Analyze DVB Programmatic Functions

4.   Analyze DVB's Current Operating Environment

5.   a.) Identify and Evaluate Improvement Opportunities

     b.) Analyze and Implement Short-term Projects

6.   Conduct Software Conversion Study

7.   Prepare Functional Requirements Document

8.   Identify and Evaluate Technical Alternatives

9.   Develop Acquisition Strategy for Selected Alternative

10. Conduct Competitive Solicitation(s)

11. Test and Implement Selected Alternative

12. Conduct Post-Implementation Review

Source: From *Use of information technology by VA's Department of Veterans Benefits*, by M.D. Quasney, 1988, Washington, DC: Government Printing Office, GAO IT-IMTEC-88-6. Reprinted by permission.

Exhibit 6-15.   Who/What/When People View.

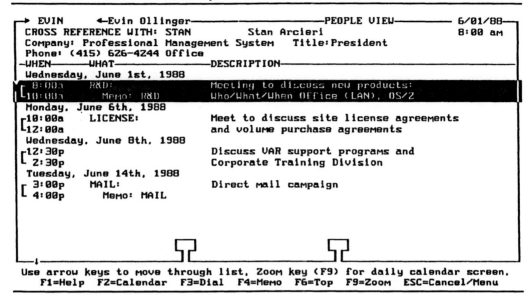

```
→ EVIN      ←Evin Ollinger──────────────PEOPLE VIEW──────── 6/01/88─
  CROSS REFERENCE WITH: STAN      Stan Arcieri              8:00 am
  Company: Professional Management System   Title:President
  Phone: (415) 626-4244 Office
─WHEN────────WHAT──────────DESCRIPTION──────────────────────────────
  Wednesday, June 1st, 1988
  ┌ 8:00a    R&D:          Meeting to discuss new products:
  └10:00a    Memo: R&D     Who/What/When Office (LAN), OS/2
  Monday, June 6th, 1988
  ┌10:00a    LICENSE:      Meet to discuss site license agreements
  └12:00a                  and volume purchase agreements
  Wednesday, June 8th, 1988
  ┌12:30p                  Discuss VAR support programs and
  └ 2:30p                  Corporate Training Division
  Tuesday, June 14th, 1988
  ┌ 3:00p    MAIL:         Direct mail campaign
  └ 4:00p    Memo: MAIL



              ┌┐              ┌┐
  ┌─┘         └┘              └┘
  └─┘────────────────────────────────────────────────────────────────
```

Use arrow keys to move through list. Zoom key (F9) for daily calendar screen.
F1=Help F2=Calendar F3=Dial F4=Memo F6=Top F9=Zoom ESC=Cancel/Menu

Source: From the WHO-WHAT-WHEN program. Reprinted with permission of Chronos Software, Inc., 1500 16th Street San Francisco, CA 94103.

Exhibit 6-16.   Who/What/When Project View.

```
┌──────────┐ ┌────
│ BROCHURE: │ │          PROJECT VIEW    Wednesday  6/01/88  8:00 am
└           └─┘
  DAY NO. 17    DAYS LEFT 61      MANAGER: Evin Ollinger
  MayJun              Jul                              Aug
  29-4    9-11   12-18  19-25  26-2   3-9   10-16  17-23  24-30  31-6   7-13
  SMTWTFSSMTWTFSSMTWTFSSMTWTFSSMTWTFSSMTWTFSSMTWTFSSMTWTFSSMTWTFSSMTWTFS
  ▓▓▓█▓▓▓▓▓▓▓▓▓▓▓▓▓▓▓▓▓▓▓▓M▓▓▓▓▓▓▓▓▓▓▓▓▓▓▓▓3▓▓▓▓▓▓▓▓▓▓▓▓▓▓▓M
  ─WHEN────────WHO──────────TASKS FOR: Brochure for new products─────
  Thursday, June 2nd, 1988
  ┌10:00a   JEFF    Others-2   * Assign art/discuss deadlines
  └11:00a
  ┌ 2:30p   MARY T  Others     Layout assignment/discuss deadlines
  └ 3:30p
  Friday, June 3rd, 1988
  ┌ 3:00p   JASON   Others     Copy writing assignment/discuss deadlines
  └ 4:00p
  Wednesday, June 15th, 1988
  TO:DO  C EVIN               MILESTONE: Brochure for new products
                             Review first drafts of copy, art, layout

  └─┘─┴─────────────────────────────────────────────────────────────
```

Use arrow keys to move through list. Press "Zoom" (F9) for daily calendar.
F1=Help F2=Calendar F3=Dial F4=Memo F6=Top F9=Zoom F10=Save ESC=Quit

Source: From the WHO-WHAT-WHEN program. Reprinted with permission of Chronos Software Inc., 1500 16th Street San Francisco, CA 94103.

Exhibit 6-17.   Who/What/When Daily Calendar.

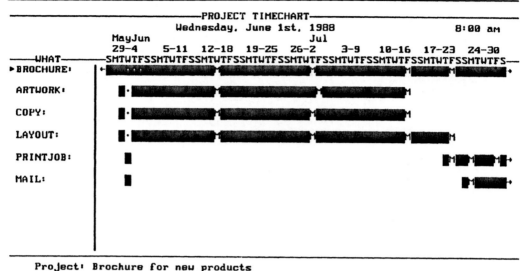

Source: From the WHO-WHAT-WHEN program. Reprinted with permission of Chronos Software Inc., 1500 16th Street San Francisco, CA 94103.

Program Evaluation and Review Technique [PERT]

As a tool, PERT enables the planner, particularly during the implementation phase, to create a road map that diagrams the flow of events toward a conclusion. Levin and Kirkpatrick [1966] list 30 methods for project planning and control using PERT. However, PERT or any other variation of this management technique, is not a panacea or mechanized answer to planning.

Exhibit 6–18 diagrams program implementation through PERT. Note that there are six steps indicated with feedback loops when clarification is required if a "no" answer is given to questions. In the section on ordering precedent events, if the PERT diagram is not logically constructed there may be inoperative loops, events that dangle in unconnected space, or events that cross over into other events. Time estimates are determined by the formula in the determination of activity time section:

$$\text{time estimate} = \frac{\text{minimum time} + 4[\text{normal time}] + \text{maximum time}}{6}$$

A critical path for the PERT network is determined by noting events that must occur before the final event. Usually, the critical path involves the greatest amount of time.

PERT's graphic network analysis consists of the following:

- Development of a model or activity network of a program or any subpart of the task.
- An evaluation of the network making adjustments to assure a minimum of risk in achieving objectives on time and within cost limitations if the implementation of the PERT plan is followed.
- Use of the network to monitor and control the project.

Exhibit 6-18. Program Implementation Using PERT [Program Evaluation and Review Technique].

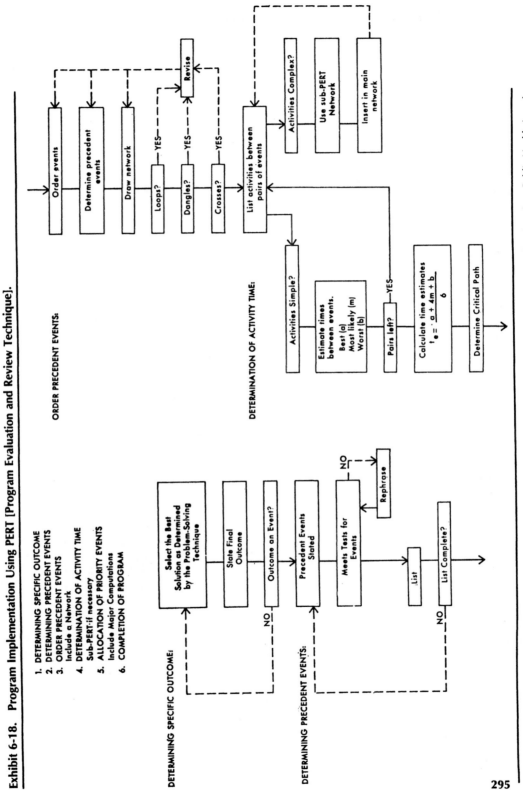

1. DETERMINING SPECIFIC OUTCOME
2. DETERMINING PRECEDENT EVENTS
3. ORDER PRECEDENT EVENTS
   Include a Network
4. DETERMINATION OF ACTIVITY TIME
   Sub-PERT: if necessary
5. ALLOCATION OF PRIORITY EVENTS
   Include Major Computations
6. COMPLETION OF PROGRAM

ORDER PRECEDENT EVENTS:

Order events

Determine precedent events

Draw network

Loops? — YES

Dangles? — YES

Crosses? — YES

Revise

List activities between pairs of events

Activities Complex?

Use sub-PERT Network

Insert in main network

DETERMINATION OF ACTIVITY TIME:

Activities Simple?

Estimate times between events.
Best (a)
Most likely (m)
Worst (b)

Pairs left? — YES

Calculate time estimates

$$t_e = \frac{a + 4m + b}{6}$$

Determine Critical Path

DETERMINING SPECIFIC OUTCOME:

Select the Best Solution as Determined by the Problem-Solving Technique

State Final Outcome

Outcome an Event?   NO

Precedent Events Stated

Meets Tests for Events

Rephrase   NO

List

List Complete?   NO

DETERMINING PRECEDENT EVENTS:

295

Source: From *Health program implementation through PERT*, edited by M.F. Arnold, 1966, pp. 44–45, San Francisco, CA: American Public Health Association, pp. 44–45. Reprinted with permission.

Exhibit 6-19. PERT Network for Developing an Open Heart Surgery Unit.

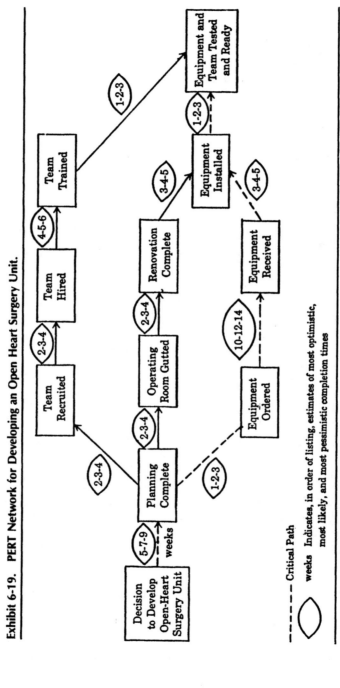

----- Critical Path

◇ weeks Indicates, in order of listing, estimates of most optimistic, most likely, and most pessimistic completion times

Source: From *Management practices for the health professional*, by B.B. Longest, Jr., 1976, p. 101. Reston, VA: Reston Publishing Company. Reprinted with permission of Appleton & Lange.

Once the decision is made, PERT is a tool that creates a structured framework with a logical, ordered plan of means to an end already agreed upon by the policy makers. Exhibit 6–19 illustrates a PERT network for the development of an open heart surgery unit. Starting with the decision to create the unit, the PERT diagram traces events related to personnel, equipment, and space. Note that the final event is having the equipment and team tested and ready to operate. This PERT network also indicates the critical path and the most optimistic, most likely, and most pessimistic completion times for each event.

Role Gridding

In a situation where power is widely diffused and public visibility high, planners need to make sure that everyone whose participation is desirable or necessary is appropriately involved in the planning process. Role gridding is a method of defining and recording that relationship among the following three elements:

1. A set of tasks to be performed.
2. A list of participants who will be contributing to one or more of these tasks.
3. The roles that the participants may exercise in relation to tasks.

Basically, this technique convenes a task-oriented committee of major participants in the planning process. That committee negotiates their own tasks and roles as well as anticipated tasks and roles for other prospective participants in the planning. A "role grid" is the written summary of the committee meeting. Exhibit 6–20 illustrates a "role grid" in a state department of mental health project re drug abuse planning. Actions are run off against the actors involved in the projects. A completed role grid shows three types of information: [a] participants involved for any given task or step in the planning, [b] involvement of any given participant in any of the tasks, [c] role of each participant in each of the planning tasks emerges as the spaces in the grid are filled in. Roles are represented by the initials as defined below:

A *prime mover* [PM] initiates the process, coordinates and facilitates activities, and follows through with implementation to completion of the task. This PM has the authority of his agency and other participants must recognize that authority as adequate and be acceptable to them.

A *contributor* [CT] suggests ideas and needs, contributes data, and points out potential problems. CTs may do task work but do not formally take part in the approval or implementation process itself.

A *major source of evaluation* [MSE] performs a review and comment function rather than contributing to the initial planning. This MSE specialist makes a detailed appraisal of material in terms of soundness, completeness, value, and relevance to specific areas of concern. An MSE may contribute ideas for improvement, reworks material as needed, and secures necessary approvals.

A *concurrer* [CC] is a person in a key position whose awareness, review, participation, and future cooperation is desired. However, CCs cannot literally stop the planning process. CCs review materials to determine their impact on their own particular areas of interest, concur with recommendations as applicable, and discuss disagreements in order to reach a final resolution.

Approvers [A] do have the authority and power to veto results of the planning process. In

Exhibit 6-20. Role Gridding Model: State Mental Health Department Drug Abuse Program.

ACTIONS

Actors & Roles	Planning Design	Leadership	Mobilize Activities	Assess Needs	Priorities & Recommendations Regional	District	State	Division	DMH Review	Gov.	A-95
										OK	OK
Local Programs and/or Services	CC			CT	CT	CT	MSE	CT			
Local Govt.	CC		CC	CT	CT	CT	MSE				
DMH Drug Plan Coordinator	CT	CC	PM/A	A	MSE	MSE	CT	MSE			
DMH Section Coordinators	CT		CT	CT	CT	CT	CT				
DMH Regional Prog. Develop. Specialists	CC		CT	PM	CT	CT	CT				
Regional Advisory Councils	CC		CC	CT	PM/A	MSE	MSE	MSE	MSE		
Planning Agencies	CC		CC	CT	CC						
District MH Boards	CC		CC	CT	PM/A	MSE	MSE	MSE	MSE		

Statewide Inter-
agency Council   CC -- CT

State Level
Data Sources   MSE --- CT

State Drug Abuse
Advisory Council   CC ------------------------------- CT -------- PM/A -- MSE ------ MSE - MSE

DMH Div. Directors PM ------ PM/A ----- MSE --------- MSE -------- MSE ------ PM/A ----- MSE - MSE

DMH Director   A ---------------------------------- MSE --------- MSE -------- PM/A -MSE ----- PM ---- PM

Attorney General   -- MSE

Governor   CT -- A

A-95 Agency   MSE ----------------------------------- MSE -------------- MSE

State Health
Coordinating
Council   CC --- CC ---- CC

US Dept. of
Health & Human
Services   CT -- A

A = Approver   CC = Concurrer   CT = Contributor   MSE = Major Source of Evaluation   PM = Prime Mover

299

this obviously critical role, As can give the final go-ahead or sanction, can send the plan back for reworking, or can flatly disapprove. When a number of agencies are involved, there may be an ad hoc committee acting as the approver as contrasted to a single approver when only one agency is involved.

In essence, the key to role gridding is negotiating and defining the role of each participant in each planning task in a mutually agreed and consistent manner.

Gaming and Simulation

In using gaming and simulation, the planner seeks to duplicate a real-world situation while still maintaining the attraction of a game or drama. Monopoly is a familiar game that imitates a real estate market as players strive to purchase Boardwalk or Park Place. Simulations can be seen regularly on TV as actors portray a news or historical event.

Gaming/simulation techniques allow planners to test a variety of alternative implementation strategies and to learn from the miniature dry run of the proposed activity. With the knowledge garnered from the game and/or simulation, the planner can then actually implement the real-life project. Importantly, gaming/simulations can reveal the glitches and bugs inherent in the activity and allow planners to prepare resolutions to the difficulties. That vital characteristic occurs whether the game/simulation is conducted with human participants or with computers.

A game is defined as any contest [play] among adversaries [players] operating under constraints [rules] for an objective [winning]. A simulation is a representation of reality wherein participants assume roles that are assigned to them and then engage in scheduled meetings to attempt to define the nature and extent of the problem and to find resolutions. Information on a wide variety of games/simulations can be secured from the American Society for Training and Development [Washington, DC], the Association for Business Simulation and Experimental Learning [Statesboro, GA], and University Associates [San Diego, CA].

Gaming/simulations have a number of common structural components such as:

- Participants cast in *roles* with written background material for each "actor's" characterization.
- *Interactions* between those participants in their *roles*.
- *Rules* governing the interaction between the participants while playing their roles.
- *Goal[s]* with respect to which the interactions occur.
- A *criterion* for determining the attainment of the goal, which also indicates the end of the game/simulation.

In discussing METRO-APEX, a gaming/simulation for exploring urban issues relating to air pollution, James and McGinty [1981] delineated the following criteria for "real-world experience" in a laboratory community during the simulation:

- Game to be comprehensive in design and content creating a dynamic simulation dealing with complex urban systems.
- "Real-world" data to be used within models allowing for system-wide effects of participant's decisions.

- Sociopolitical and technical aspects to be included to allow participants to communicate with the public. Role reversal experiences to be included so participants can play the role of the adversary.
- Simulation to contain sufficient technical, legal, and administrative information to provide self-contained system experiences and to stimulate additional research by participants.
- Game to emphasize the allocation of the limited resources of materials, money and personnel in a competitive environment.

A weakness of this technique may be that all the participants know that nothing is really at stake in the game/simulation. Nevertheless, this technique can be worthwhile by making the participants feel that their efforts will yield information that can be adapted to the real-life situation [Broadwell, 1987]. Following are examples of games and/or simulations.

Care for Patients with Renal Failure. In caring for patients with irreversible renal failure, Davies and Davies [1986] discuss the use of interactive microcomputer techniques in "time slicing" simulations, that is, discrete event simulations. Input data for the simulation could include resource restraints which could be altered as well as additional data that could be changed interactively. Simulation outputs could respond to patient numbers, resource availability, resource utilization and waiting lists with all those factors related to costs [Exhibit 6–21].

Facility Decision Support System. Beech, Brough, and Shaw [1985] describe a computerized decision support system to aid and abet planners that uses a database and a simulation model. Planning tasks included the transfer of inpatients, the reduction of a school of nursing, and the rationalization of acute care services. A simulation model gains input from questions and answers at the terminal about the following database areas: inpatient activity by speciality, opening and closing of wards, revision of operating schedules, rearrangements of beds by speciality, staffing changes, and nursing school alterations. A number of scenarios can be tested with this model that pay particular attention to feasibility and the revenue consequences for other parts of the system. In the case of the transfer of inpatients, the resolution changed from

Exhibit 6-21.   Input and Output Data from Health Services Simulation.

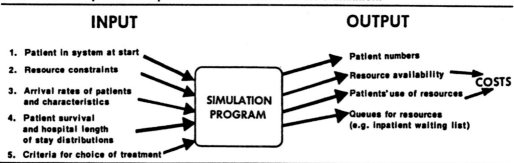

Source: From "Using simulation to plan health service resources: discussion paper," by R. Davies & T. Davies, 1986, *Journal of the Royal Society of Medicine*, 79[3], 154–157. Reprinted with permission.

extending the existing lease for the facility to closing the hospital after 20 different options were generated by the simulation model. For the nursing school problem, the simulation developed a number of scenarios linking student enrollment to patterns of ward staffing arriving at a gradual reduction of teaching staff. Regarding acute care services, the simulation indicated direct correlations between revenue reductions and modifications in the services provided and a shifting of acute care to the general hospitals. This simulation "decision support system has proved a major aid for managers and clinicians involved in planning hospital services . . . [Beech et al., 1985].

In line with decision support systems, Rash [1986] opts for using "What if . . . ?" scenarios that combine data + tools + methodologies + interpretation to yield the vital strategic information. With particular reference to health care marketing choices, Rash states that "decision support systems give planners and managers the most complete available map to find the roads that lead to success."

Child Mortality Simulation. A mathematical optimization model was used by Pradilla, Barnum, Barlow, and Fajardo [1987] to make policy choices regarding activities to reduce morbidity and mortality in three childhood age groups: neonatal, infant, and toddler. There were 42 interventions and seven socioeconomic variables used in the simulations. Intervention activities for pregnant women, mothers and children included laboratory testing for diseases, follow-up treatment, immunizations, nutritional supplements, early detection, and institutional or home care as required. After gathering information on the intervention impacts, costs, and baseline data for each specific problem, this type of mathematical simulation can be used in an analysis of the cost-effectiveness of suggested implementation activities.

Strategic Planning Computer Game for Administrators. Feldstein's [1986] computer game seeks to upgrade decision-making skills in strategic planning and forecasting for health care administrators, hospital trustees, medical staff, and students.

A game scenario includes one community served by five hospitals: a university facility, an investor-owned hospital, two voluntary nonprofit hospitals in a multihospital system controlled by a religious order, and one more voluntary nonprofit facility. This community divides into four geographic zones with varying population levels, growth rate, and uneven distribution of Medicare, Medicaid, Blues, commercial insurance, and self-pay classes of payers. All five hospitals are located in three of the zones with a fourth zone having no hospital but a rapid growth. One area has both the university hospital and one religious voluntary nonprofit facility. This area has an older population with more Medicare and Medicaid patients resulting in higher inpatient utilization. However, any of these givens can be changed by the referee at the beginning of the game.

Each team is responsible for one of the five hospitals. All participants in the game receive a Player's Guide with additional background information on the community, the hospitals, balance sheets, expenses, and a description of the decisions each team can make. It is suggested that eight rounds of play be scheduled over two days to avoid decision-making pressures placed upon the participants. After ending the game, the referee leads an evaluation session pinpointing rationales for decisions using guideline questions that emphasize strategic planning and forecasting principles.

Decisions by the participants relate to choices to be made in 14 critical strategic planning areas:

Utilization forecasts
Market research reports
Hospital inpatient prices
Outpatient prices
Fund drives, fund transfers
Constructing beds
Financing decisions
Dropping particular services
Hospital investments
Building inpatient satellites
Skilled nursing facilities
Ambulatory care clinics
Retirement centers for seniors
Home health agencies

Beginning in the third round of the game, a community newsletter will be distributed periodically to the players. Announcements about events impacting on decisions relate to Medicare DRGs, Preferred Provider Organizations [PPOs], insurance coverage for outpatient surgery, Medicare vouchers, hospices, Blue Cross HMOs, and change in Blue Cross payments to hospitals.

There is no doubt that this strategic planning computer game represents a "true life" situation. Modifications in Player Guidelines, Referee Guides and announcements provide conduits for integrating rapidly changing environmental factors into the simulation.

Computer GamePlan for Decision Making. GamePlan is a computer simulation utilizing theories on effective management regarding decision making and organizational behavior. While this particular software program deals with a business situation and an individual manager's goal of being promoted to vice-president, the applications to strategic planning are readily apparent. GamePlan works within distinct internal and external environmental variables such as differing corporate cultures, political power in organizations, personal and formal power, cooperation vs. coercion, individual credibility, and decision choices among 12 available actions.

This simulation begins with the player, a Manager of the End User Computing [EUC] group, who supervises two Analysts and who has 21 "credibility chips" to use. A Manager who amasses 50 chips gets promoted to vice president; losing all 21 chips gets the Manager fired. Based on effective management theory, actions taken by the Manager accumulate additive or subtractive chip payoffs.

There are only 12 cards [actions] that a player can take to achieve the goal. Exhibit 6–22 shows a computer frame of a traditional corporate culture with a time frame for each actor with the 12 cards for selection. This Exhibit also summarizes the actions. Note the similarity to strategic planning options as in problem identification and implementation [C], in resources assessment [B], in priority selection [F], in support for implementation [G and H], and in objective attainment [I and K]. Also note that a number of the actions may be repeated and the inferences to the planner's attention to the sociopolitical aspects of the corporate culture. Playing a card costs the Manager chips dependent upon favors requested, time, trust and budget. Chips are won when the card is complete based on the value of the action toward the ultimate goal.

A key to GamePlan is the environment of the simulated organization and four dramatically

Exhibit 6-22.   GamePlan Computer Menu and Summary of Cards.

```
Played\Complete: A0\0 B0\0 C0\0 D0\0 E0\0 F0\0 G0\0 H0\0 I0\0 J0\0 K0\0 L0\0

                |Year 1 |
Traditional     |February| March  | April  |  May   |  June  | July   |
----------------+---+---+--------------------------------------------+---+
A. Manager      |   |   | Select one of the following:               |   |
B.              |   |   |                                            |   |
----------------+---|   | ---> A.  IS Pilot                          |---+
C. Analyst      |   |   |      B.  User Implementation               |   |
D.              |   |   |      C.  Strategic Plan                    |   |
----------------+---|   |      D.  Briefing Paper                    |---+
E. Analyst      |   |   |      E.  Backbone Network                  |   |
F.              |   |   |      F.  Staff Steering Committee          |   |
----------------+---|   |      G.  User Steering Committee           |---+
Chip Counts 21    2 |   |      H.  Management Awareness Program       |
                    |   |      I.  Personal Computer Policy Statement |
                    |   |      J.  Information Center                 |
                    |   |      K.  Formal Charter                     |
                    |   |      L.  Additional Staff                   |
                    +----------------------------------------------------+
```

Play Card

```
<UP-ARROW>, <DOWN-ARROW>, or type letter; then <RETURN>
<BACKSPACE> to cancel
```

Summary of Cards

A. IS Pilot Implement systems for your EUC group and selected managers in the Information Systems department; serves as a showcase, test-bed and learning experience.

B. User Implementation Implement systems for a small group of user managers an assessment, justification of expenditures, design of systems, installation and training, and an optional evaluation of results. (May be repeated.)

C. Strategic Plan Publish a detailed document that describes the opportunities from EUC, systems architecture, implementation plans, and an image of the future. (May be repeated annually.)

D. Briefing Paper Publish a 10 to 12 page document ("white paper") that defines EUC and describes its many opportunities to corporation as a whole.

E. Backbone Network Select and install a backbone data communications network as a company-wide infrastructure to connect all existing and future user implementation sites and to distribute central information and services. (May be repeated for greater connectivity.)

F. Staff Steering Committee Form a steering committee made of representatives of the various staff groups in the Information Systems and Administration departments.

G. User Steering Committee Form a steering committee made of senior representatives of the various user groups.

H. Management Awareness Program Make a presentation to management on the potential of EUC and your progress to date. (May be repeated.)

I. Personal Computer Policy Statement Publish a document that describes purchasing, support and usage policies for personal computers.

J. Information Center Build a room where users can get help, request information from MIS systems, view demonstrations or work with EUC tools. (Provides monthly payoff.)

K. Formal Charter Request approval of an official charter statement for the EUC staff group. (Subject to approval. May be repeated to increase power. Provides monthly payoff.)

L. Additional Staff Request an additional analyst (headcount) for your EUC staff group. (May be repeated.)

Source: GamePlan software reprinted with permission of N. Dean Meyer and Associates Inc., 233 Mountain Road, Ridgefield, CT 06877.

different corporate personalities are identified: traditional, Consensus-driven, profit-center structured, and futurist. Certainly comparable with the structure of health care organizations, characteristics of those four corporate cultures are described in Exhibit 6–23.

Strategy is everything in GamePlan with rewards for the traditional player who "plans his work and works his plan" as well as for the player who practices "the politics of innovation."

A review of GamePlan in *PC Week* [DeJean, 1988], states: "It could be termed a computerized non-fiction adventure game. Or, educational software. Or, perhaps it's best described as a management textbook with all the examples taken from one's own experience. Take your pick."

SOCIOPOLITICAL INTERACTION IN IMPLEMENTATION

Since the real world does not always abide by rational logic, strategic planners must be alert to the social and political interactions that could impact upon implementation activities. Lewton [1989] cites numerous examples of the critical role of a facility's public relations personnel bridging the communication and misunderstanding gaps. Using telecommunications, Siktberg [1989] applies a high-tech tool in conjunction with community health planning and education. As shown in the gaming/simulation techniques, human factors can be integrated into planning situations.

Even though she focused on planning for mental health Mahaffey [1986] sheds light on sociopolitics as "a process of dealing with the interaction of the individuals and society and the allocation of resources in society. . . Society regulates through government in order to establish limits on how society will relate to individuals." Individual interaction in a case study of political ideology and local health planning in the United States indicated that things don't always work as anticipated. Fontana [1986] expected that there would be confrontation between consumers and professionals on a local Health Systems Agency Governing Board. However, he found that "health planning did not seem to be ideologically contentious . . . it was clear that the status of consumer or provider did not necessarily imply peculiar interests and perspectives." A generic question concerns whether or not a consumer is competent to make decisions on health care issues. Cynics may feel that the health care professional controls all the information and de facto co-opts the consumer. In any event, the inequity between the actors in sociopolitical situations does create unequal bargaining abilities.

Presenting the other side of the coin, Cherskov [1986] reported that the demise of the Health Policy and Resources Development Act of 1974 means that competing special interests will take over as federally sponsored health planning fades. An American Hospital Association official is quoted as saying that "competition will allow for the appropriate distribution of services."

Models of Health Care Governance

In discussing the goverance of health care organizations, Starkweather [1986] delineates three conceptualizations: a corporate model, a nonprofit enterprise, and an organization using exchange theory with multiple centers of bureaucratic power. Suggesting sociopolitical areas, Starkweather arrives at five issues for further investigation: relative power, accountability, composition and motivation, hierarchic roles, and performance.

Exhibit 6-23.   Four GamePlan Corporate Sociocultural Descriptions.

Traditional:
* Organized by traditional functional areas
* Staff has legitimate power
* Decision-making top-down
* Good at control: cost and product line
* Poor at innovation, risk-averse
* Medium at integration of product line
* Industries: mature, slow-growth, commodity products, price competition, regulated industries, government

Consensus-driven:
* Organized by market views, stakeholders, and matrixes
* Layers of corporate staff selling to each other
* Decision-making middle-out
* Decisions by consensus, committees
* Good at integration of product line
* Medium at cost control, innovation
* Poor at market niche response
* Industries: integrated product line; eg computer systems

Profit-center structured:
* Not holding company, but organized into independent units
* Most of staff is decentralized to profit-centers
* Decision-making middle out by independent profit-center managers
* Good at responding to market niches
* Poor at product line integration
* Medium at cost control, innovation
* Industries: niche tailoring; eg consumer marketing

Futurist:
* Organized around personalities
* Staff lean, little power
* Decision-making at top by entrepreneurs
* Good at innovation, risk-preferred
* Poor at control of costs, product line integration
* Industries: fast growth, leading edge, start-ups, personality based; (eg ventures, law firms, universities)

Traditional	Top-down Formal hierarchy Mature industries
Consensus-driven	Middle-out Matrix management Integrated product line
Profit-center structured	Middle-out Independent P/L mgt. Diverse product line
Futurist	Top-down Personality-based org. Few leading-edge products

Source: GamePlan software reprinted with permission of N. Dean Meyer and Associates Inc., 233 Mountain Road, Ridgefield, CT 06877.

Classification of Sociopolitical Actors

Regardless of the organizational structure of health care providers, Morone [1981, p. 262] provides a colorful classification of provider and consumer strategic planning participants with sociopolitical overtones:

Providers
- Neanderthal—Government has no place in medicine.
- Self-seeker—Uses planning toward their own ends.
- Tory—Urges cautious reform to avert revolutionary change.
- Renegade—Seeks to alter the organization.

Consumers
- Eminents—Too busy; don't attend; send alternates.
- Warm Bodies—Contribute little and don't understand.
- Volunteers—Advocates without a cause wanting to do good.
- Advocates—Goal-oriented with public interest view.
- Interest Group Champions—For their own constituency.
- Occupational Representatives—For their organizations.
- Statesmen/Politicians—For the agency itself.

Considering the actors in the sociopolitical strategic planning process raises a number of questions to ponder regarding the reasons that agencies and individuals participate:

- Is health a major concern of the community?
- Why upset the status quo?
- What's the role of business and industry?
- Is there a payoff for politicians?
- What's the influence of the health care professionals

Competitive vs. Cooperative Bargaining

Strategic planning in a drama with a possible cast of actors outlined by Morone could cause trepidation about ever resolving anything. To the point, Shortell and Kalunzy [1988, p. 134] chart the differences between cooperative and competitive bargaining with attention to key strategic questions. Generic stances consider juxtapositions such as firm positions vs. trust and openness; misrepresented needs vs. an understanding of all underlying needs; false issues and dummy opposition vs. sticking to the major problems; and overvaluing concessions to maximize own utility vs. expressed preferences and maximum joint utility. These opposing attitudes translate into sociopolitical stances regarding honesty, disclosure, argumentativeness, secretiveness, and true negotiation. Planners must be aware of the possibility that participants may be engaging in such approaches. Blair, Savage, and Whitehead [1989] classify their strategies into four types: collaborate, subordinate, compete, and avoid negotiating.

Techniques to improve coordination and cooperation could stress information sharing, review and comment procedures, sign-off responsibility on plans or documents, joint data analysis, joint resource allocation, and joint service delivery. If competitive organizations can engage in these activities, it may be possible to achieve a level of trust that would result in joint planning and policy making [Hagedorn, 1977, p. 52].

Three agencies—the Veteran's Administration, the National Institute on Aging and the National Institute of Dental Research—illustrate cooperative implementation working on jointly agreed goals [Loe, 1985]. Agreeing that oral health needs of the elderly require attention, the three organizations met to plan for the future dental health of older Americans. "Our intent is to extend and enrich those [Shakespeare's] seven ages of man to a century of health and zest for life of man—and woman!"

When planning funds were greatly reduced in Texas, the Texas Foundation for Human Services emerged as a regional coalition of private and government groups to decide what makes the most sense for their particular area [Carrell, 1987]. Local decision making via consensus stimulated cooperative interactions rather than competitive bickering.

Manipulation of Community Involvement

Madan [1987] uses an example of community involvement in health policy in India to direct attention to the concept of "community participation" in health planning. He states that community participation is promoted as an alternative strategy by voluntary associations and activist groups as a check on governmental agencies that may not do right by the people. Basic considerations revolve around What is a community? and What is involvement? Even settling those issues, Madan comes to a skeptical conclusion: "Available evidence suggests . . . that community involvement can be debased easily and employed to describe euphemistically the manipulation of people by politicians, bureaucrats and technocrats. . . Community involvement thus becomes a part of social rhetoric." Strategic planners must be particularly alert to an interpretation that individuals are participating merely as "window dressing." Considering the marketing and initiatives of the health care providers, this situation may require a judicious approach.

In a related area, Braithwaite and Lythcott [1989] talk about the politics of inclusion, not exclusion. They suggest community empowerment as the strategy and community-based health promotion intervention as the technique to achieve behavior changes.

One Hospital's Trials and Tribulations

Narrated in the first person by the chief executive officer [CEO] of Riley Memorial Hospital for 23 years, this case study begins when the Board Chairman fires the CEO [Johnson, 1985]. Sociopolitical actions included decisions urged by the CEO and approved by the Board to close two specialized nursing units, to lay off 134 personnel, to comingle patients on surgical and medical floors, and to do something about decreased occupancy. Board members were being required to make decisions with uncomfortable speed. Physicians had been complaining for some time about the lack of parking and the need for a private dining room. In addition, three radiologists planned to set up a competing ambulatory imaging center across the street from the hospital. Reacting, the CEO recommended that the Board terminate the radiologists' contract and the CEO sent a carefully worded letter to the radiologists on behalf of the Board. A maelstrom ensued! A special meeting of the medical staff met and a motion was passed to terminate the CEO. Confident of his value to the hospital, the CEO did not meet with individual Board members; the physicians did. After excusing the CEO from the Board meeting, the vote was seven to six to fire the CEO.

This case study contains all the events vital to a simulation on administrative decision making and strategic planning. There are defined roles to play: the CEO, the Board chairman, the Chief of the medical staff; the three radiologists, the laid-off employees, patients, supporters, and detractors of the CEO and other health care agencies in the community. Certainly, the events are vivid and in tune with current issues in health care systems. Above all, the sociopolitics of confrontation, competition, and cooperation can be integrated into a role-playing situation.

Task Forces, Work Groups, and Sociopolitics

With input from 172 organizations, more than 425 people in six work groups of 20 to 30 people each, a 37-member steering committee, an Advisory Committee and $12 million, the Health Policy Agenda for the American People [HPA] evolved with 195 recommendations [Klett, 1987]. There was an emphasis on establishing a standard so that both government and private parties could see how their benefits programs measured up; a need for Medicaid reform with uniform eligibility and coverage of the medically needy; and a suggestion for a pilot study of a patient compensation fund to reduce malpractice expenditures. Since the HPA was initiated by the American Medical Association, critics may feel that the recommendations are tainted but the input of so many organizations and individuals would tend to negate that view.

A Primary Health Care in Boston Seminar brought together a working group task force to develop state and local strategies for high risk groups [Korda, Plough, & Delbanco, 1986]. Public and private sector policymakers looked at health status, payer coverage, and the availability of health care providers to render services to persons at high risk. Planners developed strategic actions related to health insurance, reimbursement and access to providers to improve services. A special point was made of the need for collaborative efforts.

With a spotlight on national planning for locally controlled health systems in Finland, Saltman [1988] tackles the potentially explosive sociopolitical interactions involved. In the United States, the situation is akin to federal legislation that mandates state and local financial participation in the national Medicaid program. Even with strong attributes favoring national planning in Finland, problems were identified that reflect on the sociopolitical nature of the proposed implementation. Saltman found differences between the national concept and the reality at the local level. Dilemmas were noted in coping with the intermixture of variations regarding actual/official, technical/bureaucratic vs. publicly elected rational/political interactions. There was the finding that it is difficult to develop locally controlled health systems within a national planning concept.

At times, strategic planners may elect to use subgroups to resolve sociopolitical complications. Parry [1985] listed 14 reasons for using subgroups such as interaction increases synergism and ideas beget ideas; there is more feedback; there is deductive rather than inductive problem solving; tension is reduced with a varying pace; team building takes place; and participants become committed to the group's decisions.

Sociopolitical interaction usually generates an unduly large number of meetings. Miller and Popowinak [1986] identify attributes of the good meeting:

- Clear agenda distributed in advance to all participants.
- Purpose of the meeting identified in advance, i.e., briefing, information and discussion, problem solving, or decision making.
- Reports and written material distributed several days before.

- Visual aids to support the main points.
- Participants know their responsibilities beforehand.
- Sharing of views and discussion encouraged.
- Openness prevails with support for positive contributions.
- Focus on issues, not personalities.
- Primary objective is clear and thoughtful solutions emerge.
- Limit to 90 minutes or less with conclusions summarized and specific tasks and deadlines set before adjourning.

Techniques for Meetings and Presentations

If there is one constant regarding implementation activities, it is the fact that planners will be heavily involved in meetings and presentations with professional and/or lay task forces, ad hoc committees and study groups. A variety of meeting styles are detailed in Exhibit 6–24 by the purpose, the type, and relevant features of each technique. These methods and techniques can be adapted to meet the mandates of participation, sociopolitical interaction, representation and the production of the final product—the recommendations.

Sociopolitical Tradeoffs in Planning

Assuming that appropriate individuals and organizations can be identified that should take part in the planning process, how does the planner motivate the obvious participants to do so? Rational approaches may or may not provide the stimulation. Trade-offs may frequently provide the answers. What can the strategic planner tradeoff with the intended parties in return for their active participation? In his classic book espousing a theory of political influence in urban politics, Banfield [1961, pp. 3–6] delineated a variety of methods to influence people:

- *Obligation*—Individuals feel obligated to participate because it is morally right or a personal duty.
- *Friendship*—People participate because a friend asked them to do so.
- *Selling*—Individuals respond to a sales pitch.
- *Coercion*—People are politely blackmailed into activity.
- *Rational Persuasion*—Individuals are persuaded by the power of the data and the weight of the persuasion.
- *Inducement*—Either positive or negative inducements bring people over to the planner's side.

All these incentives must be tailored to fit the specific person or agency in each particular situation. One similar message does not move all people with equal force.

Inducements that create resources of influence can be vital to the implementation of any planning activity. As usual, when considering resources used to influence people, the issue of which means to what ends arises. None of these inducements are nefarious in themselves. Planners may apply the following resources to influence people in a judicious and reasonable manner:

Exhibit 6-24.   Meetings, Groupings, and Presentation Techniques.

TYPE OF MEETING

If This Is Your Purpose ▼	This Type ▼	Has These Features ▼

WORK CONFERENCE

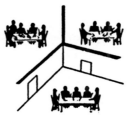

To plan, get facts, solve organization and member problems

▼ general sessions and face-to-face groups (15 or less)
▼ usually high participation
▼ provides more flexible means for doing organization's work

WORKSHOP

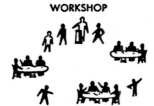

To train each other to gain new knowledge, skills or insights into problems

▼ general sessions and face-to-face groups
▼ participants are also "trainers"
▼ trainers can be brought in, too

SEMINAR

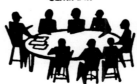

To share experience among "experts"

▼ usually one face-to-face group
▼ discussion leader also provides expert information

INSTITUTE

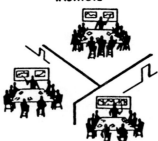

To train in one or several subjects

▼ general sessions and face-to-face groups
▼ staff provides most of training resources

(continued)

311

Exhibit 6-24. *(Continued)*

KINDS OF GROUPINGS

If This Is Your Purpose ▼	This Kind ▼	Has These Features ▼

GENERAL SESSION

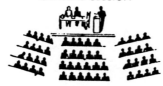

To give orientation or information to total group, transact official business

▼ includes total meeting group

▼ useful for demonstrations, speeches, lectures, films

▼ can be subdivided for limited face-to-face group activities

SPECIAL INTEREST GROUPS

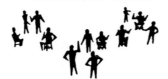

To consider special interests of various members by means of exchange of opinions, experience, and ideas

EXAMPLE:
"Let's plan our golf tournament"
"How can we get more members interested?"
"Can we get an expert on this subject t address us?"

▼ composed of those interested in subject

▼ usually no action required, but findings may be reported

▼ size varies widely; best if kept small

ORIENTATION GROUPS

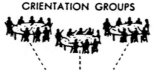

To help new members get acquainted, explain conference mechanics and plan of operation

EXAMPLES:
"What about getting mail?"
"Where can we go after hours?"
"What's the schedule?"

▼ mixed membership from total group

▼ member of planning staff as resource on all questions and to help them get acquainted

▼ exists for brief period at start of conference only

PRESENTATION METHODS

SPEAKER WITH VISUALS

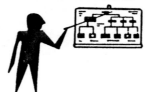

To present complex technical info, such as organization structure, processes, etc.

▼ more thorough and more certain communication but slower and more costly

▼ usually creates greater interest than speaker only

SYMPOSIUM

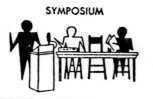

To present information from several points of view

▼ two or more speakers—each usually makes short talk

▼ speakers can help audience set full understanding of specific subject

▼ chairman summarizes and directs questions

▼ audience usually does not participate verbally

(continued)

Exhibit 6-24. *(Continued)*

If This Is Your Purpose ▼	This Method ▼	Has These Features ▼

PANEL

To present information, often controversial, from several points of view

- ▼ panel participates—each states views and holds discussion with one another
- ▼ panel members usually rehearse briefly
- ▼ discussion is guided by moderator
- ▼ questions and commentary with audience

FORUM

To develop several opposing sides of an issue

- ▼ two or more speakers take opposing sides on an issue; address audience rather than each other
- ▼ moderator summarizes points of view and leads discussion
- ▼ audience usually limited to asking questions

SITUATION PRESENTATION

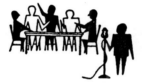

To help audience analyze individual or group action in "natural" setting

- ▼ members of group present role play, vignette or case-study (example: showing problems of coordination in staff meeting)
- ▼ commentator may call attention to specific points as play progresses
- ▼ audience gains a common experience for discussion afterwards

CONFLICT PRESENTATION

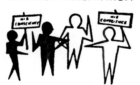

To dramatize the outer or inner forces that clash in a human situation

- ▼ members of group present role play or staged skits
- ▼ "ghost voice" or "alter ego" talks out loud to show inner thoughts of each character (example: outside pressures on two people in conflict)
- ▼ audience gains insights into problems through emotional appeal

SKILL PRESENTATION

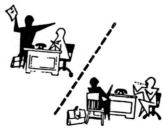

To demonstrate techniques or skills and show relative effectiveness

- ▼ members of group (or live actors) demonstrate several ways of handling a situation (example: ways to sell difficult customer)
- ▼ audience observes, discusses advantages and disadvantages of various approaches

- *Money/Credit*—It is easy to buy what you need.
- *Control of Jobs*—People that are uneasy about their jobs will be inclined to vote with the boss.
- *Control of Information*—Without all the facts, people may move in the desired direction based on the data made available.
- *Social Standing*—Some people may be influenced by those whom they regard as the "social elite."
- *Ethnic Solidarity*—There may be a compulsion to help someone of the same ethnic background.
- *Legality/Constitutionality*—Usually backed up by sanctions of some type, the power of the law may urge cooperation.
- *Personal [Human] Energy*—Over time, sheer work and ability to stay with the problem may influence others.
- *Knowledge/Expertise*—People may respond to the intellectual ability of those they admire and respect.
- *Popularity/Esteem/Charisma*—That indefinable something extra that may charm people into participating.

Having listed inducements and sources of influence in planning, it's appropriate to step back and consider the juxtaposition of the public interest versus the private interest.

Public Interests vs. Private Interests

It is doubtful that any strategic planner would believe that individuals and organizations have the public interest at heart in the majority of implementation activities. A public interest mindset seeks to further the ends of the whole public rather than the ends of some specific sector. On the other hand, private and special interests seek decisions furthering the ends of their constituents at the expense of the needs of the larger public. In a collection of case studies that consider politics, planning and the public interest, Meyerson and Banfield [1955, pp. 322–329] detail the conflicting views that participants may hold:

> community regarding *rather than* self-regarding
> general *rather than* particular in reference
> pertain to a citizen's role *rather than* to some private role
> common/statistically frequent *rather than* idiosyncratic/infrequent
> logically/morally justified *rather than* emotionally/not justified
> stable *rather than* transitory

In situations where these conflicting values are present in the individuals involved in the implementation, bitter battles and severe constraints may be imposed upon the planning outcomes. There could be prolonged debates over domains or turfs, a delay in action, a lack of consensus with a movement to retain the status quo, insufficient authority to undertake activities, and confusion regarding the exact science of planning.

Referring to the third party payers in a somewhat cynical tone, Dans [1988] comments that in the new business climate of health care, "He who has the gold makes the rules. . . This self-interest ethic leaves little room for altruism." Stivers [1987] picks up the argument at that point noting that "current health policy thinking is dominated by the language of economics."

Applying speech act theory, Stivers argues for replacing "right to health care" language with "public interest" language. Doing so would achieve a better balance between equity and efficiency concerns than mere reliance on a right to health care claim. In reviewing the literature, Stivers identifies a number of public interest terms:

social problem	social unity	legitimate public concern
social solution	common good	maximum social welfare
social decision	social responsibility	society's best interests
social investment	sense of community	feelings toward each other

"On the issue in question, we need to ask whether it is in the public interest for most U.S. health care to be delivered by profit-making corporations *before* we ask whether for-profit health care saves money. . . This article is based on the premise that, granted that hard choices must be made and that pain will result, it is still necessary to ask where the pain should fall" [Stivers, 1987].

There can be little doubt that tensions exist among health policy makers and strategic planners. Conflicting thoughts relate to the dominance of cost containment and the provision of equitable access to health care. Stivers argues that language helps to create the political reality. Redirecting health policy decisions into public interest terminology may lead to the following changes:

- Reinforcement of population-based standards of need.
- Justification of policies to address "the needs of strangers."
- Support for health services research and rational planning.

Significant or Urgent Health Problem?

In view of the spectrum of sociopolitical interactions regarding implementation of activities, how can planners determine which issues are most important? Many activities may be significant; fewer will be deemed urgent. Significant problems are no less worthy of action than urgent issues. In fact, urgent problems may be less important statistically and/or logically. Yet, the issue can be declared urgent due to a heavier loading of sociopolitical factors.

An activity may be rated as significant because of the number of people affected, the visible location of the facility, the volume of the expenditures required, the high risks or losses associated with the activity, the level of social disruption, the potential effects and/or benefits, and the identity of the participants involved in the implementation action.

For example, Canter [1986] describes planning for foot care for aging veterans as an increasingly urgent problem. Yet, for reasons that include inability to afford the service, lack of transportation, provider discrimination, and patient rejection of inferior quality services, foot care for aging veterans has not moved from a significant to an urgent problem. According to Canter, "Foot problems tend to be considered as low priority items until the patient becomes hospitalized. . . For too long, feet have been one of the most neglected parts of the anatomy."

What happens to make something an urgent problem? A number of factors can make a difference:

- Mass media communications can keep the issue in the spotlight until action is taken to meet the urgent need.
- Simply labeling the situation a crisis makes it so and a self-fulfilling prophecy prompts urgent action.

- Pressure and/or flak via letters, phone calls, personal talks, picketing, sleep-ins, and boy-cotts call attention to the need for urgent rectification of the situation.
- Moral values can be offended and an urgent demand can arise to correct the situation.
- Power brokers in "smoke-filled back rooms" can decide that something ought to be done immediately.
- Influentials having the ability to get others to think, feel or act as they wish can create an urgent situation.

Often, the U.S. health care system reacts to a crisis situation and urgent actions ensue rapidly. In fact, a Connecticut University School of Nursing [1986] study concluded that the crisis model may be the most appropriate for implementation purposes. Examples from real-life illustrate the implementation effect. When people die because harmful ingredients are mixed into a drug, the federal Food and Drug Administration is created to oversee drug safety. When both parents and five small children are killed from a faulty side-arm water heater, the New York City Health Department unleashes a massive educational and legal enforcement campaign. When a group of parents sleep-in at the Health Department's headquarters, the parents and children are given gamma globulin immunizations against hepatitis even though the treatment is not medically indicated. When patients with AIDS are burdening acute care hospitals, a comprehensive care alternative emerges [DeHovitz & Pellegrino, 1987].

It is apparent that influence is a major force in the sociopolitical interactions that cause an implementation activity to jump from being significant to being urgent. In their book on health care management, Shortell and Kaluzny [1988, p. 266] define influence as the combination of the power to affect behavior, the legitimate and/or formal authority to undertake the action, and the control of individuals to make them act as you wish.

IMPLEMENTATION IMPERATIVES

Strategic planning adds an immediate overlay of marketing principles to any implementation activity. This may translate into implementation tasks that are contained within a cadre of employees rather than the usual combination of professionals and consumers. However, even in strategic planning, implementation could involve individuals outside of the employee core because of the need to incorporate attention to the sociopolitical aspects of the task. There may be a need to grasp an idea of the community's reaction to a new service such as a wellness center or the marketing concept of securing endorsements from area leaders.

In any event, implementation requires the planner to constantly monitor the progress of events and to make appropriate changes as the unfolding outcomes dictate. Strategic planning flexibility is vital to the success of implementation activities.

REFERENCES

Ambry, R. (1988). How to forecast a medical market. *American Demographics, 10*(2), 48–50.
American Medical News. (1988). Hospital cost-containment study. *31*(34), 40.
Andren, K.G., & Rosenqvist, U. (1987). An ecological study of the relationship between risk indicators for social disintegration and use of a somatic emergency department. *Social Sciences and Medicine, 25*(10), 1121–1127.
Banfield, E.C. (1961). *Political influence: A new theory of urban politics.* Glencoe, NY: The Free Press.

Bassett, L.C., & Metzer, N. (1986). *Achieving excellence. A prescription for health care managers.* Rockville, MD: Aspen Publishers.

Beech, R., Brough, R., & Shaw, M. (1985). Aiding and abetting the planners. *Health and Social Service Journal, 95*(4958), 930–931.

Behrman, J.N. (1987). Viewpoint: The national disease: Technique over purpose. *Health Care Management Review, 12*(2), 85–91.

Bermar, A. (1988, March 8). Hospital tests smart-card marketing. *PC Week,* p. c/6.

Billings, J.S. (1889). *Opening day Address, Johns Hopkins Hospital.* Baltimore, MD: Johns Hopkins University.

Blair, J.D., Savage, G.T., & Whitehead, C.J. (1989). A strategic approach for negotiating with hospital stakeholders. *Health Care Management Review, 14*(1), 13–23.

Bonoma, T.V., & Crittenden, V.L. (1988). Managing marketing implementation. *Sloan Management Review, 29*(8), 7–14.

Braithwaite, R.L., & Lythcott, N. (1989). Community empowerment as a strategy for health promotion for Black and other minorities. *Journal of the American Medical Association, 261*(2), 282–283.

Broadwell, L. (1987). Business games: They're more than child's play. *Successful Meetings, 36*(6), 34–39.

Brown, M., & McCool, B.P. (1986). Vertical integration: Exploration of a popular strategic concept. *Health Care Management Review, 11*(4), 7–19.

Brown, S.W. (1988). *Marketing Showcase for Physicians.* Scottsdale, AZ: Health Services Marketing Ltd.

Callahan, C.B., & Wall, L.L. (1987). Participative management: A contingency approach. *Journal of Nursing Administration, 17*(9), 9–15.

Campbell, L. (1989a). Borrowed marketing strategies: A danger zone for home care. *CHAP Report, 1*(1), 4–5.

Campbell, M.I. (1989b, February 20). How could a few tasteful ads cause any trouble? *Medical Economics, 66,* 221–222, 224, 226–227.

Canter, K.G. (1986). Podiatric health planning for the aging veteran. *Journal of the American Podiatric Medical Association, 76*(1), 47–51.

Carrell, S. (1987). Health planning a private effort in Texas. *American Medical News, 30*(19), 20.

Chelimsky, E. (1988). *Reaching populations at higher risk.* (GAO, PEMD 88–35). Washington, DC: Government Printing Office.

Cherskov, M. (1986). Competition takes over as health planning fades. *Hospitals, 60*(24), 79–80.

Clark, L. (1989, February 20). A $25,000 marketing plan that any doctor can use. *Medical Economics, 66,* 159–161, 165, 168.

Clarke, R.M., & Shyavitz, L. (1987). Health care marketing: Lots of talk, any action? *Health Care Management Review, 12*(1), 31–36.

Coddington, D.C., & Moore, K.D. (1987A). Making the hard choices: A guide to board decision making. *Trustee, 40*(9), 28.

Coddington, D.C., & Moore, K.D. (1987B). Diversification offers new opportunities for health care. *Healthcare Financial Management, 41*(7), 64–71.

Collins, M.M. (1986). Shortcuts to marketing decisions. Case studies show how hospitals cut through the information overload. *Healthcare Forum, 29*(5), 96–98.

Connecticut University, Storrs School of Nursing. (1986, January 15). Development, implementation, and evaluation of a nursing center. *P–125 Government Reports, 88*(2).

Converse, P.D. (1949). New laws of retail gravitation. *Journal of Marketing, 14*(10), 379–384.

Cooper, P.D., Jones, K.M., & Wong, J.K. (1984). *An annotated and extended bibliography of health care marketing.* Chicago, IL: American Marketing Association.

Cooper, P.D. (1985A). *Health care marketing.* Rockville, MD: Aspen Systems.

Cooper, P.D. (Ed.). (1985B). *Health care marketing. Issues and trends* (2nd ed.). Rockville, MD: Aspen Systems.

Cooper, P., & Hisrich, R.D. (1987). Commentary on . . . marketing research for health services: Understanding and applying various techniques. *Journal of Health Care Marketing, 7*(1), 54–60.

Dans, P.E. (1988). The health care revolution: A preliminary report from the front. *Journal of the American Medical Association, 259*(23), 3452–3453.

Davies, R., & Davies, T. (1986). Using simulation to plan health service resources: Discussion paper. *Journal of The Royal Society of Medicine, 79*(3), 154–157.

Dawson, D.A. (1988). AIDS knowledge and attitudes: August 1988. Provisional data from the National Health Interview Survey. *NCHS Advancedata* (No. 163, DHHS Pub. No. [PHS] 89–1250).

Day, D.L., DeSarbo, W.S., & Terence, O.A. (1987). Strategy maps: A spatial representation of intra-industry competitive strategy. *Management Science, 33*(12), 1534–1551.

DeHovitz, J.A., & Pellegrino, V. (1987). AIDS care in New York City: The comprehensive care alternative. *New York State Journal of Medicine, 87,* 298–300.

DeJean, D. (1988, February 23). Game plan stimulates corporate culture, goal is to teach effective management. *PC Week, 5*(8), 117.

Dunn, H.L. (1961). *High level wellness.* Arlington, VA: R.W. Beatty, Ltd.

Eisenberg, H. (1988, May 5). Advertising works for the little guy, too. *Medical Economics,* pp. 65–79.

Emery, K.R. (1986). Developing a new or modified service: Analysis for decision making. *Health Care Supervisor, 4*(2), 30–38.

Erickson, J.L. (1987, September 21). Balancing act tough in ailing market. *Advertising Age,* pp. S1–S2, S4.

Erez, M., Earley, R.C., & Hulin, C.L. (1985). The impact of participation on goal acceptance and performance: A two-step model. *Academy of Management Journal, 28*(1), 50–66.

Feldstein, P.J. (1986). The strategic planning game: A computer game for health care administrators. *The Journal of Health Administration Education, 4*(1), 67–75.

Fontana, L. (1986). Political ideology and local health planning in the United States. *Human Relations, 39*(6), 541–556.

Freitag, E.M. (1988). Marketing in home health care. A practical approach. *Nursing Clinics of North America, 23*(2), 415–429.

Fyke, K.J. (1987). Hospital amalgamation: A practical experience. *Dimensions in Health Service, 64*(2), 28–30.

Gibbons, D.L. (1985, January). Privileges, MD surplus, costs impel hospital staff turf battles. *Medical World News,* pp. 89–93, 96.

Goodspeed, S.W., & Earnhart, S.W. (1986). Planning, developing, and implementing a freestanding ambulatory surgery center. *Health Care Strategic Management, 4*(2), 18–22.

Gostin, L.O. (1989). Public health strategies for confronting AIDS. *Journal of the American Medical Association, 261*(11), 1621–1630.

Grenell, B., & Studin, I. (1988). Strategies change—strategy paradigm cannot. *Hospitals, 62*(2), 80.

Gummer, B. (1987). There's many a slip 'twixt cup and lip: Current perspectives on implementation. *Administration in Social Work, 11*(2), 89–104.

Hagedorn, H. (1977). *A manual on state mental health planning.* (DHEW Pub. No. (ADM) 77–473). Washington, DC: Government Printing Office.

Haley, M. (1984). Positioning doctors for convenience medicine. *Hospital & Health Services Administration, 29*(4), 95–110.

Hammond, S.C., DeCenzo, D.A., & Bowers, M.H. (1987). How one company went smokeless. *Harvard Business Review, 87*(6), 44–45.

Hancock, T. (1986). Creating a healthy community: The preferred role for hospitals. *Dimensions in Health Service, 63*(6), 22.

Harrell, G.D., & Fors, M.F. (1985). Marketing ambulatory care to women: A segmentation approach. *Health Care Marketing, 5*(1), 19–28.

Holden, J.M. (1988). Target areas illustrated. AMA's map expands with graphics. *American Medical News, 31*(41), 13.

Home Health Line. (1984, March). Who will survive? *10,* 59–65.

Horgan, C.M. (1986). The demand for ambulatory mental health services from specialty providers. *Health Services Research, 21*(2), 291–319.

Ingram, T.N., & Hensel, P.J. (1985). Marketing in home health organizations: Issues in implementation. *Family & Community Health, 8*(2), 22–32.

Jaffe, E. (1985). Transition in health care: Critical planning for the 1990's, Part Two. *The American Journal of Occupational Therapy, 39*(8), 499–503.

James, J., & McGinty, R.T. (1981). A gaming-simulation system for exploring urban issues. *Perspectives in Computing, 1*(4), 10–21.

Johnson, R.L. (1985). The day after. *Hospital & Health Services Administration, 30*(6), 106–117.

Jones, W., & Loe, H. (1988). Effective policy implementation in inner city health departments. *Journal of Health and Human Resources Administration, 10*(3), 265–277.

Kannel, W.B., & McGee, D.L. (1987). Composite scoring—methods and predictive validity: Insights from the Framingham study. *Health Services Research, 22*(4), 499–535.

Keckley, P.H. (1988). *Market research handbook for health care professionals.* Chicago, IL: American Hospital Publishing, Inc.

Klegon, D.A., & Slubowski, M.A. (1985). Marketing ambulatory care centers: Assessment, implementation, evaluation. *Journal of Ambulatory Care Management, 8*(3), 18–27.

Klett, S. (1987). Health care: Of the people, for the people. *Nation's Business, 75*(2), 72–73.

Klimek-Grzesiak, I., & Stakowski, M. (1986). Computer system for hospital management. In R. Salamon, B. Blum, & M. Jorgensen (Eds.), *MEDINFO '86.* North-Holland, Amsterdam: Elsevier Sciences Publishing B.V.

Korda, H., Plough, A., & Delbanco, T. (1986). Access to primary health care: Developing state and local strategies for high risk groups. *Australian Health Review, 9*(2), 96–106.

Kotler, P. (1980). *Marketing management analysis, planning and control* (4th ed.). Englewood Cliffs, NJ: Prentice-Hall.

Kotler, P., & Clarke, R. (1987). *Marketing for health care organizations.* Englewood Cliffs, NJ: Prentice-Hall.

Lar, R. (1986). Do-it-yourself marketing for long-term care administrators. *Health Marketing Quarterly, 4*(1), 3–11.

Lewton, K.L. (1989). Health care critical conditions. *Public Relations Journal, 22*(12), 18–22.

Levin, R.I., & Kirkpatrick, C.A. (1966). *Planning and control with PERT/CPM.* New York: McGraw-Hill Book Co.

Loe, H. (1985). Dental health of older Americans: Planning for the future. *Gerodontics, 1,* 288–290.

Lutz, S. (1987). Hospitals consider product line management techniques to better meet consumers' needs. *Modern Healthcare, 17*(8), 70, 74.

MacStravic, R.S. (1987). Loyalty of hospital patients: A vital marketing objective. *Health Care Management Review, 12*(2), 23–30.

MacStravic, R.S. (1988). Outcome marketing in health care. *Health Care Management Review, 13*(2), 53–59.

Madan, T.N. (1987). Community involvement in health policy; socio-structural and dynamic aspects of health beliefs. *Social Science and Medicine, 25*(6), 615–620.

Mahaffey, M. (1986). Planning for mental health: The immediate agenda. *American Journal of Orthpsychiatry, 56*(1), 4–13.

Manassero, B. (1988a). Thorough planning is key to marketing strategy. *American Medical News, 31*(35), 15.

Manassero, B. (1988b). Four elements are key to successful plan. *American Medical News, 31*(36), 16.

McConnell, C.R. (1984). *Managing the health care professional.* Rockville, MD: Aspen Systems.

McIlrath, S. (1989). Surveys show long-term care coverage as "hot" new product. *American Medical News, 32*(11), 5.

Meyerson, M., & Banfield, E.C. (1955). *Politics, planning and the public interest.* Glencoe, NY: The Free Press.

Miller, A.R., & Popowniak, M.F. (1986). Review the meeting basics. . . *Successful Meetings, 35*(3), 128.

Morone, J.A. (1981). The real world of representation: Consumers and the HSAs. In *Health Planning in the U.S.* (Vol. 2). Washington, DC: National Academy Press, Institute of Medicine.

Mowll, C.A. (1987). Developing a care plan. *Healthcare Financial Management, 41*(3), 188–124.

Mullen, K.D. (1986). Wellness: The missing concept in health promotion programming for adults. *Health Values, 10*(3), 34–37.

National Technical Information Service. (1988). *Hospital and health care: Marketing.* Springfield, VA: Government Reports, Vol. 88, No. 8, 4(15).

National League for Nursing. (1988, December, 13). *Successful marketing strategies for home care: A "how-to" management seminar.* New York, NY.

Nauert, R.C. (1985). Review, reaction, and projection: The role of the CFO in planning. *Healthcare Financial Management, 39*(4), 54–57.

Neustadt, R.E. (1980). *Presidential power. The politics of leadership from FDR to Carter.* New York: John Wiley & Sons, Inc.

Nutt, P.C. (1986). Tactics of implementation. *Academy of Management Journal, 29*(2), 230–261.

O'Brien, K., & Roemer, D. (1989). Mergers and acquisitions: Key issues in successful transactions. *Dimensions in Health Care, 89*(2), 1–5.

Parry, S. (1985). 14 Reasons for using sub-groups. *Successful Meetings, 34*(3), 92.

Pastides, H., & Moore-Pastides, P.J. (1986). Sampling, standardization, randomized trial, and modeling: Four techniques applied to health care marketing. *Journal of Health Care Marketing, 6*(2), 57–62.

Pharmacy Practice News. (1989). Topics in administration. *16*(5), 38–39.

Porter, M. (1985). *Competitive advantage: Creating and sustaining superior performance.* New York: Free Press.

Powills, S. (1987). Diversity key to targeting women's market. *Hospitals, 61*(3), 38–39.

Pradilla, A., Barnum, H., Barlow, R., & Fajardo, L. (1987). Childhood mortality. Development of a quantitative planning model for the evaluation of policy choice. *Annals Society Belgique Medicine Tropical, 67*[Suppl.1], 105–110.

Rash, R.M. (1986). Decision support or support decision? "What data do I base my management decision upon?" *Computer Healthcare, 7*(4), 24–26.

Relman, A.S. (1980). The new medical industrial complex. *New England Journal of Medicine, 303*(17), 963–970.

Ricardo, M. (1988). *The complete medical marketing handbook.* Redondo Beach, CA: Healthcare Management Services.

Rodwin, V.G. (1984). *The health planning predicament. France, Quebec, England, and the United States.* Berkeley, CA: University of California Press.

Saltman, R.B. (1988). National planning for locally controlled health systems: The Finnish experience. *Journal of Health Politics, Policy and Law, 13*(1), 27–51.

Schillaci, C.E. (1987). Designing successful joint ventures. *Journal of Business Strategy, 8*(5), 59–63.

Schwartz, G. (1963). *Development of a marketing theory.* Cincinnati, OH: South-Western Publishing Co.

Seay, J.D., Vladeck, B.C., & Kramer, P.S. (1986). Holding fast to the good: The future of the voluntary hospital. *Inquiry, 23*(4), 253–260.

Shortell, S.M., & Kaluzny, A.D. (1988). *Health care management.* New York: John Wiley & Sons.

Siktberg, L. (1989). Community health planning and education via telecommunications. *Health Care Supervisor, 7*(3), 57–63.

Starkweather, D.B. (1986). Governance of health care organizations: A priority for scholarship. *Journal of Health Administration Education, 4*(1), 1–6.

Steiber, S., & Boscarino, J. (1985). Health care marketing: The concept is spreading. In P. Cooper (Ed.), *Health care marketing.* Rockville, MD: Aspen Systems.

Stewart, J.M. (1988). Finding the right niche for service. *Provider, 14*(6), 5–7.

Stivers, C. (1987). Reframing health policy debate. The need for public interest language. *Administration and Society, 19*(3), 309–327.

Super, K.E. (1987). Product line management needs careful implementation. *Modern Healthcare, 17*(10), 99.

Super, K.E. (1986). Nation's hospitals likely to adopt market segmentation techniques. *Modern Healthcare, 16*(16), 88–92.

Touche Ross & Co. (1988). *U.S. hospitals: The future of health care.* New York, NY.

Triolo, P.K. (1987). Marketing women's healthcare. *Journal of Nursing Administration, 17*(11), 9–14.

Tuomilehto, J., & Puska, P. (1987). The changing role and legitimate boundaries of epidemiology: Community-based prevention programmes. *Social Sciences and Medicine, 25*(6), 589–598.

Van Pelt, G. (1985). Program management and matrix reporting. *Hospitals, 59*(24), 83–84.

Vogel, G., & Doleysh, N. (1988). *Entrepreneuring: A nurse's guide to starting a business.* New York: National League for Nursing.

Wager, R.J. (1988). Approach the community as more than one public. *Provider, 14*(6), 8–10.

Waldrop, J.W. (1987). The demographics of diabetes. *American Demographics, 9*(3), 45–47.

White, E.C. (1985). Competition for healthcare markets spurs race for demographic data. *Modern Healthcare, 15*(20), 79–82.

Winter, F.W. (1986). Computerized secondary data approaches to health care location decisions. *Journal of Health Care Marketing, 6*(2), 67–75.

Yuki, G. (1981). *Leadership in organization.* Englewood Cliffs, NJ: Prentice-Hall.

7

Evaluation

In strategic planning, attention to the bottom line, as in the corporate world, may be of paramount importance. Relationships between inputs and outputs may emphasize economic factors in terms of costs and effectiveness rather than costs and benefits. Obviously, an evaluation with that focus may differ from other appraisals wherein the major thrust riveted upon health status improvement regardless of the resources expended. Furthermore, evaluation also usually marks the initiation of a new cycle of planning as the investigation reveals additional areas for programs and activities. In strategic planning, the new tasks may be considerably narrowed to concentrate upon those directly linked to the agency's goals and objectives.

Strategic planners who spend the time and effort to specify the objectives in unmisinterpretable language will find that the evaluation phase flows smoothly and directly through the entire process. Conversely, ill-defined objectives lead to frustration about unretrievable data, leaps of imagination to cover missing procedures, and unfounded conclusions.

Surprisingly, the objective need not be complex. An eminent physician attending at Boston's Massachusetts General Hospital suggested that it would be worthwhile to discover the relation between treatment received at a hospital and the patient's welfare after discharge. At the beginning of the 20th century, Dr. E.A. Codman [1914] expressed his ideas about the product of a hospital in a professional journal. However, this rather direct evaluation of treatment and outcome did not meet with enthusiastic endorsement from the hospitals. Perhaps the lack of support stemmed from the fact that Dr. Codman recommended that the information be collected in a uniform manner from all the facilities for comparative purposes. In addition, Dr. Codman noted that such evaluative data could then be used to measure management and efficiency. From a planning viewpoint, Dr. Codman sidestepped getting the approval of those individuals and organizations most directly affected by the evaluation—a fatal planning error even though the objective was straightforward, simple, and obviously beneficial to patients and professionals. In discussing practical evaluation, Patton [1982, p. 59] reinforces the principle that avoids the fatal planning error:

> The "stakeholder assumption" is the idea that key people who have a stake in an evaluation should be actively and meaningfully involved in shaping that evaluation so as to focus . . . on meaningful and appropriate issues, thereby increasing the likelihood of utilization.

WHY DO EVALUATION?

In his classic book on evaluation principles and practices, Suchman [1967, p. 31] expansively defines evaluation and clearly delineates the process and the questions with expanded descriptive wording:

> We may simply indicate the range of variation by defining evaluation as the determination [whether based on opinions, records, or subjective or objective data] of the results [whether desirable or undesirable; transient or permanent; immediate or delayed] attained by some activity [whether a program or part of a program; a drug or a therapy; an ongoing or a one-shot approach] designed to accomplish some valued goal or objective [whether ultimate, intermediate, or immediate effort of performance; long or short range].

This evaluation definition identifies the issues related to data sources, outcomes, the experimental procedure, and the relation to the objective. In another approach, Rossi, Freeman, and Wright [1979, p. 33] link four types of evaluation questions with resultant measurement outcomes:

Program planning questions → strategic compliance
Program monitoring questions → management compliance
Impact assessment questions → intervention effect
Economic efficiency questions → program impact

Considering the varied specifications assigned to evaluation, cynics could conclude that there is no *one way* to conduct an evaluation. Differential interpretations may logically lead to debates about whether the half glass of water is half full or half empty, whether the evaluator is a optimist or a pessimist, whether the statistics are not lying but the liars are using statistics. These oft-used analogies reflect the possibility that an evaluation can initiate political overtones as well as professional controversy.

A portion of the variability in evaluation interpretations can be traced to the four major perspectives [funder, provider, recipient, and public] [Windle & Neigher, 1978] and the four purposes [program amelioration or improvement, accountability, advocacy, and research] [Neigher & Schulberg, 1982]. In a similar vein while discussing quality standards in health care, Esmond and Batchelor [1988] identify the need to balance purchaser, provider, and patient expectations of quality of care evaluations. Often, the governmental agency or funding agency mandates an evaluation format requiring accountability and documentation.

Taking the positives first, evaluation can, among other things, measure the attainment of objectives; can identify strengths and weaknesses of programs; can compare alternative programs and methods; can monitor standards and quality of care; can develop innovative approaches; can assist in priority setting; can provide accountability; can suggest generalizations for the activity; and can add to the foundations of scientific knowledge [Suchman, 1967, p. 141].

Human nature being what it is, not everyone seeks an impartial evaluation. Pseudoevaluation could take place being influenced by management prerogatives that produce colorful descriptors of evaluation with the true intent in the brackets: Eyewash [choose aspects that "look good" and ignore others], Whitewash ["cover up" failures or errors], Submarine [settle internal strife by "torpedoing" a rival's program], Posture [status enhancement via a "pose of scientific research"], Postponement [used as an "excuse to gain time" while crisis subsides], and Substitution [success in one part "shifts attention" from major failure] [Suchman, 1967, p. 143].

In any event, evaluation is an integral part of strategic planning. Hopefully, planners and evaluators will be able to zero in on the measurement of specific objectives rather than the negative pseudoevaluations. Furthermore, planners should be aware that evaluation may involve more than a single method or technique. This book has many exhibits and explanations where techniques have been used to set goals, to allocate resources, to choose alternatives, to determine priorities and to implement activities. Indicators, indexes, criteria, checklists, formulas, scales, and surveys are all capable of interchangability in evaluations. Therefore, it would be appropriate to refer back to those exhibits and explanations for ideas and guidelines.

As Rossi, Freeman, and Wright [1979, p. 59] decisively commented: "If you don't care where you get to, then it doesn't matter which way you go." In strategic health planning, directions are quite clear and the use of evaluation techniques in marketing provides a concrete example of seeking which way to go.

EVALUATION AND MARKETING

Since marketing aims to sell a service or product, often the target of evaluation methodology is the consumer. Commonly, a survey is a component of the marketing information system. While Burns [1986] identifies five basic survey techniques, he does comment that there are many variations among mail surveys, telephone surveys, interview surveys, voluntary point-of-purchase surveys, and tied-to-use surveys. Mail, telephone and interview surveys are self-explanatory. Point-of-purchase refers to surveys placed at check-out counters, information desks, or other locations where consumers choose to pick them up and fill them out. Tie-to-use relates to questionnaires given to people using a service, buying a product, or upon hospital discharge. In elaborating on the collection and use of strategic data to evaluate potential markets, Boscarino [1987] adds focus groups to his discussion of mail and telephone surveys. Focus groups gather a variety of individuals together to engage in a moderator-led discussion of specific issues.

If a marketing research firm is employed to do the surveys, the price should include data collection, data processing, analysis, and a report. Focus groups range from $1,500 to $3,500 each for about 10 participants per group. Mail surveys range from $5,000 to $13,000 for 300 completed questionnaires based on a 25 percent-or-better response rate. Telephone interviews completed with 100 individuals range from $6,000 to $12,000 with a minimum 25 percent completion rate [Boscarino, 1987].

Noting that knowledge is power, Burns [1986] details the effective development of market surveys with attention to setting clear goals, creating questions, testing and reworking questions, ordering the questions, coding the responses, analysis of the results, and writing the final report. Exhibit 7–1 lists 10 tips for a successful marketing survey.

Managed Health Care Plan Market Survey

Conducting a study for a managed health care plan, Feinholz [1986] received responses to mail surveys from 599 home owners and 325 residents in the Los Angeles area relative to their judgments about the quality of health care. After three pretests, the final survey instrument emerged as a 9-point scale that rated each of the 30 items from 1 [not important] to 9 [important] with additional open-ended questions for comments and space for demographic data. Sample sizes were adequate for statistical analysis.

Exhibit 7-1.   Ten Tips for a Successful Survey.

1. Establish your goals and keep referring to them.
2. Brainstorm your questions.
3. Target your market with precision.
4. Eliminate and combine for the fewest possible questions.
5. Provide easy-to-understand response choices.
6. Polish and order questions.
7. Presentation is important: be polite, use good graphic design.
8. Write clear introductions, connectives and coding instructions.
9. Pre-test within sample population.
10. Revise, revise, revise!

Never lose track of how you intend to use the data you collect!

Source: From "Knowledge is power: how to develop effective market surveys," by J.A. Burns, 1986, *Health Marketing Quarterly*, 3 [2&3], 112. Reprinted with permission of Haworth Press Inc. Copyright 1986.

This marketing evaluation explored four areas:

• Factors consumers use to evaluate quality in health care.
• Selection of physician and health plan.
• Satisfaction with routine medical care.
• Demographic analyses of consumers.

Findings revealed that consumers were mainly concerned with the accuracy of the physician's diagnosis directly correlated with the outcome of care; the amount of information given to the patient by the physician; the physician's appearance of competence and confidence; and the physician's willingness to listen to the patient. All of these primary factors fit within the medical encounter's, mainly the physician's, interactions and relationships. There was some dissatisfaction expressed regarding obtaining appointments, waiting time, and the incompetent behavior of office staff. Age and sex of the physician were rated as least important along with lower ratings for payment methods, office location, nurses in office, and weekend/evening availability. Consumers desired to be treated as a human being whose time is valuable and not as an impersonal cog in a factory assembly line.

Feinholz advises managed health care plan providers to seek success by "positioning themselves in the market place by addressing issues of patient-physician interaction and the character and competence of office staff . . . plans incorporating the consumer evaluation factors into their benefit packages and marketing strategies will have the greatest success in positioning their product and expanding their market share."

Hospital Market Evaluation

Lourdes Hospital [Paducah, KY] surveyed the general public, recent patients, staff physicians, nonstaff physicians, and area industrial plants to evaluate the services provided, to discover what services consumers will purchase, to have consumers identify who will be providing services in the future and when the changes will occur [Schoenfeldt, Seale, & Hale, 1987]. Exhibit 7–2 details the survey method and the specific questions asked of each group of participants.

Findings showed that almost every patient wanted a greater say in their own treatment plans; more than 83 percent preferred outpatient care and 55 percent agreed even if not covered

Exhibit 7-2. Hospital Market Survey Description and Questions for General Public, Recent Patients, Physicians, and Industry.

Hospital Market Survey

Questionnaires on Lourdes Hospital were sent to the general public, recent patients, physicians on staff, area nonstaff physicians, and area industrial plants. Employees were not involved in the survey because they were included in an earlier study and are surveyed "in-house" on a regular basis.

Murray State University and Lourdes developed the survey instruments and worked out the details. The university then independently took over the sample selection process, gathering and analysis of data, and the final report. Those surveyed were informed that the hospital played no role in this part of the process. Following is a detailed explanation of how the data were gathered.

General public

Questionnaires were sent to approximately 1,600 people randomly selected from area telephone directories in western Kentucky, southern Illinois, and northwest Tennessee. The number selected from each county was based on the county's percentage of the total population. A total of 382, or 24 percent, of those selected completed and returned the questionnaires. People from 66 communities responded, with 82 percent from Kentucky, 7.6 percent from Tennessee, and 7.3 percent from Illinois.

To begin, the respondents were asked their age, sex, household income, ZIP code, and length of time they had lived in the area. In addition, they were asked the following:

1. Excluding Lourdes, which hospitals in the area come to your mind first?
2. Would Lourdes have been on the above list had it not been excluded?
3. Do you agree or disagree with the following statements concerning hospitals in general?
   a. Programs on how to prevent disease (life-style change) should be provided by hospitals.
   b. A busy hospital should be allowed to add more beds even if other hospitals in the area are not being completely utilized.
   c. The quality of care provided in a not-for-profit and a profit-making hospital is about the same.
   d. Patients and their families want to participate more fully in the decisions about the care they receive.
   e. When it comes to hospital care, most hospitals charge about the same for their services.
4. What hospital would you choose for nonemergency care?

5. How much influence (great, some, or no influence) would each of the following factors have on your choice?
   a. Convenience of location
   b. A caring attitude by employees
   c. Hospital's appearance and cleanliness
   d. Your personal physician's preference
   e. Hospital's religious affiliation
   f. Recommendation of a friend or relative
   g. Special services
   h. How soon service could be provided
6. How was the most recent choice of a hospital made in your household?
7. How do you think the choice of a hospital should be made?
8. If you had a choice, would you prefer to stay overnight in a hospital or receive outpatient services?
9. Would you prefer outpatient services even if your health insurance would not cover the entire expense?
10. For which of the following services, if any, would you be willing to pay a reasonable fee out of your own pocket?
    a. Exercise counseling program
    b. Stop-smoking clinic
    c. Diet counseling program
    d. Stress management program
    e. Health assessment clinic
11. Are hospital costs in the area too high for the level of service provided?
12. Rank the following factors in terms of their contribution to rising healthcare costs:
    a. Overall inflation
    b. New technology
    c. Government regulation
    d. Employee wages and salaries
    e. Physicians' fees
    f. Cost of malpractice insurance
    g. Influence of insurance coverage on patient charges
    h. Other (please specify)
13. How important (very important, important, not important) are each of the following sources of information concerning area hospitals and healthcare?
    a. Newspaper
    b. Radio
    c. Television
    d. Conversation with friends and relatives
    e. Your physician
    f. Other (please specify)

(continued)

by insurance; that stress management and health assessment services are desired extra offerings; and that a caring attitude, appearance, cleanliness, and availability were the most important factors in choosing a hospital.

Physicians asked for additional input regarding the evaluation of new services and equipment at the hospital; agreed that competition among providers will increase; and that more tests and procedures will be conducted in the private office.

About 70 percent of the industries in the area pay for their employee's health insurance benefits but few offer a choice of insurance plans; more than 40 percent had in-house health screening services; and only five companies encouraged use of low-cost providers. While 75

14. Indicate your level of confidence in Lourdes Hospital.
15. What two types of illness or injury does Lourdes handle with the most skill and expertise?

Recent Lourdes patients

Questionnaires were sent to 2,000 individuals who had been patients at Lourdes within the past 12 months. A total of 556, or slightly less than 28 percent, completed and returned the questionnaire.

The patients were asked the same demographic questions and questions 5 to 11, as in the survey for the general public. In addition, they were asked the following:

1. Indicate the type of treatment you received at Lourdes.
2. Rate the following areas of concern on a five-point scale from excellent to poor, with one being excellent and five being poor:
   a. Admitting
   b. Employee competence
   c. Employee attitude
   d. Food
   e. Housekeeping
   f. Parking
   g. Physicians
   h. Business office
   i. Overall patient care
3. Rate the overall quality of treatment you received at Lourdes on a six-point scale ranging from excellent to very poor.
4. Give your impression of Lourdes based on the following characteristics by using a six-point scale to determine which term best describes the hospital (with the first term being 1 and the second term being 6):
   a. Competent—incompetent
   b. Professional—unprofessional
   c. Progressive—unprogressive
   d. Quiet—noisy
   e. Concerned—unconcerned
   f. Caring—uncaring
   g. Dedicated—indifferent
   h. Responsive—unresponsive
5. Were you or any member of your immediate family a patient in any other hospital during the past three years? If so, please name the hospital, the date of admission, and the type of treatment received.
6. Rate the quality of treatment received at the other hospital on a six-point scale ranging from excellent to very poor.

7. Why did you choose the other hospital instead of Lourdes?
8. How can Lourdes improve its present services? What additional services should it offer?
9. Would you choose Lourdes if you needed to be hospitalized again?
10. Did you have any type of medical insurance? If so, approximately what percentage of the medical insurance premium did you pay out of your own pocket?

Lourdes physicians

Questionnaires were sent to the 120 physicians on staff at Lourdes Hospitals, with 42.5 percent completed and returned.

The physicians were first asked their medical specialty and whether they were on the staff at Western Baptist, the other large hospital in Paducah. They were then asked the following:

1. What approximate percentage of patients do you refer to Lourdes and to Western Baptist?
2. Rank the following reasons, in their order of frequency, for admitting patients to Western Baptist:
   a. Service unavailable at Lourdes
   b. Better quality service at Western Baptist
   c. Patient preference
   d. Physician preference
   e. Other (please specify)
3. What approximate percentage of each of the following patient types or cases did you refer out of Paducah?
   a. Burn
   b. Cardiology
   c. Oncology-hematology
   d. Ophthalmology
   e. Organ transplant
   f. Plastic surgery
   g. Other (please specify)
4. Is there a need to add or discontinue any medical specialties, subspecialties, or medical services in the Paducah area and/or Lourdes Hospital?
5. What input do you have in evaluating new services and/or equipment at Lourdes, and should you have more?
6. Rate each of the following services at the hospital on a five-point scale ranging from excellent to poor:
   a. Admitting/discharging
   b. Employee competence
   c. Employee attitude
   d. Switchboard

[*Turn page*]

(*continued*)

percent of the executives thought that wellness programs were beneficial, only three had the service and only four would be willing to purchase the service.

Responding to the market survey, the hospital restructured its planning process establishing three levels of evaluation and management input: task forces to evaluate and make recommendations; a long-range planning committee of the governing board to review the task force reports and make their own recommendations; and the Board of Directors to make the final decision. A full-time market analyst was hired to "evaluate shifts in consumer attitudes that affect services, policies, and practices." A "Health Enhancement Program," guided by a Health Promotions Director created and marketed community and employee projects on nutrition,

e. Parking facilities
f. Administration
g. Patient care
h. Laboratory/pathology
i. Radiology
j. Emergency room
k. Surgery/recovery

7. Give your impression of Lourdes on the following characteristics, indicating on a six-point scale which term best describes the hospital (with the first term being 1 and the second term being 6):
a. Professional—unprofessional
b. Quiet—noisy
c. Democratic—autocratic
d. Structured—unstructured
e. Organized—disorganized
f. Efficient—inefficient
g. Decisive—indecisive
h. Responsive—unresponsive
i. Effective—ineffective

8. Are hospital costs in general and Lourdes's costs specifically too high for the level of care provided?

9. Excluding hospitals, which setting—home, free-standing center, physician office, or other (please specify)—would be appropriate for each service listed? More than one setting per service can be chosen.
a. Surgery
b. Radiology
c. Physical therapy
d. Respiratory therapy
e. Cardiac rehabilitation
f. Kidney dialysis
g. Patient education
h. Laboratory work
i. Emergency services
j. Mental health services

10. Indicate on a five-point scale the direction each of the following healthcare areas is likely to take in the next 5 to 10 years, from decreasing greatly to increasing greatly:
a. Multispecialty group
b. Independent practicing paraprofessionals
c. Nurse practitioner or physical therapist
d. Preferred provider organizations
e. Health maintenance organizations
f. Formal preventive and wellness programs
g. Competition among individual physicians
h. Competition between physicians and other providers
i. Diagnostic tests in physician's office
j. Therapeutic procedures in physician's office

11. If you were running Lourdes Hospital, what changes would you make?

Area physicians

Questionnaires were sent to 203 area physicians who were not on staff at Lourdes Hospital, with slightly more than 17 percent responding. They included many of the questions asked of the physicians on staff. Area physicians were also asked the following:
1. In which city do you practice?
2. Do you refer some of your patients to Paducah? If so, what types of cases?
3. Of the patients referred to Paducah, what percentage is referred to Lourdes?
4. If you do not refer patients to Lourdes or Western Baptist, why not?
5. *Will* referrals from your geographic region to Paducah increase, decrease, or remain about the same over the next five years?
6. *Should* referrals from your geographic area to Paducah increase, decrease, or remain about the same?

Area industry

Questionnaires were sent to 63 area manufacturing and chemical processing plants. A total of 31, or slightly more than 49 percent, returned completed forms. Company officials were asked the following:
1. How many miles are your plants from Lourdes Hospital, and how many people do you employ?
2. How many of your emergency patients have ever been transferred directly or indirectly to Lourdes?
3. If you have used Lourdes's emergency services, could you suggest anything the hospital could do administratively to better serve your needs?
4. Should any new medical or surgical services be offered?
The plants were then asked a number of questions in 11 categories concerning their health benefit plans. The categories were outpatient surgery, health insurance premium sharing with employees, health insurance deductible amounts paid by employees, preferred provider organizations, alcohol rehabilitation, employee fringe benefit cafeteria plans (where the employee is given a choice of fringe benefits within a given cost range), insurance claim incentive plans, self-funding of health insurance coverage, competitive bidding for health benefit packages, in-house health services, and industrial preventive and wellness programs.

Source: From "Survey alerts hospital to needs of consumers," by R.C. Schoenfeldt, W.B. Seale, & A.W. Hale, 1987, *Health Progress*, 68(7), 64–66. Reprinted with permission.

smoking cessation, sports medicine, exercise, stress management, and other topics. All outpatient procedures increased including radiology, laboratory services, physical therapy, respiratory therapy, cardiac rehabilitation, and outpatient surgery. Pediatrics expanded to include overnight accommodations and direct family support in providing care. No smoking policies are now enforced and smoke-free areas expanded. Noise levels have been reduced and acoustical materials installed. Increased attention is given to a new market strategy to enhance communications with consumers via brochures, personalized visiting rules, and notices posted at nursing stations and information desks. Results of this marketing evaluation "have given direction to the hospital administration, helped shape advertising, and provided support for certificate-of-need requests."

In a related long-term care evaluation, Larkin [1988] reported on a survey of 24 demonstration projects engaged in providing elder care. Difficulties in this area related to physician resistance to geriatric programs, a lack of reimbursement, and competition from community-based providers. Acute care was identified as the key to success in the elder care market along with the management of the transfer of patients into long-term care settings.

Marketing to Industry

Ten-minute telephone interviews to 100 small- and medium-sized Midwestern firms tested the feasibility of specifically tailored health care services to be offered by a local hospital. Results revealed that the hospital could only profit from providing emergency medical care and physical exam services to medium-sized companies. There was little interest in alcohol and drug services, fitness programs, education, or screening [Boscarino, 1987].

Another industrial health care survey involved a 15-minute telephone interview to 200 benefit managers of medium and large firms in a Southeastern city. A large medical center sought information on specific products, demand estimates, pricing, and brand loyalty. Out of the potential market, 162 companies responded saying they would send employees to a hospital-sponsored fitness center. Responses ranged from very likely [22 firms], somewhat likely [63 firms], to somewhat unlikely [75 firms] and don't know [2 firms]. A follow-up survey asked about reactions to a price change, to a different sponsorship, to a more convenient location, and to an expanded service. With that data the hospital was able to develop a product attuned to the demand of local firms [Boscarino, 1987].

Marketing and Regulation

In recent years, a procompetition strategy aimed to reduce the regulatory burden on the private health care provider sector. That regulatory decrease focuses upon the removal of mandated certificate-of-need and Section 1122 reviews regarding consistency with state and local planning activities and with cost containment objectives. Hash [1986] asserts that "most studies support the contention that CON regulations are not effective in reducing or even holding down health care costs." Interestingly, deregulation of CON and 1122 activities most frequently occur in the western and southwestern states where demographic and economic growth is more rapid. O'Donnell [1987], the executive director of the American Health Planning Association, commented that "planning is antithetical to or irrelevant in a competitive health care environment." Nevertheless, Kinzer [1988] "finds little evidence that health regulation is on the decline." His view is bolstered by concepts about medical care as a right, the essential nature of the community hospital, guaranteed limitations on future health care expenditures, and the premise that the intensifying competition will engender more, and not less, regulation. Kinzer urges providers to seek a consensus on "what kinds of regulation they consider workable and acceptable."

PROCEDURES FOR EVALUATION

Regardless of the procedural steps in the evaluation process, Herzog [1959, p. 81] developed realistic guidelines that have withstood the test of time and experience [Exhibit 7–3].

With the do's and don'ts in mind as well as the realization that there is no single perfect way to do evaluation, planners can review the sequence of steps in the process. All variations of

Exhibit 7-3. Evaluation Do's and Don'ts.

Do bring in the evaluator early.
  Allow the evaluator to become fully involved. Waiting until the end of the project to employ an evaluator indicates a lack of value attached to the evaluation.
Do pre-evaluative investigation.
  It's worthwhile to secure a grass-roots feeling for what's happening.
Do engage in systematic study and exploration.
  This is an evaluation prerequisite. There is no need to reinvent the wheel; history is well known for repeating itself with regularity.
Do include other disciplines in the evaluation effort.
  Statisticians, marketing experts and others can add to the evaluation with their diversity of expertise.
Do coordinate efforts.
  This saves time, effort and wear and tear on staff members.

Don't use sophisticated evaluative techniques if other alternatives serve as well.
  Seek the simple approach first.
Don't use exciting case records as your only evaluation data source.
  An obvious bias occurs in this method and the reservations must be stated.
Don't undertake evaluation unless adequate resources are available.
  Efforts will be wasted on gerrymandered evaluations.
Don't undertake lopsided evaluations.
  It is not necessary to use a high-powered rifle to kill an ant.
Don't underestimate unpretentious evaluation techniques.
  Sometimes a simple yes or no questionnaire is powerful. Merely asking patients "why?" can be most revealing.
Don't believe in the fantasy of a neat, precise, utterly objective evaluation science.
  Reliability, validity and other variables can be questionable on numerous occasions.
Don't overvalue loosely used terms in evaluation activities.
  Jargon can cloud a study and its results in incomprehensible verbiage.

an evaluation process have much in common despite the semantic differences. Commonalties include the specifics of the objectives and/or goals; description of the program and/or activity; selection of the methods of measurement; gathering of numerical and/or anecdotal data; statistical and/or interpretive analyses; and conclusions, recommendations, limitations, and/or identification of future evaluative activities.

Goal/objective specifics require operational terms with explicit criteria, behavior, and standards noted. Gathering of data needs collection procedures, information instruments, time limits, and information storage capabilities. Analysis indicates quantitative and qualitative techniques such as statistics, frequencies, modes, verbal descriptions, log books, and interviews. Conclusions lead to adjustments in the program and a recycle.

From a health care managerial perspective, Levey and Loomba [1973, p. 424] enumerate the following evaluation steps:

1. Formulation of objectives.
2. Specification of the measures of performance.
3. Development of the model, plans, and programs.
4. Measurement of results.
5. Determination of explanation of degree of success.
6. Recommendations of appropriate actions in view of the variance between the predetermined objectives and the actual results.

These six planning steps include the process of planning [1,2,3], management control [3,4,5], and evaluation [4,5,6].

With an operations research theme akin to strategic planning evaluation, Russell and Reynolds [1985, p. 57] evolve a three-phase approach that includes problem analysis, solution development, and testing and evaluation. It may be useful to look at all three phases: [I] problem analysis defines the problem, analyzes the problem, and divides it into smaller operational units, collects data, sets priorities, and selects study problems; [II] solution developments for each operational problem specify objectives, identify decision variables and constraints, and/or facilitating factors, select and construct a model, collect required data, use the model to gain optimal solution and conduct sensitivity analysis of each solution; and [III] solution testing and evaluation designs a test, conducts the test, collects data, evaluates and modifies the solution, and merges resultant information.

Mowbray and Herman [1986] distinguish between "top-down" and "bottom-up" evaluation approaches emanating from the "New Federalism" in government. Top-down evaluation is normally mandated by an administrative body and serves an accountability or research purpose related to the public or the funding organization. In this case, the evaluation topic is a given and the process moves through the rational steps of methods and data collection to analysis and conclusions. Bottom-up evaluation results from a felt need at the local level and serves to improve programs and/or advocacy for the benefit of the provider or recipient. An evaluation area is determined locally through consensus before proceeding to the other steps in the procedure. These authors prefer the bottom-up evaluation technique since the stakeholders are more likely to be involved. However, Carr-Hill [1985] argues that although participation is vital there is a problem getting people involved, thereby making the political aspects prime. Nevertheless, the question is asked: "Can that participation ever be meaningful if structured and legislated from above?" Would the same comment apply to managerial evaluation such as monitoring?

MONITORING AS EVALUATION

In discussing the monitoring of health indices in the community, Stone [1985] defines the process:

> Monitoring is a centralized, systematic and ongoing [whether continuous or periodic] method of collecting, analyzing and interpreting health and health service data in order to detect, investigate and, where appropriate, control or ameliorate deviations from predetermined norms.

A common example of monitoring as evaluation takes place in utilization reviews. Writing in *Business—Insurance,* Drury [1984] reported about several UR monitoring successes. Caterpillar Tractor Company [Peoria, IL] employed a peer review organization to conduct utilization review of their employer funded health benefit plan. In a five-year period UR reduced hospital days per 1,000 employees from 1,000 to 700. In a two-year period, Illinois state government lowered hospital days with no acute care rendered from 23 percent of total hospital days to only nine percent. It appears that providers do better simply because they are being watched. UR trims costs via a "sentinel effect."

Monitoring components identified by Stone [1985] included the following strategic planning principle: centralization, continuous periodic measurements, data collection and analysis, recording of deviations, and action to correct deviations. A schematic monitoring flow process evolves:

Problem definition → continuous data collection → periodic analysis → rapid interpretation → recommendations for action → evaluation of impact and recommendations → new problems.

Jenster [1987] posits that Strategic Performance Indicators [SPIs] "specifically measure and monitor key individuals' short-term progress toward achieving good performance along a critical dimension." Six categories indicate that SPIs should be:

1. *Operational* and focus on action and information for control.
2. *Indicative of desired performance* to measure against desired productivity/performance levels.
3. *Acceptable to subordinates* with significant input from them into the design/review process.
4. *Reliable* and appropriate to the factor that is being measured within minimal ranges and magnitudes.
5. *Timely* and correspond to the time span of the event.
6. *Simple* and direct attention to the targeted performance results.

GENERIC MEASUREMENT CONCEPTS

Typically measurements can fall into two basic classifications as illustrated in the oft-repeated toast: "May you have a long and healthy life." *Long* is an example of a quantitative measure and *healthy* refers to a qualitative measure. Following through on the example, length is numerically quantifiable as noted by average life expectancy, mortality rate, or mortality due to a specific cause. Healthy is qualitative and can be measured by living standards, housing, job satisfaction, and neighborhood.

Ware [1987] identifies five generic health concepts for measurement purposes: physical health, mental health, social functioning, role functioning, and general health perceptions.

Physical health measures apply to abilities that assess positive aspects or to limitations that assess negative aspects. Importantly, there are individual differences regarding the levels of effort, pain, difficulty, and need for help in the measurement categories listed below:

Abilities—able to walk uphill/upstairs/engage in sports
Well being—energy/vitality/satisfaction with physical shape
Limitations—needs help bathing/dressing/eating
Bed days—number of days sick in bed in past month

Mental health measures include behavioral dysfunction along with frequency and intensity of psychological distress symptoms. Obviously, mental health measures must tap a range of differences in the following areas:

Anxiety/depression—very unhappy/nervous/depressed
Cognitive functioning—confused/forgetful/mistake-prone
Psychological well being—happy/pleased/cheerful/satisfied
Behavioral/emotional control—stable/lose control/mood changes

Social functioning refers to people networks and support systems such as the following:

Interpersonal contacts—friends visited/visits outside/calls
Social resources—number of close friends/people to talk to

Role functioning concerns the individual's ability to cope with their usual major life activity such as the following:

Work—travel to job/co-workers/supervisors/lay offs
School—attend classes/take exams/failure
Home—cook/clean/shop/children/family health

General health perceptions relate to a self-assessment of feelings of well being, energy level, and satisfaction with life such as the following:

Health outlook—expectations for good health/can cope
Pain—tolerates/interferes/incapacitates/how much?
Health rating—excellent/good/fair/poor/bad

Scrivens, Cunningham, and Charlton [1985] review available instruments and classify evaluation measures into the five Is: *i*ndividual health status, *i*ntermediate short-term health status, *i*ndicators of the population's health status, *i*ndexes of health status that are population-based, and *i*nferential health status measures that are proxy indicators. All five Is are linked to health intervention activities that are evaluated based on the regulatory ability to achieve efficient and effective performance or to promote equitable distribution of health care. In addition, Scrivens' five Is distinguish between measurements of the levels of health in populations and the measures of outputs of health services.

Regardless of the generic health concept being measured, a scale should be labeled in terms of the content of the measurement and not based upon what the evaluator wishes to measure. To be useful, instruments should represent multiple health concepts and a range of health states pertaining to general functioning and well being. Often, scales artificially restrict the range of individual differences.

Selection of a suitable measurement technique is a difficult and complex process. Consideration must be given to the purpose of the measure; the conceptual focus of what is being measured; the quality of the measure in terms of validity and reliability; and the operational approach to use to collect the data. "There is no simple formula for suggesting when ideal, intermediate, indexes, indicator or inferential measures are appropriate" [Scrivens et al., 1985].

Specific measurements could include written surveys, ratings, interviews, behavioral observations, and achievement tests with data from records, participants, staff, significant others, evaluation teams, and community level indexes [Posavac & Carey, 1985]. TIROS can be a handy classification pneumonic: *t*ests, *i*nterviews, *r*eports, *o*bservations, and *s*amples. Dr. Carlos J.M. Martini, American Medical Association Vice President for Education comments that medical education should be measured by the "final product" or "outcome." In arriving at the most valid means to do so, Martini opts for "observing what is done" rather than "knowing how to do it." Competence evaluation is pinpointed as the key education issue [*American Medical News*, 1988]. This agrees with evaluation experts who assert that knowledge can be tested and attitudes can be measured, but actually observing the desired behavior is the ultimate measurement mode.

Evaluation Terminology Classifications

Words are frequently found in the literature indicating evaluation measurements. Three of the most common terms are effort, effect, and efficiency. Effort deals with productivity such as funds expended, personnel involved, facilities used, specimens obtained, or volume of patient/provider encounters. Effect relates to observable changes such as in mortality, morbidity, health status, recovery from specific diseases/conditions, and functioning ability in activities of daily living. Efficiency adds a strategic comparative analysis of costs and benefits as to how well the activity did relative to alternative programs.

There is no difficulty measuring effort since that is a mere tabulation of inputs. To evaluate the effect and the efficiency of an activity is more difficult. Valid and reliable statistics are needed but the numbers may tend to contradict and to confuse the evaluation.

Suchman [1967, p. 60] uses five elements in his evaluation terminology: adequacy, efficiency, effort, performance, and process. Adequacy could be equated to effect or impact. An example of a bird in flight illustrates all five aspects of this evaluation technique. How many times did the bird flap its wings [effort]? How far did the bird fly [performance]? How far did the bird fly relative to the total flight distance [adequacy]? Could the bird have flow alternative routes or used air currents to get there faster [efficiency]? What aerodynamic design changes could improve the flight [process]?

Another common evaluation model groups together the five Ds: death, disease, disability, discomfort, and dissatisfaction. Definitions and problems of each measurement are noted below:

Death. Vital statistics collected universally are readily available in most states. However, records may be incomplete, the population base uncertain, and the data may not be up-to-date.

Disease. Measurements relate to deviations from appropriate age and sex physiologic and/or functional norms for acute, chronic, incurable and self-terminating diseases/conditions. Obviously, individual clinical diagnoses will differ regarding severity and the variables related to causation.

Disability. Number of days of disability and confinement to bed are common measurements that are related to acute and chronic disability and degree of impairment. Functioning measurements are linked to inability to perform usual role and responsibilities on the job, attending school, or maintaining a household. Judgment decisions regarding social functioning and differentiations between being disabled and being handicapped compound the use of this measurement.

Discomfort. Using both scientific and subjective measures, the degree of discomfort and the number of days occurring are recorded. Discomfort is usually self-reported and subjectivity and sociocultural background may bias the individual's accounting.

Dissatisfaction. A wide range of physical, intellectual, emotional, social, and environmental factors can all influence the degree and intensity of this measurement. Attitudes of health care providers and cost are common sources of dissatisfaction. Apparently, the data will be subjective and biased by a host of variables.

A number of measurable words are often grouped together to form an evaluation mechanism. However, the terms are listed alphabetically with brief comments to illustrate the aspects being measured:

Acceptability—patient satisfaction
Accessibility—public transportation, no barriers
Accountability—moral contract between provider and consumer
Adequacy—what percent of the problem was solved?
Appropriateness—the relative impact of the program
Availability—enough beds, enough providers
Adequacy—degree to which the problem is eliminated
Benefit—how much? how improved? what resources?
Content—program elements provided and why
Context—what? where? when? and who?
Continuity of care—referral system, records, case manager
Cost—affordable, insurance coverage
Effectiveness—how much of the goal was achieved?
Efficiency—ratio between input and output
         could the same results be achieved at lower cost?
Effort—comparison to accepted standards
Performance—what are the outcomes?
Process—how care is organized and delivered
Outcome—did the event take place?
Output—how many times did it happen?
Quality—structure, process and outcome factors

GENERIC STATISTICAL APPROACHES

Just as there are generic measurement concepts, there are also generic statistical approaches. Numbers can be used with hard data such as mortality and morbidity and also with soft data such as attitudes and opinions. Data usually fall into four classification scales: nominal, ordinal, interval, and ratio. Exhibit 7–4 defines each scale, notes appropriate statistical measures and tests, and illustrates each.

Nominal scales are of the lowest power and essentially are frequency counts of distinct equivalent attributes such as hair color, skin color. There is no relationship among the variables and only the specific quality is counted.

An ordinal scale adds a relationship to the equivalence with a greater than or lesser than distinction. Illness can be mild, moderate, or severe. People can be profoundly, severely, moderately, or mildly retarded.

Interval scales continues adding to equivalence and greater than with the addition of a defined difference between the measurements. Weather temperature measurements have arbitrary starting points—freezing is 0 on one and 32 degrees on the other. However, the interval between the numerical degrees are equal on the temperature scales even though there is no absolute initial starting point. It would be false to say that 20 degrees is twice as cold as 10 degrees. Soft data measurements such as attitudes are difficult to cast into interval scales since the arbitrary numerical value between "happy" and "sad" is not three times as worse. Is "liked a great deal" five times better than "disliked somewhat"? Generally, health care evaluations tend to use ratio scales since the measurement relates to a base value.

Exhibit 7-4.   Four Levels of Measurement and the Statistics Appropriate to Each Level.

Scale	Defining Relations	Examples of Apropriate Statistics	Appropriate Statistical Test	Example of Measures
Nominal	[1] Equivalence	Mode Frequency Contingency coefficient		Hair: Brown/Black/Red
Ordinal	[1] Equivalence [2] Greater Than	Median Percentile Spearman$_{rs}$ Kendall$_T$ Kendall$_W$	Nonparametric Statistical Tests	Disease: Mild/Moderate/Severe

Interval	[1] Equivalence
	[2] Greater Than
	[3] Known Ratio
	  of Any Two
	  Intervals
		Mean
		Standard Deviation
		Person Product-
		  Moment Correlation
		Multiple Product-
		  Moment Correlation
				Temperature Scales

Ratio	[1] Equivalence
	[2] Greater Than
	[3] Known Ratio
	  of Any Two
	  Intervals
	[4] Known Ratio
	  of Any Two
	  Scale Values
		Geometric Mean
		Coefficient of
		  Variation
			Nonparametric
			and
			Parametric
			Statistical Tests
				Measures:
				Pulse/Height/Weight

Source: From *Nonparametric statistics for the behavioral sciences*, by S. Siegel, 1956, p. 30, New York: McGraw-Hill. Reprinted with permission.

Ratio scales add the ability of a relation to a base of zero to the other three attributes. Pulse, visual acuity, auditory acuity, height, and weight measurements are ratio scales. Clearly, a pulse of 80 is twice as fast as a pulse of 40. Someone weighing 100 pounds is one-half as heavy as a person weighing 200 pounds. With ratio scales, sophisticated numerical manipulations can be utilized.

In considering evaluations, strategic planners should be aware of the limitations of the type of data collected. It would be erroneous to force lower power scales such as nominal measurements into a sophisticated statistical test of significance requiring ratio scale data.

EVALUATION DESIGNS—SIMPLE TO COMPLEX

A strategic health planner wishes to conduct an evaluation that is actually a research design. If so, that decision should be made early enough to be reflected in the initial objectives. Appending a research afterward or during the activity biases the outcome of the evaluation.

Exhibit 7–5 illustrates three preexperimental, four true-experimental, and four quasiexperimental research designs. Note the legend explaining the Xs, Os and Rs.

Exhibit 7-5.   Variations in Evaluation Designs.

Pre-Experimental Designs:

1. One-Shot Case Study   X   O
   [weakest but most common evaluation research design]
2. One-Group, Pre-Test/Post-Test Design .... O_1 X O_2
3. The Static Group Comparison ....   X O_1
   [affords no way of knowing that the two groups were equivalent before the program]

The Experimental Designs:
[particularly applicable to field experiments and to experimental demonstration projects]

4. Pre-Test/Post-Test, Control Group Design ....   R O_1 X O_2
   R O_3 X O_4
5. Solomón Four-Group Design ....   R O_1 X O_2
   [controls and measures the experimental and the   R O_3 O_4
   possible interaction effects of the measuring process   R O_5
   itself]   R O_6
6. Post-Test Only, Control Group Design ....   R   X O_1
   R O_2
7. Comparison of Alternative Program Strategies ....   R O_1 X_1 O_2
   R O_3 X_2 O_4
   R O_5 X_3 O_6
   R O_7 O_8

Quasi-Experimental Designs:

8. Nonequivalent Comparison Group Design .... O_1 X O_2
   [well worth using in many instances in which Designs O_3 O_4
   4, 5 and 6 are impossible]
9. Comparison of Alternative Program Strategies, O_1 X_1 O_2
   Comparison of Local Projects .... O_3 X_2 O_4
   O_5 X_3 O_6
   O_7 O_8
10. Time-Series Design .... O_1 O_2 O_3 O_4 X O_5 O_6 O_7 O_8
11. Multiple Time-Series Design .... O_1 O_2 O_3 O_4 X O_5 O_6 O_7 O_8
    [excellent quasi-experimental design, perhaps O_9 O_{10} O_{11} O_{12} X O_{13} O_{14} O_{15} O_{16}
    the best of the more feasible designs]

R = Random Group[s]   O = Observation[s]   X = Experimental Program[s]

Preexperimental Designs

One-shot case studies simply expose the target group to the activity and measure the results. There is no control or comparison group and no baseline data on the target population. In effect, the evaluation produces a "testimonial" on the pluses or minuses of a specific program.

One group pretest/posttest evaluation design does gather the baseline data prior to the experimental activity and measures changes afterward. However, the pretest measurement may prepare the group for the experimental activity and the posttest. In addition, there is no control for extraneous events and passage of time alone can account for change.

A static group design takes measurements of two groups; one exposed to the activity and the other not. Again, the lack of baseline data prohibits knowledge about the measurement and demographic equivalence of the two groups prior to the activity.

True Experimental Designs

Pretest/posttest control group design involve two randomly selected and assigned populations with baseline measurements for both groups. Only one group is exposed to the experimental activity but each group is measured for differences between the first observation and the second observations afterward. Pretest conditioning is still a question for both groups.

Solomon's four group design uses four randomly selected matched groups with baseline observations taken for only two of the groups. One pretested group and one untested group are both exposed to the experimental activity. Measurements are taken for all four groups afterward with differences noted for those groups having two observations. Comparisons among all four group measurements yields data about pretest sensitivity and extraneous variables. Obviously, this evaluation is expensive but it is a true research design.

Posttest only control group design begins with two randomly matched groups with only one group exposed to the activity and both groups measured afterward. Baseline data are omitted and there is an assumption that any difference in measurement is due to the experimental activity.

Comparison of alternative program strategies has four randomly matched groups with baseline measurements for all four groups. Three of the groups are exposed to different experimental activities while the fourth is not. All four groups are tested afterward for differences between the first and second observations. An assumption is made that any difference is the result of the different activity. Again, there may be a pretest sensitivity and a difficulty in distinguishing between the impact of each of the three differing experimental activities.

Quasi-Experimental Designs

Nonequivalent comparison group design is similar to the pretest/posttest control group design without the two random groupings.

Comparison of alternative program strategies is similar to the true experimental design described above without the four random groups.

Time-series design conducts multiple observations prior to and after exposure to the experimental activity. Observations over time can be compared to pinpoint measurements changes before or after the activity. Extraneous variables may be defined based on time of occurrence.

Multiple time series design adds a control group providing a comparison of changes over time for the two populations.

Using other terms, Rhoads [1986] talks about a cohort study, a case control approach, and a randomized clinical trial [RCT]. In a cohort study, patients receiving experimental procedures are compared to a nonparticipating comparison group. A case control study retrospectively starts with identified cases in the community to determine if those individuals participated in the experimental activity. In a randomized clinical trial, patients are randomly allocated between the experimental activity and the usual program using placebos for one and the new therapy for the other. Neither the investigators nor the patients know which individuals get which—a double-blind situation. Carr-Hill [1985] agrees that the strict scientific model RCT does apply in evaluating drug therapies, medical procedures, and in clinical situations. In fact the advantageous features of the RCT include objectives that are unequivocally specified, control over inputs, exclusion of extraneous influences, validly tests interventions against alternatives or no intervention, and the achievement of uncontroversial success. However, Carr-Hill does posit that the RCT simply does not apply in many community health care situations.

An evaluation of multihospital systems illustrates the problem of even thinking about a RCT. Howard and Alidna [1987] identify the independent variables by hospital type—multihospital versus freestanding hospital. Dependent variables include efficiency in terms of operating costs and eight measures of effectiveness: availability and quality of personnel, scope and volume of services, organization and administration, facilities, equipment, and supplies, policies and procedures, research, education, and quality assurance. Eight items are included in the control variables of the evaluation study design: management philosophy, time period, level of care, bed size, number of hospitals in system, geographical dispersion, ownership type, and organizational maturity. Simply based upon the number of effectiveness outcomes and control variables, the mere suggestion of a RCT can cause strong evaluators to cringe.

While admitting the superiority of the RCT and the cohort study, Rhoads [1986] does favor the case control method when a single outcome is to be measured; when the activity has already been used by a significant portion of the population; when the outcome of greatest importance is uncommon; and to extend and confirm clinical trial findings in lower risk populations.

Regardless of the choice of an evaluation design, there are basic issues that must be addressed such as:

- Identification of the targeted study population.
- Choosing a random group population universe.
- Selection of matched experimental and control groups.
- Assignment of individuals into each group.
- Recruiting volunteers as well as a representative group.
- Identification of factors producing measurement changes.
- Explanation of why change took place.
- Explanation of cause and effect of input or other factors.
- Specific definition of program success factors.
- Measurement of program success factors.

These evaluation design issues are closely related to additional problems in evaluation of strategic planning efforts.

PROBLEMS IN EVALUATION

Difficulties in evaluation have already been cited in earlier sections of this chapter that dealt with setting goals and objectives, with the do's and don'ts of evaluation, with evaluation procedures, with definitions of terminology, with measurement concepts, and with research designs. To achieve a worthwhile evaluation, many critical areas must be thoughtfully considered and specific decisions made and adhered to throughout the process. A number of evaluation dilemmas can be placed at the extremes of a continuum. Dilemmas following are obvious examples from the wording alone and conjure up hours of debate during economical, ethical, and moral considerations:

Spending enough vs. spending too much for evaluation
Short-term vs. long-term evaluation
Experimental vs. placebo effects in changes
Evaluation rigor vs. significance of outcomes
Cost effectiveness vs. cost benefits of activities
Risk to patients vs. payoff in health status improvement

Since health care evaluations often deal with human patients/providers/consumers common questions arise about reliability and validity. It is conceivable that patients may tell the interviewers what they want to hear so as not to displease them; providers may do likewise to ingratiate themselves with administrators; and consumers may simply wish to be in with the majority view. Inconsistency can occur in evaluations in the following generic groupings:

- Respondents—may be influenced by fatigue, mood, motivation, or nature of services received.
- Environmental factors—such as lighting, location, seating arrangements, time, and weather may cause variable responses.
- Test instruments—could be ambiguous, have double meanings, or be poorly worded and result in variegated responses.
- Data processing—outcomes may be affected by coding errors, computer glitches, mechanical breakdowns, or evaluator interpretations that yield biased results.

Reliability and Validity

To reduce the possibility of bias and error, evaluators should seek the highest levels of reliability and validity. Reliability refers to the achievement of a high level of agreement when repeated administrations of the same measurement instrument yields the same results. Validity refers to the degree to which any measure actually succeeds in measuring what it is supposed to measure. High-level reliability can occur without high validity. Respondents can answer the same way every time but the instrument may not be gathering the data it was designed to amass. Contrariwise, to be valid an instrument must be reliable. However a measurement tool may be valid in one environmental situation and not in another. Validity generates more difficulties than reliability in the following areas: basic study assumptions may be invalid and yield invalid conclusions; inappropriate or irrelevant data affect instrument validity; population sample may not be representative causing invalidity; constant observer and/or evaluator bias invalidates responses; deliberate misinformation from respondents creates invalid data; operational validity may be affected by a host of vested interests management factors; and invalid rationales applied during analysis to strengthen preconceived results obviously yields erroneous conclusions.

Furthermore, validity can be determined in a variety of ways such as face validity, consensual validity, correlational validity, and predictive validity. An illustrative example places the four methods into practice. An evaluation of special interest high schools assumes that talented students in drama and music will select the School of Performing Arts [face validity]. Entrance selection committees at the School agree [consensual validity]. Practical auditions, personal interviews, and intellectual examinations correlate with the talented students theory [correlational validity]. There is every reason to expect that the School will continue to attract talented students in the future [predictive validity].

Validity can also be classified as to the ability to create changes. Internal validity means that the evaluation revealed evidence of change. External validity allows the evaluator to make generalizations from the results that are applicable outside of the project population group. Limiting strategic planning to internal validity also prevents general applications. On the other hand, if the planning objectives focused upon general applications, the results may not always be usable for specific groups. Internal and/or external validity requires attention to the goals and objectives as well as to the political realities of the situation.

Under the federal government's prospective payment system [PPS], the Peer Review Organization [PRO] is mandated to evaluate the quality of inpatient hospital care received by Medicare beneficiaries. Pierson [1986], an official of the American Medical Peer Review Association, specifies the physician peer review indicators as "monitoring for underutilization, unacceptable short cuts and for failure to deliver adequate care." In addition, he states that a successful evaluation of the quality of care delivered by physicians depends on resolving the following problems:

- Making measurement instruments for quality of care as universal and objective as those accepted for utilization.
- Collection of primary data on the physician's quality of care by nonphysician reviewers in as efficient a manner as they collect data on utilization.
- Severe underfunding of the PROs that engenders shortcuts and borrowing from other resources.
- Support from organized medicine for the PROs to defuse the "inevitable pressures on the buddy system."
- Impact of the threat of professional liability lawsuits and the risk of exposure resulting in less than the "honest and careful record-keeping" vital to peer review.

Continuing to discuss issues related to the quality of care, Brook and Lohr [1985] specifically tackle the problem of boundary-crossing research. Their point is that terms such as efficacy, effectiveness, variations in population-based rate of use, and quality of care have all been treated as isolated evaluation subjects. A suggestion is made that a macro model is needed to focus on the continuing problems in the medical system. "Within a research framework, the quality of medical care is that component of the difference between efficacy and effectiveness that can be attributed to care providers taking account of the environment in which they work." Of course, this approach emphasizes the requirement that terminology must be defined so that everybody is talking the same language. Brook and Lohr do explicitly define and defend their semantics. Essentially, and perhaps simplisticly, efficacy refers to benefits; effectiveness to performance; variations to per capita consumption; and quality as maximization of the patient's welfare.

Even if evaluation activities do gain valuable insights that could dramatically affect health care programs, those insights may not be utilized by health care management. Brownlee [1986] investigated the "application-gap" problem between research evaluators and decision makers. Strategies suggested to improve the situation involved the training of decision makers to use applied research evaluations for problem solving, orienting decision makers to applied research, and the bolstering of the use of evaluation research in health services management.

It is obvious that considerable evaluation is undertaken and that large numbers of reports and recommendations end up gathering dust on shelves or cartons in musky basements. Organizational inertia may contribute to that situation because decision makers may resist change and opt to maintain the comfortable and convenient status quo. A related barrier to underutilization of evaluation could result from deliberate actions to keep the evaluations from being communicated and disseminated to the appropriate policy and decision makers.

While management may be more involved in strategic planning activities, the point still stands that those decision makers should comprehend the vagaries of evaluation methods and techniques to arrive at a supportable conclusion prior to taking action. Top management should be able to discern gross methodological weaknesses and irrelevant designs in evaluation undertakings.

EVALUATION MEASUREMENTS, METHODS, AND TECHNIQUES

Strategic health planners engaging in evaluation do not have to reinvent the wheel. Compilations of methods, techniques, and instruments do exist in book form. In addition, professional journals in specialty areas as well as in evaluation routinely publish articles dealing with evaluation that describe instruments, methods, and techniques. Regardless of the source, evaluators can modify and adopt existing materials for use in their own particular situation.

About 50 measures of functional disability, psychological well-being, social adjustment, quality of life, and pain are reviewed and critiqued by McDowell and Newell [1987]. This 359-page reference compendium assists evaluators to choose, administer, and score available questionnaires and rating scales by providing descriptions of the instrument's purpose and conceptual basis, a copy of the tool, reliability tests, and validity constructs.

Ward and Lindeman [1978] review 325 instruments for measuring nursing practices and other health care variables. In two volumes, the authors describe and critique 140 instruments and reproduce 135 measurement tools. Psychosocial instruments are placed in the following classifications: by health care provider and significant others as to characteristics, cognitive variables, and alternative variables; by client as to characteristics, cognitive variables, affective variables [anxiety, depression, distress, self-concept, psychological health status], physical health status, and biopsychosocial health status [sociobiological functioning]; by provider/client interaction as to provider perceptions [of client, of patient care, of health services], patient's perceptions of satisfaction with [provider, patient care, health services], and interactions regarding provider behavior, client behavior, and the quality of care; client/significant others interaction with the client and with the providers. Typical instruments titles included the following: Acting-Out Checklist, Decision Scale, Environmental Fear Scale, Health Perceptions Questionnaire, Hospital Stress Rating Scale, Older Persons Questionnaire, Patient Satisfaction with Health Care Survey, Patient's Bill of Rights Questionnaire, Quality Patient Care Scale, Semantic Differential for Health, Spouse's Perception Scale, Symptom Rating Test, Trust Scale for Nurses, and You and Death. In addition, Ward and Lindeman list other compilations of psychosocial instruments.

In more than 500 pages, Reeder, Ramacher, and Gorelink [1976] present a handbook of scales and indices of health behavior. A chapter is devoted to evaluation material in each of the following areas: preventive health behavior, health status, health observations, illness behavior, and utilization of health services. Each section assesses the technique, describes the theoretical framework, indicates relations among the variables, discusses the sampling, gives major findings, and a copy of selected instruments.

Shaw and Wright [1967] illustrate scales for the measurement of attitudes in 600 pages packed full of sample instruments. Included are scales on social practices, social issues, international issues, abstract concepts, political and religious attitudes, ethnic and national groups, significant others and social institutions. Each attitude scale is discussed and data are presented relative to reliability, validity, and results using the instrument.

There are many other collections that can be consulted including those of Corcoran [1987] on measuring clinical practice, Mueller [1986] on social attitudes, Martin [1986] on human behavior measurements, Gillion [1985] on expenditure, costs, and performance measurements in health care from 1960 to 1983, Miller [1983] on social measurement in behavioral and social sciences, Budde [1979] on performance in human service systems, and Lyerly [1973] on psychiatric rating scales. Chun [1975] provides a guide to 3,000 original sources for psychological assessment; Buros [1974] has an index to tests, test reviews, and the literature on specific tests; and Lake [1973] covers social functioning assessment.

Knowledge, Attitudes, and Behavior

Measurements could test knowledge via multiple choice questions, fill-in the blanks questions, matching questions, true or false choices, essays, or through recall questions asking the respondent to identify, describe, list, or provide attributes. Most people have experienced these knowledge-testing variations in a school environment.

Measuring attitudes raises the obvious difficulty in the evaluator's knowing whether or not true attitudes are being reflected in the responses. Unless proven otherwise, it is generally assumed that the respondent has no reason to lie and that the answer given is accurate. Attitudes can be evaluated via paper and pencil tests, interviews, observations, and facial expressions. Questionnaires can be direct response type with "yes, no, don't know" choices or can allow respondents a wider choice such as extremely satisfied/somewhat satisfied/uncertain/somewhat dissatisfied/extremely dissatisfied. Frequently, a simple duo of attitude questions such as the following provides a great deal of insight:

- What did you like about [the care, the doctors, etc.]?
- What didn't you like about [care, doctors, etc.]?

Both AIDS knowledge and attitudes are collected regularly in the National Health Interview Survey conducted by the federal National Center for Health Statistics [Dawson, 1988]. More than 60 questions are tabulated by age, sex, race, and education.

Behavior is the acid test of an evaluation. People can secure high marks when tested for knowledge and give the appropriate attitude responses on paper while still not engaging in the required behavior. Noncompliance is a staggering problem in health care as patients have the knowledge and know the correct attitude, but still do not follow the physician's regimen. Behavior can be tested using case studies, simulated situations, or questions to respond to verbally or in writing. Again, the difficulty lies in "doing what I say or doing what I do." That doubt could take place even when the individual demonstrates the appropriate behavior in a testing environment. A patient with diabetes may be able to demonstrate the correct use of a syringe on a model and still not be able to do so at home on his own body. Optimal measurement of behavior remains direct observation at the locale and time when the behavior is to occur. If a patient has to exercise at home after work, that is where and when the behavior should be observed. If pills are to be taken four times a day, there should be four observations of the actual behavior. A checklist can be prepared for data collection personnel that merely requires a checkmark under a yes or no for each behavior.

At time, evaluation measurements will combine the testing of all three attributes: knowledge, attitudes, and behavior. Nevertheless, if choices are to be made, it is better to err on testing for behavior as the ultimate objective.

In a series of eight evaluation handbooks, IOX Assessment Associates [1988] provides assessment tools to measure knowledge, affectiveness, skill, and behavior. There are 12 criterion-referenced measuring instruments for alcohol abuse, 17 for drug abuse, 8 for smoking cessation, 12 for diabetes, 18 for nutrition, 10 for stress management, 11 for physical fitness, and 7 for physiological attributes. Instrument titles in stress management include Facts About Stress, Ways to Lower Stress [knowledge], How Will You Feel?, Could You Deal With It? [affective], How to Lower Stress, Appropriate Responses to Stress [skill] and Stress Management Checklist, How You Deal With Your Stress [behavior].

STRUCTURE, PROCESS, AND OUTCOME EVALUATION

Donabedian is credited with the development of a longstanding approach to the measurement of the quality of care that involves structure, process, and outcome evaluations [Donabedian, 1966, 1980, 1988]. In fact, Donabedian's [1988] own words can be used to elaborate on the three characteristics:

Structure denotes the attributes of the settings in which care occurs. This includes the attributes of material resources [such as facilities, equipment, and money], of human resources [such as the number and qualifications of personnel], and of organizational structure [such as medical staff organization, method of peer review, and methods of reimbursement]. Basically, structural characteristics evaluate the resources and indicate the capability of providing care.

Process denotes what is actually done in giving and receiving care—the curing process. It includes the patient's activities in seeking care and carrying it out as well as the practitioners' activities in making a diagnosis and recommending or implementing treatment. That encompasses components such as diagnostic procedures, laboratory tests, surgical interventions, and level of nursing care. Both, the technical aspects and the art of care are included in process observations.

Outcome denotes the effects of care on the health status of patients and populations. Improvement in the patient's knowledge and salutary changes in the patient's behavior are included under a broad definition of health status, and so is the degree of the patient's satisfaction with care—essentially the end product of the health care system. Components of outcome include mortality, morbidity, functioning, patient/provider/community satisfaction, and wellness level.

"This three part approach to quality assessment is possible only because good structure increases the likelihood of good process, and good process increases the likelihood of a good outcome" [Donabedian, 1988]. Exhibit 7–6 illustrates the relationship in the structure-process-outcome evaluation.

Management Use of S-P-O

Using a health care management viewpoint, Shortell and Kaluzny [1988, p. 428] delineate selected structure-process-outcome measures in the areas of financial performance, quality-of-

Exhibit 7-6.   Measures of Structure, Process, and Outcome.

Structure Components	Process Components	Outcome Components
Facilities	Provider/patient encounters	Mortality
Equipment	Health care system process	Morbidity
Organization patterns	Desirable health practices	Individual physical functioning
Funding	Technical aspects of care	
Staffing	"Art" aspects of care	Provider satisfaction
Personnel qualifications		Consumer satisfaction
Personnel experience		Community satisfaction
Environmental quality		Wellness level
Risk factors		Tests and vital signs relative to norms
[Resources]	[Curing process]	[Health status]

care performance, and personnel recruitment and retention [Exhibit 7–7]. Similarities are apparent between the quality measures and the other two management evaluation areas.

Similarly, there are patient care and administrative measures in structure, process, and outcome. Structural patient care items include staff qualifications and training, special care unit availability, and accreditation. Process in patient care covers average length of stay, autopsy rate, and medical staff audit. Outcome is measured by hospital acquired infections reported and treated, adjusted death rate, and malpractice suits. In administration, structure could include personnel per bed, employee development programs, and staff qualifications. Process may focus on occupancy rate, use of management studies, and community involvement. Outcome could be in cost per unit of output, man-hours per patient day and financial stability.

Fottler [1987] examined structural [nature of organization, participation in hospital system] and process [planning procedures, power/participation processes, communication/coordination processes, human resource processes, control processes] determinants of health care organizational performance outcomes such as cost efficiency, productivity, clinical quality, patient satisfaction, and financial outcomes. This evaluative approach is crucial at this time because of the turbulent nature of the health care system as reactions occur to increased competition, prospective pricing, and the growth of multifacility systems. Based on an exten-

Exhibit 7-7.   Selected Performance Measures.

	Financial Performance	Quality-of-Care Performance	Personnel Recruitment and Retention
Structure	Use of accrual accounting	Percentage of board-certified active staff physicians	Education and qualifications of personnel office staff
	Education and qualifications of financial and accounting staff	JCAHO accreditation	Existence of an up-to-date wage and salary administration system
	Existing organization-wide cost-containment committee	Number of residency approvals	Existence of a position control system
Process	Examination of budget variances	Medication error rates	Quality of education and training programs
	Ratio of current assets to current liabilities	Postsurgical infection rates	Job satisfaction survey assessments
	Ratio of net accounts receivable to average daily operating revenue	Percentage of indicated procedures performed for specific diagnoses	Organization climate assessment
Outcome	Ratio of operating income to operating revenue	Standardized case-severity adjusted mortality rates	Employee turnover
	Ratio of long-term debt to fixed assets	Standardized case-severity adjusted morbidity rates	Employee absenteeism
	Ratio of operating income plus interest to total assets		Cost per applicant recruited
	Market share		

Source: From *Health care management,* by S.M. Shortell & A.D. Katuzny, 1988, p. 428. New York: John Wiley & Sons. Reprinted with permission.

sive evaluation of about 150 health care administration articles, Fottler discovers a host of managerial relationships between structural and process elements that engender efficiency and effectiveness outcomes [Exhibit 7–8]. In fact, Fottler contends that that either efficiency or effectiveness can be enhanced without diminution of the other in the application of the identified variables. "Some of these managerial guidelines are applicable across a wide range of organiza-

Exhibit 7-8. Structural and Process Variables Enhancing Organizational Performance.

Structural Variables Enhancing Organizational Performance
Large size of facility
Participation in a multi-institutional system
Group purchasing arrangements
Use of contract management
Provision of ambulatory alternatives to inpatient care
Little or no unionization
High degree of specialization
Structured involvement of physicians in decision making
Low proportion of indigent and/or poor patients
Low level of formalization
Management information system integrating financial and clinical data
Use of physician extenders in ancillary personnel
A close fit between technology and structure
Mechanisms to promote continuity of care
An activist governing board representing the community power structure

Process Variables Strengthening Agency Performance
Significant board involvement in institutional activities
Significant physician/nurse/department head participation in strategy development, strategy implementation and operational management
Avoidance of total physician autonomy
Constant board and management monitoring of external environment
Development and implementation of a strategic plan
Emphasis on intra- and inter-departmental communication and coordination
Use of incentive compensation
Efforts to make consequences of decisions and strategies visible
Identification of varying needs and goals of various stakeholders
Active efforts to meet expectations of key stakeholders
Use of many indicators of performance
Efforts to reward creativity and innovations
Administration and board involvement in boundary-spanning activity
Use of quality circles and other employee participation programs
Active efforts to measure and improve service quality
Development of data to measure and enhance patient and employee satisfaction
Use of flextime and flexible staffing
Provision of many opportunities for employees to voice dissatisfaction
Organizational development efforts
Confining physician services to areas of expertise
Development of physician protocols where process/outcome relationships are fairly certain
Development of a proactive managerial ideology emphasizing outcomes and the constant necessity to adapt to environmental change

Source: From "Health care organizational performance: Present and future research," by M.D. Fottler, 1987, *Journal of Management, 13*(2), 385–386. Reprinted by permission.

tions. Others may be more appropriate for health care organizations or certain types of health organizations."

S-P-O in "Soft Services"

In addition, Wilson [1987] uses the structure-process-outcome model to respond to arguments that "soft services" such as mental health, social work, chaplaincy, staff education, and psychology have little or nothing to measure in terms of quality assurance. Starting with outcomes, Wilson lists measurable program results such as reduction in inpatient days; patients holding down jobs and living independently; measurable responses from other professionals such as the number of nursing referrals to the chaplain or others; the perception of success by the referring professionals and the appropriateness of referrals between professionals; and the third outcome grouping of patient responses in satisfaction with counselors, to remaining in counseling and to changes in behavior. Process deals with therapeutic encounter procedures such as crisis intervention, marital counseling, family counseling, or vocational counseling in treating generic problems such as bereavement, acute anxiety, post-abortion reaction, attempted suicide, depression, addiction, or the trauma of sexual and/or physical abuse. Wilson does comment that "counseling is like trying to catch a fly ball with the sun in your eyes—you do your best." Nevertheless, Wilson states that process can be evaluated using the frame of reference of appropriate principles of adult education or other recommended therapeutic processes. Structure is most similar in that human, mechanical, and environmental factors are evaluated such as staff qualifications, supervision, continuing education, adequacy of budget, taping of sessions, access to patient records, freedom from interruption, privacy, and comfort. In concluding, Wilson advises that "soft services should realize that they are not much worse off than most other departments. Although their problem may not be solved, it will be brought into perspective."

Mainly Outcome Evaluations

Not every evaluation uses all three elements of Donabedian's framework. Harking back to Dr. Codman's [1914] outcome of hospitalization investigations, Schroeder [1987] asked if the health care system was ready for outcome assessment. In a responsive manner, experts comment that outcome evaluation—measurement of what happens to the patient—is clearly the foundation on which the evaluation of the quality of care should be based [Gonnella & Zeleznik, 1974; Kessner & Kalk, 1973; Kessner, Kalk, & Singer, 1973; Williamson, 1971]. Factors that contribute to outcomes are identified by Gonnella and Louis [1988] as the physician's contribution to health care; the contribution of the setting where care is rendered; the contribution of the patient in accepting appropriate responsibilities; and the contribution of the social and physical environment. These authors declare that "improvement of health care outcomes is the most important goal of a quality assurance system."

JCAHO Outcome-Oriented Clinical Indicators. Traditionally, the Joint Commission on Accreditation of Healthcare Organizations looked at structure and process measures. However, the JCAHO's [1987] "Agenda for Change" focuses on 48 proposed "outcome-oriented clinical indicators" for anesthesia, obstetrics, and hospital-wide care [Meyer, 1988a]. Pilot testing is taking place at 17 hospitals throughout the nation.

PROs and Outcomes. Peer Review Organizations [PROs] examine the process of care as recorded in random patient charts. Hospital specific mortality data is used as a quality measure by the federal Health Care Financing Administration [HCFA] and that information is released to the public and the mass media [Esmond & Batchelor, 1988]. However, the interpretation of hospital mortality data have resulted in bitter controversy, particularly from the hospitals with bad rates. Kahn, Brook, and Draper [1988] and Jencks, Daley, and Draper [1988] both address the issue of interpreting hospital mortality data as outcome measures. Both articles suggest clinical risk adjustments to the mortality outcome related to the severity of the patient's illness at admission. To increase interpretative power, Kahn et al. [1988] suggest including outcomes other than death. In patients with acute myocardial infarction, data could be collected about complications [coma, shock, pneumonia], periods on clinical instability [unstable vital signs, new onset of altered mental status], or life-threatening laboratory values [serum potassium level <2.5 mmol/L]. Jencks et al. [1988] examine the role of risk-adjusted outcomes in congestive heart failure, myocardial infarction, pneumonia, and stroke to relate to the effectiveness of care. Continuing that concept, Daley et al. [1988] explore a method of predicting hospital-associated mortality for Medicare patients with those same four conditions. Using a microcomputer-based system, patient attributes at admission are used to predict death within 30 days of hospital admission. Predictors are taken from the medical record and the results indicate a higher level of relationship than noted in prior systems.

Functional Outcomes. Wilson [1988] reports on functional outcome assessment tools that are used primarily with patients receiving intensive care at home. Areas measured included activities of daily living [ADL] functioning, psychosocial functioning, and knowledge and application for both the patient and the caregiver. Evaluations would relate to goals such as: Within eight weeks of service the patient's functional status will increase 50 percent. Observational summaries could say that "during the first quarter of 1988, 60 percent of new CVA patients increased ADL function by 50 percent within 12 nursing visits." Related to functioning, Rinke [1988] delineates the state of the art in outcome standards in home health care.

Medicare Patient Outcome Analyses. In a Government Accounting Office [GAO] study, Chelimsky [1988a] looked at Medicare patient outcome analyses and concluded that improved mechanisms would improve quality assessment. Exhibit 7–9 shows the comparison of HCFA and alternative approaches to the analysis of patient outcomes. *General purpose* summarizes the basic issues addressed as each approach has been applied. *Diagnoses included* describes the patient population covered by the approach as defined by the principal diagnosis. *Severity adjustment* gives an overall rating based on the degree to which diagnostic data were used to adjust individual patient risks and care was taken to distinguish complications from comorbidities. *Quality of measurement* rates the validity, reliability, and sensitivity of measures used in the analysis. *Appropriateness of application* rates the extent to which applications of the analytical technique used accords with its assumptions and limitations. *Data quality* summarizes the probable impact of missing or inaccurate data elements on results. *Extent of validation* sums up the available evidence on the effectiveness of the approach in identifying quality of care problems. Note the emphasis on mortality in the column on "Outcome type." A *subjective focus* encompasses diagnoses, populations and severity of illness adjustments. *Technical adequacy* includes the quality measurement, the analytical technique and its appropriateness, data quality, and the extent of validation.

There was no determination by the GAO of which approach works best because none of the methods had been fully validated. However, the GAO based their evaluation on "a logical analysis of how completely and carefully different approaches deal with specific problems faced by outcome analyses using administrative data" [Chelimsky 1988, p. 83].

Exhibit 7-9. Comparison of HCFA and Alternative Approaches for Analyzing Medicare Patient Outcomes.

Approach	General purpose	Outcome type	Diagnoses included	Discrete populations analyzed
HCFA-intramural			Substantive focus	
1986 hospital mortality analyses	Provider performance	Inpatient mortality	All	9 diagnosis-related groups
1987 hospital mortality analyses	Provider performance	Mortality within 30 days of admission	All	16 diagnostic clusters
HSQB monitoring systems	Trends over time, patient subgroups	Mortality and readmission over multiple time periods following admission; morbidity and disability based on postdischarge costs	All for trend analyses, 9 specific medical and surgical conditions for patient subgroup analyses	7 "major conditions" for trend analyses; patient subgroups defined by 9 "tracer conditions," further divided by race, sex, age, and presence of 9 comorbidities
HCFA-extramural				
Nonintrusive Outcomes Study	Provider performance	Inpatient mortality, postdischarge mortality	48 medical and surgical conditions	Individual hospitals for the 48 conditions
Risk-Adjusted Mortality Index	Provider performance	Inpatient mortality	All except neonatal conditions	Individual hospitals for 310 diagnostic groups
Disease Staging Adapted to Mortality Analyses	Trends over time	Mortality within 30 days of admission	All	31 specific disease categories plus age, sex, comorbidities, and disease stage
National Hospital Rate-Setting Study	Trends over time, patient subgroups	Mortality within 30 days and 1 year of admission	59 "urgent care" conditions and 8 elective surgical procedures	15 state programs regulating hospital revenues
Non-HCFA				
Risk-Adjusted Monitoring of Outcomes for Nonelective Surgery	Patient subgroups, provider performance	Inpatient mortality	250 higher risk surgical procedures	Hospital, physician, diagnosis, and others
Computerized Identification of Surgical Complications	Provider performance, patient subgroups	Surgical complications resulting in hospital readmissions	Hysterectomy, cholecystectomy, prostatectomy	Hospital, physician specialty, urban or rural location, and others

(continued)

GAO recommendations [Chelimsky, 1988a, p. 5] to improve patient outcome analyses suggested taking greater advantage of available diagnostic data in adjusting for patient severity of illness; employing data for several years when analyzing outcomes involving small numbers of cases; expanding comparative outcomes among demographic and diagnostic subgroups of patients; periodically assessing the relative strengths and limitations of available approaches for analyzing Medicare patient outcome data in terms of substantive focus, technical adequacy, and degree of validation relative to overall degree of effectiveness in identifying patterns of patient care with quality problems; evaluation of the data elements for completeness and accuracy based on a nationally representative sample of Medicare patients.

Disease Staging and Outcome Based Ambulatory Care. Using a disease staging methodology, Gonnella and Louis [1988] design specifications for an outcome-based ambulatory quality assurance system. Beginning with a patient assessment, the 12 specifications include an examination of the process of care and a look at all the parts of the system—physician, institution, patient, and community. Evaluation characteristics of the system aim to be

Exhibit 7-9. (Continued)

Severity adjustment	Technical adequacy		Appropriateness of application	Data quality	Extent of validation
	Quality of measurement	Analytical technique			
Rudimentary	Medium	Multiple regression, t-test for significance	Significance test not appropriate	Unknown	Fragmentary evidence based on PRO reviews employing varying approaches
Moderate	Medium	Logistic regression, formula for range of "expected" mortality incorporates both sampling variance and overall interhospital variance	Appropriate	Unknown	None based on independent data sources; consistency using alternative statistical procedures tested
Moderate	High for mortality, low for morbidity	Life table analyses, Cox proportional modeling	Appropriate	Unknown	Limited case record reviews underway
Rudimentary	High	Indirect standardization, binomial significance tests	Appropriate	Currently unknown, but under study	Extensive case record reviews underway for two conditions
Sophisticated	Medium	Indirect standardization, logistic regression, binomial and Poisson significance tests	Appropriate	Results influenced by incomplete secondary diagnosis coding	Limited number of hospital site visits; consistency of results using data from different years tested
Sophisticated	Medium	Indirect standardization, logistic regression, chi-square significance tests	Appropriate	Results influenced by random variation in coding of diagnoses in claims files	None
Moderate	Medium	Multiple regression	Appropriate	Results influenced by changes in diagnostic coding over time, but only principal diagnosis used	None
Sophisticated	Medium	Indirect standardization, recursive partitioning, chi-square and Poisson significance tests	Appropriate	Results influenced by accuracy of coding for elective and nonelective surgery	Tests for potential bias, limited number of hospital site visits
Moderate	Medium	Logistic regression, chi-square significance test	Appropriate	Results influenced by thoroughness and accuracy of coding in medical record of surgical complications	None

Source: From *Medicare improved patient outcome analyses could enhance quality assessment*, by E. Chelimsky, 1988, Washington, DC: GAO/PEMD-88-23. Reprinted by permission.

simple and inexpensive, objective and consistent, clinically sound, documentable, flexible, action-oriented, timely, compatible with inpatient evaluation and audit protocols, and allow for easy verification. According to Gonnella and Louis, disease staging meets those specifications.

Staging uses information from clinical records to measure the severity of medical problems. Traditional diagnostic classifications are redefined to produce patient clusters requiring similar treatment procedures and services measurable in quality assessment studies. Although substages are used to refine categories, disease staging involves the application of the following four major stages of severity:

Stage 1—conditions with no complications or problems of minimal severity.
Stage 2—problems limited to an organ or system, significantly increased risk of complications over Stage 1.
Stage 3—multiple site involvement, generalized systemic
Stage 4—involvement, poor prognosis.

From an evaluation point of view, the staging concept is quite direct in its progression. "Undesirable outcomes are determined; the causes of those undesirable outcomes are determined; corrective actions are instituted; and the results are monitored to ensure that the desired results are being achieved" [Louis & Gonnella, 1986].

Computer Audit of Outcome. Through computer management data collection, Gilbert, Schoolfield, and Gaydou [1987] developed a quality assurance technique for a surgical intensive care unit. A Systems Outcome Score [SOS] uses data that reflect the likelihood of death such as simple dysfunction indices for all organ systems. Those correlate with an Outcome Index [OI] that compares actual mortality with expected mortality in monitoring the quality of care.

Process, Outcome, and Impact. In another use of outcome, a scheme relates process, outcome and impact. Exhibit 7–10 illustrates the concept as applied to a drug abuse prevention program. Impact could possibly be similar to behavior measurements in other evaluation models.

Outcome Related to Structure and Process. Critics have long made the point that most of the evaluation studies concentrated on the process aspects to the detriment of the outcome observations and also to the relation between process and outcome. As the old saw goes: The surgery was a success but the patient died! A representative of the JCAHO editorially commented on Donabedian's [1988] article. O'Leary [1988] stated that "despite exhortations for self-examination from the physician community since early in this century, what we know and have done about quality assessment to date is remarkably little. A Spring 1988 issue of *Health Affairs* paid particular attention to quality evaluation with Caper [1988] defining quality, Lohr, Yordy, and Thier [1988] identifying issues, Eddy and Billings [1988] looking at medical evidence, and Roper and Hackbarth [1988] discussing HCFA's plans to promote high quality care.

To counter, Donabedian notes that outcome is influenced by a variety of personal and environmental factors in addition to the care rendered. Outcome by itself does not pinpoint what may have gone wrong [Esmond & Batchelor, 1988]. Donabedian [1988] comments:

> As a general rule, it is best to include in any system of assessment, elements of structure, process, and outcome. This allows supplementation of weakness in one approach by strength in another; it helps one interpret the findings; and if the findings do not seem to make sense, it leads to a reassessment of study design and a questioning of the accuracy of the data themselves.

INDICATORS AS MEASUREMENTS

From a management view, Escobar [1985] says that "an indicator is a way of measuring policies, plans, and actions, whose goals can be expressed as a relationship, ratio or percentage between two or more data [numbers]." Scrivens [1985] regards the level of infant mortality as the most common indicator of the general health of a nation's population. However, the interpretation of indicators is not as clear-cut as a single infant mortality rate. Validity and reliability issues becloud even those indicators so routinely used to judge the health status of a nation's population. Infant mortality and longevity levels by themselves do not explain where the health care delivery system is failing. Critics point out that the United States has a heterogeneous population as compared to countries with lower infant mortality rates and that the longevity

Exhibit 7-10.   Process, Outcome, and Impact Evaluation in Drug Abuse Prevention.

Type of Evaluation	Process ------------------------- →	Outcome ------------------------- →	Impact
Level of Evaluation	Prevention Program Effects		Aggregate or Cumulative Effects at the Community Level

Potential Indicators of Effectiveness	Description of target audience/recipients of service
	
	Prevention services delivered
	
	Staff activities planned/performed
	
	Financing resources utilized
		Changes in drug-related:
		○ Perceptions
		○ Attitudes
		○ Knowledge
		○Actions:
		   Drug use
		   Truancy
		   School achievement
		   Involvement in community activities
			Changes in:
			○ Prevalence and incidence of drug use
			○ Drug-related mortality/morbidity
			○ Institutional policy/programs
			○ Youth/parent involvement in community
			○ Accident rates

Potential Prevention Evaluative Approaches	Examples: Process Evaluation Cost accountability model Quality assurance assessment	Examples: Experimental paradigms Quasi-experimental designs Ipsative designs, e.g., goal attainment scaling	Examples: Epidemiologic studies Incidence and prevalence studies Drug-related school surveys Cost-benefit analysis

leaders are nations that have national health service schemes. Scrivens likens the use of these national indicators to a warning light signaling the need for policy innovation or reorientation.

Administrative Data Indicators

Roos, Roos, Mossey, and Havens [1988] compared administrative indicators such as hospital utilization, ambulatory utilization and market context [admissions, days per admission, diagnoses per admission], [visits for diseases/conditions, specialists seen, laboratory services used], and [beds per population, doctor/population ratio, inpatient vs. outpatient practice procedures] with data secured from health interviews. A large sample of elderly residents of Manitoba, Canada were followed to gather data about entry to hospital, nursing home, and death. In a two-year period after a health interview took place, 294 people died. One-hundred-two were admitted to a nursing home and 1,140 had hospital admissions. Claims data from health care providers generated the comparable administrative indicators. Investigators concluded that "administrative and interview data provided roughly similar predictions of nursing home entry, with the claims data generating significantly better predictions of death and future hospital entry."

BED Instead of DOC

In developing countries, Indrayan [1987] discussed the use of the infant mortality rate and the physician/population ratio as an indicator of health service availability. In India, population per physician [DOC] was discarded in favor of population per bed [BED] as a proxy measure of health service availability. "In the case of both Indian and international data, infant mortality rate showed a better correlation with the availability of beds than with the availability of physicians." BED was judged a clearly defined superior indicator with an easy and accurate count while physician accounting may be incomplete and exclude other than medical school graduates.

Poor-Quality Indicators

An Office of Technology Assessment report claims that "formal disciplinary actions by state medical boards provides the most accurate and valid information concerning poor-quality physicians" [*U.S. Medicine*, 1988]. Disciplinary action is the indicator clearly linked to poor-quality physicians. An additional eight indicators of the quality of care in the OTA evaluation included hospital mortality rates; adverse events such as infections acquired in hospitals; sanctions imposed by the USDHHS based on PRO recommendations; malpractice compensation; evaluations of physicians' treatment for certain conditions such as hypertension; volume of service in hospitals and performed by physicians; scope of hospital services such as emergency services; and patients' assessment of their care.

In the JCAHO new accreditation program, three of the 48 clinical indicators are as follows: in obstetrics—a term infant who has a clinically apparent seizure before discharge from the delivery room; in anesthesia—respiratory arrest within a specified time following anesthesia care; and a hospital-wide indicator of the development of pneumonia in patients treated in special care units [Meyer, 1988a].

In defining the essential characteristics of a program to monitor, evaluate, and improve the quality of care, Roberts [1987] a JCAHO vice-president for research and planning, selects three critical components:

- Those aspects of care that are high volume, high risk, or are believed to be problem prone are chosen for monitoring.
- Indicators of high or low quality are identified for each of these aspects of care.
- Thresholds for evaluation are established for each indicator.

Exhibit 7–11 illustrates an application of those three components to ambulatory care, inpatient care, home care, long-term care, hospice care, and alcoholism treatment. In the thresholds of evaluation note that there are numerical guidelines to accompany the indicators.

Data for Indicators

Generically, indicators could depend upon the source of data such as budgetary, demographic, educational, economic, financial, health examination surveys, health interview surveys, housing, medical records of all types, morbidity statistics, operational reports, and registries of all types. Mootz [1986] notes advantages and disadvantages of some of the available data sources for the development of health indicators: comparatively reliable and valid, but usually too specific [integral counts or registrations]; detailed record material, but information is exclusive to single institution with an unknown population at risk [institutional records]; large-scale random data, but nonresponse is usually high and method is very expensive [health examination surveys]; data varied and comprehensive allowing correlations of indicators but expensive with

Exhibit 7-11. Indicators and Criteria for Important Aspects of Care, by Type of Care.

Component of Monitoring System	TYPE OF CARE						
	Ambulatory Care	Inpatient Care	Home Care	Long-term Care	Hospice Care	Alcoholism Treatment	
Important Aspect	Adequate prenatal care	Adequate intra- and post-partum care	Adequate foot care in diabetic patients	Providing the least restrictive environment that is feasible	Effective control of the symptoms of cancer	Continuity of care	
Indicator	Initiation of prenatal care in the 1st trimester	Resuscitation with intubation in term infant	Adequate instruction in foot care	Residents are free from unnecessary restraints [chemical or physical]	Adequate control of pain	Patient receives post-discharge services	
Thresholds for Evaluation	At least 75 percent of patients have prenatal care initiated in the 1st trimester	Less than 2 percent incidence	No patients develop foot infections after admission to the home care program	Restraints are used only after less restrictive alternatives have been tried	For each patient reviewed, pain is adequately controlled or another therapeutic approach is being considered	At least 80 percent of patients initiate care as planned after discharge	

Source: From "Reviewing the Quality of care: priorities for improvement," by J.S. Roberts, 1987, Health Care Financing Review [Annual Supplement], p. 71. Reprinted by permission.

self-assessment problems and also high nonresponse rate [health interview surveys]. With the data sources and the limitations in mind, examples of indicators could include the following:

Gross income
Literacy
Total deaths
House owners
Operative costs
Rural area residents
Income from government—on welfare
Total medical consultations
Actual expenses
Occupied beds

Gross income may be associated with higher expenditures for health care; income from government may indicate more severe health problems in poverty groups; or occupied beds could be linked to an epidemic situation.

In a number of managerial processes, indicators can be of use in areas such as budgeting, decision making, diagnosis, evaluation, objective setting, planning, policy making, programming, and strategy determination. Shortell and Kaluzny [1988, p. 439] illustrate three types of management indicators: productivity indicators could include admissions per FTE, physician visits per FTE, and ancillary service units per FTE; efficiency indicators such as cost per patient, cost per admission, or cost per physician visit; financial viability indicators include cash flow ratios, market share, debt/equity ratio, current assets/current liabilities, and profit margin.

Using 32 minimum requirement performance indicators, HCFA inspectors evaluated all 15,000 Medicare certified nursing homes in the U.S. between January 1987 and July 1988. Their work resulted in a 75 volume report that found 40 percent of the facilities to be substandard. Meyer [1988b] reported a sampling of the indicators and the percentage of skilled nursing facilities [SNF] and intermediate care facilities [ICF] failing on that specific indicator:

Indicator	SNF	ICF
• Administration of drugs per physician's prescription	29%	25%
• Food handling	43	45
• Isolation techniques	25	-
• Resident personal hygiene	30	25
• Rehabilitative nursing care	22	14
• Care to prevent skin breakdown	18	12

Policy determinations can be illustrated in a few examples:

• Government and politicians can use indicators to show the community what they want to accomplish such as a reduction in the infant mortality rate.
• Hospitals can use the geographic bed census ratio to project their probable future patient case mix.
• Alternative ambulatory care services could estimate the percentage of people with specific ailments likely to use their facilities based on the percent of costs covered by insurance.

Objectives of Indicators

Health indicators generally provide insight into the prevalence and incidence patterns of specific diseases/conditions and into the health status of a population. With those health indicators, international infant mortality rates and longevity can be compared, improvement or deterioration in morbidity from heart disease can be noted, and resources can be allocated based on areas with the most illness. Furthermore, indicators can provide insight into the relation of medical and social phenomena contributing to illness, to individual behavior and to the subjective meaning of illness. Other phenomena could include personal characteristics [age, sex, socioeconomic status], life habits [smoking, drinking, eating, exercise], environmental factors [air pollution, traffic safety, work conditions], social networks [friends, family, lay referrals], and the occurrence of stress at work, at home, or at school. Medical-related dimensions such as the clarity of the diagnosis, the duration or frequency of symptoms, the restriction of daily activities, and the anticipated prognosis can interact with the other phenomena to aggravate the situation.

Health Concept and Indicators

Considering the objectives of health indicators, there is an obvious need to clarify the health concept. Positive health has been defined by the World Health Organization as not merely the absence of disease or infirmity but the state of complete physical, mental, and social well-being of the individual. Most of the positive health concepts are expansive and in the same idealistic atmosphere. However, three characteristics are distinguished in negative health concepts [Mechanic, 1982]:

Disease = medical biological view of illness
Sickness = subjectively perceived illness
Illness behavior = going to bed, visit to doctor, take medicine

In this framework, the disease concept is considered an objective indicator of directly observable phenomena. On the other hand, the sickness concept is considered a subjective indicator of the of the perceptions of people as to their situation and their satisfaction with it. Mootz [1986] distinguishes between the objective health indicators and the subjective social indicators. His definition states that social indicators relate "to the quantitative presentation of information regarding social phenomena, their development and correlation. . . The social indicator movement is closely connected with policy and planning." Exhibit 7–11 lists 30 social indicators that are highly correlated with the need for mental health services. Obviously, many of the indicators can be directly associated with nationwide policy decisions and program planning activities. Phenomena evaluated include poverty, unemployment, education, overcrowding, mobility, disability, working mothers, aged living alone, female headed households, ethnicity, and race.

Obviously, there could be an unlimited number of indicators and strategic planners need to make selections. It should be apparent that indicators should be selected that are few in number and that reveal a proven relationship between the variables. Criteria that come into play could include accuracy, cost, feasibility, necessity, opportunity, and ease of understanding. Importantly, indicators can certainly change over time and therefore a comparison with a standard is helpful. Existing standards may include an historic average of indicators, statistical trends,

Exhibit 7-12. Social Indicators Highly Correlated with Need for Mental Health Services.

1. Median income of families and unrelated individuals.
2. Percent of all families below poverty level.
3. Percent of employed males 16 and over who are operatives, service workers, and laborers, including farm laborers.
4. Percent of labor force 16 and over who are unemployed.
5. Median number of school years completed by persons 25 and over.
6. Percent of population 14 to 17 not enrolled in schools.
7. Persons under 18 in households per 100 persons 18 to 64.
8. Percent 65 or older in households per 100 persons 18 to 64.
9. Percent of persons in household in housing units with 1.01 or more persons per room.
10. Percent of population who moved last year.
11. Percent of population who live in group quarters.
12. Percent of persons 16 to 64, not inmates of institutions and not attending school, who are disabled or handicapped.
13. Percent females 14 and over who are divorced or separated.
14. Percent of households with only one person.
15. Percent of population 14 to 17 not enrolled in school.
16. Percent of women 16 and over in labor force having their own children under 6 years old.
17. Percent of persons 65 and over below poverty level.
18. Percent of related children under 18 below poverty level.
19. Percent of all households headed by one person 65 or over.
20. Percent of occupied housing units with 1.51 or more persons per room and without complete plumbing facilities.
21. Percent of families with at least one related child under 18 that are female headed below poverty level.
22. Percent of persons 16 to 64, not inmates of institutions and not attending school, who are disabled or handicapped and who are unable to work.
23. Percent of households with 6 or more persons that have an annual income of less than [$ value poverty related income].

Sources: USDHHS, National Institute of Mental Health. 1975. *A typological approach to doing social area analysis.* Series C, No. 10 Washington, DC: Government Printing Office. DHEW Pub. No. [ADM] 76-262.

USDHHS, NIMH. 1975. *Catchment areas with unusually high proportions of some "high risk" groups: Region X.* MHDPS Working Paper No. 20, Bethesda, MD.

Hagedorn, H. 1977. *A manual on state mental health planning.* Washington, DC: Government Printing Office, DHEW Pub. No. [ADM] 77-473.

indicators from similar institutions or programs, work measurement standards, and set targets for accomplishment.

Shortcomings of Poverty Indicators

Poverty indicators were examined by Datta [1988] relative to the U.S. Census Bureau's method of valuing noncash benefits as part of the measurement of poverty. Three points were made:

1. People can be reclassified or misclassified in or out of poverty by the valuation methods.
2. Valuation methods can be systematically assessed and the magnitude and direction of the impact can be empirically determined.

3. There is no adequate warning of the magnitude of differences in poverty estimates resulting from conceptual, operational, and computational concerns with the valuation of noncash benefits.

Five questions aided in the evaluation of the poverty indicators and are guidelines for considerations about indicators in general:

1. What is the basis for defining income?
2. Are the methods valid?
3. Do the values assigned accurately represent the benefits?
4. What is the quality of the data and data analytic procedures used to derive benefit values?
5. Are definitions used consistently across key steps of poverty measurement?

Using the five questions, an empirical investigation looked at changes in poverty rates over time, subgroups affected differentially, an index of the dispersion of changes in poverty-gap distributions and the average benefit assigned. Among the 32 conceptual concerns identified were the use of a market method, the recipient value method, official minimum needs standards, and lifetime income projections. Operational concerns included using questionable HCFA Medicaid data, underreporting of income, and household versus family as income unit in the 27 problems. Seven technical computational concerns dealt with items such as low regression values, use of central tendency instead of average, mean medical benefit, and negative values of housing subsidies.

Quality of Life Indicators

Measurement of the quality of life is frequently a major factor in medical decisions for patients with end stage renal disease [ESRD] as with other complex diseases or conditions. Decisions to use a special procedure or to expend a large volume of scarce resources can be linked to indicators of the quality of life. In a HCFA study [USDHHS, 1987, p. 81] investigators used two objective indicators [ability to work and functional impairment] and three subjective indicators [psychological affect, well-being, and life satisfaction] to evaluate the quality of life for ESRD patients. Even after statistical adjustments for case mix and treatment modalities, significant differences persisted in both the objective and subjective indicators of the quality of life. Transplant patients consistently reported a higher quality of life than patients on dialysis, although home dialysis patients were similar in many respects; patients on continuous peritoneal dialysis [COPD] and in-center hemodialysis patients both reported being worse off than either the transplant or the home dialysis group. Additional subjective quality of life indicators included the following:

General Well-Being Index
Positive Affect Scale
Negative Affect Scale
Affect Balance Scale
General life satisfaction
Satisfaction with savings/investments
Satisfaction with standard of living
Satisfaction with sex life

Feeling about present life [hard vs. easy]
Feeling about present life [tied down vs. free]

Utility Value of Life

Speedling and Rose [1985] raise the issue of a utility scale in assessments of the quality of life. A utility value is the individual's quantification of personal perceptions about an outcome. An elderly patient with angina pectoris must choose between surgery or medical therapy. Surgery can result in 10 years of pain-free life with a 10 percent chance of immediate death. Medical therapy assures survival and 10 years of life with continued angina. If the elderly person indicates that life with angina has a utility value of 95 percent, then each of the 10 years is valued at 9.5 "quality adjusted years" and medical therapy is the preferred choice. If the elderly persons says that life with angina is worth 80 percent of normal, then surgery results in a preferred outcome since each year is worth 9.0 quality adjusted years [90 percent of 10 years with 100 percent quality plus 10 percent chance of 0 percent quality]. Obviously, the utility value indicator is subject to a weighting factor relative to the individual's attitude toward risk; high- or low-risk takers.

Using the four program effect evaluation criteria of targeting success, achievement of intended objectives, cost-effectiveness and other effects, Chelimsky [1988b, p. 55] reviewed Medicaid eligibility extension indicators. In this comparative evaluation framework of children's programs, Exhibit 7–13 relates the indicators to measures and analyses for each of the four program effect classifications. While the measures and analyses appear to be objective for the most part, the specific numerical reductions or increases are not given. Taken as directions for the states, the actual numbers can be supplied to meet anticipated differences among the states.

Access to Services Indicators

Even prior to the provision of care, individuals must have access to the services. Aday [1986] identifies four monitoring activities relative to the access to medical care: indicators of need reflected in mortality and morbidity; discrepancies in the use of services; existence of a regular source of care; and public or private health insurance coverage. Those four indicators indicate that the United States has made tremendous progress toward the provision of equity of access to health care. In the case of ambulatory services for economically disadvantaged children, Newacheck and Halfon [1986] also found substantially improved access attributed to Medicaid programs. Nevertheless, children with substantial health problems still lagged behind their cohorts in health status in higher income families. Three health status indicators included average annual bed disability days; self-reported health status among excellent, good, fair or poor; and long-term limitation in usual activities.

Sentinel Health Events [Occupational]

A Sentinel Health Event [SHE] indicator was discussed in Chapter 2 in relation to needs assessment and illustrated in Exhibit 2–11. Carr, Szapiro, Heisler, and Krasner [1989] applied SHEs to hospitalized patients in New York State in 1983. They found more than 17,000 possibly avoidable deaths and more than 336,000 disease cases that were potentially preventable.

Exhibit 7-13.   Medicaid Eligibility: Criterion, Indicators, and Measures.

Evaluation criterion	Indicators	Measures and analyses
Targeting success	Enrollment of eligible population, for the options each state adopted	Relationship of family income to poverty level
		Eligibility category
		Family structure and employment status
		Prior insurance coverage
		Homelessness
		State and local area
		Urban or rural residence
	Increased participation rates over time	
Achievement of intended objectives	Improved access to health care among the newly enrolled, by relationship of family income to poverty level	Earlier receipt and extended continuity of care
		Receipt of medically-recommended frequency and timing of prenatal, well-baby, and well-child care, by maternal age and marital status
		Treatment of problems identified in EPSDT screening
	Improved quality of care received	Decreased use of hospital emergency rooms as source of nonemergency care
Cost-effectiveness	Costs of prenatal care versus reductions in expenditures for treating complicated births and for neonatal intensive care	Full federal, state, and local costs of financing such care
	Costs of preventive health care for children versus reductions in expenditures for treating childhood chronic diseases	Full federal, state, and local costs of financing such care
	Costs of incorrectly granting presumptive eligibility versus effects of improving early access to prenatal care	
	Full costs and effects of expanding Medicaid eligibility versus subsidizing more clinics and health centers through federal health care block grants	
Other effects	Improvement in health status of low-income pregnant women and children among newly enrolled	Reduced incidence of poor pregnancy outcomes (low birthweight and preterm birth)
		Reduced incidence of perinatal mortality and morbidity
		Reduced length of neonatal hospital stays
		Reduced incidence of chronic illness and disability
	Reduced Medicaid expenditures in the long term for infants and children	More frequent use of less expensive preventive services
		Reduced incidence and duration of neonatal intensive care
		Reduced use of acute services in an inpatient setting
	Reduced expenditures for other programs	Long-term institutional care
		Special education
		Early intervention programs for infants and toddlers
	Redirection of block grant and Community and Migrant Health Centers funds	Decreased expenditures on primary health care
		Increased outreach and support services (e.g., transportation)
		Expanded service to persons ineligible for Medicaid
	Increased federal Medicaid expenditures in the short term	
	Increased work incentives by detaching eligibility from welfare receipt	Increased participation in workfare programs offering Medicaid eligibility
	Societal goals	Increased reliance on the government for health insurance coverage
		Contribution to the nation's progress toward the Surgeon General's goals for reducing infant mortality and low birthweight

Source: From *Children's programs. A comparative evaluation framework and five illustrations*, by E. Chelimsky, 1988, Washington, DC: GAO/PEMD-88-28BR.

As a precursor to the next set of SHEs, Rutstein [1981] commented that both communicable and man-made disease are amenable to intensive preventive efforts. In an article with 190 references, Rutstein, Mullan, and Frazier [1983] unveiled their SHE[O]—Sentinel Health Event [Occupational]—as a basis for physician recognition and public health surveillance [Exhibit 7-14]. An SHE[O] could be eye cataracts caused by pesticides with dinitrophenol. Rutstein [1984]

Exhibit 7-14. Sentinel Health Events—Occupational.

ICD-9	CONDITION	A	B	C	INDUSTRY/OCCUPATION@†	AGENT
011	Pulmonary Tuberculosis (O)*	P*	P,T*	P,T	Physicians[21], medical personnel[143], med lab workers[69]	Mycobacterium tuberculosis.[21,69,143]
011, 502	Silicotuberculosis	P	P,T	P,T	Quarrymen, sandblasters, silica processors, mining, metal foundries, ceramic industry.[33]	SiO₂ + Mycobacterium tuberculosis.[33,82,15]
020	Plague (O)	P	—	P,T	Shepherds, farmers, ranchers, hunters, field geologists.[17]	Yersinia pestis.[17]
021	Tularemia (O)	P	—	P,T	Hunters, fur handlers, sheep industry workers[69], cooks, vets, ranchers, vet pathologists.[169]	Francisella tularensis.[69,159]
022	Anthrax (O)	P	—	P,T	Shepherds, farmers, butchers, handlers of imported hides or fibers[30], veterinarians, veterinarian pathologists, weavers.[118]	Bacillus anthracis.[30,118,170]
023	Brucellosis (O)	P	P	P,T	Farmers, shepherds, veterinarians, lab workers[132], slaughterhouse workers.[118,170]	Brucella abortus, suis.[118,132,170]
037	Tetanus (O)	P	—	P,T	Farmers, ranchers.[169]	Clostridium tetani.[169]
056	Rubella (O)	P	P	P	Medical personnel[61,113,142], intensive care personnel[143].	Rubella virus.[61,113,142]
070.0.1	Hepatitis A (O)	P	P	P	Day care center staff[65,171], orphanage staff[37], mental retardation institution staff[71,164], medical personnel[62].	Hepatitis A virus.[37,62,65,71,164,171]
070.2.3	Hepatitis B (O)	P	P	P	Nurses and aides,[54,67,96] anesthesiologists[38], orphanage and mental institution staff[54], med lab personnel[96,102,106], general dentists[124] and oral surgeons[55], physicians[67,96,102]	Hepatitis B virus.[38,54,55,67,96,102,106]
070.4	Non-A, Non-B Hepatitis (O)	P	P	P	As above for hepatitis A and B	Unknown.
071	Rabies (O)	P	—	P	Veterinarians, animal and game wardens, lab researchers, farmers, ranchers, trappers.[169]	Rabies virus.[163]

					Occupation	Agent
073	Ornithosis (O)	P	—	P,T	Psittacine bird breeders, pet shop staff, poultry producers, veterinarians, zoo employees.[119]	Chlamydia psittaci.[119]
155M*	Hemangiosarcoma of the Liver	P	P	P	Vinyl chloride polymerization industry.[42] Vintners.[53]	Vinyl chloride monomer.[42,86,87,168,184] Arsenical pesticides.[53,86]
160.0	Malignant Neoplasm of Nasal Cavities (O)	P	P,T	P,T	Woodworkers, cabinet, furniture makers.[12,14,34,107,151] Boot and shoe industry.[11,12] Radium chemists and processors[52], dial painters[141] Chromium producers, processors, users.[86] Nickel smelting and refining.[48,85,176]	Hardwood dusts.[12,14,34,107,151] Unknown.[11,12] Radium.[52,141] Chromates.[86] Nickel.[48,65,86,175]
161	Malignant Neoplasm of Larynx (O)	P	P,T	P,T	Asbestos industries and utilizers.[149]	Asbestos.[86,149]
162	Malignant Neoplasm of Trachea, Bronchus, and Lung (O)	P	P	P	Asbestos industry and utilizers.[24,49,99] Topside coke oven workers.[104,145,146] Uranium and fluorspar miners.[45] Chromium producers and processors[51], users.[108,172] Nickel smelters, processors, users.[48,85] Smelters.[175] Mustard gas formulators.[182] Ion exchange resin makers, chemists.[57,185]	Asbestos.[24,49,86,99,159] Coke oven emissions.[104,145,146] Radon daughters.[45] Chromates.[51,86,106,172] Nickel.[48,85,86] Arsenic.[86,175] Mustard gas.[182] Bis(chloromethyl)ether, chloromethyl m ether.[57,86,135]
158, 163	Mesothelioma (MN of Peritoneum) (MN of Pleura)	P	—	P	Asbestos industries and utilizers.[24,99]	Asbestos.[24,82,86,99,159,150]
170	Malignant Neoplasm of Bone (O)	P	—	P	Dial painters[109], radium chemists and processors.[52]	Radium.[52,109]
187.7	Malignant Neoplasm of Scrotum	P	—	P,T	Automatic lathe operators[72,91], metalworkers[150].	Mineral/cutting oils.[72,86,91] Soots and tars, tar distillates.[72,66]

(continued)

Exhibit 7-14. (Continued)

ICD-9	CONDITION	A	B	C	INDUSTRY/OCCUPATION@†	AGENT
188	Malignant Neoplasm of Bladder (O)	P	—	P	Coke oven workers, petroleum refiners, tar distillers.[72] Rubber and dye workers.[39,40,183]	Bendizidine[158,189], alpha and beta naphthamine[39,86], auramine[40,86], magenta[40,6], aminobiphenyl[116], 4-nitrophenyl[56,178]
189	Malignant Neoplasm of Kidney, Other, and Unspecified Urinary Organs (O)	P	P	P	Coke oven workers.[145,146]	Coke oven emissions.[145,146]
204	Lymphoid Leukemia, Acute (O)	P	—	P	Rubber industry.[114,115] Radiologists.[110,111]	Unknown.[114,115] Ionizing radiation.[41,110,111]
205	Myeloid Leukemia, Acute (O)	P	—	P	Occupations with exposure to benzene Radiologists.[110,111]	Benzene.[16,43,54,86,180,181] Ionizing radiation.[41,110,111]
207.0	Erythroleukemia (O)	P	—	P	Occupations with exposure to benzene.[110,111]	Benzene.[16,83,84,86,180,131]
283.1	Hemolytic Anemia, Non-autoimmune (O)	P	—	P,T	White washing and leather industry.[44] Electrolytic processes, arsenical ore smelting.[78]	Copper sulfate.[44] Arsine.[78,892,134,139]
284.8	Aplastic Anemia (O)	P	—	P	Plastics industry.[15] Dye, celluloid, resin industry.[59] Explosives manufacture.[81,162] Occupations with exposure to benzene. Radiologists[111], radium chemists and dial	Trimellitic anhydride.[15] Naphthalene.[59] TNT.[70,81,152] Benzene.[16,130,181] Ionizing radiation.[41,111,163]
.0	Agranulocytosis or Neutropenia (O)	P	—	P	Occupations with exposure to benzene.[32] Explosives and pesticide industries.[32] Pesticides, pigments, pharmaceuticals.[93]	Benzene.[16,180,181] Phosphorus.[32] Inorganic arsenic.[93]
.7	Methemoglobinemia (O)	P	—	P,T	Explosives and dye industries.[66,70,125,188]	Aromatic amino and nitro compounds (eg, aniline, TNT, nitroglycerin).[66,70,81,125,188]
.7	Toxic Encephalitis (O)	P	P	P	Battery, smelter, and foundry workers.[19,31] Electrolytic chlorine production, battery	Lead.[19,31] Inorganic and organic memory.[22,31,56]

Code	Condition			Industries/Occupations	Agents
				makers, fungicide formulators.[22,31]	
332.1	Parkinson's Disease (Secondary) (O)	P	P	—	Manganese processing, battery makers, welders.[154]	Manganese.[154,167]
334.3	Cerebellar Ataxia (O)	P	P	—	Internal combustion engine industries.[60] Chemical industry using toluene.[28] Electrolytic chlorine production, battery makers, fungicide formulators.[31,43]	Carbon monoxide.[60] Toluene.[26] Organic mercury.[31,43]
357.7	Inflammatory and Toxic Neuropathy (O)	P	P,T	P,T	Pesticides[75], pigments, pharmaceuticals.[46] Furniture refinishers, degreasing operations.[74] Plastic-coated-fabric workers.[26] Explosives industry.[7■] Rayon manufacturing[56,179] Plastics, hydraulics, coke industries.[121] Battery, smelter, and foundry workers.[19,31] Dentists[88,161], chloralkali workers[166] Chloralkali plants, furgicide makers, battery makers.[43] Plastics industry[127], paper manufacturing[100].	Arsenic and arsenic compounds.[46,75] Hexane.[74,155] Methyl n-butyl ketone.[26] TNT.[70] CS$_2$.[56,155,177,179] Tri-o-cresyl phosphate.[121,155] Inorganic lead.[19,31,56,155] Inorganic mercury.[88,161,166] Organic mercury.[43,56] Acrylamide.[100,127,155]
366.4	Cataract (O)	P	P,T	—	Microwave and radar technicians.[90] Explosives industries.[70] Radiologists.[120] Blacksmiths, glass blowers, bakers.[120] Moth repellant formulators, fumigators.[59] Explosives, dye, herbicide and pesticide industries.[130]	Microwaves.[90] TNT.[63,70] Ionizing radiation.[63,120] Infrared radiation.[63,120] Naphthalene.[59,63,120] Dinitrophenol[120], dinitro-o-cresol.[130]
388.1	Noise Effects on Inner Ear (O)	P	P		Exposure.[131]	Excessive noise.[131]
443.0	Raynaud's Phenomenon (Secondary) (O)	P	—	—	Lumberjacks[97,144], chain sawyers, grinders, chippers.[173]	Whole body or segmental vibration.[97,144,173]

(continued)

Exhibit 7-14. (Continued)

ICD-9	CONDITION	A	B	C	INDUSTRY/OCCUPATION@†	AGENT
495 to 495.6. .8	Extrinsic Allergic Alveolitis	P	P	P,T	Vinyl chloride polymerization industry.[47,98,103] Farmer's lung, baggassosis, bird fancier's lung, suberosis, malt worker's lung, mushroom worker's lung, maple bark disease, cheese washer's lung, coffee worker's lung, fish-metal worker's lung, furrier's lung sequoiosis, wood worker's lung, miller's lung.[147,187]	Vinyl chloride monomer.[47,87,96,103] Various agents.[147,187]
493.0. 507.8	Extrinsic Asthma (O)	P	P,T	P,T	Jewelry, alloy and catalyst makers.[35,135] Polyurethane, adhesive, paint workers.[35,138] Alloy, catalyst, refinery workers.[35] Solderers.[35] Plastic, dye, insecticide makers.[35] Foam workers, latex makers, biologists.[35] Printing industry.[35] Nickel platers.[35] Bakers.[35,174] Plastics industry.[35,139] Woodworkers, furniture makers.[35] Detergent formulators.[35]	Platinum.[35,135,137] Isocyanates.[35,137,138] Chromium and cobalt.[35] Aluminum soldering flux.[35] Phthalic anhydride.[35,137] Formaldehyde.[35] Gum arabic.[35] $NiSO_4$.[35] Flour.[35,174] Trimellitic anhydride.[35,136,137] Red cedar and other wood dusts.[35] Bacillus-derived exoenzymes.[35]
500	Coalworkers' Pneumoconiosis	P	P	P	Coal miners.[76,122]	Coal dust.[76,82,122]
501	Asbestosis	P	P		Asbestos industries and utilizers.[24,99,126]	Asbestos.[24,82,99,126,159]
502M	Silicosis	P	P		Quarrymen, sandblasters, silica processors[20], mining, metal, and ceramic industries.[129,190]	Silica.[20,82,129,156,190]
	Talcosis				Talc processors.[95]	Talc.[95]
503M	Chronic Beryllium Disease of the Lung	P	P	P	Beryllium alloy workers, ceramic and cathode ray tube makers, nuclear reactor workers.[68,163]	Beryllium.[68,183]

Code	Disease	Type	Industry/Occupation	Agent
504	Byssinosis	P	Cotton industry workers.[29,117,128]	Cotton, flax, hemp, and cotton-synthetic dusts.[117,29,128]
506.0, 506.1	Acute Bronchitis, Pneumonitis, and Pulmonary Edema Due to Fumes and Vapors (O)	P	Refrigeration, fertilizer[101], oil refining industries.[123]	Ammonia.[101,123]
			Alkali and bleach industries.[123]	Chlorine.[123]
		P,T	Silo fillers, arc welders, nitric and industry.[58]	Nitrogen oxides.[58,123]
			Paper and refrigeration industries, oil refining.[123]	Sulfur dioxide.[123]
		P	Cadmium smelters, processors.[123]	Cadmium.[123]
			Plastics industry.[73]	Trimellitic anhydride.[73]
570, 573.3	Toxic Hepatitis (O)	P	Solvent utilizers, dry cleaners,[23] plastics industry[105].	Carbon tetrachloride[140], chloroform[27], tetrachloroethane[105], trichloroethylene.[18,23]
		P	Explosives and dye industries.[32,70]	Phosphorus[32], TNT.[70,162]
			Fire and waterproofing additive formulators.[79,94]	Chloronaphthalenes.[79,94]
			Plastics formulators.▪	Methylenedianiline.[112]
			Fumigators, gasoline, fire extinguisher formulators.[133]	Ethylene dibromide.[133]
			Disinfectant, fumigant, synthetic resin formulators.[80]	Cresol.[80]
584, 585	Acute or Chronic Renal Failure (O)	P	Battery makers, plumbers, solderers.[157]	Inorganic lead.[157]
		P,T	Electrolytic processes, arsenical ore smelting.[78,139]	Arsine.[78,134,139,157]
		P,T	Battery makers, jewelers, dentists.[157]	Inorganic mercury.[157]
			Fluorocarbon formulators, fire extinguisher makers.[157]	Carbon tetrachloride.[164,157]
606	Infertility, Male (O)	P	Antifreeze manufacture.[25]	Ethylene glycol.[25]
		P	Formulators.[36]	Kepone.[36]
		—	DBCP producers, formulators, and	Dibromochloropropane.[50,152,186]

(continued)

Exhibit 7-14. (Continued)

ICD-9	CONDITION	A	B	C	INDUSTRY/OCCUPATION@†	AGENT
692	Contact and Allergic Dermatitis (O)	P,T	P,T	—	applicators.[50,152,186] Leather tanning, poultry dressing plants, fish packing, adhesive and sealants industry, boat building and repair.[13]	Irritants (e.g., cutting oils, solvents, phenol, acids, alkalis, detergents); Allergens (e.g., nickel, chromates, formaldehyde, dyes, rubber products).[148]

External causes of injury and poisoning (occupational) include accidents and are classified in the ICD-9 under the E codes.

A = Unnecessary disease
B = Unnecessary disability
C = Unnecessary untimely death
@ = INDUSTRY/OCCUPATION listings are examples only

†Industry/Occupation reference numbers inside commas and inside periods apply only to the immediately preceding category, those outside of periods apply to all prior categories pertaining to a particular agent or process.

+ (O) = Only where an occupational exposure can be established
*P = prevention, T = treatment
*M = Modified ICD rubric

Source: From "Sentinel health events (occupational): A basis for physician recognition and public health surveillance," by D.D. Rutstein, R.J. Mullan, & T.M. Frazier, 1983, *American Journal of Public Health, 73*(9), 1056–1058. Reprinted with permission.

states that the SHE[O]s are limited to conditions documented in the scientific literature for agent, industry, and occupation.

Comparison of National Health Indicators

In a comparison of selected health indicators from Denmark, the Federal Republic of Germany, the Netherlands, and the United Kingdom, Mootz [1986] points out existing difficulties with using health/social indicators for comparative purposes. Data came from a variety of governmental reports on health problems, bed disability, vision problems, hearing problems, and current physical problems. No health problems were reported by 84 percent of the Germans and 58 percent of the Dutch while only 19 percent of the English population had no health problems. That health status gap appears to be implausible and is attributed to differences in the definitions and formulations of the questions in the survey. Bed disability shows the English and the Dutch both reporting about 18 percent while the Germans only report 6 percent. Permanent physical problems are reported by both 9 percent of the Dutch and the Germans as compared to about 27 percent for the Danes and the English. Even on the supposedly more objective indicators, there are differences although closer. Vision problems equaled 9 percent for the Danes, 11 percent for the English, and 3 percent for the Dutch. Hearing problems came out as 15 percent for the English, 10 percent for the Danes, and 7 percent for the Dutch. Rationales could include population base determinations, time of survey, age distribution, double counting, and mechanical counting errors. Nevertheless, Mootz still feels that the indicators are valuable and can be made comparable through repeated measurements using the same instruments, relation of the indicators to data other than survey data, and use of an adequate random sample. Three conclusions emerge from Mootz's analysis:

- There are many different definition of health and social indicators and expectations are usually too high regarding their usability for policy goals.
- Selection of health/social indicators is always arbitrary and inevitably dependent on the research problems and available sources.
- There is no point in trying to develop one single health indicator or one health index since this disregards the various dimensions of the health concept within a given research problem.

MEASUREMENT USING INDEXES

Strategic planners may not distinguish between indicators and indexes as evaluation measurements. Basically, an indicator is a single specific dimension related to elements such as education, income, or social status. An index is a measure which summarizes data from two or more components to reflect the health status or status quo of an individual or defined group. Usually, an arbitrary numerical weighting converts the data into a single numerical score allowing for statistical manipulations. Solon's [1974, p. 263] definition of a health status index emphasizes the distinctions:

> A quantified, standardized, weighted composite of a set of selected indicators of an individual's or a population's health status, which together—on some kind of scale—presumes to give a broad-spectrum representation of an individual's or a population's general health and well-being.

Stone [1985] reports on four primary health field divisions with potentially suitable indices for each area: human biology [demographic, mortality, morbidity, health status, risk factor status], environment [pollution, housing, transport, climate], lifestyle [smoking, alcohol use, drug use, diet, sexual behavior, employment, income, recreation], and health care organization [public health services, social services, legislation, health care at all levels].

Years Lost, Well Years and Healthy Days

In the G health status index model, Chen [1973] uses indicators of mortality, life expectancies at the mean age of death from specific diseases, abridged life tables, and disease specific hospitalization to calculate the years of life lost in a population. Bush, Chen, and Patrick [1973] use the index technique to derive the number of well years produced by the cost effectiveness analysis of a PKU screening and treatment program. In a similar vein, Barnum [1987] use the index of healthy days of life gained to evaluate health projects. This quantitative index has four components to calculate days of healthy life lost from premature death; acute illness; disability before premature death; and chronic disability. Discounting is used to equate present and future values, productivity weights are assigned by age to the days lost, and aggregate disease groupings tend to diminish inequities in the index. An index of healthy days lost could provide directions for the selection of activities.

Functional Status Index for ESRD

A Karnofsky Index [USDHHS, 1987, p. 108] classifies a patient's overall functional status. There are three classifications: able to carry on normal activity, unable to work, and unable to care for self. Each of the three classifications has three alphabetical designations—A, B or C. There is a further division based upon 11 categories that cover all possible function levels from completely normal to dead. Each of the 11 categories is tied to a percent of performance status from 100 percent for normal decreasing by 10 percent for each lower functioning level to 0 percent for dead. In the unable-to-care-for-self classification, the A classification has two categories: disabled [40 percent] and severely disabled [30 percent]; B has hospitalization necessary [20 percent]; and C has moribund [10 percent] and dead [0 percent].

Cross National Index Comparisons

In moving away from a single index of health care for cross national comparisons, Larson [1986] developed a three-part index measuring inputs, outputs, and hospital system variables. Each index used a five-point ranking from least favorable to most favorable for each data indicator. Six input measures included per capita health expenditures, health expenditures as a percentage of the Gross National Product, annual percentage increase in health expenditures, population per hospital bed, population per physician, and population per nurse and midwife. Five output indicators included life expectancy at birth, life expectancy at age 65, infant mortality rate per 100 live births, death rate from heart disease per 100,000, death rate from cancer per 100,000. Three hospital system variables included patient days per capita, admissions per capita, and average length of stay. In the five countries studied from 1980 to 1982 using this index, Canada's health care system was the best with the Federal Republic of Germany the worst. In between the extremes were Sweden, the United Kingdom, and the

United States. Obviously, critics may take issue with the choice of indicators, the weighting of indicators, and the limited time period. Nevertheless, Larson's cross national index of health care does provide a starting point.

Rehabilitation Index

This example illustrates the use of indicators to discover quality of life aspects and the evolution of an index to measure the individual's ability to readjust to society. Using the Reintegration to Normal Living index [RNL] as a proxy measure for the quality of life index [QLI], Wood-Dauphinee and Williams [1987] evaluated the individual's functional status. Reintegration can be judged by societal expectations for normal people, by before and after functioning evaluations, or by a utility value on the lifestyle.

Investigators began with a vignette as the basis for developing the RNL. That vignette described a young, married, active, and successful man involved in an accident that resulted in multiple fractures, a prolonged hospital stay, and an above-the-knee amputation followed by rehabilitation and discharge. Two questionnaires were developed by the researchers to gather information on behavior related to reintegration to normal living patterns: one unstructured and the other more structured. Both questionnaires were examined by experts and found to be acceptable, precise, and comprehensive. Three advisory panels were set up using a pool of 126 matched groups of professionals, patients and lay people. Each 42-member panel contained patients with cancer, myocardial infarction, rheumatoid arthritis or diabetes, relatives of the patients, healthy people, physicians, social workers, physical and occupational therapists, vocational counselors, psychologists, and clergy. Panel 1 was interviewed by trained interviewers using the first unstructured questionnaire. Panel 2 members received the more structured questionnaire in the mail to fill out and return. Information from those two panels was used to construct a third questionnaire in which respondents had to rank the importance of factors specifically identified in the first two questionnaires. Results from all three questionnaires showed the following areas to be most important in reintegration:

Mobility
Self-care activities
Daily activities
Recreational activities
Social activities
Family roles
Personal relationships
Presentation of self
General coping skills

On the basis of the evaluative procedures followed and the data gained, an 11-item RNL index evolved and was pretested. With minor modifications, similar instruments were developed for professionals and significant others. Exhibit 7–15 shows the patient version statements with visual analog scale [VAS] phrases providing specific cues as to the responses. Further analysis yielded two logical subscales to comprise the RNL index: Daily Functioning [items 1 through 8] and Perception of Self [items 9 through 11].

Each item is scored one for minimal reintegration and 10 for complete reintegration with the total of 110 points proportionally converted to a 100-point scale. While the quality of life

Exhibit 7-15.   Reintegration to Normal Living Index: Survey Statements.

1. I move around my living quarters as I feel is necessary. [Wheelchairs, other equipment or resources may be used.]
2. I move around my community as I feel is necessary. [Wheelchairs, other equipment or resources may be used.]
3. I am able to take trips out of town as I feel are necessary. [Wheelchairs, other equipment or resources may be used.]
4. I am comfortable with how my self-care needs [dressing, feeding, toileting, bathing] are met. [Adaptive equipment, supervision and/or assistance may be used.]
5. I spend most of my days occupied in a work activity that is necessary or important to me. [Work activity could be paid employment, housework, volunteer work, school, etc. Adaptive equipment, supervision and/or assistance may be used.]
6. I am able to participate in recreational activities [hobbies, crafts, sports, reading, television, games, computers, etc.] as I want to. [Adaptive equipment, supervision and/or assistance may be used.]
7. I participate in social activities with family, friends, and/or business acquaintances as is necessary or desirable to me. [Adaptive equipment, supervision and/or assistance may be used.]
8. I assume a role in my family which meets my needs and those of other family members. [Family means people with whom you live and/or relatives with whom you don't live but see on a regular basis. Adaptive equipment, supervision and/or assistance may be used.]
9. In general, I am comfortable with my personal relationships.
10. In general, I am comfortable with myself when I am in the company of others.
11. I feel that I can deal with life events as they happen.

Source: "Reintegration to normal living as a proxy to quality of life," by S. Wood-Dauphinee 8,. J.I. Williams, 1987, *Journal of Chronic Diseases, 49*(6), 491–499, Copyright 1987 by Pergamon Press Inc. Reprinted by permission.

was not mentioned in the questionnaires, a comparison with seven QLI instruments showed similarities indicating the reliability of the RNL index in measuring what it is supposed to measure. Wood-Dauphinee and Williams conclude that the RNL is applicable to patients with cancer, myocardial infarction, and a few additional chronic diseases.

Tracer Method as Index

By selecting appropriate characteristics of care in specific situations, evaluators can trace the process to determine if standards are being met or if guidelines are being followed. This "tracer method" [Kessner, Kalk, & Singer, 1973; Rhee, Donabedian, & Burney, 1987] has been used to measure the quality of care rendered to patients with particular ailments. If a chest X-ray is judged by experts to be an integral and significant part of a treatment program, then the medical record should indicate that "tracer" or the therapy would be considered poor quality care. Obviously, the tracer could be applied in any situation as a index of a variety of measures. However, it is vital that the identified tracer be vital in the opinion of qualified experts.

Measurement By Criteria, Checklist, Guidelines, Standards, and So On

Criteria could involve the use of checklists, standards, norms, guideposts, or a number of other words indicating that an evaluation is being conducted via a comparison with existing, predetermined measurements. A *Health Standards Directory* [ECRI, 1989] lists more than 4,000 published standards, guidelines, and recommendations by organization, by name and address, by laws, legislation and regulations, by abbreviations, and by key words.

A simple example that most people will be familiar with is looking for a new job. Let's suppose that your definitions of good climate, entertainment variety, adequate housing, good salary, and low taxes comprise your criteria to evaluate job offers in Boston, District of Columbia, and New York City. Counting each plus or minus as one, your job criteria chart could look like this:

Criteria	Boston		DC		NYC	
	+	−	+	−	+	−
Climate		X		X		X
Entertainment	X		X		X	
Housing	X			X		X
Salary	X			X	X	
Taxes		X	X			X
Total	3	2	2	3	2	3

Based on your criteria, Boston would be your first choice despite the bad marks on climate and taxes.

What is evident from this example is the need to be quite specific in choosing criteria and also in exactly defining the criteria. Assessment criteria can be either explicit or implicit. Commonly, explicit criteria are in writing, specific in nature, developed in advance, may be derived by experts and have withstood the test of time. By contrast, implicit criteria is unspoken, perhaps in the mind of the evaluator and based upon personal experiences and individual knowledge. Donabedian [1988] also notes that there are intermediate variations and combinations between these two extremes.

Some time ago, the following six elements common to all criteria were developed by Lembcke [1956] for medical record auditing by the scientific method:

1. *Objectivity*—Written criteria in precision and detail to avoid varying interpretations.
2. *Verifiability*—Criteria verified by laboratory examination, diagnostic procedures, consultation, or documentation.
3. *Uniformity*—Regardless of variables such as size and location, the criteria should stand independently.
4. *Specificity*—In evaluation, the criteria must be specific for each disease/condition and related diseases and operations in the same patient considered as a unit.
5. *Pertinence*—Criteria based on results and pertinent to the ultimate aim of the care being rendered.
6. *Acceptability*—Criteria conforms with recognized levels of good quality based on professional textbooks and literature.

In regard to productivity, efficiency, and profitability in health care, Bennett [1985] states that there are three broad areas relative to costs: direct labor standards, direct material and supply standards, and operational overhead standards. Labor standards can deal with items such as hourly rates and time efficiency by various employees to do specific tasks. Material and supply standards concern the expected prices of supplies and the amount and kinds of material. Overhead includes fixed costs and fluctuating expenses. Bennett notes that standards can be classified in four groupings: basic standards that are constant over time; theoretical ideal standards are set assuming best possible outcome with existing conditions and equipment; currently attainable standards that is a step down from ideal making allowances for breakdowns, losses, and idle time; and average past performance standards that project outcomes based on prior experience. Currently attainable standards are used most frequently since basic, ideal, and average past performance all fall short in unrealistically limiting productivity expectations.

Checklists for Evaluation

Many checklists consist of a series of questions to be asked by individuals or by evaluators. Questions may call for a positive or negative response or for an explanation.

Strategic Planning Checklist in Retardation

Exhibit 7–16 illustrates a 14-point checklist used to evaluate the planning process related to the prevention of retardation and related disabilities. If the response to the first question indicates that no written plan exists, it could be the intention of the evaluators to discontinue the process

Exhibit 7-16.   Checklist for Evaluating Mental Retardation Planning.

1. Is there a written plan for preventing retardation and related disabilities?

2. Does the written plan address:
   — Philosophy of Prevention
   — Planning Responsibilities
   — Implementation and Coordination Responsibilities
   — Role of Executive Branch
   — Role of Legislative Branch
   — Relationships between Federal, State and Local Governments
   — Relationships between Government and the Private Sector
   — Role of Private Service Providers [Physician, therapist, etc.]
   — Data Collection and Analysis
   — Evaluation and Program Success
   — Cost Benefits
   — Protection of Human Rights

3. Who is responsible for the coordination and implementation of prevention programs? Is there a governmental Office of Prevention?

4. Who is responsible for dissemination of information about available prevention strategies and services?

5. Is information given to the proper agencies, service providers, and the public?

6. Who is responsible for evaluating the effectiveness of the prevention efforts?

7. Is the prevention plan comprehensive and does it provide direction for developing policy in service delivery?

8. Does the plan define the role of governmental agencies?
   — At the state level
   — At the local level
   — At the regional level
   — At the federal level

9. How does the plan include the institutions of higher learning, including federally funded university affiliated programs?

10. How does the plan involve the private sector?
    — Does it include parent, advocacy, and consumer organizations?
    — Does it include professional organizations?
    — Does it include the primary consumer?

11. Does the private sector participate in the planning, the implementation, and the evaluation of services?

12. Does the plan address economic issues such as available resources, regionalization, cost/benefit ratios and long term effectiveness?

13. Are lines of authority and responsibility clearly defined?

14. How effective has prior planning for prevention services been?

Source: From *A guide for state planning for the prevention of mental retardation and related disability*, by President's Commission on Mental Retardation, 1987, Washington, DC: Government Printing Office, Pub. No. [OHDS] 87-21034. Reprinted by permission.

until such a written plan does exist. Almost all the other checklist questions refer back to or should be specified in the written plan for the answers. For example, question number two asks if the written plan addresses 12 issues considered critical to the prevention activity. Note that this checklist covers lines of authority, coordination, evaluation, community participation, and strategies.

In a reference guide for area board members [Spiegel, 1960, p. 40], a self-questioning criteria list ranks planning components on a five-point Likert scale from "inadequate" to "excellent." Following are the 10 questions with critical words for the respondent's consideration underlined:

1. Is your plan based on *clearly defined* objectives that are in accord with organizational goals?
2. Is your plan as *clear and simple* as the task permits?
3. Does your plan provide for the *involvement* of all *appropriate personnel*?
4. Is your planning based on *realistic analysis* of forces interacting in the situation.
5. Does your plan have *stability* and still allow for flexibility?
6. Is your planning *economical* in use of human and financial resources needed to implement it?
7. Can your plan be *divided and delegated* for efficient implementation?
8. Are the *methods* to be used reliable and up to appropriate standards?
9. Does your plan provide for adequate *training* of personnel needed for accomplishing the task?
10. Does your plan provide for continuous *review and re-evaluation*?

Using both an overall score and an item-by-item analysis of this criteria planning checklist, strategic planners are able to discover self-defined weakpoints in their planning strategy.

Corporate Critical Success Factors

Jenster [1987] posits that critical success factors [CSF] "relate to the internal or external conditions for the firm's strategy or those competencies or resources it must attain." In auditing the CSFs relevant to planning for the agency's present and future position, the following strategic areas should be evaluated:

*   General environment such as sociodemographic trends.
*   Industry characteristics such as ethics and mores.
*   Competitive forces such as quality, case mix, and costs.
*   Company specific attributes such as management style.
*   Personal values of key players such as major stockholders.
*   Resource availability in money, material and manpower.

This list of criteria and the minimal examples merely indicate the scope of the evaluation. It should be apparent that considerable effort must go into pinpointing the specifics of each of the six criterion.

Nursing Care for Long Stay Patients

Taking minimal criteria from a gerontological nursing assessment, Wells and Adolphus [1987] included six general items, 13 physical status items, 15 functional status items, 7 psychosocial items, and 2 economic items [Exhibit 7–17]. This criteria was used at the Sunnybrook Medical Centre, a teaching facility with 1130 beds divided into 620 acute, 400 extended, and 110 domiciliary. Evaluation data came from the nursing kardex, the patient care plan, the bedside nursing notes and from the primary nurse or caregiver. Results revealed that the 13 basic physical care criteria were met at a satisfactory level, but that the other criteria were not always met. In the functional status criteria, there was little self-care and regular ambulation in the patient's plan. Social activities and financial support criteria rarely received attention. In fact, patients frequently were relocated to inappropriate higher level of care units than needed because their maximum functional level was not being achieved. Four recommendations emerged from the application of evaluation criteria to this long stay care facility:

- Establish a long stay unit with adequate support services.
- Employ a recreational therapist to offer activity programs.
- Urge volunteer agencies to provide services.
- Develop a program for the long stay patient.

Relative to long-term care, Nelson, Wasson, and Kirk [1987] created a patient assessment of physical condition that uses line drawings as well as words. Exhibit 7–18 illustrates five criteria for classification of physical activity into very heavy, heavy, moderate, light, and very light. Each classification lists three or four descriptive phrases and two line drawings.

Computer and Manual Criteria for Auditing Quality of Care

McCoy, Dunn, and Borgiel [1987] developed a portable computer system for auditing the quality of ambulatory care based on comprehensive process criteria. Software packages interface with standard commercial word processing software such as ASCII in a "criteria compiler" allowing for descriptive language editing. Data and information structures are based on dBaseIII file formats. Each criteria description has three sections: alternative search terms for a diagnosis; an input screen format where the auditor enters data; and the scores for each section. This data abstraction program is menu-driven providing multiple windows that the auditor traverses with single keystrokes. Evaluations could involve 10 to 20 screens with several hundred questions.

Computer auditing using criteria has been tested at 120 sites in Ontario, Canada using 3,000 medical charts. "Objectively, these abstracters have shown approximately a 50 percent productivity increase when using the computer; subsequently, they report less stress and fatigue than when doing manual chart auditing." Investigators estimated a computer cost of $15 per chart as compared to $46 as noted in the medical literature.

Computer criteria-compiled data are similar to manual criteria data. Starting with medical members of a quality assurance committee and criteria taken from the professional literature, the Missouri Patient Care Review Foundation [Akhter, 1985] developed a 15-item quality screening criteria list [Exhibit 7–19]. A quality review coordinator uses the list when evaluating a random sample of medical records.

Reacting to this type of quality review by PROs, Dehn [1988], a practicing physician, predicts that the PROs will adopt national practice standards for common Medicare procedures.

Exhibit 7-17. Criteria for Evaluating Nursing Care.

GENERAL CRITERIA

1. A comprehensive assessment is conducted before deciding that long-term care is required. A member of the geriatric service has been involved in assessing a geriatric patient. [A functional assessment of a patient who is acutely ill is likely to be invalid.]
2. The termination of acute care treatment includes rehabilitating the functional abilities to preadmission/premorbid levels to ensure relocation or discharge to the lowest level of care.
3. The patient's social support system is assessed for potential discharge to the community.
4. Patients are reassessed monthly regarding any change in status and the appropriateness of discharge plans.
5. Application for long-term care is submitted to the appropriate facility for the required level of care. [Simultaneous submission of several applications to a number of facilities offering different levels of care shows a lack of clarity, internally and externally, regarding actual discharge needs.]
6. The label "placement" or "placement problem" is not on the record. [This label is derogatory: It reflects ageism that results in a lack of staff interest and involvement and often the discontinuation of active/acute treatment and rehabilitation.

SPECIFIC CRITERIA

1. Physical Status
- skin integrity is normal
- weight is recorded monthly [a noninvasive measure of nutritional status]
- vital signs are taken and recorded no more than weekly
- laboratory investigations, in the absence of specific doctor's orders, are conducted no more than monthly, e.g. blood work, chest X-ray
- a podiatrist is available to do foot care monthly
- if the patient wears dentures, effort should be taken to ensure the best possible fit and that they are worn when the patient is awake
- the diet is appropriate to the dental and nutritional status of the patient
- the patients sleeps approximately eight of 24 hours per day
- vision and hearing are assessed; follow-up for aids is arranged
- sensory aids are in place and functional
- if the patient is restrained, restraints are removed

2. Functional Status
- The patient spends no more than eight to 10 hours in bed per day
- the patient is assessed for and provided with the necessary aids for independent ambulation
- the patient is walked in the corridor at least four times a day
- the patient is dressed in street clothes
- nonambulatory patients are moved from bed to chair at least twice a day
- the patient sits in a chair for at least two meals
- range of motion exercises are provided to all limbs at least twice a day
- tub baths are given twice weekly
- the patient is up for basic hygiene activities and is encouraged to do as much self-hygiene as possible
- the patient is helped to the commode or toilet three times a day during the day, every three to four hours at night as needed for micturition purposes, until the patient's own routine is established
- the patient is assisted to the commode or toilet after meals and as needed for bowel movements, until the patient's own routine is established
- the etiology of bowel or bladder incontinence is established
- the etiology of cognitive impairment is established
- cognitive status is reassessed monthly
- physical function is reassessed monthly

3. Psychosocial Status
- the patient and family are involved in the decision for long-term care
- personal belongings, such as clock, calendar and radio, are available
- 10 minutes or more per day is allotted by staff or volunteer to sit, walk with, or talk to the patient
- the patient is taken to the lounge or common room at least once a day
- friends/family take the patient out once a week or at least monthly, if the patient's and/or family's condition permits
- the patient/family is satisfied with the care provided
- the patient/family is informed of the patient's status at least monthly and is prepared for relocation

4. Economic Status
The patient's financial status is assessed; if funds are available, the family is encouraged to

(continued)

Exhibit 7-17. *(Continued)*

every two hours when range of movement, skin care, and change of position are provided
- if medications are used for restraint, the need for ongoing restraint is assessed as per institutional policy
- progress and treatment, including drug therapy, are reviewed weekly by the multidisciplinary team as per institutional policy; medication counseling is available to patient and/or family

- arrange for the patient to return home with adequate supports while awaiting transfer to long-term care
- provide support for the patient while in hospital awaiting transfer to long-term care, e.g. hair appointments, care of street clothes

Source: From "Evaluating the care provided to long-stay patients," by D.L. Wells & P.D. Adolphus, 1987, *Dimensions in Health Services,* 64[10], 21. Reprinted with permission of the Canadian Hospital Association.

His article in *Medical Economics* was entitled, "PRO will soon mean 'Policing Reduced Options.'" Physicians often equate practice standards with "cookbook medicine" and as an affront to their professional judgment. Nevertheless, Dr. Dehn doubts that national standards would change most practice behaviors or interfere with physicians providing the best possible care for their patients. He comments that "standards simply outline the *minimums* required for acceptable care. . . Clearly, the kind of "maverick medicine" practiced by some of our peers is at risk. . . Nobody wants to see standards etched in stone" [author's emphasis].

Exhibit 7-18. COOP Chart to Measure Physical Function.

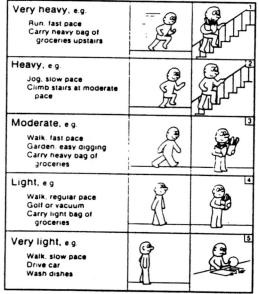

PHYSICAL CONDITION

During the past 4 weeks . . .
What was the most strenuous level of physical activity you could do for at least 2 minutes?

Very heavy, e.g. Run, fast pace Carry heavy bag of groceries upstairs		1
Heavy, e.g. Jog, slow pace Climb stairs at moderate pace		2
Moderate, e.g. Walk, fast pace Garden, easy digging Carry heavy bag of groceries		3
Light, e.g. Walk, regular pace Golf or vacuum Carry light bag of groceries		4
Very light, e.g. Walk, slow pace Drive car Wash dishes		5

Exhibit 7-19. Quality Screening Criteria.

1. Admission for complication of or recurrence of problem of previous hospitalization.
2. Readmission for progress of illness due to possible incomplete treatment.
3. Inappropriate antibiotic usage.
4. Hospital-incurred incidents.
5. Infection not present on admission [nosocomial].
6. Surgery without documented medical necessity.
7. Death: Unexpected
8. Transfer to another acute-care facility.
9. Transfer from general-care unit to special-care unit.
10. Neurological deficit present at discharge which was not present on admission.
11. Acute myocardial infarction and a surgical procedure on same admission.
12. Unplanned return to the operating room.
13. Unplanned removal, or injury requiring corrective action, or repair of an organ or structure during surgery, or any invasive procedure.
14. Cardiac or respiratory arrest.
15. Others.

Source: From "Quality assurance under the Missouri PRO program," by M.N. Akhter, 1985, *Mississippi Medicine*, 82(6), 297–299. Reprinted with permission.

Continuing with quality concepts from the consumer's viewpoint, a survey of nursing home residents across the nation by the National Citizen's Coalition for Nursing Home Reform came up with criteria to evaluate the quality of life at the facilities [Carrell, 1988]. Using that data, Koren [1988] reported that protocols adopted by the New York Quality Assurance System [NYQAS] included structured guidelines in the following areas: environment, activities, facility philosophy, privacy, choice, informed decision making, interactions, personal, social, spiritual life, and security. These guidelines are to be evaluated via observation and interview rather than on record review.

Effectiveness
1. Are patients randomized by treatment and control groups?
2. Were sources of bias considered?
3. Were all relevant outcomes measured?
4. Do the results apply to your problem?

Diagnosis
1. Technological capability to perform as expected?
2. Range of possible uses delineated?
3. Diagnostic accuracy demonstrated?
4. Impact on health care provider's diagnostic confidence?
5. Therapeutic impact in treatment decisions?
6. Patient outcome benefits from technology?

Criteria numbers five and six in the diagnosis grouping are suitable for application of the four effectiveness criteria.

In an earlier article, Guyatt, Drummond, and Feeney [1986] considered economic evaluation guidelines. Since an evaluation without cost calculations is like meat without potatoes the 10 criteria are listed:

1. Choice of level of approach: service [micro] or system [macro]
2. Identification of the viewpoint[s] for the analysis: society, institution, or individual
3. Consideration of a relevant range of alternatives: choices to resolve the same problem
4. Selection of the appropriate form of economic evaluation: cost-effectiveness, cost-benefit, or cost-utility
5. Identification of the relevant range of costs and benefits
6. Estimation of the costs and benefits
7. Distinction between average and marginal costs and benefits: per diem rates, additional costs, and incremental costs
8. Allowing for differential timing of costs and benefits: use of discounting
9. Allowing for uncertainty in costs and benefits: sensitivity analysis
10. Appropriate presentation of results: complete information needed for decisions

Combining criteria for diagnosis, effectiveness, and economics, Feeny [1987] cites an evaluation of a neonatal intensive care unit for very low birth-weight infants. A comparison, in 1978 dollars, of the net economic cost per quality-adjusted life-year gained follows:

500– 999 grams	$17,500
1000–1499 grams	1,000

Importantly, the higher cost for the lower-weight babies is due to increased treatment expenditures and to the lower level of effectiveness in prolonging life. Is that huge difference in costs worth the life-years gained for the lower weight infants? That is a tough decision for any administrator. Feeny [1987] comments: "Fundamental ethical and social value judgments are not avoided through the use of economic evaluation; mechanisms for social choice are still needed."

Technology Assessment Criteria Illustrations. To assess the clinical efficacy of magnetic resonance imaging [MRI], Cooper, Chalmers, and McCally [1988] evaluated 54 professional articles published in the first four years after the technology was introduced [1981–1984]. These 54 articles came from 12 journals, but 34 [63 percent] came from *Radiology* and *American Journal of Radiology.* Cooper et al. [1988] list all 54 articles in an appendix to the article.

Ten commonly accepted criteria of research methodology were used in the evaluation as follows:

1. Evidence of research planning in protocol and/or institutional review board approval.
2. Appropriate use of the terms sensitivity, specificity, positive or negative predictive value, false-positive or false-negative and accuracy.
3. Appropriate presentation of data described by each term.
4. Appropriate calculation of the values for each of the described terms.
5. Presentation of a "gold standard" by tissue diagnosis by biopsy or autopsy was considered fully satisfactory with other imaging procedures rated partially satisfactory.
6. Random order of imaging tests when comparing MRI with another procedure.
7. Blinding of interpreter with regard to clinical history or other test results.

8. Measurement of interobservor variability in reading images.
9. Presentation of quantitative data.
10. Appropriate statistical analysis of quantitative data.

"All of the articles evaluated in this assessment scored poorly. . . As evaluations of diagnostic efficacy, these studies are of poor quality. . . Not one evaluation contained an appropriate statistical analysis of the distributions of quantitative readings. . . " Therefore, the authors found it extremely disturbing that an editorial in the *Mayo Clinic Proceedings* took a wayward course. DiChiro [1985] stated: "The data . . . are presented unencumbered by statistics. The crystal-clear facts are listed in simple, accessible tables. The mumbo-jumbo rituals often associated with pseudostatistical analyses have been avoided. . . We should not succumb to the 'curse of Lord Kelvin' and quantify at any cost."

In an editorial comment on the Cooper et al. study in the *Journal of the American Medical Association,* Sheps [1988] notes the "gloomy results" and "suggests that the proliferation of MRI technology is based on inadequate evidence that MRI does more good than harm." Sheps goes on to even more damming remarks: "Until physicians [as well as editors] demand that appropriate evaluations be undertaken [and hinder publication of methodological poor research], the mindless 'Don't-confuse-me-with-the-facts' attitude displayed by the comments cited by Cooper et al. will continue to have a pervasive and unhealthy effect on patient care and health care costs."

According to Cooper et al., "Proper quantitative methods *do* need to be used in the evaluation of new technology" [author's emphasis].

In a related MRI evaluation, Hughes [1988] lists "choosing a vendor" criteria to be used to prepare requests for proposals [RFP] from mobile MRI vendors prior to purchasing equipment. There has to be agreement on three MRI choices, requested start date, number of moves per week, term or length of lease, and with or without staffing. A simple weighted value is assigned to each criterion based upon the relative importance to the purchaser. A decision matrix would list all the suppliers against all the criteria with total scores calculated for an evaluative decision. Hughes does note the rapid diffusion of MRI but there is no discussion of efficacy. This analysis is concerned with the financial viability of a mobile MRI project.

What Are Clinical Trials All About? Questions?

Often, people are given the opportunity to participate in a clinical trial of a new drug or procedure. To enhance the individual's decision-making ability, 18 questions were compiled from the Better Business Bureau, Biotherapeutics Inc., private physicians and the federal National Cancer Institute. Sample questions from the checklist follow:

*   What is the study's purpose? What does it involve?
*   What costs will the patient have?
*   Who has approved the study? Who is sponsoring this study?
*   How does the study affect daily life? Are there side effects?
*   Is there a written protocol? Can I see it?
*   Is the study being conducted mainly for the patients' benefit or the researcher's?

It should be apparent that a well-informed participant should desire answers to these type of checklist questions. Even if the participant does not ask the questions, the information should be provided to meet informed-consent requirements. Health care providers could use these guidelines to assure that the information is provided.

Business Checklists

Since health care is adapting corporate methods and techniques, checklists are a common corporate tool. Finkel [1984] details a National Conference Center checklist for evaluating a training facility. Using a weighed point system for the characteristics, the checklist covers eight areas of concern: the main meeting room environment [13 items, 39 maximum points], break-out room environment [5 items, 11 points], environment for informal socializing and breaks [5 items, 12 points], dining facilities [5 items, 10 points], sleeping rooms [8 items, 15 points], recreation and exercise [7 items, 7.5 points], overall environment [5 items, 100 points], and the staff [7 items, 100 points]. A superior rating is 85 to 100 while below 49 is considered poor. Staff are rated separately on the scale and the other components are totaled for a score.

A budget and administration checklist for agencies that participate in exhibits comes from Joseph E. Seagram & Sons, Inc. [*Successful Meetings*, 1987]. Budget items include space size, trim, exhibit material, transportation drayage, furniture rental, salaries, promotion, storage, and labor. Each item requires a description and actual or estimated cost. Among the 46 administration checks are electrical outlets, waste disposal, security protection, theft insurance, directory listing, souvenirs, telephone, traffic bait, rest rooms, advertising supplies, photography, spare parts, dictating machine, and roster of invited guests.

Hospitalization for Suicide

Even in an area of high-intensity emotional behavior, Riedel, Tischler, and Myers [1974, p. 79] established criteria for the hospitalization of patients exhibiting suicidal behavior. If any of 10 specific behaviors occur, it is recommended that that person be confined. In addition to the explicit suicide attempt, the stated lethal plan, a history of medically serious attempts, the criteria relate to suicidal thoughts and gestures, expectations of hospitalization, unchangeable precipitating factors, lack of change in significant others and high-risk social circumstances.

SCALES AS MEASUREMENT TOOLS

While not completely distinguished from an index, a scale is considered to evaluate a single dimension of a concept and may even be thought of as a special type of index. As the variety of scales are explained, the instrument technique should emerge clearly and most likely will be familiar to everyone.

Four questions need to be answered when selecting the appropriate scales: What information is required? How much will the technique cost? How well does the method fit with the proposed administration technique? And most importantly, how easy is the scale to use by respondents? Commonly used types of scales include the Likert scale, semantic difference scale, the Stapel scale, the percentage scale, the categorical scale and the graphic scale.

Types of Scales

A Likert scale usually allows the respondent to choose from a continuum of reactions to the question that range from one extreme to the other. Generally, Likert scales are relatively easy to devise and administer. Respondents may be given as few as three choices [yes/don't know/no] to five or more [agree completely/somewhat agree/unsure/disagree somewhat/disagree completely]. Choices can also be given arbitrary numerical designations such as 1,0,2 in the first example to 5,4,3,2,1 in the second example. Adding numbers allows for the scale to be used in statistical tests of significance. In addition, evaluators can test for significance in the five point scale for each answer separately or can collapse the 5 and 4 answers and the 1 and 2 answers and test for significance on agreement and disagreement. Using the five-point choice Likert scale, questions could look like the following:

Circle your answer

Physician costs are reasonable.	AC	SA	U	SD	DC
Hospitals charge too much.	AC	SA	U	SD	DC
Insurance doesn't cover costs.	AC	SA	U	SD	DC

A semantic differential scale allows individuals to indicate their opinion on as many as seven bipolar descriptive words or phrases. Again, this type of scale is simple to construct and to administer. However, respondents may have difficulty distinguishing between the extremes. In addition, evaluators should be aware that if too many questions are asked of respondents, there may be a tendency toward "respondent set" as people get tired, bored or whatever and tend to mark the middle choice of no opinion or neutral. Again, this scale can be scored using arbitrary number assignments to choices. In a management area, Bassett and Metzger [1986, p. 186] illustrate a 28-item scale on which employees can be asked to rate themselves or supervisors. Using a five-point scale [Very/Quite/Slightly/No Opinion/Slightly/Quite/Very] items include the following:

	V	*Q*	*S*	*NO*	*S*	*Q*	*V*	
competent	:	:	:	:	:	:	:	: incompetent
leader	:	:	:	:	:	:	:	: follower
closed-minded	:	:	:	:	:	:	:	: open-minded
emotional	:	:	:	:	:	:	:	: objective

A Stapel scale is a modified version of a semantic differential scale with six nonverbal unipolar choices that measure direction and intensity simultaneously. Unlike the semantic differential scale, the Stapel scale uses one word or phrase with positive and negative values to assure true bipolarity. Construction and administration are easy but there may be questions based on semantic consistency. An example relating to the attitudes of physicians might look like this:

Physicians are [circle your choice]

+3	+3	+3	+3	+3
+2	+2	+2	+2	+2
+1	+1	+1	+1	+1
Caring	Too busy	Money Hungry	Friendly	Competent
−1	−1	−1	−1	−1
−2	−2	−2	−2	−2
−3	−3	−3	−3	−3

A percentage scale allows respondents to reply using a familiar 0 percent to 100 percent agreement or disagreement. While the scale is easy to devise and to administer, can the respondents really differentiate between 50 and 60 percent? It is possible to choose the extremes and the middle but the percentages in-between may be doubtful. Think about the following examples:

Circle the percentage of your agreement

Nurses are helpful   0   10   20   30   40   50   60   70   80   90   100

Hospitals require too   0   10   20   30   40   50   60   70   80   90   100
    many forms

Doctors give too many   0   10   20   30   40   50   60   70   80   90   100
    lab tests

A categorical scale has responses positioned in a series of boxes and the respondent simply checks their choice. Sometimes, this scale is called a closed-end scale since all the choices are delineated. Even where there may be a choice labeled other or comments, that is a closed end choice because the individual checks that box and then writes in additional data. People could be asked about the value of statistics such as:

Hospital mortality statistics reveal the quality of care at the facility:

To a very great extent   [ ]
To a great extent   [ ]
To a moderate extent   [ ]
To some extent   [ ]
To little or no extent   [ ]

A graphic scale could use some form of pictorial matter to indicate the continuum of choices. This technique may appeal to respondents and ease the decision-making process. Variations of the round happy face to the sad face could indicate agreement or disagreement at various stages. Clues about hospital patient education activities could be discerned from the following question at discharge:

Do you have questions   *Circle a question cluster*
about your therapy?   ?   ??   ???   ????   ?????

Based on his own research, Elbeck [1987] suggests strongly that the elderly prefer a graphic scale while the middle-aged show an equal preference for the Likert, percentage and categorical scales. Since factors such as pre- and post-therapy anxiety, medication use, and a strange environment may influence those answering scaled measurements, it is usually advisable to select the simplest, most common, and easiest format.

Performance Appraisal Systems

In as health care is a labor-intensive industry, the evaluation of personnel is a routine part of administration. There are a number of methods that can be used singly or in combination including behaviorally anchored rating scales [BARS]. These scales stress ongoing behaviors, are designed for specific job classifications, are unique in that behavior is measured and do confront the issue of effectiveness in performance. Wiatrowski and Palkon [1987] enumerate five distinct steps as detailed below:

1. Develop a behavioral job classification system.
2. Analyze the jobs and break them down into discrete dimensions or components describing the skills needed to perform those functions.
3. Based on the job descriptions, supervisors develop statements detailing observable behaviors signifying effective performance relative to 10 to 15 major functions.
4. Descriptions range from highly effective to effective to marginal to ineffective setting up an ordinal scale which requires the agreement of 75 percent of the supervisors.
5. Item values are determined by standard psychometric scaling processes and a completed BARS may have 10 to 15 job dimensions with each dimension having 7 to 9 written behavior examples rated from poor to superior or low to high.

In an evaluation of a registered nurse's work in the dimension of patient and family education, the BARS examples could be as follows:

- *Highly effective performance with a rating of 9 or 8*—Consistently begins patient and family education at admission. Refers patients to community agencies as additional resource.
- *Effective performance with a rating of 7 or 6*—Consistently does preoperative teaching based on patient's needs. Uses established patient education programs.
- *Marginal performance with a rating of 5 or 4*—Fails to discontinue teaching when patient is anxious. Discusses posthospital care with patient/family only if requested.
- *Ineffective performance with a rating of 2 or 1*—Consistently postpones patient education until discharge day. Provides no patient/family education to deal with an illness.

Additional performance appraisal methods utilizing scales include a graphic rating scale, a forced choice scale, and a comparison scale.

A graphic rating scale is commonly used in the health care field. An employee may be compared with a standard for the specific position. Using a five- or seven-point scale, the supervisor reviews each items on the standard and can rate the employee as outstanding, satisfactory, average, poor, or unsatisfactory. A number value for each item can be totaled to yield a total numerical performance score.

While this graphic scale is simple and inexpensive, there can be difficulties with consistent supervisor objectivity in the standards, with real values for the choices on the scale and with feedback to average employees yearning to become superior.

In the forced choice scale, the supervisor selects words or phrases describing job behavior or personal qualities that are most and least applicable to each employee. None of the choices can be changed or modified. While each descriptive word or phrase has a numerical value, the supervisor is not given that information. Consequently, the forced choice scale fails to secure the specific information to improve performance, does not help in human resource planning and could easily not reflect actual performance.

A comparison scale ranks all employees against each other in numerical order along specific dimensions such as efficiency, effectiveness, promptness and accuracy. Regardless of the differing jobs, employees may be rank-ordered on only one dimension and not take into account their multiple skills. If an employee is ranked fifth on accuracy, how can that person move up higher? This technique may cause dissension in the ranks or even result in peer pressure to lower performance standards.

Both BARS and PAS should aim to resolve criteria such as goal inclusion, equity, motivation, planning, communication, and legality.

Ward Atmosphere Scale

If health care providers truly believe in the "milieu therapy" approach, then the healing benefit of the atmosphere of the facility and/or service can not be ignored. Although Milne [1986] used the ward atmosphere scale [WAS] in a psychiatric day hospital, the applications are general in nature. Initial assumptions realize that there is a defined social environment, that as many people as possible from that environment should be included in any changes, that individual goals must also be considered, and that evaluation can be used to facilitate the change. Six nurses and about 50 patients responded to a WAS that contained 40 items within the following 10 key dimensions in the underlined subscales of the WAS:

- *Involvement* in day-to-day social functioning
- *Support* actions of patients and staff in helping others
- *Spontaneity* in acting openly and freely expressing feelings
- *Autonomy* in independent and self-sufficient actions
- *Practical orientation* toward discharge and return to society
- *Personal problem orientation* toward resolution of difficulties
- *Anger and aggression* capable of being expressed without fear
- *Order and organization* looks at schedules, planned activities, appointments, and general demeanor
- *Program clarity* deals with explicit expectations and routines
- *Staff control* examines rules, regulations, and restrictions

Results from the use of the WAS indicated that a facility or service can be regarded as a client and does have a personality, that the atmosphere can be defined and measured in a simple but sensitive manner, and that there is a positive relationship between the WAS and clinical outcomes.

Scales Rate Doctors Who Use Computers

From a marketing viewpoint, health care providers must be concerned about the possibility that the use of computers and high technology may make medicine appear to be "dehumanized." Cruickshank [1985] reports on an evaluation of physicians who used a computer program known as "First Aid" to help to diagnose gastrointestinal problems.

Using a 38-item seven choice semantic differential scale, 140 new outpatients compared their doctor to an ideal doctor. Almost half of the patients were treated by a physician who used a computer in the encounter. "All doctors were rated as less than ideal on more characteristics when using the computer." With a maximum score of 3 and a minimum score of −3, several examples of the semantic scale follow:

Unsympathetic	I I I I I I I	sympathetic
Warm	I I I I I I I	cold
Not listening	I I I I I I I	listening

Patients said that the ideal doctor must listen [2.91] and pay attention [2.91]. Other characteristics rating higher than 2.8 included asking questions, thoroughness, helpfulness, explaining, usefulness, and professionalism. Cruickshank [1985] concludes that "patients put professional competence above the more human skills." With the computer, the physician was rated as less than ideal on thoroughness, decisiveness, and convincingness. Could it be that the patients thought that the doctor was not clever enough without the computer? However, all three doctors in this study rated lower than the ideally confident, reassuring, listening, and explaining physician. This semantic scale could be used to discover what patients want from their health care providers and those aspects could be marketed.

Arthritis Impact Measurement Scale

Displaying a high reliability, validity, and generalizability, Meenan [1986] reports on the Arthritis Impact Measurement Scales [AIMS]. This scale consists of nine dimensions and a total of 45 items for all aspects: mobility [4], physical activity [5], dexterity [5], household activities [7], activities of daily living [4], anxiety [6], depression [6], social activity [4], and pain [4]. Each item requires a choice of frequency, a gradation of ability or an estimate of effort. Scales could be numerical, could range from a great deal to little or none or always able to never able. Typical measurements include the following examples:

Are you able to use public transportation?
Do you have trouble bending, stooping, or lifting?
Can you easily open a jar of food?
Do you handle your own money?
How often have you had severe pain from your arthritis?
How much of the time have you felt tense or high strung?
How much of the time have you felt downhearted and blue?
How much help do you need in getting dressed?
How often were you on the phone with close friends?

SURVEY TECHNIQUES IN EVALUATION

In selecting a survey for the desired evaluation, strategic planners could incorporate aspects of methods using indicators, indexes, criteria, scales, and elements of a structure/process/outcome approach as well as others. A. Cartwright [1987] reviews more than 50 different public health surveys illustrating the practical application of the technique and the potential for contributing to understanding health and health care. In a book on the design and use of questionnaires, the major tool utilized in surveys, Berdie, Anderson, and Niebuhr [1986] annotate almost 500 references in a 137-page section. In addition, that book contains sample questionnaires, suggestions on stimulating responses, and a discussion of reliability and validity. Keeping up to date, Frerichs and Tar [1989] even explain how to use portable computers to assist in rapid surveys in developing countries.

Surveys are an extremely popular method of evaluation and the professional literature is replete with articles reporting the outcomes of surveys. Many articles include copies of the instruments and can provide planners with suggestions and ideas for their own investigations. Therefore, while the evaluator certainly has no need to reinvent the survey technique, there is definitely a need to apply the methodology with accuracy to attain reliable and valid results.

Types of Surveys

Initially, planning procedures identify the problem, establish goals and objectives, collect data, amass resources, consider alternatives, set priorities, and implement the activity. If a survey is selected as the evaluation mechanism, a questionnaire is usually developed. That questionnaire could be used in a personal interview or the instrument could be self-administered. If a personal interview with the target audience or significant others is chosen, the interview could be on a one-to-one basis at home or some other site, could be via telephone or in group multiples such as a focus group technique. If self-administered, the survey could be conducted by mail, by group meetings at a central location where respondents fill out the forms at the same time, or by people responding to a menu driven computer questionnaire.

Selection of a particular survey mode may be influenced by factors such as cost, time limitations, content of the questionnaire, statistical response rate requirements, and the target population. In telephone surveys, Marcus and Crane [1986] cite the following advantages: less expensive, reaching people in secure locations or high-risk areas, central location and supervised interviewers can reach nationwide target audience, and a possible reduction in interviewer bias.

Regardless of the type of survey, generic problems afflict all the evaluations and must be resolved or accommodated. Roos, Roos, Mossey, and Havens [1988] point out that survey participants are likely to be healthier than the general population, possibly because of self-selection. In addition, surveys may rely on self-reports of service utilization and medical conditions and the range of memory recall is substantial. Furthermore, surveys tend to be expensive, logistical-difficult, and sporadic in nature. To add to the problem list, Marcus and Crane [1986] focus on the target audience sampling selection, the doubts about the quality of the data collected, the difficulty in questionnaire development, the scheduling of interviewers, the burden upon the respondent in time and energy and the potential interviewer effects that could bias responses.

Taking direct aim at the overwhelming problem of nonresponse to direct mail surveys, Tatter [*Successful Meetings*, 1986] offers tips to improve responses. Personalize the survey with a signed cover letter accompanying the questionnaire in a typed envelope with a first-class postage stamp rather than a metered third-class envelope. This letter should tell the audience how long it should take to fill out the questionnaire and when the responses are due. A reminder of the response deadline can be included in a box on the questionnaire itself. Response may increase with a survey announcement card seven to 10 days prior to the actual survey preparing receptive individuals for the questionnaire. People are urged to respond even if they do not wish to participate so their name can be removed from the survey list. Additionally, obvious coding or labeling on the first page is better than secreting the code number under the pasted on stamp. Blue ink on white paper appears to be more acceptable than black ink. Questions that offer a range of response choices may supply more definitive data than a simple yes or no answer. Dividing the questionnaire into logical sections may also maintain interest in the survey and reduce boredom. Deliberately varying question lengths and the number of questions in each section also may keep the respondent attentive. Paying attention to timing can increase responses. Questionnaires that arrive on a Friday tend to attract fewer responses than those arriving on Monday or during the week.

Mail, Telephone, and Personal Survey Comparison

In a study of the exposure of Australian Vietnam veterans to Agent Orange type herbicides and subsequent health outcomes, O'Toole, Battistvita, Long, and Crouch [1986] compared a self-administered mail questionnaire, a telephone interview, and a personal interview. These three survey modes were compared for survey costs, adequacy of completion, test-retest reliability, validity of responses to medical questions, and estimates of morbidity. Respectively, costs per household were $A42.75, $A74.33, and $A71.89. Overall, telephone and home interviews cost about twice as much as mailed surveys with most of the differential being actual interview costs that were two and one-half times higher for the telephone and home interviews. Inadequate completion occurred mainly in the mailed questionnaire with about a six percent average item omission among the 84 questions as compared to 0.4 percent for telephone and 0.2 percent for home interviews. Despite the fact that the survey asked about events that took place 10 to 15 years ago, "don't know" responses were virtually absent expect for precise details such as names of chemicals and code names of operational sites with no differences among all three modes. Reliability to medical questions was high, particularly to conditions requiring a medical diagnosis, and no mode differences were observed. Validity of medical information responses varied by mode and type of question. Underreporting and overreporting were both highest and lowest in the mail mode depending on whether a medical diagnosis or medical opinion was required. Overall, the army records of the 600 veterans listed 936 medical conditions but the subjects only reported 526 of those, less than 50 percent. On the other hand, the respondents did report 655 conditions of which only 232 were verified. Obviously, false negatives and false positives compounded the validity. Variability could possibly be related to the passage of time, the seriousness of the event, and the sensitivity of the questions.

Computer-Assisted Telephone Interview

Using the technology of random-digit dialing [RDD], a computer-assisted telephone interview [CATI] generates telephone numbers based on an estimate of all possible combinations in the target audience, including unlisted numbers. While RDD reduces sample bias, negative design effect and fieldwork costs, the technique may yield a large number of telephone numbers that are not in service, businesses, or out of the target area. There may be as many as five or more ineligibles for every eligible number. Waksberg [1978] suggests cluster designs to minimize that problem.

Proceduraly, the questionnaire is programmed into the CATI system and is visible on the computer terminal screen during the telephone call. Interviewers read from the screen and record responses directly into a data file. A dozen useful survey management functions can be provided by a CATI system according to Marcus and Crane [1986]:

* Generation of random telephone numbers and automatic dialing.
* Scheduling of initial and follow-up calls.
* Online display of current numbers and final disposition.
* Random interviewer assignment to reduce bias.

- Random question location and/or sequence reducing order effects.
- Automatic branching of responses to subsections.
- Online identification of responses beyond preset valid range.
- Internal consistency check on similar appropriate questions.
- Response retrieval to insert or refer to in later questions.
- Open-end responses sent to separate file or added in online.
- Online monitoring of interviews by supervisors.
- Immediate input of completed interview into raw data file expediting initial data processing.

To be somewhat equitable, four potential drawbacks to CATI are also indicated: CATI may be time-consuming to implement and evidently initially costly; interviewers require several days more training because of the technical skills required; data quality checking is often overestimated and may disrupt the interview's flow and timing; and a highly skilled computer programmer has to be on hand at all times to insure the reliability and efficiency of the hardware and software.

Based on a review of research findings, Marcus and Crane arrive at four main conclusions about CATIs:

- CATIs are a viable alternative to costly face-to-face surveys in cross-sectional studies of the general population.
- CATIs offer a viable alternative to expensive and time-consuming follow-up face-to-face interviews.
- In survey groups having both low telephone coverage and high nonresponse rates such as low income and low education respondents, CATIs should be used cautiously with perhaps a dual sampling framework combining face-to-face and telephone interviews.
- "CATI represents one of the most important and innovative technologic advances in health survey research in recent years."

Marcus and Crane's conclusion is equally strong and enthusiastic. "The advantages of CATI in improving survey management are noteworthy and ideally suited for moderate-to-large sample surveys. CATI also provides an attractive [and largely untapped] resource for testing and refining other methodologic protocols in survey research."

Surveys of Health Status

A health status survey could apply to the common greeting of friends who ask "How're doing today?" Responses range from great to fine to poorly to terrible indicating a subjective analysis of your own health status. Of course, the computerized Patient Health-Illness Profile [H-IP] developed by Yusim and Vallbona [1986] takes the health status concept into areas such as patient care, administrative decision making, and primary care research. Data are entered using a minimum of keystrokes as the H-IP includes the following health status elements of data: patient identification, demographic data, treatment site and date, vital signs of height, weight, blood pressure, fasting plasma glucose, and frontal occipital circumference, family history of heart disease, cancer, diabetes, hypertension, and obesity, personal risk factors such as alcohol or drug abuse, smoking, drug allergies, food allergies, and improper eating habits, active problems with dates and attending physician, inactive problems with resolution or inactivity dates, pharmacy data, laboratory data, and free text medical memos. Analysis of the H-IP data revealed the five most common health status problems to be hypertension, obesity, acute upper respiratory tract infection, osteoarthritis and diabetes mellitus. For each of these problems, Yusim and Vallbona noted that the Casa de Amigos Neighborhood Clinic in Houston, Texas initiated interventions gathering guidance from the computerized health status network data.

As the H-IP indicates, health status evaluation can secure data on physical or mental health, social and role functioning and general health perceptions [Ware, 1987]. Putting it into only two classifications, Scrivens [1985] opts for the components of clinical symptoms and social functioning to determine health status. Actually, both groupings probably aim to secure similar information.

In selecting measurements of health status, attention must be given to the following evaluation factors since a combination of methods and techniques may be used in the survey:

- Reliability and validity of the survey responses.
- Purpose of the survey such as health outcomes.
- Conceptual focus of the instrument's content related to definitions of health utilized.
- Operational approach re interviewers or self-reporting.
- Sensitivity in distinguishing micro and macro changes.
- Utility weighting via combining and values of items.
- Amenability of quantitative statistical manipulation.

In an application, Fink [1989] notes methodologic and substantive problems in measuring the health status of children.

Health status survey measurements could result from an instrument with a single aggregated score on all aspects. Alternately, there could be a single survey instrument with subscores on each aspect of health status. Still another survey could use separate instruments that are specific to each such as mobility or anxiety levels. Scrivens, Cunningham, and Charlton [1985] states that health status measurements tend to be weighted producing an index based upon standard scaling techniques, standard gambles, or time tradeoffs. An overall health status index is usually lengthy and time-consuming to complete.

Health Status Instruments in Evaluation. A number of health status evaluation instruments have developed over the years and there have been comparative studies of the effectiveness of some of the following tools:

Duke-UNC Health Profile [DUHP]	[Parkerson, Gehlbach, & Wagner, 1981]
Functional Status Index [FSI]	[Jette, Davies, & Cleary, 1986]
General Health Questionnaire [GHQ]	[Tennant, 1977]
General Health Rating Index [GHRI]	[Davies, & Ware, 1981]
Index of Well-Being [IWB]	[Fanshel, & Bush, 1970; Kaplan, Bush, & Berry, 1976; Patrick, Bush, & Chen, 1973]
McMaster Health Index Questionnaire [MHIQ]	[Chambers, McDonald, & Tugwell, 1982]
Medical Outcomes Study [MOS]	[Stewart, Hays, & Ware, 1988]
Nottingham Health Profile [NHP]	[Hunt, McKenna, & McEwen, 1981]
Quality of Life Index [QLI]	[Spitzer, 1981]
Rand Health Experiment Measures [RHIEM]	[Brook, Ware, & Davies, 1979a, 1979b; Ware, 1988]
Sickness Impact Profile [SIP]	[Bergner, Bobbitt, & Pollard, 1976; Bergner, Bobbitt, & Carter, 1981]

These health status instruments combine the use of interviews, self-reporting, indexes, and the emphasis on physical, mental, and social well-being.

Health Status Measures Compared. Stressing relevance as the priority criterion in selecting a health status measure, Hall and Masters [1986] compared five health status measures—SIP, RAND, NHP, DUHP, and IWB. These five instruments are not disease-specific and focus on more than death and illness in addition to being sensitive to low morbidity levels allowing for discrimination among asymptomatic populations. In addition, the reliability and validity of all the instruments have been studied. Descriptive summaries of each instrument by Hall and Masters follow:

- SIP . . . focuses on sickness/dysfunction . . . questions in physical dimension [ambulation, mobility, body care and movement], psychosocial dimension [social interaction, alertness behavior, emotional behavior, communication], and independent categories [sleep and rest, eating, work, home management, recreation and pastimes . . . is a well-validated and reliable measure . . . gives a single summary score of health status . . . is appropriate in many contexts . . . may be of limited sensitivity in "healthy" populations due to its focus on dysfunction related to sickness.
- RAND measures physical, mental, and social health along with general health perceptions . . . developed as an outcome measure appropriate for general populations . . . validity and reliability investigated extensively . . . sensitive to changes in ostensibly health groups . . . may be difficult to discriminate among "healthy" people on the basis of physical function . . . provides a profile rather than a single index.
- NHP measures self-perceived health problems in areas such as energy, pain, emotional reactions, sleep, social isolation, and physical mobility . . . requires "yes" or "no" responses to each item . . . should only be used when measuring self-perceived health status of disabled people . . . not investigated as extensively as SIP and RAND but represents a promising development for use in a limited area.
- DUHP measures symptom status and functioning in physical, emotional and social activities . . . primarily an outcome measure in the evaluation of primary care services . . . developers note use as day-to-day clinical assessment tool in primary care . . . reliability of symptom status, physical and emotional function measures good . . . demonstrated reliability and validity in a fairly young group of people with transient health problems . . . further testing needed with older or more disabled groups . . . shortcoming in lack of explicitly derived weights and apparent insensitivity.
- IWB measures ability to carry on activities of daily living . . . uses mobility, physical activity, and social activity scales . . . no coverage of mental health status or social and psychological aspects . . . application limited by need for an interviewer . . . scaling method yields reliable and valid weights that are amenable to sophisticated statistical manipulation.

Exhibit 7–20 shows Hall and Masters' comparison of the five health status measures including the number of items, mode of administration, rating of reliability and validity, population applicability, sensitivity, statistical level of movement, and ease of scoring.

In conclusion, Hall and Masters state that the "SIP is widely applicable but will measure low level sickness dysfunction." Similarly, the RAND has wide applicability "but with better discrimination in well populations. . . The NHP has been shown to work in elderly populations with disabilities. . . The DUHC appears applicable to younger age groups but again with

Exhibit 7-20. Comparisons of Five Health Status Measures.

Instrument	No. of Items	How Administered	Reliability	Validity Converg.	Validity Discrim.	What Groups	Sensitivity	Level of Movement	Ease of Scoring
SIP	136	Self Interviewer Mail	000	000	000	General population to chronically disabled	00	Interval	00
RAND	94	Self	000	000	000	General population only [over 15]	000	Ordinal-interval	0
NHP	38	Self	0	00	0	Disabled only	0	Ordinal	00
DUHP	63	Self Interviewer	0	000	000	General population under 50 years	0	Nominal	00
IWB	116	Interviewer	00	00	00	General	0	Interval	00

0 = Poor evidence   00 = Fair evidence   000 = Good evidence

Reliability occurs when the instrument repeatedly results in similar responses.
Validity occurs when the instrument measures what it is supposed to measure.
Convergent validity occurs when the proposed measure is highly correlated with another measure of the same construct.
Discriminant validity occurs if the new measure correlates less well with measures from which it was supposed to differ.
Sensitivity refers to the ability to register the changes that are expected to occur.
Level of movement refers to statistical definitions [see Exhibit 7-4 for further explanation].

Source: From "Measuring outcomes of health services: a review of some available measures," by J. Hall & G. Masters, 1986, *Community Health Studies, 10*(2), 154. Reprinted with permission.

definite health problems . . . the IWB has been tested in general populations; it has wide applicability but is a more complicated instrument to administer."

Testing health status measures in a Sydney, Australia population of 160 patients in two general practice settings, Hall, Hall, Fisher, and Killer [1987] compared the RAND, SIP, and the GHQ. In comparison to the RAND and the SIP, the GHQ seeks to identify probable cases of nonpsychotic psychiatric illness in screening of general populations. A 20-item instrument does appear to detect transient emotional episodes and responses to physical illness as well as psychological disturbance. While the GHQ has been used extensively in Australia, rarely have validation studies been conducted. These investigators conclude that the SIP appears to measure different aspects than the other two and that "the RAND measures appear to have the best discriminative ability in this population . . . patients visiting their general practitioner are prepared to complete questionnaires about all aspects of their health."

Looking for practicality and validity, Read, Quinn, and Hoefer [1987] evaluated three measures of overall health—SIP, GHRI [Davies & Ware, 1981] and QWB [Kaplan, Bush, & Berry, 1976; Patrick et al., 1973]—using 400 patients from a suburban VA medical center. Practicality evaluation investigated interviewer training time, administration difficulty, coding and scoring difficulty, difficulty and comprehension for subjects as rated by interviewers and the time of administration.

GHRI dimensions measure prior health, current health, health outlook, health worry/concern, resistance/susceptibility and sickness orientation. QWB measures symptoms/problems, mobility, physical activity and social activity.

Read et al. [1987] find strong evidence supporting the validity of all three instruments. Therefore, the choice is related to available resources, the proposed intervention, the target group, and the priority of dimensions of the instruments. However, there were considerable differences in the use of resources to administer the surveys. GHRI was the easiest to use taking 20 minutes to complete and requiring little interviewer training. Both the SIP and the QWB require considerable interviewer training. In addition, the complexity of the QWB precludes self-administration.

"Where resources are most limited, in situations where brief, self-administered forms are required, or when controversy regarding standardized weighting schemes pose a problem, the GHRI would be preferred. The SIP is the most versatile measure of overall health, dealing with a wide range of specific dysfunctions in a manner easy to understand [and communicate]. It also has strength in the area of mental functioning. The QWB incorporates complexities necessary in a measure intended to provide data for cost-effectiveness analysis and resource allocation decisions."

Commenting that most of the existing health status measures contain too many questions and take too long to complete for practical use in the clinic setting, Stewart et al. [1988] tested a short 20-item Medical Outcomes Study [MOS] instrument that satisfied standards of acceptability, reliability, and validity in a general population [Ware, Sherbourne, & Davies, 1988]. Their short health status form was used with more than 11,000 patients in various practice settings in Boston, Chicago, and Los Angeles between February and October of 1986. Six health concepts are included in the short 20-item instrument: Six physical functioning items assess strenuous to basic physical activity limitations due to health. Two role functioning and one social functioning item ask about interference, usual daily activities and with social activities. Five mental health items assess psychological distress and well-being. Five health perceptions items ask the respondent to rate their own current health in general. One pain item assesses physical discomfort and bodily pain. Physical functioning, mental health, and health perceptions examine both positive and negative aspects of health. Exhibit 7–21 shows the MOS instrument.

Exhibit 7-21.   Short Form Health Survey: Medical Outcomes Study.

2. In general, would you say your health is: ___ Excellent ___ Very Good ___ Good ___Fair ___ Poor
                                                  1   2   3   4   5

16. For how long [if at all] has your health limited you in each of the following activities?
    CHECK ONE CHOICE ON EACH LINE.

	Limited For More Than 3 Months	Limited For 3 months Or Less	Not Limited At All
	1	2	3
a. The kind or amounts of vigorous activities you can do, like lifting heavy objects, running or participating in strenuous sports	___	___	___
b. The kinds or amounts of moderate activities you can do, like moving a table, carrying groceries or bowling	___	___	___
c. Walking uphill or climbing a few flights of stairs	___	___	___
d. Bending, lifting or stooping	___	___	___
e. Walking one block	___	___	___
f. Eating, dressing, bathing, or using the toilet	___	___	___

17. How much bodily pain have you had during the past 4 weeks?
    ___ None ___ Very Mild ___ Mild ___ Moderate ___ Severe
     1   2   3   4   5

18. Does your health keep you from working at a job, doing work around the house or going to school?
    ___ Yes, for more than 3 months ___ Yes, for 3 months or less ___ No
     1   2   3

19. Have you been unable to do certain kinds or amounts of work, housework or schoolwork because of your health?
    ___ Yes, for more than 3 months ___ Yes, for 3 months or less ___ No
     1   2   3

FOR EACH OF THE FOLLOWING QUESTIONS, PLEASE CHOOSE THE ONE ANSWER THAT COMES CLOSEST TO THE WAY YOU HAVE BEEN
FEELING DURING THE PAST MONTH.   [CHECK ONE CHOICE ON EACH LINE]

	All of the Time	Most of the Time	A Good Bit of the Time	Some of the Time	A Little of the Time	None of the Time
	1	2	3	4	5	6
20. How much of the time, during the past month, has your health limited your social activities [like visiting with friends or close relatives]?	___	___	___	___	___	___
21. How much of the time, during the past month, have you a very nervous person?	___	___	___	___	___	___
22. During the past month, how much of the time have you felt calm and peaceful?	___	___	___	___	___	___
23. How much of the time, during the past month, have you felt downhearted and blue?	___	___	___	___	___	___
24. During the past month, how much of the time have you been a happy person?	___	___	___	___	___	___
25. How often, during the past month, have you felt so down in the dumps that nothing could cheer you up?	___	___	___	___	___	___

PLEASE CHOOSE THE ANSWER THAT BEST DESCRIBES WHETHER EACH OF THE FOLLOWING STATEMENTS IS TRUE OR FALSE FOR YOU.
[CHECK ONE ANSWER ON EACH LINE]

	Definitely True	Mostly True	Not Sure	Mostly False	Definitely False
	1	2	3	4	5
26 a. I am somewhat ill	___	___	___	___	___
b. I am as healthy as anybody I know	___	___	___	___	___
c. My health is excellent	___	___	___	___	___
d. I have been feeling bad lately	___	___	___	___	___

NOTE: Item numbers indicate the order in which the questions appeared in the questionnaire.

Source: From "Communication. The MOS short-form general health survey. Reliability and validity in a patient population," by A.L. Stewart, R.D. Hays, & J.E. Ware, Jr., 1988, *Medical Care, 26*[7], 733–735. Reprinted by permission of Lipincott/Harper & Row.

This MOS "survey achieves breadth and depth of measurement while permitting self-administration in only 3–4 minutes . . . reliabilities observed were not substantially lower than those observed for long-form measures." Validity was indicated by "excellent item discrimination" . . . correlations among and between the measures similar to those observed in the longer forms [Ware, Davies, & Brook, 1980] . . . "and substantial differences in health between the patient and general population samples were observed and the pattern of differences [across measures] was consistent with previous research" [Nelson et al., 1983].

Moving in the same direction toward short, easy-to-administer survey instruments, Broadhead, Gehlbach, DeGruy, and Kaplan [1988] created the Duke-UNC Functional Social Support [DUFSS] questionnaire [Exhibit 7–22]. DUFSS is a two-scale, eight-item instrument that measures affective [displaying affection] and confidant [displaying confidence] types of support. Construct, concurrent, and discriminant validity are demonstrated on 400 patients in a Family Medicine Center in Durham, North Carolina although use with black, male, and elderly populations may be limited. Investigators suggest adding scales to measure instrumental [help] support and affirmation or praise. In summary, Broadhead et al. say that "the DUFSS does not satisfy all the needs of a new instrument . . . it is a beginning and may be useful in further

Exhibit 7-22. Duke–UNC Functional Social Support Questionnaire.

HERE IS A LIST OF SOME THINGS THAT OTHER PEOPLE DO FOR US OR GIVE US THAT MAY BE HELPFUL OR SUPPORTIVE. PLEASE READ EACH STATEMENT CAREFULLY AND PLACE AN X IN THE BLANK THAT IS <u>CLOSEST</u> TO YOUR SITUATION.

HERE IS AN EXAMPLE:

	As much as I would like	Much less than I would like
I get enough vacation time	. . X . . .	

If you put an X where we have it, it means that you get <u>almost</u> as much vacation time as you would like, but not quite as much as you would like.

ANSWER EACH ITEM AS BEST YOU CAN. THERE ARE <u>NO</u> RIGHT OR WRONG ANSWERS.

	As much as I would like	Much less than I would like
I get		
1.* visits with friends and relatives		
2.* help around the house		
3.* help with money in an emergency		
4.* praise for a good job		
5. people who care what happens to me		
6. love and affection		
7.* telephone calls from people I know		
8. chances to talk to someone about problems at work or with my housework		
9. chances to talk to someone I trust about my personal and family problems		
10. chances to talk about money matters		
11. invitations to go out and do things with other people		
12. useful advice about important things in life .		
13.* help when I need transportation		
14. help when I'm sick in bed		

* = Items deleted from final questionnaire.

Source: From "The Duke–UNC functional social support questionnaire. Measurement of social support in family medicine patients," by W.E. Broadhead, S.H. Gehlbach, F.V. DeGruy, & B.H. Kaplan, 1988, *Medical Care*, 26[7], 722. Reprinted with permission of Lippincott/Harper & Row.

studies of the effects of social support on health and the interaction of social support with other determinants of health."

With a stress on a humanistic philosophy, Liang and Robb-Nicholson [1987] discuss health status and quality of life measurements based on experiences caring for people with rheumatic diseases. Several of their comments are particularly relevant: "Most important decisions in medicine are not completely rational and come colored with emotions and experience. . . Clinical medicine needs to be more quantitative but also more humanistic . . . patient care is humanistic and the emphasis is on differences . . . there are no perfect measures of function or health status." That last comment reflects their examination of 11 quality of life and health status measures used in rheumatic disease. These investigators suggest that the following six simple screening questions can measure change, assess patient preferences and determine priorities:

How does your condition affect you?
Which activity is most difficult for you?
Worse, better, or same as before?
Can't do, but could do before?
Can't do, but need to want to do?
What's the most important thing for us to improve?

Without loss of sensitivity, these simple clinical-based questions account for relativity of function, changing of values, personal circumstances and for the dynamic state of learning, adjusting and accommodation over the course of an illness.

In view of the accelerated concern with health promotion, Breslow [1989] raises the issue of determining health status. Measures could fall along a continuum that ranged from "perfect" harmony with the environment to the extreme invalidism in the premorbid state.

Surveys of Mental Illness

In a study of the problems and options in estimating the numbers and trends of homeless mentally ill persons, Chelimsky [1988c, p. 40] delineated prevalence assessment measures used in 13 studies. Exhibit 7–23 lists the four mental health status measures: self-reported psychiatric history, standardized scales in symptoms and in level of function, structured interviewing, and clinical evaluation, the various instruments used with a brief description and the study references. In addition, the four types of measures are rated for seven operational factors important in the selection of an appropriate instrument.

Also in the mental health area, Burnam, Wells, Leake, and Landsverk [1988] developed an 8-item self-reporting instrument to screen for depressive disorders such as major depression and dysthymia. Exhibit 7–24 lists all eight items with the specific values calculated for each using an equation including the differential coefficient values for each item and a natural logarithm. A departure from other screening instruments is that the individual items are weighted differentially and that two of the items [7 and 8] concern diagnostically relevant durations of depressed mood. Analysis of more than 3,000 survey participants from a general population and from primary care and mental health patients indicated high sensitivity and good positive predictive value for the brief screening instrument. This tool worked especially well for depressive disorder that is current and active.

Some time ago, Blau [1977] used quality of life indicators to evaluate the impact of care provided to psychiatric patients. Lately, quality of life measures are applied to chronic illness

Exhibit 7-23. Measures Used in 13 Studies to Assess Prevalence of Mental Illness Among Homeless Persons.

Measure	Instrument	Description	Study
Self-reported psychiatric history	—	Respondents asked about previous psychiatric hospitalization	Struening (1986)
Standardized scale			
Symptom	Center for Epidemiologic Studies Depression Scale (CES-D)	Self-report of depressive symptoms and current distress; number and content of items modified for use with homeless persons	Farr et al. (1986), Robertson et al. (1985), Struening (1987)
	Psychiatric Epidemiology Research Interview (PERI)—psychoticism scale	Self-report of psychotic beliefs, feelings, and perceptions; modified for use with the homeless	Struening (1987)
	Schedule of Affective Disorders and Schizophrenia change version (SADS-C)	Respondents rated by trained interviewers on 7 dimensions of psychopathology	Barrow and Lovell (1984)
	Brief Symptom Inventory (BSI)	Self-report on 9 psychological and social dimensions	Morse (1984), Morse and Caslyn (1984), Solarz and Mowbray (1985)
	Psychiatric Evaluation Form (PEF)	Rating of respondents on 19 symptoms, using clinical records and brief interviews	Chafetz and Goldfinger (1984)
	Psychiatric Status Schedule (PSS)	Self-report on 10 symptom areas	Roth et al. (1984)
	General Health Questionnaire (GHQ)	Self-report on 20 items covering current distress	Fisher et al. (1986)
Level of functioning	Global Assessment Scale (GAS)	Respondents rated on overall functioning and symptomatology	Mulkern et al. (1985)
	Structured Level of Functioning (SLOF)	Respondents rated on 6 dimensions, including social acceptability, skills, personal care	Schneider and Struening (1983)
Structured interview that yields diagnoses	Diagnostic Interview Schedule (DIS)	Respondents interviewed by lay interviewers on substance abuse, schizophrenic disorders, affective disorders, anxiety and somatoform disorders, antisocial personality, cognitive impairment; generates DSM-III diagnoses	Farr et al. (1986), Fisher et al. (1986)
	Structured Clinical Interview for DSM-III (SCID)	Respondents interviewed by trained clinicians on schizophreniform, schizoaffective-depressed, schizoaffective-bipolar, depression with psychotic features, other psychotic disorders; generates DSM-III diagnoses	Struening and Susser (1986)
	Schedule of Affective Disorders and Schizophrenia Lifetime Version (SADS-L)	Respondents interviewed by clinically trained interviewers on schizophrenia, schizoaffective, anxiety, and personality disorders, alcoholism and drug abuse; generates research diagnostic criteria (RDC) diagnoses	Barrow and Lovell (1984)
Clinical evaluations	—	Respondents interviewed and DSM-III or other clinical benchmark criteria are applied	Arce et al. (1983), Bassuk et al. (1984)

Measure	Reliability	Concurrent validity	Expresses duration or periodicity	Potential confounding with effects of homelessness	Identifies the dually disordered	Practical for field surveys	Observer bias
Self-reported psychiatric history	Low	Low	Yes	Low	No	Yes	Low
Standardized scale							
Symptom	High	Moderate	No	High	No	Yes	Low
Level of functioning	High	Moderate	No	High	No	Yes	Moderate
Structured interview yielding diagnoses	High	High	Yes	Low	Yes	No	Low
Clinical evaluation	Low to moderate	No data	Yes	High	Yes	No	Moderate

*The ratings in this table were based primarily on two review of the literature on the measurement of mental disorders among homeless persons: Koegel and Burnham (forthcoming) and Lovell et al. (forthcoming).

Source: From *Homeless mentally ill. Problems and options in estimating numbers and trends of homeless mentally ill persons*, by E. Chelimsky, 1988, pp. 40–41, Washington, DC: GAO/PEMD-88-24. Reprinted by permission.

References Cited in Exhibit 7-23

Arce, A. et al. 1983. A psychiatric profile of street people admitted to an emergency shelter. *Hospital and Community Psychiatry* 34:812–812.

Barrow, S. and A.M. Lovell. 1982. *Evaluation of Project Reach Out, 1981–1982*. New York State Psychiatric Institute.

Bassuk, E., L. Rubin and A. Lauriat. 1984. Is homelessness a mental health problem? *American Journal of Psychiatry* 141:1546–1549.

Chafetz, L. and M. Goldfinger. 1984. Residential instability in a psychiatric emergency setting. *Psychiatric Quarterly* 56:20–34.

Farr, R., P. Koegel and A. Burnham. 1986. *A study of homelessness and mental illness in the skid row area of Los Angeles*. Los Angeles County Department of Mental Health, Los Angeles.

Fisher, P.J. et al. 1986. Mental health characteristics of the homeless: a survey of mission users. *American Journal of Public Health* 76(5):519–524.

Morse, G. and R.J. Caslyn. 1986. Mentally disturbed homeless people in St. Louis: needy, willing, but under-served. *International Journal of Mental Health* 14:73–94.

Mulkern, V. et al. 1985. *Homelessness needs assessment study: findings and recommendations of the Massachu-setts Department of Mental Health*. Massachusetts Department of Mental Health. [August].

Robertson, M.J., R.H. Ropers and R. Boyer. 1985. *Emergency shelter for the homeless in Los Angeles County*. Basic Shelter Research Project, School of Public Health, University of California, Los Angeles [July].

Roth, D. et al. 1985. *Homelessness in Ohio: a study of people in need*. Department of Mental Health, Columbus, Ohio [February].

Solarz, A., C. Mowbray and S. Dupuis. 1986. *Life in transit: homelessness in Michigan*. Lansing, MI: Michigan Department of Mental Health.

Struening, E.L. 1987. *A study of residents of the New York City Shelter System*. New York, NY: New York City Department of Mental Health, Mental Retardation, and Alcoholism Services [April].

Struening, E.L. and E. Susser. 1986. *First time users of the New York City Shelter System*. New York State Psychiatric Institute, New York.

Exhibit 7-24. Short Screening Instrument for Depression

Screener Item	Possible Values	Coefficient
1. I felt depressed	0–3	1.078
2. My sleep was restless	0–3	0.185
3. I enjoyed life [reverse scored]	0–3	−0.269
4. I had crying spells	0–3	0.329
5. I felt sad	0–3	−0.280
6. I felt that people disliked me	0–3	0.288
7. In the past year, have you had 2 weeks or more during which you felt sad, blue, or depressed, or lost pleasure in things that you usually cared about or enjoyed?	0–1	2.712
8. Have you had 2 years or more in your life when you felt depressed or sad most days, even if you felt okay sometimes? [If yes] Have you felt depressed or sad much of the time in the past year?	0–1	2.182

Souce: From "Development of a brief screening instrument for detecting depressive disorders," by M.A. Burnam, K.B. Wells, B. Leake, & J. Landsverk, 1988, *Medical Care*, 26[8], 775–789. Reprinted by permission of Lippincott/Harper & Row.

situations, rehabilitation, geriatrics, and other conditions where the question is raised, "Is life worth living?" Chubon [1987] developed a "Life Situation Survey" tool to use in health care evaluation. This self-administered instrument consists of 20 items with a seven-rating interval scale: agree very strongly/agree strongly/agree/disagree/disagree strongly/disagree very strongly with the midpoint omitted and used as a noresponse score. Questions are divided equally in being phrased positively or negatively with a random dispersment to avoid bias. About 20 minutes are needed to complete the Life Situation Survey and to add the usual demographic data. Total scores can range from 20 to 140. Examples of the items follow:

	AVS	AS	A	D	DS	DVS
My future is hopeless.	[ ]	[ ]	[ ]	[ ]	[ ]	[ ]
I am a happy person.	[ ]	[ ]	[ ]	[ ]	[ ]	[ ]
My health is good.	[ ]	[ ]	[ ]	[ ]	[ ]	[ ]
My sleep is restful and refreshing.	[ ]	[ ]	[ ]	[ ]	[ ]	[ ]

Studies indicate support for reliability and validity, and internal consistency is acceptable. There is substantial discriminant validity with sensitivity to health and nonhealth factors, population distinctions, and measuring treatment impacts.

PATIENT SATISFACTION SURVEYS

Patient satisfaction is somewhat akin to concepts about marketing surveys in that the responses are likely to be subjective and may or may not be related to the actual technical capabilities of the health care delivery system. Cleary and McNeil [1988] relate patient satisfaction to the quality of care. Donabedian [1988] comments that "it is futile to argue about the validity of patient satisfaction as a measure of quality . . . information about patient satisfaction should be as indispensable to assessment of quality as to the design and management of health care systems." Likewise, in marketing health care, should the adage apply, "The customer is always right?" Furthermore, the possibility exists that a satisfied patient may recover quicker [Summers, 1985]. In fact, Elbeck [1987] puts it bluntly that "client satisfaction is now a core issue to the survival of health care institutions. . . The degree of satisfaction is not necessarily a reflection of what *actually* happened, but is more a reflection of what the client *perceived* as happening [author's emphasis]." Hays and Ware [1986] support the perception emphasis in an article telling why "my medical care is better than yours."

Ethics and Philosophy in Patient Satisfaction

There are ethical considerations and philosophical changes for including patients in evaluation efforts. Ethically, the Hippocratic ideal commands that the well-being of the patient comes first [primum noli non nocere]. In addition, there is a democratic value that believes that those affected by a decision should have a voice and participate in that decision. Furthermore, consumerism supports the right of consumers to decide what they want. Philosophically, there is a movement to introduce social accountability into health care with a utilitarian focus of doing the greatest good for the greatest number of people. There is also some movement from an exclusively biological concept of disease to an experiential concept of disease wherein subjective feelings are as real as objective clinical findings in influencing illness and treatment.

Vuori [1987] suggests that these ethical and philosophical rationales indicate three ways to measure patient satisfaction with the quality of care:

- As an *attribute*: Care cannot be high quality unless the patient is satisfied.
- As an *indicator*: Views of patients on the care received are a proxy measure of qualitative perceptions.
- As a *prerequisite*: Satisfied patients cooperate, follow regimens and seek care again when needed.

Measurement Components of Satisfaction

Three attitudinal components of measurements are identified by Elbeck [1987] as cognitive or perceptual [Physicians exist to cure disease], affective or feeling, [I prefer nurses to physicians], and conative or intentions [I would respond more readily to the physician's order than to the nurses]. In addition, Elbeck notes the use of evaluative beliefs in comparative measures of attributes [Nurses are friendlier than doctors] and of similarities [Nurses and doctors both work in hospitals].

If there are ethical and philosophical reasons for evaluating patient satisfaction and modes of measurement, what should be measured? Based on a review of the literature, Spiegel and Backhaut [1980] identify the following three aspects of health care that consumers value:

- Science of medicine: technical competence, knowledge, and skills to resolve the problem.
- Art of care: interpersonal, expressive, and communicative attributes of "caring" for the individual.
- Amenities of care: comfort, courtesy, privacy, and promptness in the setting in which care is rendered.

Contrary to a marketing approach where the customer is considered king, health care evaluators are reluctant to include patient satisfaction among quality of care measurements.

Common rationales include the following five: patients lack the technical and scientific knowledge to evaluate health care; patient's physical and/or mental status may make them incapable of judgments; rapid pace of events inhibits patient's comprehensive view of care; physicians and patients may have different care goals; and because it is difficult to impossible to define what quality of care means to patients. Vuori [1987] comments that these arguments may not be raised out of genuine concern but rather out of professional self-interest to avoid any inroads toward external control of the profession.

Taking all of the above into consideration, Vuori [1987] concludes: "In spite of admitted methodological difficulties, it is possible to measure patient satisfaction in a valid and reliable way."

Components of patient satisfaction have been identified and instruments designed to measure the following dimensions: personal qualities, professional competence, cost, convenience, physician conduct, availability of services, continuity of care, access to care, physician interactions, nonphysician interactions, and ancillary services. In a comparison of the main components of patient satisfaction, Roberts and Tugwell [1987] used the well accepted Ware, Snyder, and Wright [1976] and Hulka, Kupper, and Daly [1975] questionnaires with 59 people hospitalized for acute myocardial infarction in Ontario, Canada. Out of a total of 40 items, Hulka's questionnaire contained 14 dealing with professional competence, 14 evaluating the professional qualities of the provider and 12 on cost and convenience. Ware's 50 items fell into eight groupings: 8 on access/convenience, 3 on finances, 5 on availability of resources, 3 on continuity of care, 9 on the quality/competence of the physician, 8 on the humaneness of the physician, 4 on general satisfaction, and 10 on the efficacy of care. Results indicated that both patient satisfaction instruments were reliable, valid and acceptable to the patients. Both tests were easy to administer and interpret yielding comparable scores. Both instruments allow for specific documentation of satisfaction and/or dissatisfaction. "This study supports the use of either of these patient satisfaction questionnaires to measure the main components of satisfaction with medical care as constructed by Hulka and Ware."

Satisfaction with the Hospital

Using a 31-item questionnaire with almost 500 hospital patients in Beer-Sheva, Israel, satisfaction with medical, nursing, and supportive hospital services was evaluated [Carmel, 1985]. Sociodemographic, psychosocial, situational, and attitudinal characteristics were correlated to satisfaction levels. A single question measured overall satisfaction: "In general, are you satisfied or dissatisfied with your present hospitalization?" Respondents could choose from six classifications ranging from "not at all satisfied" to "very satisfied." Conclusions indicated the following:

- Combining the "very satisfied" and "satisfied" choices, 83 percent were generally satisfied with physicians, 80 percent with nurses and 52 percent with supportive services.
- Older age is a significant predictor of satisfaction with physicians and supportive services, but not of satisfaction with nurses.
- Surgical ward patients are most satisfied followed by medical wards and least satisfied with orthopedic wards.
- Patient's improvement in health best explains satisfaction with physicians and nurses.
- Perceived improvement in health is found to be the best predictor of patients' general satisfaction with *all* the studies hospital services [author's emphasis].

Carmel's major conclusion "is that when a client feels that he is achieving his goal, he adapts to the deficiencies in the process of achieving it by attaching less importance to the process."

Employing a market research firm, the New York Hospital used a telephone survey to analyze the satisfaction levels of 841 discharged patients. Abramowitz, Cote, and Berry [1987] developed an instrument containing 35 items with four-scaled choices plus two open ended questions. Attributes evaluated included 10 sets of services: admission, attending physicians, house staff, nurses, nurse's aides, housekeeping, food services, escort services, other staff, and miscellaneous services. After the study, researchers found that the questions could be reduced to 10 measurements: overall satisfaction with medical care, house staff, nursing care, and nurse's aides; for satisfaction with the noise level in the hospital and with escort services, adequacy of the food served and the staff explanations of procedures/treatments, for cleanliness of the hospital, and expectations about the quality and kind of services. On the basis of the survey results, New York Hospital initiated a guest relations program called "Hospital-ity." Abramowitz et al. conclude by commenting on the following strategies hospitals can use to maximize limited resources and improve patient satisfaction:

- Improve management's recognition of nurses who play a central role in the patient's positive perception of hospital care by being attentive to the patient's needs.
- Educate patients about staff responsibilities and hospital services to alleviate dissatisfaction caused by erroneous expectations of specific staff members.
- Institute a guest relations program to address patient concerns proactively. A commercial business newspaper reported that Beth Israel Hospital [New York City] employed 14 persons from customer services industries to do exactly that [Moss, 1986].
- Strengthen housekeeping services even though curtailment may save money in the short run and not diminish the quality of care. Reductions are likely to be costly relative to patient satisfaction.

These survey results of satisfaction with hospitals could be subsumed under the rubric of perceptions on the quality of life. Importantly, the attributes of quality of life are not static and reflect a process of living. Holder and Frank [1988] report on a survey of 450 residents by the National Citizens' Coalition for Nursing Home Reform [NCCNHR]. Some of the specific factors mentioned include the following and could be a summation of facility/care satisfaction expectations of patients:

- Maintenance of the best possible physical condition with discomfort and pain minimized.
- Movement of body, exercise, action, continued functioning at maximum potential.
- Self-determination, personal comfort, involvement in group efforts and group decision making, participation in civic affairs.
- Kindness, cheerfulness, laughter from and with others, as well as good listening, empathy, and sympathy.
- Supportive, positive, constructive attitudes of individuals one lives with or who are always around.

In addition, there are other contributors to the quality of life concept that deal with quietness, privacy, personal grooming, communication, learning opportunities, physical surrounding, outdoor areas, tasty food, and interaction with nature.

Obstetrical Care Satisfaction

In a study of patient satisfaction with obstetric care, Zweig, Kruse, and LeFevre [1986] used a five-point agree-or-disagree scale with a number of questions and three open-ended questions about feeling toward medical care, desired changes in care, and things that doctors should know. About one-half of the 258 respondents to the mailed survey questionnaire were critical of the physician/patient relationship and particularly communication. Expressed desires suggested that "physicians spend more time with patients, listen better, provide more information and respect the patient and the pregnancy as unique." Anderson [1982] reinforces the satisfied consumer aspects relative to benefits in a study of service return behavior in the hospital obstetrics market. Incidentally, the next highest critical comment only involved 16 percent of the respondents and dealt with the discomforts of pregnancy and labor.

Satisfaction with Family Practice

A survey questionnaire was mailed to patients who received care at a family practice residency teaching center. Patients could evaluate eight dimensions of care: art of care, technical quality, accessibility, efficacy, cost, physical environment, availability, and continuity of care. Gerace and Sangster [1987] found four variables to be significant to patient satisfaction:

* Adequate time spent with the family physician and provision of clear explanations regarding the patient's care.
* Feeling that the family physician was available.
* A positive attitude regarding the teaching program.
* Felt comfortable in expressing concerns about the teaching program.

These authors noted difficulties in the evaluation: patient satisfaction is a vague and ill-defined concept; patients tend not to give negative ratings; and perceptions of patient satisfaction can change.

In a similar study, Cohen, Breslau, and Porter [1986] found patient perceptions of satisfaction to remain high after reorganization of the traditional medical clinic into a academic group practice. Patients perceived an increased access to physicians, a decrease in waiting time for an appointment, and a decrease in charges and utilization.

Nursing Care Satisfaction

A total of 1,357 [39 percent] ex-patients from seven British acute care hospitals returned mailed questionnaires asking for information about the nursing care [Moores & Thompson, 1986]. Questions dealt with the following 10 nursing areas:

* adequate bathrooms/toilets; privacy
* help from nurses
* have to ring bell for nurse; speed in responding
* are nurses under pressure?
* favoritism by nurses
* staff attitudes toward nurses
* attitudes of nurses to others
* nursing team spirit

- form of information given—book/leaflet/spoken/nothing
- discharge care

Response patterns revealed wide disparities between the seven hospitals and pinpointed specific areas requiring additional study. In fact, four of the hospitals commissioned surveys of 1,200 ex-patients to gather additional information. Typical response ranges among the seven hospitals to specific questions are illustrated below:

No information given before admission: 7 to 39 percent
Lack of bathroom facilities: 2 to 32 percent
Had to ring bell for nurse: 26 to 74 percent
There was nurse favoritism: 6 to 15 percent
Nurses treat doctors as superiors: 66 to 74 percent
Prefer different hospital if needed again: 2 to 21 percent

Simpson [1985] used a consumer opinion survey questionnaire of nursing care that contained 27 items with a four-point Likert scale and scoring with unequally weighted numerical values. Questions concerned the patient environment [use of call button and equipment], basic needs [grooming and exercise help], nursing care planning [participated in daily schedule], patient teaching [taught to care at home], discharge planning [financial aid and self-care activities], and evaluation of nursing care [explanations and adjustments to preferences]. Coded questionnaires along with a self-addressed and stamped return envelope were mailed to 850 patients during two and one-half years and about one-third were returned. Results indicated that a large percentage of the elderly were dissatisfied; that a large percentage of all ages were not given the chance to participate in planning their own care; and male patients seemed more satisfied than females. Improvements were made to patient teaching and discharge planning reflecting the patients' perceptions.

In a comparison of three separate studies, La Monica, Oberst, Madea, and Wolf [1986] sought to develop and test an instrument to measure the satisfaction of hospitalized patients with nursing care. Study 1 surveyed 75 patients being treated for cancer using an instrument consisting of 50 randomly ordered nurse behaviors with a five point Likert rating scale. Study 2 surveyed 100 cancer patients using a 42-item questionnaire describing nurse behaviors with a seven point Likert rating scale. Study 3 surveyed 710 patients with the same instrument used in study 2—the La Monica-Oberst Patient Satisfaction Scale [LOPSS]. LOPSS contains 17 items relative to dissatisfaction, 13 items on interpersonal support, and 11 related to good impressions. One item was dropped from the 42. Typical dissatisfaction questions concerned attentiveness, friendliness, keeping promises, thoroughness, organization, explanations and reluctance to assist. Interpersonal support asked about following the treatment program, emergency situations, availability for support, gentleness, and a feeling of security. Good impression dealt with respect, caring attitude, freedom to ask questions, and pleasantness. While the LOPSS instrument did not achieve greater sensitivity, the tool was similar to existing instruments in score ranges, location of mean, skewness and variability.

EVALUATION OF PROGRAMS

Program evaluation helps to answer questions and make decisions about what services to provide, for whom, and how. Specific subject areas for program evaluation could include the following: client outcomes, utilization of services, quality of care review, impact upon the community, assessment of needs, citizen participation, cost-benefit analysis, cost-effective analysis, cost-utility analysis, and costs to produce income. Economic evaluations of health care programs including methods, techniques, appraisals and training are thoroughly covered by Drummond, Stoddard, and Torrance [1987] with particular attention to cost and utility analysis.

Distinctions Between Evaluation and Research

Sometimes program evaluation and evaluative research are regarded as synonymous. Helper [1988] clarifies the distinction: "Evaluative research is carried out for the purpose of contributing to general knowledge available to society, while program evaluation is carried out for the purpose of supporting specific decisions for individual organizations." Criteria of time, level of confidence, audience, and scope also highlight differences. Program evaluation has time constraints for decisions, uses available evidence based on beliefs, management is the audience and the scope is local. In evaluative research, time is not a factor, knowledge provides confidence, mankind is the audience and there is a global scope.

Steps in Program Evaluation

Since program evaluation is an integral part of a business approach to health care, Helper [1988] details the six steps in the planning process.

1. *Defining the objective of the evaluation*—Keeping in mind that the program evaluation is probably being undertaken in support of a management decision, an examination of benefits is the most likely objective. Outcomes from this evaluation then allows management to allocate resources in funding and personnel.

2. *Choosing and defining the program to be evaluated*—Management has to fit all the pieces together and therefore the relationship of the program to the corporation's objectives will be a major consideration in choice. In all likelihood, a priority for program evaluation will emerge from management deliberations. Other factors in selection can include probable program costs and benefits, availability of indicator variables for measurements, and the threat and relation to existing programs. In addition, the program to be evaluated should be mature and stable to avoid unreliable results.

3. *Choosing indicator variables*—Evaluation measurements should be relevant to corporate objectives and professional values, data should be accessible, and the indicators must be reliable and valid. If the corporate objective is to increase market share, opinions and attitudes of patients may be most relevant. Management can seldom afford the time and effort required for original data collection, so information should be on hand or easily secured. Available reliable and valid indicators could include management specific items such as length of stay, cost per admission, advertising cost per new patient, or number of patients seen per physician. It is also possible that several indicators could be used together.

4. *Designing the program evaluation*—A program evaluation design should not result in a "So what?" response when the outcomes are discussed. Therefore, an evaluation design must consider interpretability, generalizability, and appropriateness. Keeping the facts simple along with a basis for comparison allows for facile interpretation. If a realistic representative sample of the target audience is in the design, there should be predictive generalizability to the larger population universe. Appropriateness looks at the costs of right or wrong decisions and who is to make the decision.

Designs could use standards such as "tracers" or "sentinel events" or "professional guidelines" to compare with the evaluation results. Another variation involves controlled designs such as those detailed in Exhibit 7–5. Obviously, management input into the choice of the evaluation design will take into account the relative inexpensiveness of the use of standards as compared to the expense of controlled designs.

5. *Presenting the results*—As a management tool, the program evaluation report should be written in the frame of reference of the decision maker. That may mean an emphasis on the bottom line and fewer internal nitty gritty details. Commonly, a one-page executive summary may be the only part of the report that is fully digested by the decision maker. Strategic planners must prepare the report specifically for the designated decision maker.

6. *Planning follow through*—Since most planners always believe that their projects will be approved, an implementation plan should also be ready for that event. However, it is critical to keep track of the evaluation report as the approval process goes on. Learn who is reading the report and listen to what is being said about the proposal. Online information allows planners to make adjustments for contingencies such as partial approval, budget changes and personnel allocations. If the proposal is rejected, ask how to improve the evaluation for next time rather than an outright "why?" which may antagonize top management.

Evaluation of Utilization Review Program

From a management orientation, Feldstein, Wickizer, and Wheeler [1988] analyzed a large private insurance carrier's claims data on 222 groups of employees and dependents for 1984 and 1985. Utilization review [UR] is considered an effective tool in cost containment efforts and that was a major management objective of this program evaluation. Preadmission certification, on-site review and concurrent review were the three UR activities in this comparative study of 555 insured groups with UR and 668 without UR. Administrative data examined included admissions per 1000 insured persons, length of stay days, patient-days per 1000 insured, total hospital expenditures per insured and total medical expenditures per insured. An additional 24 variables were included in the multivariate analysis such as age and sex distributions [males under 19 and over 50, females under 19, 20, to 50, over 50]; expenditures on various diseases/conditions [pregnancy and childbirth, ischemic heart disease, other heart disease, hypertension, urinary system, female genital system]; coordination-of-benefits expenditures [Medicare coordination, carve-out savings and subtraction savings]; and health care market factors [HMO penetration rate, physicians per 1,000 market area residents, charges covered, coinsurance rate].

Controlling for various factors, this program evaluation indicated significant benefits for UR. Admissions were reduced by 12 percent, inpatient days by 8 percent, hospital expenditures by 12 percent, and total medical expenditures by 8 percent. In insured groups having a relatively high admission rate before UR, results were respective reductions of 35, 34, 31 and 24 percent. Overall, $8 was saved for every $1 expended for UR. A comparison of costs and savings for average use and high use typical 1,000 employee firms emphasizes the value of program evaluation in this situation:

Measures	Average Use	High Use
Annual UR cost	$ 18,960	$ 18,960
Savings per year	$165,312	$536,097
Net savings per year	$146,352	$517,137
Savings of total medical costs	7.3%	23.4
Savings to cost ratio	8.7:1	28.3:1
Discounted net savings 5 year UR program	$633,558	$2,238,686

Even considering the smaller and more easily understood expenditures per employee, the data are dramatic. Annual UR cost per employee is $189.60 for either firm. Net annual savings per employee were $146 and $517 respectively. Obviously, there is information here for employers, providers and insurance companies to ponder relative to the value of UR.

Self-Care Program to Reduce Utilization

Using a randomized controlled trial [RCT], Stergachis [1986] evaluated the use of a self-care pamphlet about upper respiratory infections [URI] by an HMO, the Group Health Cooperative of Puget Sound in Seattle, Washington. There were 2,365 people in the experimental group and 2,358 control enrollees. In January 1982, the control group was sent a postcard reminder about the upcoming cold and flu season, the lack of effective treatment and the self-limiting nature of the illness. Simultaneously, the experimental group was sent a 10-page pamphlet on cold and flu care that included information about self-care symptoms, criteria for calling a consulting nurse, and appropriate home treatments. In addition, a medicine request form was included allowing members to secure cold and flu medication directly from the HMO pharmacy. Evaluation measurements included the telephone encounters, cold/flu drugs and the use of the pamphlet from data in nurse consultation forms, pharmacy patient profiles and a random subsample patient survey. Results indicated that the distribution of the simple self-care pamphlet significantly reduced the nurse telephone consultations and the use of drug prescriptions the pamphlet sought to control. There was no impact upon the appropriateness of the nurse consultant telephone calls and no secondary bacterial infection harm as indicated by the equality of antibiotic prescriptions among the two groups. Importantly, effective treatment was not withheld from the experimental group. Less than one-half of the targeted group was effectively reached by the pamphlet based on the patient survey responses on remembrance and reading the material. Management decisions emanating from this program evaluation included the availability of a modified pamphlet for distribution at all the hmo primary care centers and an additional RCT study on service utilization for URI.

Utilization Focused Evaluation

Calling their approach utilization focused evaluation, Durland [1987] reports on an investigation of the activities engendered by the 1981 implementation of the Colorado legislature's passage of the Alternatives to Long-Term Nursing Home Care Act. That Act came about because of the burgeoning Medicaid costs in general and long-term nursing home costs in particular. A program evaluation was specifically designed to address the obligatory legislative programmatic decisions aimed at reducing costs and improving the living environment of clients.

An evaluation team consisting of three individuals from unrelated state agencies: a health administration faculty member from the University of Colorado Medical School, a health economist in the Health Department's Policy Planning and Evaluation Unit, and a program evaluator from the Governor's Planning and Budget Office. Initial efforts related to the involvement of the program administrators and service providers since they would ultimately apply the evaluation results. A 31 member Evaluation Advisory Committee was established and the members were actively involved. Noting that the body was *advisory* rather than a *steering* committee, Durland comments that the evaluation team was "able to use good ideas and discard bad ones without ever having to obtain agreement to proceed" [author's emphasis].

Beginning with the assumption that alternatives to a nursing home were desirable and less costly, evaluators found the concepts valid and economical. Based on the team evaluation, three procedural administrative actions took place:

- Nursing home admission processes examined all possible alternatives earlier in the process.
- Hospital discharge planners greatly increased their participation in the alternatives program.
- County case workers moved to become true case managers utilizing all available community resources rather than just county delivered services and with much greater use of home health agencies.

In summary, Durland [1987] states that the utilization focused evaluation allowed the three member evaluation team to do the tasks required by the legislature. "We were able to 'stay clean' and do the pure data analysis needed for the research and cost comparisons and 'get our hands dirty' by opening appropriate portions of the evaluation to the opinions of individuals who could assist in identifying problems, developing solutions, and interpreting results." It is possible that those involved felt a moral obligation to implement the recommendations since they participated in the process of making them. Designing an evaluation with the end users in mind results in a cost-effective evaluation.

Technology Assessment Iterative Loop [TAIL]

All the decisions in the TAIL approach to the evaluation of technology aim to reduce the burden of illness. At each of the seven steps in the process, different evaluation questions are raised that may necessitate securing new information with varying methods and techniques. Bennett and Tugwell [1986] contend that TAIL is a practical guide to decision makers considering the acquisition of new technology and to planners implementing evaluations. This following process is iterative since repeated cycles of the loop may be required to really make a dent in reducing the burden of illness:

1. *Burden of illness*—Identification and quantification of the illness burden with a focus on specific technologies' ability to reduce the burden at all care levels: primary, secondary and tertiary.
2. *Efficacy*—Responds to basic question: "Does this technology do more good than harm to patients who are diagnosed accurately, appropriately cared for, and fully compliant with treatment recommendations?"
3. *Screening and diagnosis*—Refers to the accurate detection of those who will and/or will not benefit from efficacious use of the technology.
4. *Community effectiveness*—Deals with burden of illness reduction in realistic operational conditions as measured by five factors: efficacy; diagnostic accuracy; health provider compliance; patient compliance; and coverage,
5. *Efficiency*—Involves the application of cost-effectiveness, cost-utility and cost-benefits analysis of technology options within and across specific clinical conditions.
6. *Synthesis and implementation*—Integrates the burden of illness, feasibility, effect, and efficiency into a plan for the diffusion and use the technology along with performance criteria for assessment.
7. *Monitoring and reassessment*—Selection and application of indicators of success as well as identification and correction of factors inhibiting success. Reassessment of the burden of illness and reiteration of the loop.

"TAIL subdivides the spectrum of information into groups that constitute a logical progression from quantifying the burden of illness [or need for health care technology], through identifying those in need and applying the technology, to determining whether the burden of illness has been reduced."

National Long-Term Care Channeling Demonstration

From 1982–1984, the federal government funded 10 channeling demonstration sites that sought to substitute community care for nursing home care through case management and expanded community services. All told, there were 18 detailed technical evaluation reports covering the study design and methods, operational experiences, comparisons of alternatives, formal and informal care, and a spectrum of outcomes. With a mostly negative overtone relative to objectives and outcomes evaluations, Kemper [1988] details 14 of the findings as follows:

1. Channeling served a very frail population, but the population turned out not to be at high risk of nursing home placement.
2. Program elements were implemented largely as desired.
3. Technical evaluation design was implemented successfully.
4. Channeling was tested in service environments that already provided community care.
5. Channeling did not substantially reduce nursing home use.
6. Channeling increased formal community service use.
7. Neither model had a major effect on informal caregiving, although the financial model led to small reductions in some areas.
8. Channeling did not affect longevity, hospital use, or use of physicians and other medical services.
9. Channeling increased total costs.
10. Channeling reduced unmet needs, increased clients' confidence in receipt of care, and increased their satisfaction with life.
11. Channeling did not affect measures of client functioning, with the possible exception of physical functioning [ADL] under the financial model.
12. Channeling increased informal caregivers' satisfaction with service arrangements and satisfaction with life.
13. Results may have differed between models.
14. Channeling's effects were generally similar across sites and subgroups of the population.

"There is, in our judgment, little doubt about the basic conclusions. . ." Kemper's confidence is supported by three pieces of evidence: consistency of results across the sites; consistency with other community care demonstrations; and that "changes of any plausible magnitude . . . would not alter the basic conclusion about costs."

This evaluation yields to the surfacing of an age-old ethical dilemma in the health care field. Massive results show that costs are not reduced but that benefits are increased. Can decision makers justify the continuation of channeling initiatives merely because the activities reduced unmet needs, increased in-home care, and improved satisfaction with life among clients and informal caregivers? Professional opinions aim at both sides of the issue. Some say that the channeling efforts should be redirected with intensified attention to enrolling the appropriate target population. On the other hand, some opt for keeping the program going since people should not be denied the laudatory benefits that far outweigh the financial drawback.

In adding to the long-term care dilemma, Joshua Wiener and Alice Rivlin of the Brookings Institution evaluated 50 funding options during a three-year study [Wagner, 1988]. In estimates, they anticipated an increase in private long-term care insurance; by 2020 between 26 to 45 percent of the elderly would have coverage. Wiener and Rivlin urged improved Medicare coverage and increased taxes for funding. Their estimates: an increased 1.6 percent payroll tax to maintain the system and a 3 percent increase between now and 2050 to fund comprehensive long term care. Being an intellectual advocate for the elderly, Wiener contends that society can, and should, ensure their long-term care. Labeled a liberal, one colleague aptly describes Wiener: "He's one of the few people I know who actually gives money to the homeless."

Access to Primary Care at Lower Cost

Through a Municipal Health Services Program [MHSP], five city governments [Baltimore, Cincinnati, Milwaukee, St. Louis, and San Jose] created networks of primary care clinics. Major concerns dealt with reaching populations in need, reducing fragmented care and rendering care at lower cost than alternatives. HCFA granted Medicare and Medicaid waivers to make the services attractive to that covered population. Fleming and Andersen [1986] evaluated a number of the program's aspects by responding to the following questions:

How needy were the service areas? MHSP communities have greater minority representation, more low-income people, more publicly insured people, and more people with less appropriate regular sources of care. However, they did not have more uninsured people. Thus, the MHSP communities do contain the populations the program was designed to reach.

Are people with special needs served? MHSP stresses services to children and to people with public insurance or no insurance. Some of the MHSP centers do emphasize services to blacks and Hispanics while others do not. No concentration was found for the elderly, for persons in poor health, or for those without a regular source of care.

Did MHSP improve utilization patterns? There was no significant differences between the MHSP users and people receiving care at the public hospital clinic, the private doctor and other hospitals. However, a higher ratio of physician visits by the MHSP users suggests their emphasis on ambulatory care may be substituting for inpatient care.

Did MHSP patients receive appropriate care? MHSP users are just as likely to receive preventive physical examination and appear to have somewhat lower continuity of care than patients of private physicians. In response to symptoms, MHSP and private doctors behave more appropriately than public facility and other hospital providers.

Were MHSP patients as satisfied as users of other facilities? MHSP patients were less satisfied than other hospital and private doctor users with appointment waiting time, office waiting time, provider interaction and the total satisfaction scale. These patients were the second least satisfied with travel time and with cost.

What was the expenditure per visit at each source of care? MHSP patient expenditures were lower than the public and other hospital for both the user status [$48 to $53 and $67] and source [$54 to $56 and $86]. However, MHSP costs were higher than the private doctor for both measures [$48 to $40 and $54 to $35].

Did MHSP reduce overall expenditures? Adjusted total annual expenditures comparisons showed no statistically significant differences among the users. However, MHSP total yearly adjusted expenses was $875, other hospital $1,117, private doctor $969 and public hospital $832 with possibly substantive respective differences of +$242, +$96, and −$43.

Did MHSP reduce expenditures by public payers? Adjusted per capita savings were significant for Medicare patients at MHSP than at other providers [$989 to $1,705]. Similar Medicaid costs were lower but not significant [$1,084 to $1,193].

In conclusion, Fleming and Andersen [1986] state that "we are relatively certain that MHSP did not result in *increased* expenditures. In an earlier time period the gains of MHSP in access and coverage without concurrent expenditure *increases* would have been viewed as a success" [author's emphasis]. An implication is made that in the cost containment era, the evaluation success is doubtful.

EVALUATION REPORTS DO SPREAD THE WORDS

No matter how superb your evaluation design, implementation, and results are, a poorly prepared project report can doom the communication to a dust-filled basement carton. Strategic planners should start thinking about the final report at the beginning of the evaluation. If funds are available, an amount should be included in the budget for hiring a writer and for preparation, production, and distribution of the report. Notes should be kept during the progress of the project along with samples of materials, instrument, computer printouts, or documents used. There should be a complete and comprehensive file should any questions arise. In addition, it is better to err on the conservative side and save more until the activity is concluded and the report written.

Juzwishin and Boates [1987] synthesize their suggested components for writing effective program proposals into a compact checklist. Not every report will cover all the elements and circumstances will dictate deletions or additions. Nevertheless, a perusal of the items should start the evaluator thinking. There could be a cover or title page, a table of contents, an executive summary, a statement of the problem, background information, alternative courses of action, program descriptions [operations, staffing, costs, supply costs, space requirements, capital costs], multiyear budget projections, implementation methodology, evaluation outcomes, community/regional and/or other implications, marketing strategies and appendices. Incidentally, Juzwishin and Boates note that the executive summary is written last but placed at the beginning emphasizing major points clearly and concisely and listing recommendations.

In colorful language, Frank [1986] tells how to get your point across in 30 seconds or less with a one-page executive summary consisting of a hook, body, and close. A hook may be one or two brief sentences that outline the scope and importance of the report. Like the fish, the management has to be enticed by the bait to read the report. In the body, the summary sketches the project and the projected outcomes, and refers to supporting evidence in data in the report itself. In the close, the evaluation executive summary specifies alternatives for decisions, existing time constraints and recommends the suggested action for management to take. Moving from this tight and focused executive summary, the other parts of the report are broader and expansive in supporting documentation for the suggested management action. Importantly, the details are there for all who wish to scrutinize them. Yet, the details do not detract from the overall message.

A management consultant in business communication, MacMillan [1985] enumerates three common mistakes in report preparation:

- *Failure to think ahead*—Advance thinking creates a solid base for forming the message. With an appropriate skeleton, the flesh can be added with written notes, priorities, transitions, and actions in a format that is well organized, easy to read, and easy to understand.
- *Failure to edit after writing*—Nothing is as irritating as misspelling somebody's name. Your report may be wonderful but the person whose name is wrong may vote against it. Obviously, there should be checks for typos, spelling, and grammar. There are a number of computer word processing programs that automatically check documents for these such as Word Perfect and Word Star. However, editing should also look at unnecessary words, sentence length, active verbs rather than passive, slang and jargon, wasted words, and staring sentences with "the." Computer software such as Grammatik III [Williams & Wilkins, 1989a], RightWriter [RightSoft 1989] and Steadman's Medical Dictionary [Williams & Wilkins, 1989b] can help with the task. A caution not to overedit is appropriate since your end product may be dull and boring.
- *Failure to listen for tone*—Here, it's not what you say but how you say it. Reports should fit the message, the personality, and the manner of doing business. Tips include visualizing the report recipient, using personal pronouns when appropriate, and using language that harmonizes with the tone. Tone could be direct, friendly, stilted, or humorous.

Exhibit 7-25.   Checklist for Better Written Communications.

1. **ANALYZE**
   __ What are the facts?
   __ Which are relevant?
   __ What is the problem?
   __ Can I offer a solution?

2. **ORGANIZE**
   __ Have I properly defined the WHO, WHAT and WHY in the opening sentences?
   __ Does my lead generate enough reader interest for follow-through?
   __ Can my reader follow my development?
   __ Did I use an inverted pyramid approach?

3. **STYLIZE**
   __ Does it sound like me?
   __ Does it express or impress?
   __ Is it clearly understandable?

4. **VITALIZE AND HUMANIZE**
   __ Have I used active voice and action verbs?
   __ Did I use personal words?
   __ Have I used concrete words?
   __ Did I overqualify or hedge?

5. **FORMALIZE**
   __ Can it be misinterpreted?
   __ Did I really make a point?

6. **FINALIZE**
   __ Is my meaning clear?
   __ Have I removed redundancies and superfluous words?
   __ Can I tighten my writing without making it too dense?
   __ Did I define my terms?
   __ Is my message "in focus"?
   __ Was I forceful?
   __ Was I tactful?

According to MacMillan [1985], resolving these three common writing errors can assure your report of the successful basic building blocks of tone, clarity and organization.

Exhibit 7–25 is a six-point checklist for better written communications that covers items linked to analyze, organize, stylize, vitalize and humanize, formalize and finalize. An oft-condemned bastardization of common nouns with an "ize" ending is intentionally used for "effect."

A NEW CYCLE OF EVALUATION

As demonstrated throughout this book and particularly in this chapter, strategic planning and evaluation are cyclical in nature. It should be apparent that an evaluation raises as many questions as it answers and sets in motion a new round of activity. Likewise planning can start at any phase and go backward or forward to gather the missing elements. Feeny [1986] specifically asks a relevant question for these times: "Is there any way to harness the methods of clinical and economic evaluation to facilitate and improve the decision making process?" A like question could be phrased about the potential of strategic planning and decision making.

There is no doubt that decisions are going to be made in reaction to the constantly changing currents and tides in the health care delivery system. Strategic planners must strive to provide a rationale for those decisions while providing clinical, economical, political, and social components that complement each other. According to T.J. Cartwright [1987]: "The key to success in planning lies in the fine art of balancing what you really want and need with the ways and means actually available for achieving it."

REFERENCES

Abramowitz, S., Cote, A.A., & Berry, E. (1987). Analyzing patient satisfaction: A multianalytic approach. *Quality Review Bulletin, 13*(4), 122–130.

Aday, L. (1986). Access in the 1980s: Progress, problems and prospects. *The Internist, 27*(2), 16–19.

Akhter, M.N. (1985). Quality assurance under the Missouri PRO program. *Missouri Medicine, 82*(6), 297–299.

American Medical News. (1988). Growing demand seen for accountability. Competence evaluation key education issue. *31*(32), 23.

Anderson, D. (1982). The satisfied consumer: service return behavior in the hospital obstetrics market. *Journal of Health Care Marketing, 2*(4), 25–33.

Barnum, H. (1987). Evaluating healthy days of life gained from health projects. *Social Science and Medicine, 24*(10), 833–841.

Bassett, L.C., & Metzger, N. (1986). *Achieving excellence.* Rockville, MD: Aspen Publishers Inc.

Bennett, J.P. (1985). Standard cost systems lead to efficiency and profitability. *Healthcare Financial Management, 39*(5), 46–53.

Bennett, K.J., & Tugwell, P. (1986). Iterative loop gives framework for assessing technology. *Dimensions in Health Service, 63*(8), 68–71.

Berdie, D.R., Anderson, J.F., & Niebuhr, M.A. (1986). *Questionnaires: Design and use* (2nd ed.). Metuchen, NJ: Scarecrow Press.

Bergner, M., Bobbitt, R.A., & Pollard, W.E. (1976). The sickness impact profile: Validation of a health status measure. *Medical Care, 14*(1), 57–67.

Bergner, M., Bobbitt, R.A., & Carter, W.B. (1981). The sickness impact profile: Development and final revision of a health status measure. *Medical Care, 19*(8), 787–805.

Blau, T.H. (1977). Quality of life, social indicators and criteria of change. *Professional Psychology, 8*(4), 464–473.

Boscarino, J.A. (1987). Collecting and using strategic market data. *Health Care Strategic Management, 5*(7), 14–17.

Breslow, L. (1989). Health status measurement in the evaluation of health promotion. *Medical Care, 27*(3), S205–S216.

Broadhead, W.E., Gehlbach, S.H., DeGruy, F.V., & Kaplan, B.H. (1988). The Duke-UNC functional social support questionnaire. Measurement of social support in family medicine patients. *Medical Care, 26*(7), 709–723.

Brook, R.H., & Lohr, K.N. (1985). Efficacy, effectiveness, variations, and quality. Boundary-crossing research. *Medical Care, 23*(5), 710–722.

Brook, R.H., Ware, J.E., & Davies, A.R. (1979a). *Conceptualization and measurement of health for adults in the health insurance study: Volume VIII, overview.* Santa Monica, CA: Pub. No. R–1987/8-HEW.

Brook, R.H., Ware, J.E., & Davies, A.R. (1979b). Overview of adult health status measures fielded in RAND health insurance study. *Medical Care, 17*(Suppl), 1–131.

Brownlee, A.T. (1986). Applied research as a problem-solving tool: Strengthening the interface between health management and research. *The Journal of Health Administration Education, 4*(1), 31–44.

Budde, J.F. (1979). *Measuring performance in human services systems: Planning, organization, and control.* New York: AMACOM.

Burnam, M.A., Wells, K.B., Leake, B., & Landsverk, J. (1988). Development of a brief screening instrument for detecting depressive disorders. *Medical Care, 26*(8), 775–789.

Burns, J.A. (1986). Knowledge is power: How to develop effective market surveys. *Health Marketing Quarterly, 3*(2&3), 99–112.

Buros, O.K. (1974). *Tests in print II: An index to tests, test reviews, and the literature on specific tests.* Highland Park, NJ: Gryphon Press.

Bush, J.W., Chen, M.M., & Patrick, D.L. (1973). Health status indexes in cost effectiveness: analysis of a PKU program. In R.L. Berg (Ed.), *Health status indexes.* Chicago, IL: Hospital Research and Educational Trust.

Caper, P. (1988). Defining quality in medical care. *Health Affairs, 7*(1), 49–61.

Carmel, S. (1985). Satisfaction with hospitalization: A comparative analysis of three types of services. *Social Science and Medicine, 21*(11), 1243–1249.

Carr, W., Szapiro, N., Heisler, T., & Krasner, M.I. (1989). Sentinel health events as indicators of unmet needs. *Social Science in Medicine, 29*(6), 705–714.

Carrell, S. (1988). Questions to ask of treatment programs. *American Medical News, 31*(34), 35.

Carr-Hill, R.A. (1985). The evaluation of health care. *Social Science and Medicine, 21*(4), 367–375.

Cartwright, A. (1987). *Health surveys in practice and in potential.* New York: Oxford University Press.

Cartwright, T.J. (1987). The lost art of planning. *Long Range Planning, 20*(2), 92–99.

Chambers, L.W., McDonald, L.A., & Tugwell, P. (1982). McMaster health index questionnaire as a measure of quality of life for patients with rheumatoid disease. *Journal of Rheumatology, 9*(5), 780–784.

Chelimsky, E. (1988a). *Medicare: Improved patient outcome analyes could enhance quality assessment.* (GAO/PEMD-88-23). Washington, DC: Government Printing Office.

Chelimsky, E. (1988b). *Children's programs. A comparative evaluation framework and five illustrations.* (GAO/PEMD-88-28BR). Washington, DC: Government Printing Office.

Chelimsky, E. (1988c). *Homeless mentally ill. Problems and options in estimating numbers and trends of homeless mentally ill persons.* (GAO/PEMD-88-24). Washington, DC: Government Printing Office.

Chen, M.K. (1973). The G index for program priorities. In R.L. Berg (Ed.), *Health status indexes.* Chicago, IL: Hospital Research and Educational Trust.

Chubon, R.A. (1987). Development of a quality-of-life rating scale for use in health-care evaluation. *Evaluation and The Health Professions, 10*(2), 186–200.

Chun, K. (1975). *Measure in psychological assessment: A guide to 3,000 original sources and their applications.* Ann Arbor, MI: Survey Research Center.

Cleary, P.D., & McNeil, B.J. (1988). Patient satisfaction as an indicator of quality care. *Inquiry, 25*(1), 25–36.

Codman, E.A. (1914). The product of a hospital. *Surgery, Gynecology and Obstetrics, 18*(4), 491–496.

Cohen, D.I. et al. (1986). Academic group practice—the patient's perspective. *Medical Care, 24*(11), 990–998.

Cooper, L.S., Chalmers, T.C., & McCally, M. (1988). The poor quality of early evaluations of magnetic resonance imaging. *Journal of the American Medical Association, 259*(22), 3277–3280.

Corcoran, K. (1987). *Measures for clinical practice: A sourcebook.* New York: Free Press.

Cruickshank, P.J. (1985). Patient rating of doctors using computers. *Social Science and Medicine, 21*(6), 615–622.

Daley, J., Jencks, S., & Draper, D. (1988). Predicting hospital-associated mortality for Medicare patients. A method for patients with stroke, pneumonia, acute myocardial infarction, and congestive heart failure. *Journal of the American Medical Association, 260*(24), 3616–3624.

Datta, L. (1988). *Evaluation of poverty indicators.* (GAO/T-PEMD–88–1). Washington, DC: Government Printing Office.

Davies, A.R., & Ware, J.E. (1981). *Measuring health perceptions in the health insurance experiment.* (Pub. No. R–2711.) Santa Monica, CA: The RAND Corporation.

Dawson, D.A. (1988). AIDS knowledge and attitudes: August 1988. *NCHS Advancedata* No. 163. DHHS Pub. No. (PHS) 89–1250.

Dehn, T.G. (1988). PRO will soon mean "policing reduced options." *Medical Economics, 65,* 20–25.

DiChiro, G. (1985). Magnetic resonance imaging: A time for assessment. *Mayo Clinic Proceedings, 60*(2), 135–136.

Donabedian, A. (1966). Evaluating the quality of medical care. *Milbank Quarterly, 44,* 166–203.

Donabedian, A. (1980). *The definition of quality and approaches to its assessment. Volume I: Explorations in quality assessment and monitoring.* Ann Arbor, MI: Health Administration Press.

Donabedian, A. (1988). The quality of care. How can it be assessed? *Journal of the American Medical Association, 260*(12), 1743–1748

Drummond, M.F., Stoddard, G.L., & Torrance, G.T. (1987). *Methods for the economic evaluation of health care programs.* New York: Oxford University Press.

Drury, S.J. (1984). Employers say utilization reviews work. *Business Insurance, 18*(2), 3, 27.

Durland, E.N. (1987). Colorado's nursing home alternatives program: An evaluation designed to be used. *New England Journal of Human Science, 7*(1), 35–37.

ECRI. (1989). *1990 Health Care Standards Directory.* Plymouth Meeting, PA: ECRI.

Eddy, D.M., & Billings, J. (1988). The quality of medical evidence: Implications for quality of care. *Health Affairs, 7*(1), 19–32.

Elbeck, M. (1987). An approach to client satisfaction measurement as an attribute of health service quality. *Health Care Management Review, 12*(3), 47–52.

Escobar, W.A. (1985). An introduction to indicators. *World Hospitals, 21*(1), 32–34.

Esmond, T.H., & Batchelor, G. (1988). Setting quality standards in health care: Balancing purchaser, provider, and patient expectations. *Dimensions in Health Care, 88*(3), 1–5.

Fanshel, S., & Bush, J.W. (1970). A health status index and its application to health services outcomes. *Operations Research, 18*(6), 1021–1066.

Feeny, D. (1986). Clinical and economic evaluation of new health care technology. *Dimensions in Health Service, 63*(7), 25.

Feeny, D. (1987). The economic evaluation of health care technology. *Dimensions in Health Service, 64*(3), 41–42.

Feinholz, L.S. (1986). Using consumer evaluations of health care quality to identify marketing opportunities. *Health Marketing Quarterly, 3*(4), 73–81.

Feldstein, P.J., Wickizer, T.M., & Wheeler, J.R.C. (1988). Private cost containment. The effect of utilization review programs on health care use and expenditures. *New England Journal of Medicine, 318*(20), 1310–1314.

Fink, R. (1989). Issues and problems in measuring children's health status in community survey research. *Social Science in Medicine, 29*(6), 715–719.

Finkel, C. (1984). A checklist for evaluating a training facility. *Successful Meetings, 33*(6), 94.

Fleming, G.V., & Andersen, R.M. (1986). The Municipal Health Services Program. Improving access to primary care without increasing expenditures. *Medical Care, 24*(7), 565–577.

Fottler, M.D. (1987). Health care organizational performance: Present and future research. *Journal of Management, 13*(2), 385–386.

Frank, M.O. (1986). *How to get your message across in 30 seconds or less.* New York: Simon and Schuster.

Frerichs, R.R., & Tar, K.T. (1989). Computer-assisted rapid surveys in developing countries. *Public Health Reports, 104*(1), 14–23.

Gerace, T.M., & Sangster, J.F. (1987). Factors determining patient's satisfaction in a family practice residency teaching center. *Journal of Medical Education, 62*(6), 485–490.

Gilbert, J., Schoolfield, J., & Gaydou, D. (1987). Improved medical quality assurance in special care areas through computer management data collection. In *Symposium on computer applications in medical care.* Washington, DC: Computer Society Press.

Gonnella, J.S., & Zeleznik, C. (1974). Factors involved in comprehensive patient care evaluation. *Medical Care, 12*(11), 928–934.

Gonnella, J.S., & Louis, D.Z. (1988). Evaluation of ambulatory care. *Journal of Ambulatory Management, 11*(3), 68–83.

Guyatt, G.H., Drummond, M., & Feeny, D. (1986). Guidelines for the clinical and economic evaluation of health care technologies. *Social Science and Medicine, 22*(4), 393–408.

Guyatt, G.H. (1987). The clinical evaluation of health care technology. *Dimensions in Health Service, 64*(1), 42–44.

Hall, J., & Masters, D. (1986). Measuring outcomes of health services: a review of some available measures. *Community Health Studies, 10*(2), 147–155.

Hall, J., Hall, N., Fisher, E., & Killer, D. (1987). Measurement of outcomes of general practice: comparison of three health status measures. *Family Practice, 4*(2), 117–122.

Hash, M.M. (1986). Health planning and the CON: Changing directions. *Michigan Hospitals, 22*(7), 27–32.

Hays, R.D., & Ware, J. (1986). My medical care is better than yours. *Medical Care, 24*(6), 519–523.

Helper, C.D. (1988). Economic aspects of clinical decision making: Evaluative clinical programs. *American Journal of Hospital Pharmacy, 45*(3), 554–560.

Herzog, E. (1959). *Some guidelines for evaluative research.* (USDHEW Children's Bureau, Pub. No. 375–1959). Washington, DC: Government Printing Office.

Holder, E.L., & Frank, B. (1988). Residents speak out on what makes quality. *Provider, 14*(12), 28–29.

Howard, J.W., & Alidina, S. (1987). Multihospital systems increase costs. . . and quality. *Dimensions in Health Services, 64*(3), 20–24.

Hughes, C.M. (1988). The evaluation process for mobile MRI vendors. *Administrative Radiology, 7*(4), 36–38.

Hulka, B.S., Kupper, L.L., & Daly, M.B. (1975). Correlates of satisfaction and dissatisfaction with medical care: A community perspective. *Medical Care, 13*(8), 648–658.

Hunt, S.M., McKenna, S.P., & McEwen, J. (1981). The Nottingham health profile: Subjective health status and medical consultations. *Social Science and Medicine, 15A*(3,pt.1), 221–229.

Indrayan, A. (1987). Proxy measure of adequacy of health care in developing countries: Doctors vs. beds. *International Journal of Epidemiology, 16*(1), 137–138.

IOX Assessment Associates. (1988). *Program evaluation handbooks for health promotion and health education.* Culver City, CA.

Jencks, S.F., Daley, J., & Draper, D. (1988). Interpreting hospital mortality data. The role of clinical risk adjustment. *Journal of the American Medical Association, 260*(24), 3611–3616.

Jenster, P.V. (1987). Using critical success factors in planning. *Long Range Planning, 20*(4), 102–109.

Jette, A.M., Davies, A.R., & Cleary, P.D. (1986). The functional status questionnaire: Reliability and validity when used in primary care. *Journal of General Internal Medicine, 1*(3), 143–149.

Joint Commission for the Accreditation of Healthcare Organizations (JCAHO). (1987). The agenda for change. *Update, 1*(1), 1–2.

Juzwishin, D.W.M., & Boates, L.J. (1987). Writing effective program proposals. *Dimensions in Health Service, 64*(10), 58–59.

Kahn, K.L., Brook, R.H., & Draper, D. (1988). Interpreting hospital mortality data. How can we proceed? *Journal of the American Medical Association, 260*(24), 3625–3628.

Kaplan, R.M., Bush, J.W., & Berry, C.C. (1976). Health status: Types of validity and the index of well being. *Health Services Research, 11*(4), 478–507.

Kemper, P. (1988). The evaluation of the National Long Term Care Demonstration. Overview of the finding. *Health Services Research, 23*(1), 161–174.

Kessner, D.M., & Kalk, C.E. (1973). A strategy for evaluating health services. *Contrasts in health status* (Vol. 2). Washington, DC: Institute of Medicine.

Kessner, D.M., Kalk, C.E., & Singer, J. (1973). Assessing high quality—the case for tracers. *New England Journal of Medicine, 288*(4), 189–194.

Kinzer, D. (1988). The decline and fall of deregulation. *The New England Journal of Medicine, 318*(2), 112–116.

Koren, M.J. (1988). Quality assurance in New York State. Resident-centered protocols the basis. *Provider, 14*(12), 21–22.

Lake, D.C. (1973). *Measuring human behavior: Tools for the assessment of social functioning.* New York: Teachers College Press.

La Monica, E.L., Oberst, M.T., Madea, A.R., & Wolf, R.M. (1986). Development of a patient satisfaction scale. *Research in Nursing & Health, 9,* 43–50.

Larkin, H. (1988). Acute care is key to success in elder market. *Hospitals, 62*(10), 92.

Larson, J.S. (1986). A cross-national index of health care. *Journal of Health and Human Resources, 9*(2), 200–212.

Lembcke, P.A. (1956). Medical auditing by scientific methods illustrated by major female pelvic surgery. *Journal of the American Medical Association, 162*(7), 646–655.

Levey, S., & Loomba, N.P. (1973). *Health care administration. A managerial perspective.* Philadelphia, PA: J.B. Lippincott.

Liang, M.H., & Robb-Nicholson, C. (1987). Health status and utility measurement viewed from the right brain: experience from the rheumatic diseases. *Journal of Chronic Diseases, 40*(6), 579–583.

Lohr, K.N., Yordy, K.D., & Thier, S.D. (1988). Current issues in quality of care. *Health Affairs, 7*(1), 17.

Louis, D.Z., & Gonnella, J.S. (1986). Disease staging: Applications for utilization review and quality assurance. *Quality Assurance and Utility Review, 1*(1), 13–18.

Lyerly, S.B. (1973). *Handbook of psychiatric rating scales* (2nd ed.). Rockville, MD: National Institute of Health.

MacMillan, B.B. (1985). Good writing skills can advance your career. *Successful Meetings, 34*(5), 102–103.

Marcus, A.C., & Crane, L.A. (1986). Telephone surveys in public health research. *Medical Care, 24*(2), 97–112

Martin, P. (1986). *Measuring behavior: An introductory guide.* New York: Cambridge University Press.

McCoy, J.M., Dunn, E.V., & Borgiel, A.E. (1987). A portable computer system for auditing quality of ambulatory care. In *Symposium on computer applications in medical care.* Washington, DC: Computer Society Press.

McDowell, I., & Newell, C. (1987). *Measuring health. Guide to rating scales and questionnaires.* New York: Oxford University Press.

Mechanic, D. (1982). *Symptoms, illness behavior, and help-seeking.* New York: Prodist.

Meenan, R.F. (1986). New approaches to outcome assessment: the AIMS questionnaire for arthritis. *Advances in Internal Medicine, 31,* 167–185.

Meyer, H. (1988a). Outcome data won't be used in accreditation of hospitals. *American Medical News, 31*(44), 5–6.

Meyer, H. (1988b). Nursing home report flaws cast doubt on quality findings. *American Medical News, 31*(47), 37–38.

Miller, D.C. (1983). *Handbook of research design and social measurement: A text and reference book for the general and behavioral sciences* (4th ed.). New York: Longman Pub.

Milne, D. (1986). Planning and evaluating innovations in nursing practice by measuring the ward atmosphere. *Journal of Advanced Nursing, 11*(2), 203–210.

Moores, B., & Thompson, A.G.H. (1986). What 1357 hospital inpatients think about aspects of their stay in British acute hospitals. *Journal of Advanced Nursing, 11*, 87–102.

Mootz, M. (1986). Health indicators. *Social Science and Medicine, 22*(2), 255–263.

Moss, L. (1986, November 17). Beth Israel competes by pampering patients. *Crain's New York, 2*(52), 11.

Mowbray, C.T., & Herman, S.E. (1986). Evaluation approaches in mental health: implications of the new federalism. *Evaluation and Program Planning, 9*(4), 335–344.

Mueller, D.J. (1986). *Measuring social attitudes: A handbook for researchers and practitioners.* New York: Teachers College Press.

Neigher, W.D., & Schulberg, H.C. (1982). Evaluating the outcomes of human service programs: A reassessment. *Evaluation Review, 6*(6), 731–752.

Nelson, E.C., Wasson, J., & Kirk, J. (1987). Assessment of function in routine clinical practice: The COOP project. *Journal of Chronic Diseases, 40*(Suppl 1), 55S–63S.

Newacheck, P.W., & Halfon, N. (1986). Access to ambulatory care services for economically disadvantaged children. *Pediatrics, 78*(5), 813–818.

O'Donnell, J.W. (1987). The evolution of health planning in a competitive health care era. *The Journal For Hospital Admitting Management, 13*(2), 10–11.

O'Leary, D.S. (1988). Quality assessment. Moving from theory to practice. *Journal of the American Medical Association, 260*(12), 1760.

O'Toole, B.I., Battistutta, D., Long, A., & Crouch, K. (1986). A comparison of costs and data quality of three health survey methods: Mail, telephone and personal home interview. *American Journal of Epidemiology, 124*(2), 317–328.

Parkerson, G.R., Gehlbach, S.H., & Wagner, E.H. (1981). The Duke-UNC health profile: An adult health status instrument for primary care. *Medical Care, 19*(8), 806–828.

Patrick, D.L., Bush, J.W., & Chen, M.M. (1973). Toward an operational definition of health. *Journal of Health and Social Behavior, 14*(1), 6–23.

Patton, M.Q. (1982). *Practical evaluation.* Beverly Hills, CA: Sage.

Pierson, R.N. (1986). Will physician peer review succeed? *The Internist, 27*(6), 13–14.

Posavac, E.J., & Carey, R.G. (1985). *Program evaluation methods and case studies* (2nd ed.). Englewood Cliffs, NJ: Prentice-Hall.

Read, J.L., Quinn, R.J., & Hoefer, M.A. (1987). Measuring overall health: An evaluation of three important approaches. *Journal of Chronic Diseases, 40*(Suppl 1), 7S–21S.

Reeder, L.G., Ramacher, L., & Gorelnik, S. (1976). *Handbook of scales and indices of health behavior.* Pacific Palisades, CA: Goodyear Publishing Co. Inc.

Rhee, K.J., Donabedian, A., & Burney, R.E. (1987). Assessment of the quality of care in a hospital emergency unit: A framework and its application. *Quality Review Bulletin, 13*(1), 4–16.

Rhoads, G.G. (1986). Use of case-control studies for the evaluation of preventive health care. *Journal of Ambulatory Care Management, 9*(4), 53–64.

Riedel, D.C., Tischler, G.L. & Myers, J.K. (1974). *Patient care evaluation in mental health programs.* Cambridge, MA: Ballinger.

RightSoft, Inc. (1989). *RightWriter.* Sarasota, FL.

Rinke, L.T. (1988). *Outcome standards in home health: State of the art.* New York: National League for Nursing.

Roberts, J.S. (1987). Reviewing the quality of care: Priorities for improvement. *Health Care Financing Review* (Annual Supplement), pp. 69–74.

Roberts, J.S., & Tugwell, P. (1987). Comparison of questionnaires determining patient satisfaction with medical care. *Health Services Research, 22*(5), 637–654.

Roos, N.P., Roos, L.L., Mossey, J., & Havens, B. (1988). Using administrative data to predict important health outcomes. *Medical Care, 26*(3), 221–239.

Roper, W.L., & Hackbarth, G.M. (1988). HCFA's agenda for promoting high quality care. *Health Affairs, 7*(1), 91–98.

Rossi, P.H., Freeman, H.E., & Wright, S.R. (1979). *Evaluation. A systematic approach.* Beverly Hills, CA: Sage Publishers.

Russell, S., & Reynolds, J. (1985). *Operations research issues: Community financing.* Chevy Chase, MD: Primary Health Care Operations Research Center for Human Services.

Rutstein, D.D. (1981). Controlling the communicable and the man-made diseases [Editorial]. *New England Journal of Medicine, 304*(23), 1422–1424.

Rutstein, D.D., Mullan, R.J., & Frazier, T.M. (1983). Sentinel health events (occupational): A basis for physician recognition and public health surveillance. *American Journal of Public Health, 73*(9), 1054–1062.

Rutstein, D.D. (1984). The principle of the sentinel health event and its application to the occupational diseases. *Archives of Environmental Health, 39*(3), 158.

Schoenfeldt, R.C., Seale, W.B., & Hale, A.W. (1987). Survey alerts hospital to needs of consumers. *Health Progress, 68*(7), 61–66.

Schroeder, S.A. (1987). Outcome assessment 70 years later: Are we ready? *New England Journal of Medicine, 316*(3), 160–162.

Scrivens, E., Cunningham, D., Charlton, J., & Holland, W.W. (1985). Measuring the impact of health interventions: A review of available instruments. *Effective Health Care, 2*(6), 247–261.

Shaw, M.E., & Wright, J.M. (1967). *Scales for the measurement of attitudes.* New York: McGraw-Hill.

Sheps, S.B. (1988). Technological imperatives and paradoxes. *Journal of the American Medical Association, 259*(22), 3312.

Shortell, S.M., & Kaluzny, A.D. (1988). *Health care management: A text in organizational theory and behavior.* New York: John Wiley & Sons.

Simpson, K. (1985). Opinion surveys reveal patients' perceptions of care. *Dimensions, 62*(7), 30–31.

Solon, J.A. (1974). Measurement of health status. In R. Taffe & D. Zalkind (Eds.), *Evaluation of health services delivery.* New York: New York Engineering Foundation.

Speedling, E.J., & Rose, D.N. (1985). Building an effective doctor-patient relationship: From patient satisfaction to patient participation. *Social Science and Medicine, 21*(2), 115–120.

Spiegel A.D. (1960). *Reference guide for area board members.* Boston, MA: Massachusetts Department of Mental Health.

Spiegel, A.D., & Backhaut, B. (1980). *Curing and caring.* Jamaica, NY: Spectrum.

Stergachis, A. (1986). Use of a controlled trial to evaluate the impact of self-care on health services utilization. *Journal of Ambulatory Care Management, 9*(4), 16–22.

Stewart, A.L., Hays, R.D., & Ware, J.E., Jr. (1988). Communication. The MOS short-form general health survey. Reliability and validity in a patient population. *Medical Care, 26*(7), 724–735.

Stone, D.H. (1985). Suggested guidelines for monitoring health indices in the community. *Community Medicine, 7*(4), 295–298.

Successful Meetings. (1987). Checklist. Exhibiting: Budget and administration checklist. *36*(13), 124.

Successful Meetings. (1986). Improve direct-mail survey performance. *35*(1), 112–113

Suchman, E.A. (1967). *Evaluation research. Principles and practice in public service and social action programs.* New York: Russell Sage Foundation.

Summers, J. (1985). Take patient rights seriously to improve patient care and to lower costs. *Healthcare Management Review, 10*(4), 55–62.

Tennant, C. (1977). The general health questionnaire: A valid index of psychological impairment in Australian populations. *Medical Journal of Australia, 2*(12), 392–394.

USDHHS, Health Care Financing Administration. (1987). *Findings from the National Kidney Dialysis and Kidney Transplantation study.* (HCFA Pub. No. 03230). Washington, DC: Government Printing Office.

U.S. Medicine. (1988). Report examines measures for publicizing care quality. *23*(13&14), 41.

Vuori, H. (1987). Patient satisfaction—an attribute or indicator of the quality of care? *Quality Review Bulletin, 13*(3), 106–108.

Wagner, L. (1988). Evaluating the options. *Modern Healthcare, 18*(19), 56.

Waksberg, J. (1978). Sampling methods for random digit dialing. *Journal of American Statistical Association, 73*(361), 40–46.

Ward, M.J., & Lindeman, C.A. (Eds.). (1978). *Instruments for measuring nursing practice and other health care variables* (Vol. 1 & Vol. 2). (DHEW Pub. No. HRA 78–53). Washington, DC: Government Printing Office.

Ware, J.E., Jr., Sherbourne, C.A., & Davies, A.R. (1988). *A short-form general health survey.* (Pub. No. P-7444). Santa Monica, CA: The RAND Corporation.

Ware, J.E., Jr. (1987). Standards for validating health measures: definition and content. *Journal of Chronic Diseases, 40*(6), 473–480.

Ware, J.E., Davies, A.R., & Brook, R.H. (1980). *Conceptualization and measurement of health for adults in the health insurance study: Volume VI, analysis of relationships among health status measures.* (Pub. No. R-1987/6-HEW). Santa Monica, CA: The RAND Corporation.

Ware, J.E., Snyder, M.K., & Wright, W.R. (1976). *Development and validation of scales to measure patient satisfaction with health care services.* Carbondale, IL: University of Southern Illinois.

Wells, D.L., & Adolphus, P.D. (1987). Evaluating the care provided to long-stay patients. *Dimensions, 64*(10), 20–22.

Wholey, J.S., Scanlon, J.W., & Duffy, H.G. (1970). *Federal evaluation policy.* Washington, DC: The Urban Institute.

Wiatrowski, M.D., & Palkon, D.S. (1987). Performance appraisal systems in health care administration. *Health Care Management Review, 12*(1), 71–80.

Williams & Wilkins. (1989a). *Grammatik III.* Baltimore, MD.

Williams & Wilkins. (1989b). *Steadman's medical dictionary.* Baltimore, MD.

Williamson, J.W. (1971). Evaluating quality of patient care. A strategy relating outcome and process assessment. *Journal of the American Medical Association, 218*(4), 564–569.

Wilson, A.A. (1988). Measurable patient outcomes: Putting theory into practice. *Home Healthcare Nurse, 6*(6), 15–18.

Wilson, C. (1987). Assessing quality in the "soft services." *Dimensions in Health Care Services, 64*(5), 29–30.

Windle, C., & Neigher, W. (1978). Ethical problems in program evaluation: Advice for trapped evaluations. *Evaluation and Program Planning, 1*(2), 97–108.

Wood-Dauphinee, S., & Williams, J.I. (1987). Reintegration to normal living as a proxy to quality of life. *Journal of Chronic Diseases, 49*(6), 491–499.

Yusim, S., & Vallbona, C. (1986). Use of health-illness profile data base in health services research. *MEDINFO 86,* pp. 731–735.

Zweig, S., Kruse, J., & LeFevre, M. (1986). Patient satisfaction with obstetric care. *The Journal of Family Practice, 23*(2), 131–136.

Author Index

A

Aaron, H.J., 104, *153*
Abanobi, O.C., 37, 38, *99*
Abraham, L., 125, *153*
Abramowitz, S., 403, *414*
Abramson, J.H., 88, *99*
Adams, S., 212, *248*
Aday, L., 39, *99, 360, 414*
Adolphus, P.D., 376, 378, *421*
Agovino, T., 144, *153*
Akhter, M.N., 376, 379, *414*
Albrecht, K., 164, 165, 169, *199*
Alexander, J.A., 133, *153*
Alidina, S., 339, *417*
Altimont, T.J., 12, *25*
Ambry, R., 272, *316*
Andersen, R.M., 39, *99, 411, 412, 417*
Anderson, D., 404, *414*
Anderson, G.M., 55, *99*
Anderson, J.F., 387, *414*
Anderson, J.P., 55, *99*
Andren, K.G., 253, *316*
Aram, J.D., 128, *153*
Ashbaugh, J.W., 70, 71, *99*
Ashton-Tate, 96, *99*
Attinger, E.O., 143, *156*
Auth, J.B., 135, *157*

B

Backhaut, B., 401, *420*
Baine, D.P., 115, *153*
Banfield, E.C., 310, 314, *316, 319*
Banta, H.D., 206, 207, *248*
Barer, M.L., 124, 125, 126, *153, 156*
Barkholz, D., 134, *153*
Barlow, R., 302, *320*
Barnett, R., 134, 136, *155*

Barnum, H., 302, *320*, 370, *414*
Barrett, F.D., 162, *199*
Bass, R., 121, *157*
Bassett, L.C., 129, *153*, 255, *317*, 383, *414*
Batchelor, G., 324, 349, 352, *416*
Battistutta, D., 389, *419*
Beaves, R.G., *199*
Beech, R., 301, 302, *317*
Beeson, P.G., 135, *154*
Behrman, J.N., 261, 262, *317*
Belsky, M.S., 172, *199*
Benjamin, M., 104, 108, *154*
Bennett, A.C., 162, 163, 164, 168, 169, *199*
Bennett, J.P., 129, 131, *154*, 373, *414*
Bennett, K.J., 409, *414*
Bentzen, N., 97, *99*
Berdie, D.R., 387, *414*
Berenberg, W., 61, 62, 69, *101*
Bergner, M., 37, 59, 60, *99*, 391, *414*
Bergthold, L.A., 243, 244, *248*
Bergwall, D.F., 23, *25*
Bermar, A., 265, *317*
Bernard, B., 105, *154*
Berry, C.C., 391, 394, *418*
Berry, E., 403, *414*
Billings, J.S., *317*, 352, *416*
Birch, S., 187, *199*
Black, P.V., 94, *101*
Blades, C.A., 182, 183, 185, 191, 196, 197, *199*
Blair, J.D., 307, *317*
Bland, M., 88, *99*
Blank, R.H., 104, 108, *154*
Blau, T.H., 397, *415*
Blayney, K.D., 126, 127, *154*
Blevins, L., 95, *100*
Blischke, W.R., 55, *99*
Blum, H.L., 221, *248*

Boates, L.J., 412, *418*
Bobbit, R.A., 37, 59, 60, *99*, 391, *414*
Bodson, P., 118, 120, *157*
Bolley, H., 181, *199*
Bonoma, T.V., 252, 263, *317*
Bonstein, R.G., 88, 98, *100*
Boone, M.E., 94, *100*
Borgiel, A.E., 376, *418*
Boscarino, J.A., 259, *320*, 325, 330, *415*
Bowers, M.H., 254, *318*
Bowsher, C.A., 187, 188, 189, *199*
Bowskey, C.A., 138, 139, 141, *154*
Boyer, E.G., 210, *250*
Bradley, S., 125, *154*
Braithwaite, R.L., *317*
Brandt, E.N., Jr., 205, *248*
Breslow, L., 205, *248*, 397, *415*
Brewster, A.W., 181, *199*
Broadhead, W.E., 396, *415*
Broadwell, L., 301, *317*
Brook, R.H., 342, 349, 391, 395, *415*, *418*, *421*
Brooks, J., 121, *157*
Brough, R., 301, 302, *317*
Brown, M., 262, *317*
Brown, S.W., 259, *317*
Brownlee, A.T., 342, *415*
Brozovich, J., 5, *26*
Bruhn, J.G., 144, *154*
Budde, J.F., 343, *415*
Budrys, G., 3, *25*
Buehler, J.W., 93, *100*
Burnam, M.A., 397, 400, *415*
Burney, R.E., 372, *419*
Burns, J.A., 325, 326, *415*
Buros, O.K., 343, *415*
Burt, U.L., 92, *99*
Bush, J.W., 51, 55, *99*, 370, 391, 394, *415*, *416*, *418*, *419*
Buyer, L.S., *199*

C
Cabin, W., 196, *199*
Califano, J.A., 108, *154*
Callahan, C.B., *317*
Callahan, D., 108, *154*
Campbell, L., 274, *317*
Campbell, M.I., 263, *317*
Canter, K.G., 315, *317*
Caper, P., 352, *415*
Carey, R.G., 334, *419*
Carlyn, M., 210, *248*
Carmel, S., 402, *415*
Caro, J., 5, 6, *26*
Carr, W., 61, 62, 70, *99*, 234, 360, *415*
Carrell, S., 308, *317*
Carr-Hill, R.A., 332, 339, *415*
Carter, W.B., 37, 59, 60, *99*, 391, *414*
Cartwright, A., 387, *415*

Cartwright, T.J., 5, *25*, 414, *415*
Chalmers, T.C., 69, *101*, 380, *416*
Chambers, L.W., 37, 61, 62, *101*, 391, *415*
Champagne, F., 6, *25*
Charles, G., 62, *100*
Charlson, M.E., 59, 61, 86, 88, 89, *100*
Charlton, J., 334, 391, *420*
Charny, M.C., 185, 186, 197, 198, *199*
Chelimsky, E., 98, *99*, 279, 280, 281, *317*, 349, 350, 351, 360, 397, *415*
Chen, M.K., 39, 51, *99*, 370, 391, *415*
Chen, M.M., 370, 394, *415*, *419*
Cherskov, M., 204, *248*, 305, *317*
Cho, W.H., 229, *250*
Christiansen, T., 97, *99*
Chubon, R.A., 400, *415*
Chun, K., 343, *416*
Churchill, L.R., 104, 108, *154*
Clapp, N.E., *100*
Clark, H., 163, 165, *199*
Clark, L., 259, *317*
Clarke, R.M., 263, *317*, *319*
Cleary, P.D., 391, 400, *416*, *417*
Clemenhagen, C., 6, *25*
Coddington, D.C., 262, 269, *317*
Codman, E.A., 323, 348, *416*
Cohen, A.B., 121, *154*
Cohen, D.I., 404, *416*
Cohen, S.B., 92, *99*
Cole, J.R., 95, *99*
Coleman, B., 30, *99*
Collins, M.M., 269, 272, *317*
Conlin, D.W., 183, *199*
Conlin, J., 161, 172, *199*
Conner, D.R., 29, *99*, 128, *154*
Converse, P.D., 274, *317*
Cooper, L.S., 380, *416*
Cooper, P.D., 260, 269, 271, *317*
Cooper, T., 209, *248*
Corcoran, K., 343, *416*
Corman, H.E., 193, *200*
Cote, A.A., 403, *414*
Cowart, R., 10, *25*
Cox, P., 108, *154*
Crandall, L.A., 146, *156*
Crane, L.A., 388, 389, *418*
Cretin, L.G., 82, 83, 84, 85, *100*
Crittenden, V.L., 252, 263, *317*
Cross Dunham, N., 125, *155*
Crouch, K., 389, *419*
Crowell, A., 136, *154*
Cruickshank, P.J., 386, *416*
Crystal, R.A., 181, *199*
Culbertson, R.A., 127, *156*
Culyer, A.J., 182, 183, 185, 191, 196, 197, *199*
Cummings, S., 10, *25*
Cunningham, D., 334, 391, *420*

Cutter, G.R., 196, *201*
Cwikel, J., 105, *157*

D
Daley, J., 349, *416, 417*
Dalkey, N.C., 176, *199*
Daly, M.B., 402, *417*
Dans, P.E., 314, *318*
Datta, L., 358, *416*
Davies, A.R., 391, 394, 395, *415, 416, 417, 421*
Davies, R., 301, *318*
Davies, T., 301, *318*
Dawson, D.A., 280, *318*, 344, *416*
Day, D.L., 274, *318*
Deber, R.B., 210, *248*
de Bono, E., 162, *199*
DeCenzo, D.A., 254, *318*
DeGeus, A.P., 15, *25*
DeGruy, F.V., 396, *415*
Dehn, T.G., 376, *416*
DeHovitz, J.A., 12, *25*, 316, *318*
DeJean, D., 305, *318*
De La Rosa, M., 38, *99*
Delbanco, T., 309, *319*
Delbecq, A.L., 172, *199*, 207, 217, *248, 250*
DeSarbo, W.S., 274, *318*
Dever, G.E., 241, 243, *248*
Deyo, R.A., 59, 61, *99*
DiChiro, G., 380, *416*
DiGioia, D., 59, 61, 86, 88, 89, *100*
Digman, L.A., 3, 6, *27*
Dinkel, R.H., 184, 187, 188, *199*
Dobie, J., 104, *156*
Doleysh, N., 277, *321*
Donabedian, A., 345, 352, 372, 373, 400, *416, 419*
Donaldson, C., 187, *199*
Drake, J., 212, *248*
Draper, D., 349, *416, 417, 418*
Drew, E.B., 192, *199*
Drucker, P.F., 5, *25*, 126, *154*
Drummond, M.F., 181, 182, 197, *199*, 380, 406, *416, 417*
Drury, S.J., 16, *25, 416*
Duffy, H.G., *421*
Dufour, R.G., 74, *99*
Duggan, J.M., 104, *154*
Dumas, M.B., 4, *26*
Duncan, P., 146, *156*
Dunn, E.V., 376, *418*
Dunn, H.L., 276, *318*
Dunne, M., 192, *200*
Durland, E.N., 408, 409, *416*
Dyson, R.G., 6, *25*

E
Earley, R.C., 252, *318*
Earnhart, S.W., 254, *318*
Eberle, R., 168, *199*

Eddy, D.M., 352, *416*
Eichler, R.J., 207, *249*
Eisenberg, H., 259, 266, *318*
Elbeck, M., 384, 401, *416*
Elliot, L.B., 164, *199*
Emery, K.R., 253, 265, *318*
Erez, M., 252, *318*
Erickson, J.L., 259, *318*
Escobar, W.A., 352, *416*
Esmond, T.H., 324, 349, 352, *416*
Evashwick, C.J., 4, *25*
Evashwick, W.T., 4, *25*

F
Fackelmann, K.A., 191, *199*
Fahs, M.C., *200*
Fajardo, L., 302, *320*
Falkenburger, A.J., *154*
Fanshei, S., 391, *416*
Farber, N.J., 210, *250*
Farel, A.M., 103, *154*
Feeny, D., 380, 414, *416, 417*
Fein, R., 105, *154*
Feinholz, L.S., 325, *416*
Feldstein, P.J., 302, *318*, 407, *416*
Ferris, N.B., 7, *26*
Fifer, W.R., 11, *25*, 124, *154*
Files, L.A., 16, *25*
Fink, R., 391, *417*
Finkel, C., 382, *417*
Fisher, E., 394, *417*
Fleming, G.V., 411, 412, *417*
Fogel, R.L., 188, 190, 191, *199*, 211, *248*, 284, 291
Folmer, H.R., 116, *154*
Fontana, L., 241, *248*, 305, *318*
Ford, W.E., 135, *154*
Fors, M.F., 267, *318*
Foster, M.J., 6, *25*
Fottler, M.D., 121, *154*, 346, 347, *417*
Frank, B., 403, *417*
Frank, M.O., 412, *417*
Frazier, T.M., 361, 368, *420*
Freeman, H.E., 324, 325, *420*
Freitag, E.M., 260, 261, 275, *318*
Frerichs, R.R., 387, *417*
Freudenheim, M.H., *25*
Fuchs, M., 210, *248*
Fuchs, V.R., 104, 107, *154*, 181, *199*
Fulcher, J.H., 120, 121, *156*
Fyke, K.J., 256, *318*

G
Gallina, J.N., 121, *154*
Gallivan, M., 143, *154*
Garfunkel, J.M., 205, *249*
Gaydou, D., 352, *417*
Gehlbach, S.H., 36, 56, 58, *100*, 391, 396, *415, 419*
Gelberg, L., 208, *249*

Gerace, T.M., 404, *417*
Geschka, H., 174, *199*
Gesler, W., 117, *154*
Gianelli, D.M., 125, 126, *154*
Gibbons, D.L., 258, *318*
Gilbert, J., 352, *417*
Gildea, J., 196, *199, 200*
Gill, S.L., 207, *248*
Ginzberg, E., 1, *26*
Giordano, R., 95, *99*
Gold, B., *99*
Goldsmith, C.H., 37, *101*
Goldsmith, H.F., 237, *249*
Gonnella, J.S., 348, 352, *417, 418*
Goodall, R., 94, *99*
Goodes, M.R., 21, 23, *26*
Goodspeed, S.W., 254, *318*
Goplerud, E.N., 70, *99*
Gordon, W.J.J., 175, *200*
Gorelnik, S., 343, *419*
Gostin, L.O., 279, *318*
Gottlieb, S.R.V., 31, *99*
Grad, J.H., 98, *100*
Graham, R.G., 128, *154*
Grant, A.A., 229, 230, *250*
Grant, M.M., 70, 81, 82, *100*
Greenfield, S.S., 82, 83, 84, 85, *100*
Grenell, B., 260, *318*
Gross, J., 104, *155*
Gross, L., 172, *199*
Grossman, M., 193, *200*
Grumet, G.W., 108, *155*
Gummer, B., 252, *318*
Gunn, R.A., 128, *155*
Gustafson, D.H., *199*, 217, *248*
Guyatt, G.H., 380, *417*

H
Hackbarth, G.M., 352, *420*
Hagedorn, H., 308, *318*
Hagman, E., 208, *249*
Haig, T.H.B., 55, *100*
Hale, A.W., 326, 329, *420*
Haley, M., 273, *318*
Halfon, N., 360, *419*
Hall, J., 392, 393, 394, *417*
Hall, N., 394, *417*
Hammond, S.C., 254, *318*
Hancock, S.H., 163, *200*
Hancock, T., 211, *249*, 258, *318*
Hanlon, J.J., 224, *249*
Hannan, E.L., 134, 136, *155*
Harrell, G.D., 267, *318*
Harris, L., 104, *155*
Hash, M.M., 330, *417*
Havens, B., 353, 388, *419*
Hawley, C., 9, *26*, 29, 33, 34, *100*
Hays, R.D., 391, 394, 395, 401, *417, 420*

Heineken, P.A., 61, *100*
Heisler, T., 360, *415*
Helper, C.D., 406, *417*
Henderson, J., 118, 119, *156*, 211, *249*
Henry, K., 206, *249*
Hensel, P.J., 274, *319*
Herman, S.E., 332, *419*
Hernandez, S.R., 121, *154*
Herzlinger, R.E., 31, *100*
Herzog, E., 330, *417*
Hiatt, H.H., 104, 108, *155*
Hickman, C.R., 165, *200*
Hicks, R.S., 210, *248*
Higgins, C.W., 184, 185, 192, *200*
Hinton, C.L., 253, *318*
Hisrich, R.D., 259, 269, 271, *317*
Hoefer, M.A., 394, *419*
Holden, J.M., 266, 274, *318*
Holder, E.L., 403, *417*
Holland, W.W., *420*
Holloman, J.L.S., Jr., 206, *249*
Hoque, C.J.R., 93, *100*
Horgan, C.M., 274, *318*
Howard, J.W., 339, *417*
Howe, A.L., 151, 153, *155*
Hsueh, W.A., 208, *249*
Hudak, J., 7, *26*
Hughes, C.M., 381, *417*
Hulka, B.S., 402, *417*
Hunt, S.M., 391, *417*
Hyman, H.H., 7, 20, *26*, 148, 152, 288

I
Iglehart, J.K., 124, *155*
Indrayan, A., 353, *417*
Ingram, J.J., 72, *100*
Ingram, T.N., 274, *319*
Inui, T.S., 59, 60, *99*
Ireys, H.T., 207, *249*
Isaacs, J., 212, *248*
Isaacs, M.R., 135, 137, *155*

J
Jackson, B., 208, *249*
Jacobs, H.M., 7, 8, *26*
Jacobson, E.A., *154*
Jaffe, E., 256, *319*
Jager, J.C., 89, *100*
James, J., 300, *319*
James, S.A., *100*
Jemison, T., 115, *155*
Jencks, S.F., 349, *416, 417*
Jennett, B., 107, *155*
Jensen, J., 208, *249*
Jenster, P.V., 333, 375, *417*
Jette, A.M., 391, *417*
Johnson, R.L., 308, *319*

Joiner, C.L., 121, *154*
Jones, K.M., 259, *317*
Jones, L., 104, *155*
Jones, R.B., 194, 195, *200*
Jones, W., 258, *319*
Joseph, A.E., 118, 120, *157*
Joseph, H., 181, *199*
Joyce, T., 193, *200*
Juzwishin, D.W.M., 412, *418*

K
Kahn, A.A., 117, *155*
Kahn, H.A., 88, *100*
Kahn, K.L., 349, *418*
Kalk, C.E., 348, 372, *418*
Kaluzny, A.D., 129, *157*, 307, 316, *320*, 345, 346, 356, *420*
Kannel, W.B., 253, *319*
Kaplan, B.H., 396, *415*
Kaplan, R.M., 55, *99*, 394, *418*
Katz, M., 204, *249*
Kaufman, J.L., 7, 8, *26*
Kavaler, F., 14, *26*
Kazemek, E.A., 128, *155*
Keckley, P.H., 269, *319*
Keil, A., 96, *100*
Kelley, K., 59, 61, 86, 88, 89, *100*
Kelliner, M.E., 128, *155*
Kemper, P., 410, *418*
Kennedy, L., 4, *26*
Kessner, D.M., 348, 372, *418*
Killer, D., 394, *417*
Kindig, D.A., 125, *155*
Kinnis, C., 126, *153*
Kinzer, D., 330, *418*
Kirk, J., 376, 395, *419*
Kirkpatrick, C.A., 294, *319*
Kitzhaber, J., 108, *155*
Klafehn, K.A., 116, *155*
Klarman, H.E., 181, *200*
Klegon, D.A., 273, 274, *319*
Klein, D.A., 146, *156*
Kletke, P.R., 241, 242, *249*
Klett, S., 309, *319*
Klimek-Grzesiak, I., 282, *319*
Knauf, J.W., 128, *153*
Koek, K.E., 132, *155*
Korda, H., 309, *319*
Koren, M.J., 379, *418*
Korpman, R.A., 95, *100*
Kosterlitz, J., 206, *249*
Kotler, P., 259, 263, *319*
Kramer, P.S., 257, *320*
Kramon, G., 30, *100*
Krasner, M.I., 360, *415*
Kriegel, M.H., 164, *200*
Kriegel, R., 164, *200*
Kruse, J., 404, *421*

Kupper, L.L., 402, *417*
Kushner, J.W., 95, *100*

L
Labelle, R., 143, *155*
Lake, D.C., 343, *418*
Lamm, R.D., 2, *26*, 107, *155*
LaMonica, E.L., 405, *418*
Landsverk, J., 397, 400, *415*
Lane, D., 76, 77, 78, *100*
Langstaff, J.H., 121, 122, 123, *155*
Lapin, L.L., 75, *100*
Lar, R., 275, *319*
Larkin, H., 106, *155*, 330, *418*
Larson, E.B., 106, *157*
Larson, J.S., 370, *418*
Leake, B., 397, 400, *415*
LeBailly, S.A., 241, 242, *249*
LeFevre, M., 404, *421*
Leiken, A.M., 129, *155*
Lembcke, P.A., 373, *418*
Lemon, R.B., 94, *100*
LeTouze, D., 72, *100*
Levey, S., 8, 15, *26*, 331, *418*
Levin, R.I., 294, *319*
Levkoff, S.E., 105, *157*
Lewis, F., 92, *100*
Lewton, K.L., 305, *319*
Liang, M.H., 397, *418*
Lincoln, T.L., 95, *100*
Lindblom, C.D., 15, *26*
Lindeman, C.A., 343, *421*
Linn, L.S., 208, *249*
Linton, R., 176, 177, *200*
Liss, A., 117, *155*
Liu, K., 128, *156*
Lloyd-Jones, J., 5, 6, *26*, 163, 185, *200*
Loe, H., 258, 308, *319*
Lohr, K.N., 342, 352, *415*, *418*
Lomas, J., 124, 125, *156*
Long, A., 389, *419*
Loomba, N.P., 331, *418*
Lord, K.S., 204, *249*
Louis, D.Z., 348, 352, *417*, *418*
Lowman, C., 232, 239, 240, 243, 245, 246, *250*
Lund, D.S., 106, 107, *156*
Lutz, S., 264, *319*
Lyerly, S.B., 343, *418*
Lythcott, N., 308, *317*

M
Mackensie, C.R., 59, 61, 86, 88, 89, *100*
MacMillan, B.B., 412, 414, *418*
MacPherson, A.S., 37, *101*
MacStravic, R.S., 103, *156*, 266, 267, *319*
Madan, T.N., 241, *249*, 308, *319*
Madea, A.R., 405, *418*
Mager, R.F., 24, *26*

Mahaffey, M., 209, *249*, 305, *319*
Malin, H., 232, 239, 240, 243, 245, 246, *250*
Manassero, B., 260, *319*
Manassuzin, H., 125, *155*
Mandelblatt, J.S., 200
Manderscheid, R.W., 70, 71, *99*
Manoukian, L.M., 95, *101*
Marcus, A.C., 388, 389, *418*
Martin, P., 343, *418*
Mason, G.O., 204, *249*
Masters, D., 392, 393, *417*
McCally, M., 380, *416*
McCann, P., 212, *248*
McCauley, R.G., 37, *101*
McConnell, C.R., 255, 256, *319*
McCool, B.P., 262, *317*
McCormick, B., 125, *156*
McCoy, J.M., 376, *418*
McDevitt, P., 4, *26*
McDonald, C.J., 95, *100*
McDonald, L.A., *415*
McDowell, I., 343, *418*
McEwen, J., 391, *417*
McGee, D.L., 253, *319*
McGinty, R.T., 300, *319*
McGregor, M., 106, *156*
McIlrath, S., 275, *319*
McKenna, S.P., 391, *417*
McNeil, B.J., 400, *416*
McTernan, E.J., 129, *155*
Mechanic, D., 357, *418*
Meehan, R.H., 164, *200*
Meenan, R.F., 387, *418*
Meiners, M.R., 128, *156*
Melville, K., 104, *156*
Metzer, N., 255, *317*
Metzger, N., 129, *153*, 383, *414*
Meyer, H., 348, 354, 356, *418*
Meyer, N.D., 94, *100*
Meyerson, M., 314, *319*
Mick, S.S., 2, *26*
Millar, J.D., 205, *249*
Miller, A.R., 309, *319*
Miller, D.C., 343, *419*
Milne, D., 386, *419*
Moller, T., 117, *155*
Monetti, C.H., 34, *101*
Moore, K.D., 262, 269, *317*
Moore, W.B., 208, *249*
Moore-Pastides, P.J., 270, *320*
Moores, B., 404, *419*
Mootz, M., 354, 357, 369, *419*
Morone, J.A., 307, *320*
Morrisey, M.A., 133, *153*
Morrow, R.C., 232, *249*
Moscovice, I., 121, *157*
Moss, L., 403, *419*

Mossey, J., 353, 388, *419*
Mowbray, C.T., 332, *419*
Mowll, C.A., 255, *320*
Mueller, D.J., 343, *419*
Mueller, K.J., 2, *26*
Muhlbaier, L.H., *100*
Mullan, R.J., 361, 368, *420*
Mullen, K.D., 275, *320*
Myers, J.K., 382, *419*
Myers, M.L., 205, *249*

N
Nardone, D.A., 106, *156*
Nauert, R.C., 262, *320*
Neigher, W.D., 324, *419*, *421*
Nelson, E.C., 376, 395, *419*
Nelson, S.H., 207, *249*
Nettleman, M.D., 194, 195, *200*
Neuman, B.S., 88, 94, 98, *100*, 128, *154*
Neustadt, R.E., 251, *320*
Newacheck, P.W., 360, *419*
Newell, C., 343, *418*
Newman, J.A., 29, *99*
Niebuhr, M.A., 387, *414*
Nolan, R.L., 98, *100*
Norton, D.P., 94, 98, *100*
Nutt, P.C., 252, *320*

O
Oberst, M.T., 405, *418*
O'Brien, K., 257, *320*
O'Donnell, J.W., 330, *419*
Ojala, M., 94, *100*
Olchanski, V., 95, *101*
O'Leary, D.S., 352, *419*
Olson, S., 144, *156*
Oreglia, A., 146, *156*
Orsay, E.M., 192, *200*
Osborn, A.F., 159, 161, 166, 167, *200*
O'Toole, B.I., 389, *419*
Owens, D.L., 116, *155*

P
Padilla, G.V., 79, 81, 82, *100*
Page, L., 125, 126, *156*
Palkon, D.S., 385, *421*
Panerai, R.B., 143, *156*
Parkerson, G.R., Jr., 36, 56, 58, *100*, 391, *419*
Parkin, D., 118, 119, *156*
Parry, S., 309, *320*
Pastides, H., 270, *320*
Patel, M., 203, *249*
Patrick, D.L., 51, *99*, 370, 394, *415*, *419*
Patton, M.O., 323, *419*
Pearson, A.E., 162, *200*
Pearson, C., 92, *101*
Peasant, C., 81, 82

Pederson, K.M., 97, *99*
Pellegrino, V., 316, *318*
Perloff, J.D., 241, 242, *249*
Perrone, J., 104, 107, *156*
Peterkin, K., 94, *101*
Peters, J., 4, *26*
Petrovski, A.M., 95, *101*
Philips, B.U., 144, *154*
Phillips, C., 151, 153, *155*
Pickett, G.E., 224, *249*
Pierson, R.N., 342, *419*
Pillemer, K., 39, *101*
Pinchot, G., III, 163, *200*
Pinkney, D.S., 14, *26*
Plough, A., 309, *319*
Poizner, S.L., 117, *156*
Pollard, W.E., 391, *414*
Pomrinse, S.D., 3, *26*
Popowniak, M.F., 309, *319*
Porter, M., 266, *320*
Posavac, E.J., 334, *419*
Powills, S., 267, *320*
Pradilla, A., *320*
Preston, G., 151, 153, *155*
Pushka, P., 255, *321*

Q
Quinn, J.B., 164, 165, *200*
Quinn, R.J., 394, *419*

R
Rada, R.T., 210, *249*
Rall, D.P., 205, *249*
Ramacher, L., 343, *419*
Rash, R.M., 302, *320*
Raudsepp, E., 159, 160, 165, *200*
Read, J.L., 394, *419*
Reeder, L.G., 343, *419*
Reeves, P.H., 23, 24, *25*
Rehnstrom, T., 208, *249*
Reid, R.A., 120, 121, *156*
Reinhardt, U.E., 105, *156*
Relman, A.S., 16, *26*, 262, *320*
Renz, L., 144, *156*
Reynolds, J., 332, *420*
Rhee, K.J., 372, *419*
Rhoads, G.G., 339, 340, *419*
Ricardo, M., 259, *320*
Riedel, D.C., 382, *419*
Ries, D.A., 206, *249*
Rifkin, S.B., 103, *156*
Rinke, L.T., 349, *419*
Robb-Nicholson, C., 397, *418*
Roberts, C.J., 185, 186, 197, 198, *199*
Roberts, J.S., 254, 255, 402, *419*
Roddy, P.C., 128, *156*
Rodwin, V.G., 258, *320*

Roemer, D., 257, *320*
Rohrer, J.E., 8, 15, *26*, 181, *199*
Roos, L.L., 353, 388, *419*
Roos, N.P., 353, 388, *419*
Roper, W.L., 352, *420*
Rose, D.N., 360, *420*
Rosen, B.M., 237, *249*, *250*
Rosenqvist, U., 253, *316*
Rossi, P.H., 324, *420*
Roswell, R.H., 109, *156*
Rouse, R.L., 134, 136, *155*
Ruitenberg, E.J., 89, *100*
Rusnak, J.E., 94, *101*
Russell, S., 332, *420*
Rutstein, D.D., 61, 62, 69, *101*, 361, 368, *420*

S
Sackett, D.L., 37, *101*
Salipante, P.F., Jr., 128, *153*
Salmon, M.E., 127, *156*
Saltman, R.B., 309, *320*
Sandblad, B., 117, *155*
Sangster, J.F., 404, *417*
Sarll, D.W., 229, 230, *250*
Satin, M.S., 34, *101*
Savage, G.T., 307, *317*
Sayles, L.R., 171, *200*
Scanlon, J.W., *421*
Schillaci, C.E., 262, *320*
Schlicksupp, H., 174, *199*
Schoenfeld, G., 172, *200*
Schoenfeldt, R.C., 326, 329, *420*
Schoolfield, J., 352, *417*
Schroeder, S.A., 17, *26*, 348, *420*
Schulberg, H.C., 324, *419*
Schwartz, G., 274, *320*
Schwartz, W.B., 104, *153*
Schwaude, G.R., 174, *199*
Scott, D.A., 55, *100*
Scotti, D.J., 32, 35, *101*
Scrivens, E., 334, 352, 391, *420*
Seale, W.B., 326, 329, *420*
Seay, J.D., 257, *320*
Seiden, D., 107, *156*
Sempos, C.T., 88, *100*
Shaw, M.E., 301, 302, *317*, 343, *420*
Sheps, S.B., 381, *420*
Sherbourne, C.A., 394, *421*
Shortell, S.M., 129, *157*, 307, 316, *320*, 345, 346, 356, *420*
Showstack, J.A., 17, *26*
Shyavitz, L., 263, *317*
Siktberg, L., 305, *320*
Silva, 165, *200*
Simpson, K., 405, *420*
Simyar, F., 5, 6, *26*, 163, 185, *200*
Singer, J., 348, 372, *418*

Sisk, J.E., 191, 197, *200*
Sleet, D.A., 207, 243, *250*
Slubowski, M.A., 273, 274, *319*
Smeeding, T.M., 104, 108, *157*
Smith, D.P., 4, *26*
Smith, H.L., 120, 121, *156*
Smith, J.C., 93, *100*
Snow, B., 94, *101*
Snyder, M.K., 402, *421*
Solon, J.A., 369, *420*
Sorkin, D.L., 7, *26*
Speedling, E.J., 360, *420*
Spiegel, A.D., 7, 12, 14, 20, *26*, 148, 152, 196, *200*, 288, 375, 401, *420*
Stakowski, M., 282, *319*
Stark, A.L., 76, 77, 78, *100*, 126, *153*
Starkweather, D.B., 305, *320*
Steiber, S., 259, *320*
Stergachis, A., 408, *420*
Stewart, A.L., 391, 394, 395, *420*
Stewart, J.M., 275, 276, *320*
Stimson, D.H., 62, *100*
Stivers, C., 314, 315, *320*
Stoddard, G.L., 124, 125, *156*, 406, *416*
Stoline, A., 3, *26*
Stone, D.H., 332, 370, *420*
Strauss, L.T., 93, *100*
Stroot, P., 204, *250*
Studin, I., 260, *318*
Suchman, E.A., 324, 335, *420*
Sullivan, L.W., 206, *250*
Summers, J., 401, *420*
Super, K.E., 264, 267, *320, 321*
Szapiro, N., 360, *415*

T
Tabatabai, C., *157*
Talbott, J.A., 207, *250*
Tar, K.T., 387, *417*
Tarlov, A.R., 122, *157*
Taylor, J.W., 164, 165, 167, 171, *200*
Tennant, C., *420*
Terence, O.A., 274, *318*
Thier, S.D., 352, *418*
Thompson, A.G.H., 404, *419*
Thompson, J.D., 2, *26*
Thompson, L.H., 153, *157*
Thouez, J.M., 118, 120, *157*
Tibbitts, S.J., 162, 163, 164, 168, 169, *199*
Tierney, W.M., 94, *100*
Timmel, N., 5, *26*
Tischler, G.L., 382, *419*
Tolchin, M., 11, *26*, 125, *157*
Tomich, N., 140, 142, *157*
Toole, J.E., 94, *100*
Torrance, G.T., 406, *416*
Triolo, P.K., 259, 265, 266, *321*
Trivedi, V., 121, *157*

Trochim, W.M.K., 176, 177, *200*
Tugwell, P., 402, 409, *414, 415, 419*
Tuomilehto, J., 255, *321*
Turnbull, T.L., 192, *200*

U
Unger, E.L., 237, *249*
Uppal, P., 134, 136, *155*
Uyeno, D., 76, 77, 78, *100*

V
Vallbona, C., 390, *421*
Van de Ven, A.H., 172, *199*, 217, *248, 250*
VanGundy, A.B., 166, 168, *200*
Van Pelt, G., 264, *321*
Vladeck, B.C., 257, *320*
Voelker, R., 12, *27*
Vogel, G., 277, *321*
Von Fange, E.K., 171, 174, *200*
Vuori, H., 401, 402, *420*

W
Wager, R.J., 265, 266, 268, *321*
Wagner, E.H., 36, 56, 58, *100*, 391, *419*
Wagner, L., 411, *421*
Wagstaff, A., 31, *101*, 241, *250*
Waksberg, J., 389, *421*
Waldrop, H., 96, *101*
Waldrop, J.W., 272, *321*
Walker, A., 182, 183, 185, 191, 196, 197, *199*
Wall, L.L., 253, *317*
Walling, M.F., 96, *101*
Walt, G., 103, *156*
Ward, M.J., 343, *421*
Ware, J.E., Jr., 333, 391, 394, 395, 401, 402, *415, 416, 417, 420, 421*
Warheit, G.J., 135, *157*
Warner, K.E., 196, *201*
Wasson, J., 376, 395, *419*
Weaver, R.L., 164, *201*
Weiner, J.L., 210, *250*
Weiner, J.P., 3, *26*
Welch, H.G., 106, *157*
Wells, D.L., 376, 378, *421*
Wells, K.B., 397, 400, *415*
Wetle, T., 105, *157*
Wheeler, J.R.C., 407, *416*
White, E.C., 265, *321*
Whitehead, C.J., 307, *317*
Whiting, C.S., 174, *201*
Whitman, J.J., 6, 7, 9, *27*
Whittle, J.W., 229, 230, *250*
Wholey, J.S., *421*
Wiatrowski, M.D., 385, *421*
Wickett, L.I., 55, *100*
Wickizer, T.M., 407, *416*
Wilensky, G.R., 104, 106, *157*
Willbern, J.A., 96, *101*

Williams, A., 203, *250*
Williams, J.I., 371, 372, *421*
Williamson, J.W., 348, *421*
Wilson, A.A., 349, *421*
Wilson, C., 348, *421*
Wilson, R., 232, 239, 240, 243, 245, 246, *250*
Windle, C., 324, *421*
Windom, R.E., 205, *250*
Windsor, R.A., 196, *201*
Winter, F.W., 274, *321*
Wolf, R.M., 405, *418*
Wong, J.K., 259, *317*
Wood-Dauphinee, S., 371, 372, *421*
Woodside, N.B., 23, 24, *25*
Worthington, H.V., 229, 230, *250*
Worthman, L.G., 82, 83, 84, 85, *100*
Wright, J.M., *420*
Wright, S.R., 324, 325, 343, *420*
Wright, W.R., 402, *421*

Y
Yang, J.M., 229, *250*
Yasnoff, W.A., 96, *101*
Yoo, S., 3, 6, *27*
Yordy, K.D., 353, *418*
Young, A., 38, *101*
Yu, S.M., 229, *250*
Yuki, G., 253, *321*
Yusim, S., 390, *421*

Z
Zeckhauser, R., 181, *199*
Zeitler, R.R., 181, *199*
Zeleznik, C., 348, *417*
Zimmerman, M., 191, 192, *201*
Zoghlin, G.G., 248, *250*
Zones, J.S., 17, *26*
Zweig, S., 404, *421*
Zylke, J.W., 38, *101*, 206, *250*

Subject Index

A

AARP, 14
Access to services, 362
Access, to primary care, 411–412
Accreditation, 3, 354
Accuracy (of management techniques), 36–37
Acute care (RAM model), 110
Affiliation arrangements (hospital), 120
Aged, 30, 106, 411; *see also* Elderly
AIDS, 12, 89, 92, 206, 279–281
Alcohol mortality, 239–240
Allocation of research planning, 109, 142
Alphabetical evaluation, 370
Alternative care settings, 11
Alternatives, 159
   creativity, 159
   examining, 180
   generating, 161, 166
   ground rules, 161
Alternatives to Long-Term Nursing Home Care Act, 408
Ambulatory Care
   JCAHO indicators, 354, 360
   marketing, 273–274
   model, 110
   outcome based, 350
   quality of care, 376
   surgery, 254–255
American Hospital Association, 3
American Medical Association, 266
Ancillary personnel, 104
Appropriate data analysis techniques, 41–42
Appropriate disposition, 84
"Approver", 297, 300
Arthritis measurement, 387

Attitude measurement, 344
Availability of care, 8, 14
Average costs, 183
Averted costs, 183

B

Bargaining, competitive vs. cooperative, 307–308
B.E.D., 353, 354
Bed needs, 34, 125, 135, 136
   formula approach to, 135–136
   market health, 136
Behavior change, *see* Change
Behaviorally anchored rating scales (BARS), 384–386
Board of Executives, 207, 262
Board of Trustees, 207, 262
Boundary crossing research, 342
Brainstorming, 166–167
British rationing, 107
Business
   health care costs and, 31, 32
   HMO and, 31, 32
Business groups
   costs and, 31
   on health, 9
   HMO and, 31, 32

C

California Community Mental Health Program Model, 136
Canadian system, 1
Cancer
   breast, 272
   cervical, 196
   trachea, bronchus, and lung, 246–247

Capital and hospital failure, 3
  resources, 134, 135
Cardiovascular product line, 265
Cartographic analysis, 117
Case mix management, 94
Catastrophic medical plan, 14, 30
Categorical Scale, 384
Categories of evaluation
  words used in, 335, 336
Census, 89
Centers for Disease Control (CDC), 12
Centrographic analysis, 117
Certificate of Need [CON], 134, 330
  regulation and, 330
Cervical cancer, see Cancer
Change
  barriers to, 255–258
  behavior, 255
  character of, 255
  in hospital environment in '80s, 2–3
  implementing, 255
Channeling, 410
Charting, 169–171
Checklists
  for business, 382
  for evaluation, 374, 413
  for mental retardation planning, 374–375
  for questions, 167–168
Chest pain and criteria mapping, 84
Chief Executive Officer [CEO], 122, 262
  priorities of, 208
Chief Financial Officer [CFO], 262
Child mortality simulation, 302
Citizen committees, 96–97
Civilian Health and Medical Program of the Uniformed
    Services (CHAMPUS), 142
Clinical Trials, 381–382
Cluster method prioritizing, 233–235
Colostomy and quality of life index, see Quality of life
    index
Community assessment, 34–36
  components of, 32
  and criteria mapping, 84–85
Community care, 411–412
Community involvement in planning, 308
Community and marketing assessment, see Community
    assessment
Community survey, 42–45
Comparison scale, 385
Competition, 10
  professional, 11
Composite Health Care system, 187
Comprehensive health planning, 7–9, 15
  disjointed incrementalism and, 15–16
  See also Strategic planning
Computer-assisted telephone interview (CATI), 389–390

Computers
  allocation of technology and, 143
  auditing outcomes (SPO/cr) and, 352
  auditing quality of care, 376
  creativity (innovator) and, 176–180
  data and, 94–96
  decision making (GamePlan) and, 303–305
  doctors who use, 386–387
  ER CEA and, 196
  gaming, 302–305
  implementation and, 289
  LANS, 10
  management decisions and, 94
  mapping, 117–118
  planning software and, 43, 95–96
  priority graphic mapping and, 243–247
  project management and, 289
  simulation, 116–117
  smart card, 265
  software, 95–96, 289
  strategic planning and, 95–96, 302–303
  telephone interview, 389
  visual graphics and, 95–96
Concepts of health, 37–38
Conceptualization, 176
Concurrer, 297
Congress, 14, 30
Consumers, 307
  involvement in health planning, 17
  priorities, 208
  self-care, 11
Content validity, of health concepts, 37–38
Continuity of care, 336
Contributor, 297
Cooperative bargaining, 307
Coronary care, criteria mapping for chest pains, 82–86
Corporate market planning, 4, 261
Cost (measurement technique)
  average, 183
  averted, 183
  containment, 3, 14
  discounting, 183
  incremental, 183
  marginal, 183
  measurement terminology, 182–183
  opportunity, 183
  projections, see GAO
Cost-Benefit Analysis (CBA), 181–183, 183–191
  examples of, 185–188
  GAO application of, 189–190
  limitations, 184
  purposes, 184
  steps in, 185
Cost—standard cost of activities, 129–130
Cost-effectiveness analysis (CEA), 181–183, 191–196
  examples, 192–196

limitations, 191
steps in, 192
Cost-utility analysis, 181–183, 196–197
Creativity, 159–160, 163
  barriers to, 164–165
  behavior, 163–164
  conformity and, 162–163
  elements of, 163–164
  exercises, 160, 198
  guidelines, 159, 161
  lateral thinking, 162
  techniques, 166–171
  vertical thinking, 162
Crisis models, 316
Criteria definition, 82
  for audits, 376
  calculations, 84
  checklists and, 374–375
  for chest pains, 82–86
  for corporate success, 370–371
  decision, 212
  elements common to, 373
  key factors, 84
  long-term care in, 376–377
  mapping, 82–86
  for priority determination, 210–211
  retardation and, 374–375
  technical assessment and, 143
  weighting method, 221–224
Critical success factors, 375
Cross national index comparisons, 370–
  371

D
Data
  census data, 89
  collection of, 16, 146–147
  considerations and, 96–98
  demographics, 45–47, 266
  epidemiology and, 88
  for indicators, 354–356
  indicators for administration, 353
  interpretation of, 88
  obstacles and, 98
  research studies and, 97
  sources of, 88–93, 96
  statistics and, 88, 94, 98–99
Databases, 16, 94
Death as evaluation measurement, 335
Decision criteria, 212
Decision elements, 211
Decision making in rationing, 104–106
  by external factors, 31–32
  values and, 197
Delphi technique, 41
  alternative generating, 176

Demand
  assessment methods, 72–88
  criteria mapping, 82
  formula approach, 72–74
  Functional Status Index, 86–88
  Markov chain, 75–78
  quality of life index, 79–82
  Stochastic method, 74–75
    defined, 38
    need and, 38
Demographics, see Data
Demographic analysis, 45–47
Diabetes, 272–273
Diagnosis Related Groups [DRG], 2, 104, 106, 120
Diagnosis Related Groups + Peer Review Organization
  [PRO] + cost containment, 14
Directories, 132–133, 144
Disability as evaluation instrument, 335
Discomfort as evaluation instrument, 335
Discounting, see Cost
Disease as evaluation instrument, 335
  vs. sickness, 357
Dissatisfaction as evaluation instrument, 335
DOC, 353–354
Drug Abuse Prevention Program, 115–116
Duke-UNC Health Profile, 56, 391–392
Duke UNC Functional Social Scale, 396–397

E
Education modification component [RAM], 111
Effectiveness analysis, see Cost effectiveness
Effort, Effect, Efficiency, 335
Elderly and rationing, 105–106
Emergency care
  computer simulation of, 116–117
  coronary care and, 82–84
  cost-effectiveness analysis, 196
  criteria mapping and, 82–84
Emergency Room simulation, see Emergency care
Employees, see also Personnel, Staff
  performance indicators, 128
Endstage renal disease (ESRD), 359, 370
Environmental assessment, 29, 32, 33
Environmental dynamics, 29–30
Equipment and supplies, 103, 143
  hi-tech issues, 143
  hi-tech trends, 144
  routine supplies, 144
Evaluation
  of attitudes, 344
  of behavior, 344
  checklist, 374
  cycle, 414
  defined, 324
  designs, 337–340
  of family practice care, 404

of knowledge, 344
of managed health care plan, 325–326
marketing and, 325, 330
measurements and, 333–334, 343
methods, 343
monitoring and, 332–333
of personnel, 384
problems in, 340–341
procedures in, 330–332
of programs, 405–406
reliability and, 341
reports, 412–414
research and, 406
statistics applied to, 336–337
survey techniques, 387–400
terminology, 335–336
validity and, 341
Evolution of health planning from early 1900, 3
Exhibits (business), 382
Experimental designs, 338–340
    pre-experimental, 338
    true experimental, 338–339
    quasi-experimental, 339–340
Expert interviews, 96
Explain the difficulty, 171
External environment assessment, 9

F
Facilities, 103, 132–133
Facility decision support system, 301
Federal Government
    data, 92
    involvement of in health planning, 14
Federal Legislation
    influence of on health planning, 30
    Social Security, 70–72
Federation of Nurses and Health Professionals (FNHP),
    126
Flow diagrams, 282–285
Focus Group, 172
Forced association, 173
Forecasting bed need methodologies, see Bed
    needs
Formula for bed need, see Bed needs
For-Profit Hospitals, 133
Free Association, 171
Freestanding ambulatory surgery centers, 254
Functional evaluation and outcome, 349
Functional Status Index, 85–88, 391
Funding, 144
Funds, see Costs, financing

G
GamePlan, 303
Gaming, 300
    examples, 301

Gantt charts, see Time lines
GATOR, 95
General Accounting Office [GAO], 115, 138–140,
    188–191
General Health Questionnaire [GHQ], 391, 394
General Health Rating Index (GHRI), 391, 394
Genital infections, 194
Goals
    priority determination and, 209
    setting of, 255
Graduate Medical Education National Advisory Com-
    mittee [GMENAC] Study, 122–125
Graphic scale, 384
Greater Detroit Health Council, 31

H
Hanlon Method, 224–229
Health care
    governance, 305, 307
    plans, 120, 121
Health concept, 37–38, 333–334
    and indicators, 357–358
Health diaries, 97
Health-Illness Profile, 390–391
Health Maintenance Organization [HMO], 1, 2, 31,
    120, 123, 408
Health planning, see Strategic planning
Health planning trends, 17
Health Policy Agenda [HPA], 204
Health Status Index, 37
    dimensions, 37
Health status measures, 391–396
    a comparison of, 392–397
    Duke-UNC Health Profile, 391–392
    Quadrant Method, 70–72
    Sentinel health events, 61–70, 360–369
    Sickness Impact Profile, 59–61, 86, 391, 392
    Well-being Index, 359, 391, 392
Health status surveys, 390–391
    instruments in evaluation, 391
Health Systems Agencies [HSAs], 2
    demise of, 209
Healthy People, 204–205
High technology, 10, 143
Historic trends, 17–18
Home Health Care, 12–13
    CEA, 196
    marketing, 274–275
    parenteral nutrition, 187
Hospital Corporation of America (HCA), 134
Hospital market survey, 326–330
Hospitals
    closures, 4
    marketing and, 326
    occupancy, 11
    satisfaction with, 402

sociopolitics, 308–309
suicide criteria, 382
ward atmosphere, 386
HSRI's Quadrant Method, 70–72

I
Idea generation
  by brainstorming, 166–167
  Delphi technique for, 176
  by forced association, 173
  think tank method, 175
Implementation
  in action, 254–255
  AIDS education, 279–281
  and behavior change, 255, 273, 281
  and goal setting, 255
  imperatives, 316
  and marketing, 259–261, 263–277
  methods, 277–305
  and product lines, 264
  and risk factors, 253
  and sociopolitics, 305–316
  strategies, 252–253
Index
  calculation, 2–44
  defined, 369
  function status, 2–44
  functional status, 370, 391
  healthy days, 370
  national comparison of, 370
  rehabilitation, 371
  scales, 2–44
  and tracer method, 372
  of well-being (IWB), 359, 391, 392
  and well years, 370
  and years lost, 370
India, indicators BED, DOC, 353–354
Indian Health Services, 111
Indian Reservation Public Health Clinic, 232
Indicators
  access to service, 360
  administrative, 353
  clinical, 348
  data for, 354–356
  defined, 352
  and health concepts, 357
  as measurement, 352
  national comparison of, 369
  objectives of, 357
  poor quality, 354
  poverty, 358–359
  of priority, 240
  quality of life, 359–360
  and sentinel health events, 360–369
  utility value of life, 360
  welfare, 360
Individual practice associations, 120

Infant mortality, 193–194
Inferential indicators, 47–49
Innovator, 176, 178–180
Intermediate Care Facilities [ICFs], 356
Internal environment assessment, 9
  SWOT, 9
Investigative reports, 97

J
Joint Commission on Accreditation of Healthcare
    Organizations [JCAHO], 3
  clinical indicators and, 348

K
Key informant survey, 39–42
Key word technique, 147–148

L
LaMonica-Oberst Patient Satisfaction Scale (LOPSS),
    405
Lateral thinking, 162
Life situation survey, 400
Likert scale, 383
Local Area Networks (LANs), 10, 94
Long-Term Care [LTC], 410
  assessment, 410
  evaluation, 410
  and marketing, 275
  and Markov chain, 75
  Resource Allocation Method [RAM], 110–111

M
Magnetic Resonance Imaging [MRI], 380–381
Major Source Evaluation, 297
Managed Health Care Plans, survey, 325
Mapping, 243–247
Market research, applications of, 272–273
Market segment, 264
Marketing, 259
  basics, 259–261
  behavior change and, 255, 273, 281
  and CEO, 262
  and culture of corporate business, 261–262
  evaluation and, 325
  hospital, 325
  to industry, 330
  Market Area Profile, 266
  market messages, 266–267, 280
  problems, 263
  regulation and, 330
  research and, 269, 325
  samples, 267
  segmentation, 264
  surges, 259
  and survey methods, 325
Markov Chain, 75–79
McMaster Health Index Questionnaire (MHIQ), 391

Measurement concepts, 333
Media-driven humanitarianism, 106–107
Medicaid, 30
  abuse control, 188–190
Medical Outcomes Study (MOS), 391, 394–395
Medical Planning and Impact Analysis [MPIA], 122
Medicare, 30
  evaluation, 349
  and DRGs, 13
  and HHC, 12
Meeting techniques, 310
Mental health
  bed projection, 135–140
  system for District of Columbia, 138
Mental illness, 70
  estimated need, 70–72
  facilities in California, 136–137
  facilities in D.C., 138
  facilities in Nebraska, 135–136
  and social area analysis, 237–239
  surveys of, 397, 400
Mind mapping, 169–171
Mission statement, 17
MOSAIC Assessment, 32–34
Municipal Health Services Program [MHSP], 411–412

N
National Center for Health Statistics [NCHS], 37, 344
National Citizen's Coalition for Nursing Home Reform,
  379, 403
National Health Indicators, 369
National Health Planning and Resources Act [NHPRA],
  = PL 93-641, 2, 17, 209
  demise of, 2
National Health Service (NHS), 119
Nebraska MHS model, 135–136
Need vs. demand, 38
Needs assessment, 34
  accuracy, 36
  attributes, 36
  community survey, 42–45
  demographic analysis, 45–47
  Duke-UNC health profile, 56–59
  index of well-being, 51, 55–56
  inferential analysis, 47–49
  key informant, 39–42
  MOSAIC, 32–34
  programmatic data, 49–51
  quadrant method, 70–72
  reliability, 36
  sensitivity, 36
  sentinel health events (SHEs), 61–70, 360–369
  sickness impact profile (SIP), 59–61, 86, 391,
    392
  validity, 36
Negative health, 2–49
New York Quality Assurance System (NYQAS), 379

Nominal Group Technique, 172, 217–221
  creativity and, 172
  priorities and, 217
Nottingham Health Profile (NHP), 391–392
Nurse, entrepreneurship, 277
Nursing care evaluation, 376
Nursing shortage, 13, 140–141

O
Objectives
  criteria, 23
  development, 24
  examples, 24
  as linchpins, 23
  importance of, 25
  in SHP, 23–25, 323
Obstacles, to technical information, 98
Obstetric services, 404
Office of Technology Assessment, 354, 380
Opinion polls, 96
Outcome evaluations, 345, 348
  and JCAHO, 348
  and PROs, 348–349

P
Pan American Health Organization, 203
Patient Care Unit (PCU), 130
Patient satisfaction, 400ff
  components of, 401–402
  and ethics, 401
  with family practice, 404
  with hospital, 402
  with nursing care, 404
  with obstetric care, 404
  and philosophy, 401
  surveys, 400
PEARL, 228; see also Hanlon
Peer Review Organization (PRO), 342
Percentage scale, 384
Performance appraisal systems, 384–386
Performance indicators (employee), 128
Personnel, 103, 121, 128
  and alternative uses, 126
  performance, 128
  productivity, 128
  and shortage impact, 125, 126
  and standard costs, 129
  supply and demand, 127
  utilization, 128
PERT [Program Evaluation and Review Technique],
  294–297
Phillips 66, 172–173
Physicians
  changing roles of, 13
  and computers, 386, 387
  and GMENAC study, 122–125
  and hiring process, 121

rating, 386–387
surplus, 1, 13
Pitfalls, 21–23
Planning, *see* Strategic planning
Policy areas
    AIDS, 12
    cost containment, 14
    home health care, 12–13
    nurse shortage, 13
    physician surplus, 13
Position papers, 96
Potentially Productive Years of Life Lost [PPYLL], 241–243
Pre-experimental designs, 338
Preference surveys, 235–236
Pregnancy, smoking and, 194–196
Prevention, 1
Primary care, 7–137
Prime mover, 297
Priority, 203ff.
    AIDS, 206
    consumer, 208
    federal, 206
    determination, 209–212
    individual and irrational, 208
    public health, 205
    state health, 207
    technology, 206–207
Priority-setting methods
    clustering, 233–235
    computer graphic mapping, 243–247
    criteria weighting, 221–224
    Delphi, 229–232
    Hanlon, 224–229
    indicators, 240
    nomimal group, 217–221
    PPYLL, 241–243
    preference survey, 235–236
    simplex, 212–217
    size-of-need gap, 232–233
    social area analysis, 237–241
    timing of implementation, 236–237
Private interest, 314
Product line, 264
    cardiovascular, 265
    management, 264
    and new product, 265
Program evaluation, 405
Professional Review Organization [PRO], 3
    and outcomes, 348–349
Program Evaluation Review Technique [PERT], 294
Promotion, *see* Marketing
Prospective Payment System [PPS], 9, 342; *see also* DRGs
Public health priorities, *see* Priorities
Public hearings, 96

Public interest, 314
Public Interest vs. Private Interest, 314

Q
Quadrant Needs Assessment, 70–72
Quality of care, 9–10
Quality of Life Index (QLI), 79–82, 391
    and colostomy patients, 79–81
    components, 79
    defined, 79
Quantophrenia, 182
Quasi-experimental designs, 339–340
Questionnaires
    key informant, 39–42
    patient satisfaction, 400
    self-administered, 118
    simplex, 212, 214–216

R
RAM, *see* Resource Allocation Model
RAND Corporation, 176, 392–394
Rand Health Experiment Measures, 391, 392
Randomized Clinical Trial [RCT], 339, 408
Rationing, 104–109
    and attitudes, 108
    decisions, 104–106
    in England, 107
    guidelines, 107–108
    and the media, 106–107
Reagan, 2
Records, 351
Referral and Decision Network, 285–289
Referral Network Diagram, 285
Registered Care Technologist [RCT], 126
    and the AMA, 126
Reliability, 341
Renal failure, 301
Representative interviews, 96
Research, *see also* Marketing research
    evaluation vs., 406
    studies, 97
Resource Allocation Model [RAM], 109–115
    acute, 110
    ambulatory, 110
    components of, 110–111
    critics of, 114–115
    in Indian Health Services, 111–114
    simulation, 116
    in Veteran's Administration, 110
Resources
    and allocation methods, 109, 116
    capital, 134, 135
    checklist for, 148–150
    policies, 151, 153
    and rationing, 104–109
    simulation, 116
    and taxonomies, 145

types of, 103
  unusual, 151
  utilization groups (RUGs), 111
Resources/sources checklist, 148–150
Retardation, checklist for prevention of, 374–375
Role gridding, 297–300

S

Scales as measurement tools, 382
  and arthritis, 387
  performance appraisal, 384
  to rate doctors, 386
  types of, 382–384
  ward atmosphere, 386
SCAMPER, 168
Segmentation
  in marketing, 265
  messages, 266
Self
  administered questionnaire, 118
  care, 11, 408
Sentinel health events, *see* Needs assessment
Sickness Impact Profile [SIP], *see* Needs assessment
Simplex questionnaire, 212, 214–216
Simulation
  and RAM, 116
  and gaming, 300
Skilled Nursing Facility, 356
Slip writing, 171–172
Smoking, cessation, 254
  for pregnancy, 194–196
Social area analysis, 237
  strengths, 239–241
Socioeconomic indicators, 237–238
Sociopolitics, 305
  actors in, 307
  bargaining in, 307
  and governance, 305
  in hospital, 308–309
  and manipulation, 308
  planning tradeoffs, 310, 314
  and private concerns, 314
  and public interest, 314
  and study groups, 310
  and task forces, 309
  and urgency, 315
  and work groups, 309
Software, 95, 96, 289
Spidergram, 169–171
SPO, *see* Structure, Process, Outcome
Staff, *see* Personnel
Standard Deviational Ellipse (SDE), 117
Stapel Scale, 383
Statistics, 98
  application to evaluation, 336–337
  SUPERSTAT program, 95
  value of, 98

Strategic management, 1–5, 1–11
Strategic Performance Indicators (SPIs), 333
Strategic planning
  characteristics of, 6, 8
  and comprehensive planning, 7
  and computers, 302
  defined, 4
  pitfalls, 21–23
  steps in, 6
  and strategic management, 3, 4
Structure, process, outcome (SPO), 345
  in evaluation, 345
  and management, 345–348
  and outcome examples, 348–352
  in soft services, 348
Suicidal behavior, 382
SUPERSTAT, 95
Surveys
  comparisons, 389
  computer-assisted, 389–390
  of health status, 390–397
  of mental illness, 397
  mail, 325, 389
  and obstetric care, 404
  personal interview, 388–389
  problems with, 388
  telephone, 389–390
  types of, 388–389
Synetics, 175

T

Technology
  allocation of, 143–144
  assessment, 380
  assessment iterative loop [TAIL], 409–410
  trends, 144
Text retrieval, GATOR Program, 95
Thinking
  lateral and vertical, 162
  synetics and, 175
  think-tanks and, 175
Thought stream, *see* Free association
Time of implementation, as criteria for priority setting, 236–237
Time line, 289
Tracer method, 372

U

United States Department of Health and Human Services (USDHHS), 145
Urgent issues, 315–316
Utility value of life, 360
Utilization review program, 407–408

V

Validity, 341
  in evaluation, 341
  types of, 341

Value distinctions and choices, 197–198
Vertical thinking, 162
Veterans' Administration [VA], 109, 142, 181
Visual synetics, 174–175
Vital statistics, 96
Volunteers (hospitals), 132

W
Ward atmosphere scale, 386
Wellness centers, 275–277
WHO plan for health, 203
Who, what, when computer program, 289
Worksheets for implementation, 277
World Health Organization [WHO], 203
    and plan for health, 203